T0319253

NEURONAL AND SYNAPTIC DYSFUNCTION IN AUTISM SPECTRUM DISORDER AND INTELLECTUAL DISABILITY

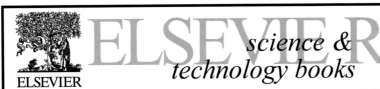

Companion Web Site:

http://booksite.elsevier.com/9780128001097

Neuronal and Synaptic Dysfunction in Autism Spectrum Disorder and Intellectual Disability
Carlo Sala and Chiara Verpelli, Editors

Available Resources:

- Abstracts
- Figures in .jpg format
- Figures in PowerPoint presentation
- Tables in PowerPoint presentation

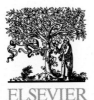

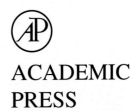

ACADEMIC
PRESS

NEURONAL AND SYNAPTIC DYSFUNCTION IN AUTISM SPECTRUM DISORDER AND INTELLECTUAL DISABILITY

Edited by

CARLO SALA
CHIARA VERPELLI

CNR Neuroscience Institute, Milan, Italy
Department of Medical Biotechnology and
Translational Medicine, University of Milan, Milan, Italy

AMSTERDAM • BOSTON • HEIDELBERG • LONDON
NEW YORK • OXFORD • PARIS • SAN DIEGO
SAN FRANCISCO • SINGAPORE • SYDNEY • TOKYO
Academic Press is an imprint of Elsevier

Academic Press is an imprint of Elsevier
125 London Wall, London EC2Y 5AS, UK
525 B Street, Suite 1800, San Diego, CA 92101-4495, USA
50 Hampshire Street, 5th Floor, Cambridge, MA 02139, USA
The Boulevard, Langford Lane, Kidlington, Oxford OX5 1GB, UK

Notices
Knowledge and best practice in this field are constantly changing. As new research and experience broaden our understanding, changes in research methods, professional practices, or medical treatment may become necessary.

Practitioners and researchers may always rely on their own experience and knowledge in evaluating and using any information, methods, compounds, or experiments described herein. In using such information or methods they should be mindful of their own safety and the safety of others, including parties for whom they have a professional responsibility.

To the fullest extent of the law, neither the Publisher nor the authors, contributors, or editors, assume any liability for any injury and/or damage to persons or property as a matter of products liability, negligence or otherwise, or from any use or operation of any methods, products, instructions, or ideas contained in the material herein.

British Library Cataloguing-in-Publication Data
A catalogue record for this book is available from the British Library

Library of Congress Cataloging-in-Publication Data
A catalog record for this book is available from the Library of Congress

ISBN: 978-0-12-800109-7

For information on all Academic Press publications
visit our website at https://www.elsevier.com/

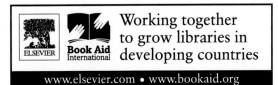

www.elsevier.com • www.bookaid.org

Publisher: Mica Haley
Senior Acquisition Editor: Natalie Farra
Senior Editorial Project Manager: Kristi Anderson
Production Project Manager: Lucía Pérez
Designer: Vicky Pearson

Typeset by TNQ Books and Journals
www.tnq.co.in

Contents

III

EXPERIMENTAL MODELS, CLINICAL AND PHARMACOLOGICAL ASPECTS OF MAJOR ASDS, AND INTELLECTUAL DISABILITY SYNDROMES

List of Contributors

Stephanie A. Barnes Centre for Integrative Physiology/Patrick Wild Centre, University of Edinburgh, Edinburgh, UK

Silvia Bassani CNR Neuroscience Institute, Milan, Italy; Department of Medical Biotechnology and Translational Medicine, University of Milan, Milan, Italy

Àlex Bayés Molecular Physiology of the Synapse Laboratory, Biomedical Research Institute Sant Pau (IIB Sant Pau), Barcelona, Spain; Universitat Autònoma de Barcelona, Cerdanyola del Vallès, Spain

Elizabeth Berry-Kravis Department of Pediatrics, Rush University Medical Center, Chicago, IL, USA; Department of Neurological Sciences, and Biochemistry, Rush University Medical Center, Chicago, IL, USA

Luigi Boccuto JC Self Research Institute Greenwood Genetic Center, Greenwood, SC, USA

Thomas Bourgeron Institut Pasteur, Human Genetics and Cognitive Functions Unit, Paris, France; CNRS UMR3571 Genes, Synapses and Cognition, Institut Pasteur, Paris, France; University Paris Diderot, Sorbonne Paris Cité, Human Genetics and Cognitive Functions, Paris, France; FondaMental Foundation, Créteil, France; Gillberg Neuropsychiatry Centre, Sahlgrenska Academy, University of Gothenburg, Gothenburg, Sweden

Jamel Chelly IGBMC, Department of Translational Medicine and Neurogenetics, Inserm U964, CNRS UMR 7104, Université de Strasbourg, Illkirch Cedex, France; Pôle de biologie, Hôpitaux Universitaires de Strasbourg, Strasbourg, France

Bice Chini National Research Council, Institute of Neuroscience, Milan, Italy; Humanitas Clinical and Research Center, Rozzano, Italy

Jérôme Ezan INSERM, Neurocentre Magendie U1215, Bordeaux, France; University of Bordeaux, Bordeaux, France

Jozef Gecz School of Medicine, University of Adelaide, Adelaide, Australia; Robinson Research Institute, University of Adelaide, Adelaide, Australia

Valentina Gigliucci National Research Council, Institute of Neuroscience, Milan, Italy

Xiaohong Gong School of Life Sciences, Fudan University, Shanghai, China; Institute of Science and Technology for Brain-Like Intelligence, Fudan University, Shanghai, China

Seth G.N. Grant Genes to Cognition Programme, Centre for Clinical Brain Science, University of Edinburgh, Edinburgh, UK

Anne Hoffmann Department of Pediatrics, Rush University Medical Center, Chicago, IL, USA

Claire Homan Robinson Research Institute, University of Adelaide, Adelaide, Australia

Elaine Y. Hsiao Division of Biology and Biological Engineering, California Institute of Technology, Pasadena, CA, USA

Guillaume Huguet Institut Pasteur, Human Genetics and Cognitive Functions Unit, Paris, France; CNRS UMR3571 Genes, Synapses and Cognition, Institut Pasteur, Paris, France; University Paris Diderot, Sorbonne Paris Cité, Human Genetics and Cognitive Functions, Paris, France

Lachlan Jolly School of Medicine, University of Adelaide, Adelaide, Australia; Robinson Research Institute, University of Adelaide, Adelaide, Australia

Eunjoon Kim Center for Synaptic Brain Dysfunctions, Institute for Basic Science (IBS), Daejeon, South Korea; Department of Biological Sciences, Korea Advanced Institute of Science and Technology (KAIST), Daejeon, South Korea

Peter C. Kind Centre for Integrative Physiology/Patrick Wild Centre, University of Edinburgh, Edinburgh, UK

Jaewon Ko Department of Biochemistry, College of Life Science & Biotechnology, Yonsei University, Seoul, South Korea

Janine M. Lamonica Department of Genetics, Perelman School of Medicine, University of Pennsylvania, Philadelphia, PA, USA

Marianna Leonzino National Research Council, Institute of Neuroscience, Milan, Italy; Dipartimento di Biotecnologie Mediche e Medicina Traslazionale, UNIMI, Milan, Italy

Natalia V. Malkova Division of Biology and Biological Engineering, California Institute of Technology, Pasadena, CA, USA

Carla Marini Neurology Unit, Meyer Children's Hospital, Florence, Italy

Caterina Michetti Department of Cell Biology and Neuroscience, Istituto Superiore di Sanità, Rome, Italy

Caterina Montani CNR Neuroscience Institute, Milan, Italy; Department of Medical Biotechnology and Translational Medicine, University of Milan, Milan, Italy

Mireille Montcouquiol INSERM, Neurocentre Magendie U1215, Bordeaux, France; University of Bordeaux, Bordeaux, France

Maïté M. Moreau INSERM, Neurocentre Magendie U1215, Bordeaux, France; University of Bordeaux, Bordeaux, France

Edoardo Moretto CNR Neuroscience Institute, Milan, Italy; Department of Medical Biotechnology and Translational Medicine, University of Milan, Milan, Italy

Alysson Renato Muotri Department of Pediatrics, University of California San Diego, School of Medicine, Rady Children's Hospital San Diego, San Diego, CA, USA; Department of Cellular & Molecular Medicine, Stem Cell Program, University of California San Diego, La Jolla, CA, USA

Emily K. Osterweil Centre for Integrative Physiology/Patrick Wild Centre, University of Edinburgh, Edinburgh, UK

Maria Passafaro CNR Neuroscience Institute, Milan, Italy; Department of Medical Biotechnology and Translational Medicine, University of Milan, Milan, Italy

Olga Peñagarikano Department of Pharmacology, School of Medicine, University of the Basque Country, Leioa, Spain

Alan K. Percy University of Alabama at Birmingham, Birmingham, AL, USA

Duyen Pham School of Medicine, University of Adelaide, Adelaide, Australia; Robinson Research Institute, University of Adelaide, Adelaide, Australia

Katy Phelan Hayward Genetics Program and Department of Pediatrics, Tulane University School of Medicine, New Orleans, LA, USA

Laura Ricceri Department of Cell Biology and Neuroscience, Istituto Superiore di Sanità, Rome, Italy

Yoann Saillour Institut Cochin, Université Paris Descartes, CNRS (UMR 8104), Paris, France; INSERM U1016, Paris, France

Carlo Sala CNR Neuroscience Institute, Milan, Italy; Department of Medical Biotechnology and Translational Medicine, University of Milan, Milan, Italy

Nathalie Sans INSERM, Neurocentre Magendie U1215, Bordeaux, France; University of Bordeaux, Bordeaux, France

Sara Sarasua Greenwood Genetic Center, Greenwood, SC, USA; Clemson University, Clemson, SC, USA

Maria Luisa Scattoni Department of Cell Biology and Neuroscience, Istituto Superiore di Sanità, Rome, Italy

Michael J. Schmeisser Institute for Anatomy and Cell Biology, Ulm University, Ulm, Germany; Department of Neurology, Ulm University, Ulm, Germany

Charles E. Schwartz JC Self Research Institute Greenwood Genetic Center, Greenwood, SC, USA

Yiping Shen Department of Pathology, Harvard Medical School, Boston, MA, USA; Department of Laboratory Medicine, Boston Children's Hospital, Boston, MA, USA; Guangxi Maternal and Child Health Hospital, Nanning, GuangXi, China; Shanghai Jiao Tong University School of Medicine, Shanghai, China

Chuan Tan School of Medicine, University of Adelaide, Adelaide, Australia

Daniel C. Tarquinio Emory University, Children's Healthcare of Atlanta, Alanta, GA, USA

Sophie R. Thomson Centre for Integrative Physiology/Patrick Wild Centre, University of Edinburgh, Edinburgh, UK

Chiara Verpelli CNR Neuroscience Institute, Milan, Italy; Department of Medical Biotechnology and Translational Medicine, University of Milan, Milan, Italy

Kazuhiro Yamakawa Laboratory for Neurogenetics, RIKEN Brain Science Institute, Saitama, Japan

Zhaolan Zhou Department of Genetics, Perelman School of Medicine, University of Pennsylvania, Philadelphia, PA, USA

Preface

Autism spectrum disorders (ASD) and intellectual disability (ID) are lifelong neurodevelopmental disorders with clinical presentation in children that affects how individuals communicate and relate to others and their surroundings.

The term "autism" came from the Greek word *autós*, meaning "self," and was used for the first time by psychiatrist Eugen Bleuler in 1908 to describe a schizophrenic patient who had withdrawn into his own world. However, the first accurate description of children with autism comes from the work of American child psychiatrist Leo Kanner in 1943 and Austrian pediatrician Hans Asperger in 1944. Both independently described a number of children with similar impaired social skills, with different severities.

For a long time it was debated whether autism was caused by an affective education of the mother or the deterioration of neuronal development. Only in the 1980, when Asperger's work was translated into English and published and came into knowledge, did it became increasingly clear that autism is not caused by the parents' education but by neurological alterations and other genetic disorders such as tuberous sclerosis, metabolic defects, or chromosomal abnormalities such as Fragile X syndrome.

It has taken decades to recognize autism as a disease and methods of classification and diagnosis have progressively improved; however, ID, which was previously defined as mental retardation, is a pathological condition recognized since antiquity and its diagnosis has developed over time as societies became more complex and psychological testing became more sophisticated and popular.

ASD and ID are often connected because three-quarters of ASD patients also manifest severe ID and epilepsy as major comorbidities.

Together these neurodevelopmental disorders have an incidence of 1–2% in all countries where they have been accurately identified and monitored. ASD and ID greatly affect and limit quality of life for those who experience their effects, both the affected patients and their families. Moreover, considering that most patients are affected since birth, these developmental disorders create a huge cost to society.

In the past 2 decades a lot of work has been done to understand the pathogenesis mechanisms for both ASD and ID. Indeed there is full consensus among the scientific community that correct functioning of the synapses is a fundamental prerequisite for a healthy brain. Thus, it is unsurprising that altered synaptic function and morphology are implicated in the molecular pathogenesis of so-called synaptopathies including ASD and ID.

A number of mutated genes that code for proteins concerned with brain synapse function and circuit formation have been identified in patients affected by ASD and ID syndromes over the past 15 years. Most of these genes are involved in synapse formation and plasticity, the regulation of dendritic spine morphology, organization of the synaptic cytoskeleton, synthesis and degradation of specific synapse proteins, and the control of correct balance between excitatory and inhibitory synapses.

Even in the presence of a genetic predisposition to ASD and ID, a number of nongenetic-like environmental triggers appear to increase a child's risk further. For example, immune system dysfunctions are also strongly correlated to the development of ASD.

In synthesis we know some genes and pathogenic mechanisms and we can correlate these gene mutations to specific syndromes and clinical manifestations. Thus some therapeutic interventions have been developed, although there remains much more to do.

In this book we summarize major advances in the study of ASD and ID, describing the genetic and nongenetic tools we used, and future tools for use in discovering pathogenesis mechanisms. Then we discuss how, studying the function of mutated genes, we can identify new pharmacological and therapeutic targets. Finally we present the disease model we use and, importantly, the clinical aspects and available therapeutic tools for some of the most frequent and studied syndromes with a clear link between genetic mutations and disease.

Thus our book is a cultural journey in how to discover genetic or nongenetic causes, through an understanding of the function of a mutated gene, and finally, how physicians can use all of this information to understand the diseases and treat them. For these purposes, the book was written by internationally recognized geneticists, neurobiologists, and pediatricians, each of whom helped us to understand better how these complex neurodevelopmental diseases are investigated, and hoped to help find new and effective therapies.

Our thought goes to all of the children and families who are dealing with the disease every day and to the hope that we researchers and physicians can give them a better future.

Carlo Sala and Chiara Verpelli

Acknowledgments

We thank all the authors who dedicated their time to realize this book.
A special thank you to all the children and parents
who inspired and motivated the entire work.

AUTISM SPECTRUM DISORDERS AND INTELLECTUAL DISABILITY: GENETIC AND NON-GENETIC CAUSES

1

Experimental Tools for the Identification of Specific Genes in Autism Spectrum Disorders and Intellectual Disability

Yiping Shen[1,2,3,4], *Xiaohong Gong*[5,6]

[1]Department of Pathology, Harvard Medical School, Boston, MA, USA; [2]Department of Laboratory Medicine, Boston Children's Hospital, Boston, MA, USA; [3]Guangxi Maternal and Child Health Hospital, Nanning, GuangXi, China; [4]Shanghai Jiao Tong University School of Medicine, Shanghai, China; [5]School of Life Sciences, Fudan University, Shanghai, China; [6]Institute of Science and Technology for Brain-Like Intelligence, Fudan University, Shanghai, China

POSITIONAL MAPPING

Linkage Mapping

Genetic linkage is the tendency of genes that are located proximally to each other on a chromosome to be inherited together during meiosis. For most neuropsychiatric diseases whose underlying pathomechanisms are largely unknown, linkage analysis is a powerful tool to detect the chromosomal location of disease genes. Genome-wide linkage studies generally use 300–500 microsatellites evenly spanning the entire genome, with an average resolution of 5–10 centimorgans (cM) (1 cM ≈ 1 million base pairs [Mbp]). A centimorgan is defined as the distance between chromosome positions for which the expected average number of intervening chromosomal crossovers in a single generation is 0.01. Microsatellites, or short tandem repeats, are repeat sequences of two to five base pairs (bp). Microsatellites are good markers for linkage studies because they have high heterozygosity. Although single nucleotide polymorphisms (SNPs) are biallelic and not as highly polymorphic as microsatellites, they are the most common type of genomic variation (about 1 SNP in 1000 bp) and have better coverage for small chromosomal regions.

Linkage analysis could be either parametric or nonparametric. Parametric linkage analysis is the most powerful statistical method to test for linkage. It requires prior knowledge of the inheritance model, the allele frequency, and the penetrance. The test statistic is called the logarithm of odds (LOD) score. An LOD score higher than 3.0 is generally accepted as the evidence supporting linkage, whereas an LOD score lower than −2.0 is considered evidence against linkage. Nonparametric linkage analysis is a model-free approach that studies the probability of an allele being identical by descent (IBD) in pairs of relatives with same phenotype. Many computer programs for linkage analysis are available: for example, LIPED, LINKAGE, FastLINK, MENDEL, GENEHUNTER, MapMaker and CRI-MAP for parametric linkage analysis, and ANALYZER for nonparametric linkage analysis.

The X chromosome spans about 155 Mbp and contains 800−900 genes out of 20,000−25,000 total genes in the human genome. X-linked intellectual disability (XLID) is a common cause of monogenic intellectual disability (ID), accounting for 8−12% of all ID cases in males.[1–4] X-linked gene defects usually lead to severe clinic symptoms in males because they have only one X chromosome, whereas female carriers may have no or milder symptoms. The hemizygosity of males in X chromosome makes the linkage mapping strategy especially successful in the identification of X-linked genes. In the review of Lubs et al. in 2012, 102 XLID genes were associated with 81 XLID syndromes and with 35 families with nonsyndromal XLID.[5]

Linkage analysis is a useful tool as the first step to map the disease gene to a refined region; the actual causal gene is then usually identified after sequencing analysis of appropriate candidate genes within this region. For example, in a three-generation Norwegian family with XLID, a panel of 48 polymorphic microsatellite markers with an average distance of 3.9 cM on the X chromosome was genotyped in three affected males and seven unaffected relatives.[6] Multipoint parametric linkage analysis achieved a maximum LOD score of 1.50 at the Xq24-q27.3 interval. Candidate gene sequencing identified a deletion in the *SLC9A6* gene, which is located to Xq26. The deletion segregated with affected males and carrier females.[6] A genome-wide parametric linkage analysis using 524 microsatellites was performed for a large consanguineous ID family with four affected individuals. There was evidence of linkage on chromosome 19p13 (LOD score ranging from 1.2 to 3.5).[7] Exome sequencing eventually identified homozygous pathogenic variants in the *TECR* gene located at the linkage interval.[8]

Although autism spectrum disorders (ASDs) are highly heritable neurodevelopmental disorders, the application of linkage analysis to localize autism genes has achieved limited success to date. The genetic heterogeneity of ASD, reduced penetrance of pathogenic variants, and relatively small size of pedigrees have contributed to the situation. More than 10 linkage studies have been performed and a series of chromosome regions were found to be linked with ASDs in at least two independent studies.[9–17] The most consistent linkage region for ASD is chromosome 7q22-32. In a meta-analysis, 7q22-q32 reached genome-wide significance and the neighboring region 7q32-qter reached suggestive significance.[18]

Balanced Translocation Breakpoint Mapping

Genome structural variants (SV) have a substantial role in the susceptibility of ASD and ID. Balanced chromosomal abnormalities (BCAs) include inversions, insertions, and translocations. Inversions are the breakage and reinsertion of a piece of a chromosome in reversed manner at the same breakage location. Insertions refer to the insertion of a large sequence into a chromosome. Translocations involve the breakage and rejoining between nonhomologous chromosomes. Translocations can be balanced with an even exchange of material or unbalanced with the gain or loss of genes. Most BCA carriers have no symptoms. However, some have a range of symptoms including ASD, ID, or neurodevelopmental disorders (NDD). Balanced chromosomal abnormalities are usually identified by cytogenetic karyotyping, with an estimated frequency of 1.3% in ASD. Genes disrupted at the breakpoint of the structure variant or dysregulated owing to their proximity to the breakpoint (positional effect) are likely causes of the symptoms.

Applying this strategy, in one study, Talkowski et al. mapped the breakpoints of 38 subjects with neurodevelopmental abnormalities using next-generation sequencing (NGS). They identified more than 20 genes that were further supported by other evidence to be associated with ASD or NDD.[19] Next-generation sequencing strategies now enable the routine detection of BCAs for clinical diagnostics and genetic researches.[20]

Autozygosity Mapping

It has been estimated that several hundred genes are likely to be associated with autosomal recessive ID (ARID).[21] However, efforts to identify ARID genes have been hampered by the extensive genetic heterogeneity of ARID and the relatively small sizes of affected families. Lander and Botstein provided conceptual insights and statistical methods for using polymorphic markers to track the disease haplotype that harbors the disease-causing mutation through homozygosity mapping.[22]

Autozygosity mapping, a productive form of homozygosity mapping, takes advantage of the increased odds of unmasking rare recessive mutations in consanguineous pedigrees.[23] It is predicted that unaffected individuals in a general population carry a number of heterozygous disease-causing recessive alleles at a low frequency. In first-cousin unions, a carrier will have a 1:8 chance of mating with another carrier regardless of how rare the disease is in the general population. In consanguineous families, there is high probability that an affected individual has inherited both copies of the mutated allele from a common ancestor, a special form of founder effect. This chromosomal region surrounding the mutated gene is homozygous because they segregate from a common ancestor (identical by descent [IBD]). Autozygome is the complete set of IBD segments in an individual.

To detect these runs of homozygosity (ROH), informative markers are required that range from microsatellites to SNPs. Although a SNP is less informative than a microsatellite, the advantages of biallelic and high-density spanning over the genome (1 per kilobyte) make SNP-based microarrays a powerful tool for autozygosity mapping. Two commonly used mapping tools are autoSNPa and HomozygosityMapper.[24,25] Carr et al. developed two programs, IBDfinder and SNPsetter, that facilitate the identification of autozygous regions within a heterogeneous SNP dataset and the detection of putative IBD regions, independently of allele frequencies and pedigree information.[26] Using Affymetrix human 500K SNP arrays, Morrow et al. screened 88 consanguineous pedigrees with ASD.[27] A locus-exclusionary approach was taken assuming a model of autosomal recessive inheritance and high penetrance. Several families showed one or two long segments of IBD with support for linkage (multipoint LOD scores ranging from 2.41 to 2.96). Interestingly, five rare homozygous deletions were found in 78 consanguineous pedigrees (6.4%) and ranged in size from 18 to >880 kilobase pairs (kbp). The largest homozygous deletion (~886 kbp) was identified in a boy diagnosed with autism and seizures, located in a 74-cM segment of IBD within 3q24. The deletion completely removes the *c3orf58* gene, which encodes an uncharacterized protein. The second large homozygous deletion (>300 kbp) is located next to the *PCDH10* gene on 4q28, which is involved in axon outgrowth. Both deletions were not present in more than 2000 individuals. The study demonstrated the effectiveness of autozygosity mapping for ASD genes.

Although every autozygous block represents homozygous haplotypes that are IBD, the reverse is not true. Homozygous blocks can also represent identical haplotypes that arise independently in the population (identical by state [IBS]). A critical issue in autozygosity mapping is the distinction between IBD and IBS. Usually, 2 Mb (1 Mb is roughly estimated as equal to the linkage distance of 1 cM) is set as a size cutoff during the autozygous mapping of offspring of first cousin mating. Alkuraya mentioned that rarely, an IBD segment with causative variants is less than 2 Mb in the hundreds of first cousin pedigrees analyzed to date.[28] On the other hand, IBS segments less than 2 Mb occasionally occur. Obviously, the more ancient the disease-causing variant, the smaller the IBD region is likely to be owing to more recombination events. Thus, it is important to emphasize that no cutoff value is perfect to distinguish IBD from IBS. Published results of autozygosity mapping have a bias toward large IBD regions, which may lead to a misleading impression that disease genes are to be found within large IBD segments. Linkage analysis could assign a statistical significance to this ROH using LOD. An LOD score of >3 is used as the reference standard for linkage in the statistical context, which means that this ROH interval is 1000 times more likely to be linked to the disease locus rather than shared by chance. In practice, if an IBD is shared exclusively by two or more affected individuals, the causative variant is likely to reside within this block regardless of the LOD score assigned. Therefore, the emphasis in autozygosity mapping is on the exclusive sharing of ROH between affected members in a pedigree.

After narrowing down the recessive disease loci to a few autozygous intervals, the identification of actual causal variant is still a major challenge by Sanger sequencing. The autozygous region is usually too large to directly sequence all the genes in this region. This bottleneck is now largely solved by performing NGS after target capturing. As reviewed by Alkuraya, more than 100 novel autosomal recessive genes were identified in January 2013 using an NGS-based autozygosity mapping approach, of which 54 genes were linked with ARID.[28] Carr et al. developed two computer programs, AgileGenotyper and AgileVariantMapper, to identify autozygous regions from exome sequencing data.[29] There are two ways to perform autozygous mapping combined with NGS: a two-step strategy using SNP arrays for autozygous mapping followed by NGS for the identification of disease genes, or a one-step strategy using only NGS. Exome sequencing could provide sufficient markers to identify most autozygous regions found by SNP-based microarrays.[30] Compared with SNP microarray data, exome data contain numerous gaps because of the uneven distribution of coding sequences across the genome. Thus, short autozygous segments could be missed in exome sequencing. The low read depth in some regions caused by GC bias may lead to miscalling. In a family with multiple affected individuals, it is much cheaper to run SNP arrays in multiple members to determine the autozygous interval than to perform exome sequencing in a single case to identify the causative homozygous variants. With the advancement of sequencing techniques and further reductions in cost, it is predicted that one-step exome sequencing or whole-genome sequencing (WGS) will replace SNP arrays for autozygosity mapping.

An extended version of homozygosity mapping strategy, called homozygous haplotype mapping, was developed and applied to study low-frequency recessive variants contributing to ASD.[31] This novel strategy is based on the observations suggesting that, even for complex disorders such as ASD, we expect to find an unusually high number of affected individuals to have the same haplotype in the region surrounding a disease mutation. This approach aims to detect homozygous sequences of identical haplotype structures that are shared at a higher frequency among ASD patients compared with parental controls. In so doing, haplotypes within shared ROH regions are identified and homozygous segments of identical haplotype that are present uniquely or at a higher frequency in ASD probands compared with parental controls are identified to be candidate regions. Applying this strategy to 1402 Autism Genome Project trios, Casey et al. identified 25 known and 1218 novel ASD candidate genes. A replication studying using 1182 independent trios validated 10 known and 300 novel ASD genes. This method added a significant number of new ASD candidate genes that are otherwise difficult to be identified.

CANDIDATE GENE APPROACH

Before the advent of high-throughput and low-cost technologies such as microarray and NGS, Sanger sequencing for candidate genes following linkage or other clues has been the major strategy to identify causative genes. Both positional and functional information is usually used to select candidate genes. Positional information could be derived from linkage analysis, autozygosity mapping, balanced translocation breakpoint mapping, and copy number variant detection. Genes within these regions may be affected either directly by altering the protein structure or indirectly by altering the expression level. Functional candidate genes could be selected based on prior knowledge of the gene's biological functions and its impact on the trait or disease.

The core question that the candidate gene approach is trying to answer is: Are the variants in the candidate genes more frequent in cases than in controls? Different genotyping methods will be used for different types of variants such as SNP or copy number variations (CNVs). Traditional genotyping methods for SNP include restriction fragment length polymorphisms, Sanger sequencing, Sequenom MassARRAY, etc. Single nucleotide polymorphisms localized in exons or regulatory regions with potential functional effects or tag SNPs, which are sufficient to capture the full haplotype information, are usually chosen for genotyping. Detection methods of CNVs of candidate genes will be discussed in the following section. Sanger sequencing for exons and exon—intron junction regions of a candidate gene is the main method for screening small variants including single nucleotide variants (SNV) and insertions and deletions (indels). According to their impacts on protein sequences, variants that occur within the coding region are categorized as frameshift, nonsense, missense, and synonymous. According to their effects on protein function, variants can also be classified into three main classes: loss-of-function variants, gain-of-function variants, and dominant negative variants. Frameshift variants lead to a different translation and nonsense variants lead to a truncated product, both of which are considered highly pathological mutations. For missense mutations, their possible impacts on the structure and function of the protein could be predicted using different types of software. SIFT uses sequence homology from multiple sequence alignments (MSAs) to predict amino acid substitutions that could be tolerated or damaging.[32] Disease-associated missense mutations typically occur at evolutionarily conserved regions that have an essential role in the structure and function of the protein. Assessing this conservation in MSAs can highlight the degree of amino acid divergence that can be tolerated. PolyPhen-2 is an online tool to predict the effect of variants using sequence- and structure-based information (http://genetics.bwh.harvard.edu/pph2/).[33] PMut uses supervised-learning method (neural networks) to analyze missense mutations (http://mmb2.pcb.ub.es:8080/PMut/). Neural networks are trained using two sets of data: disease-associated mutations and neutral mutations.[34] All of these bioinformatics tools are summarized in Table 1.

A special example of the candidate gene approach for identifying XLID genes was carried out by Tarpey et al.[35] They systematically examined the sequences of coding exons for 718 X-chromosome genes in 208 X-linked ID individuals prescreened for known X-linked ID gene mutations. This global X-chromosome exon-sequencing approach offers a strategy unbiased by assumptions concerning the nature of the genes but fulfilling the positional condition that the genes are on the X chromosome. This candidate approach led to the identification of nine X-linked ID genes.

Abnormal synaptic formation and function is a converging pathophysiological mechanism for ASD. Many syndromic and monogenic ASDs are known to be caused by mutations in genes that are part of the synaptic complex. Kenny et al. took a candidate gene approach and sequenced 215 genes in 147 ASD cases.[36] Genes were primarily selected for their function in the synapse, in categories such as neurexin and neuroligin interacting proteins, postsynaptic glutamate receptor complexes, and neural cell adhesion molecules. The study identified 31 novel truncating mutations that are

TABLE 1 Summary of Bioinformatics Tools for Genomic Analysis Mentioned in This Chapter

Tools	URL	Comments
AutoSNPa	http://dna.leeds.ac.uk/autosnpa/	Visual analysis of SNP data for autozygosity mapping
Homozygo-sityMapper	http://www.homozygositymapper.org/	Analysis of SNP data and NGS data for autozygosity mapping
IBDfinder	http://dna.leeds.ac.uk/ibdfinder/guide/	Identify IBD using Affymetrix SNP data
SNPsetter	http://dna.leeds.ac.uk/snpsetter/	Graphical presentation and collation of SNP counting results
SIFT	http://sift.jcvi.org/	Predict whether an amino acid substitution affects protein function based on degree of conservation of amino acid residues in multiple sequence alignments
Polyphen-2	http://genetics.bwh.harvard.edu/pph2/	Predict possible impact of amino acid substitution on structure and function of human protein
PMut	http://mmb2.pcb.ub.es:8080/PMut/	Annotation and prediction of pathological mutations using supervised-learning method to analyze missense mutations

excess in cases compared with controls, particularly among neurexin and neuroligin interacting proteins.

COPY NUMBER VARIATIONS

Genome-wide CNV Detection Methods

Copy number variation is a form of structural variation ranging from 1 kb to several megabases in size. Two types of platforms are widely used to detect genome-wide CNVs: array comparative genomic hybridization (CGH) and SNP arrays. For CGH arrays, test deoxyribonucleic acid (DNA) and reference DNA are hybridized to the array and the copy number of test DNA can be directly counted by comparison with reference DNA. Comparative genomic hybridization arrays have high sensitivity and accuracy for CNV calling. Comparative genomic hybridization arrays cannot detect balanced inversions and translocations. The calling of copy number by array CGH is relative to the reference (the copy number status of the control DNA). For example, if there is a loss in the control sample, it appears as a gain in the case. For SNP arrays, only test DNA is hybridized to the array and the reference baseline should be created from other experiments. Single nucleotide polymorphism arrays can identify ROHs that may indicate consanguinity relationships or uniparental disomy, and the SNP information can also help to differentiate parental origin of any genomic changes. The SNP plus CGH array is also able to provide SNP information to identify ROH.

Commercial genome-wide microarrays for CNV analysis are provided mainly by the following companies: Affymetrix, Illumina, and Agilent. The Affymetrix CytoScan HD array offers high-density resolution of the entire genome using more than 2.6 million markers for copy-number analysis and 750,000 SNPs. The Illumina Omni family of microarrays includes six different BeadChips featuring a variety of content and formats, providing wide flexibility to study genetic variation. The Illumina Omni2.5 BeadChip is the first commercial product optimally designed around 1000 Genomes Project data. It features about 2.5 million markers that capture variants down to 2.5% of minor allele frequencies (MAF) and delivers exceptional genomic coverage rates across diverse populations. The Omni5 BeadChip provides the most comprehensive coverage of common and rare variants, with 4.3 million whole-genome variants down to 1% of MAF, combined with novel functional exonic variants taken from over 12,000 sequenced exomes. Agilent SurePrint G3 CGH microarrays 1×1M, 2×400K, 4×180K, and 8×60K, scanned at 3 μm using the Agilent SureScan Microarray Scanner, provide high sensitivity, specificity, and resolution to map copy number aberration breakpoints and identify smaller CNVs in whole genome. Agilent SurePrint G3 Human CGH Microarray Kit, 1x1M, contains 961,035 probes with an average probe spacing of 3118 bp.

Next-generation sequencing has become a powerful tool for CNV detection. Compared with array-based methods, NGS enables the accurate definition of CNV breakpoints and copy number estimation. Short read alignment to a reference sequence is the first step in CNV detection using NGS data. The tools Maq, BWA, Bowtie, BFAST, and SHRiMP are widely used for Illumina and ABI data, whereas SSAHA2 and BWASW are used for the Roche/454 platform.[37−43] Sequence alignment/map format and its compressed binary equivalent form (binary alignment/map [BAM]) enable storing huge numbers of sequence reads, as well as their alignments to a reference genome, in a single file. Sequence alignment/map/BAM files are compatible with multiple NGS data types and algorithms.

After the alignment of sequence reads to a reference sequence in paired-end sequencing, three datasets are produced: correct read pairs mapped uniquely to the genome with correct spacing and orientation; discordant read pairs in terms of distance and/or orientation, or in which only one read is mapped; and reads that are not mapped at all. For SV detection, most approaches test discordant reads, which suggests the presence of underlying variation. In contrast to SV detection, copy number estimation usually use correct read pairs.

It is possible to generate CNV and SV from NGS data. Multiple tools and algorithms have been developed for this purpose. These have been reviewed extensively by Zhao et al.[44] Next-generation sequencing-based CNV detection methods can be categorized into five different strategies including paired-end mapping (PEM), split read (SR), read depth (RD), de novo assembly of a genome, and a combination of these approaches (CB). Most PEM-, SR-, and CB-based tools are not specific to CNV detection, but rather to SVs identification, whereas most RD- and AS-based tools are developed to detect CNVs instead of SVs. Read depth—based methods are major approaches to estimate copy numbers. The underlying hypothesis of RD-based methods is that the read depth in a genomic region is correlated with the copy number of the region. For example, a gain of copy number should have a higher intensity than expected. Thirty-seven tools to detect CNV using WGS data, including 14 RD-based tools and 11 tools specific to whole-exome sequencing data, were listed and discussed in detail by Zhao et al.[44] It is anticipated that NGS will eventually replace microarray for CNV detection; the sensitivity and specificity of CNV detection by NGS need to be further improved.

Targeted CNV Detection Methods

Many methods have been introduced to screen and valid targeted CNVs. Conventional chromosomal analysis (karyotyping) could detect large chromosomal aberrations (more than 3 Mb). Fluorescence in situ hybridization (FISH) increases the resolution to 1 Mb or even smaller (50 kb) by hybridizing fluorescently labeled DNA probes to metaphase chromosome spreads or interphase nuclei. The main limitations of FISH are that it is relatively costly, it is time-consuming, and it has low-throughput. However, it is still an accurate technique in clinical diagnostics, especially for the detection of balanced translocation.

Real-time quantitative polymerase chain reaction (qPCR) combines standard PCR with fluorescent detection technologies to detect and measure the amplicons in real time during each cycle of the PCR process, which are directly proportional to the amount of template. Two common methods in qPCR are nonspecific fluorescent dyes that intercalate with any double-stranded DNA (e.g., SYBR green) and sequence-specific DNA probes

consisting of oligonucleotides that are labeled with a fluorescent reporter that permits detection only after hybridization of the probe with its complementary sequence (e.g., TaqMan). The main limitation of qPCR is that the number of loci is no more than four in a single tube.

Multiplex ligation-dependent probe amplification (MLPA) is a widely used method for CNV analysis based on multiplex PCR. Each MLPA probe consists of two separate oligonucleotides, each containing a target-specific sequence and a universal PCR primer sequence. One of the oligonucleotides also contains a stutter sequence that allows each probe set to have different fragment lengths and that can be separated by capillary electrophoresis. After hybridization of the MLPA probes to genomic DNA, the two probes are ligated proportionally related to the number of target sequence. Because only ligated probes will be amplified during the subsequent PCR reaction, the number of target sequence could analyzed through the number of probe ligation products. Multiplex ligation-dependent probe amplification can screen up to 50 loci simultaneously for a large sample. More than 300 probe sets are now commercially available from MRC-Holland (https://mlpa.com/).

Multiplex amplifiable probe hybridization (MAPH) is a method based on hybridization and multiplex PCR, like MLPA. However, MAPH does not need the step of ligation and the hybridization of the probes to genomic DNA happens in solid membranes. In brief, a set of amplifiable probes is hybridized to targeted genomic DNA that is fixed to a membrane. Then the probes are washed from the membrane, amplified using a universal primer pairs, and separated by capillary electrophoresis. A large amount of genomic DNA (>1 μg) is needed to fix on the solid membrane. Multiplex amplifiable probe hybridization can test up to 40 probes simultaneously. Improvements in MAPH, such microarray-based MAPH and quadruplex MAPH, are produced to analyze a much higher number of probes (about 700) in a reaction.

Genomic imbalances detectable by the CNV analysis tools discussed earlier contribute to a significant fraction of patients with ID and ASD. Many of these genomic imbalances represent contiguous gene deletion and duplication syndromes in which not a single gene is responsible for the condition. Because of the high rate of genomic imbalance in patients with ID and ASD, CNV detection by chromosomal microarray is currently recommended as the first-tier test for patients with ID and ASD.[45]

NEXT-GENERATION SEQUENCING

The arrival of commercial NGS technology, also known as second-generation sequencing or massively parallel sequencing, has led to a comprehensive change in genomic researches. Next-generation sequencing technology has been widely used in many fields of life science including large-scale transcriptome sequencing, chromosome immunoprecipitation sequencing, methylation of genomic sequencing, metagenomic sequencing, de novo genome sequencing, exome sequencing, and WGS.

Compared with Sanger sequencing, second-generation DNA sequencing are massively parallel, leading to high throughput, and cost-effective; the accuracy is also significantly improved owing to repeated sampling. It also provides more quantitative measures for mosaicism and is able to detect many types of variants including SNV, indel, CNV, and SV. The output of the Illumina HiSeq 2500 system is 50—1000 gigabytes per run. The Illunima HiSeq X* sequencing system can reach 1.6—1.8 Tb per run and finish in 3 days. According to data from the National Human Genome Research Institute Genome Sequencing Program, costs associated with DNA sequencing have changed greatly since the arrival of commercial NGS platforms. The costs of generating DNA sequence using Sanger-based first-generation sequencing methods were $397 per megabyte and $7,147,571 per genome (the assumed genome size was 3000 Mb) in October 2007. By July 2014, the costs of generating DNA sequence using NGS platforms were $0.05 per megabyte and $4905 per genome.

The major disadvantages of next-generation DNA sequencing include short read length and low raw accuracy compared with Sanger sequencing. However, these technologies continue to improve rapidly.

Next-Generation Sequencing Platforms

Roche 454 sequencing, Illumina Solexa technology, and the Applied Biosystems (AB) SOLiD platform are three most typical NGS platforms. Although these platforms are diverse in sequencing biochemistry and array generation, their work flows are similar in the DNA library, generation of polony array, cyclic array sequencing, imaging, and data analysis.[46—50]

The 454 system was the first commercially available NGS platform. The DNA libraries with a mixture of short, adapter-flanked fragments are denatured into a single strand and captured by amplification beads followed by emulsion PCR. Each clonally amplified bead bears PCR products corresponding to the amplification of a single molecule from the template library. Roche 454 uses pyrosequencing technology for sequencing, which relies on the detection of pyrophosphate (PPi) released during nucleotide incorporation. In brief, one dNTP complements the bases of the template strand and releases PPi, which equals the amount of incorporated nucleotide on a microfabricated array of

picoliter-scale wells. The ATP transformed from PPi drives the luciferin into oxyluciferin and generates visible light, which is detected by the CCD as corresponding to the array coordinates of specific wells. The pattern of detected incorporation events reveals the sequence of templates represented by individual beads.

Compared with other NGS platforms, the key advantage of the 454 platform is read length. In the GS FLX Titanium XL+System, its read length can reach up to 1 kb with an accuracy of 99.9% and a throughput of 0.7 Gb per run. A major limitation of the 454 is that it has a relatively high error rate in terms of homopolymers (that is, consecutive instances of the same base, such as AAA or CCC), especially when poly-bases are longer than 6 bp. The per-base cost of sequencing with Roche 454 is much higher than that of other platforms. The Roche 454 system is a good choice for metagenomic sequencing and de novo genome sequencing in which long read lengths are critical.

The Illumina Genome Analyzer/HiSeq platform relies on bridge PCR to amplify sequencing features. In brief, both forward and reverse PCR primers are tethered to a solid substrate by a flexible linker. The library with fixed adapters is denatured to single strands and amplified to form clonal DNA fragments. Each cluster contains about 1000 copies of a single template molecule and remains immobilized on an array. The technology of sequencing by synthesis is used for sequencing. Each sequencing cycle includes the simultaneous addition of four modified kinds of nucleotides that contain different cleavable fluorescent labels and a reversibly terminating moiety. A modified DNA polymerase drives a synchronous extension of primed sequencing features. After a single-base extension and acquisition of images in four channels, both the fluorescent labels and the terminating moiety are cleaved for the next cycle. The current routine read length is up to 150 bp. Read lengths are limited by multiple factors such as incomplete cleavage of fluorescent labels or terminating moieties, which cause signal decay and dephasing.

The AB SOLiD system generates clonal sequencing features by emulsion PCR on the surface of paramagnetic beads. After breaking the emulsion, beads bearing amplification products are immobilized to a solid planar substrate to generate a dense, disordered array. The AB SOLiD system uses the technology of two-base—encoded probes based on sequencing by ligase. The two-base probes contain the first two interrogation bases, followed by three degenerate bases and three universal bases, with four different fluorescent dyes. The fluorescent signal is recorded in four channels and cleared by the cleavage of last three bases. Several such cycles will iteratively interrogate an evenly spaced, noncontiguous set of bases, and a different set of noncontiguous bases is interrogated when the system is reset and the process is repeated at a different position. SOLiD has a high accuracy of 99.9% owing to the two-base probes sequencing method.

Whole-Genome Sequencing Studies in ID and ASD

Whole-genome sequencing provides the most complete view of genomic variations and can detect single nucleotide substitutions, indels, translocations, inversions, and CNVs in a genome-wide fashion, although the power to detect events across the genome is not uniform based on local genomic composition. High costs and difficulty in interpreting noncoding variants are bottlenecks in applying WGS.

Gilissen et al. performed WGS in 50 patients with severe ID and in their unaffected parents, who had been prescreened by microarray-based CNV studies and exome sequencing, with no conclusive causes.[51] A total of 84 de novo SNVs in the coding region were identified, which showed a statistically significant enrichment of loss-of-function mutations as well as enrichment for genes previously implicated in ID-related disorders. Mutations in these known ID genes included four insertion/deletion events, two nonsense mutations, and three highly conserved missense mutations. In addition, eight de novo CNVs were identified and validated, of which four de novo deletions encompassed a known ID gene and one a candidate ID gene, representing a significant enrichment for CNVs affecting known ID genes. Taken together, a conclusive genetic diagnosis was made in 21 of 50 patients with severe ID in this well-studied cohort, reaching a diagnostic yield of 42% and 62% as a cumulative estimate in an unselected cohort. These results suggested that de novo SNVs and CNVs affecting the coding region are a major cause of severe ID. Three de novo SNVs occurring in candidate ID genes were detected by WGS in a mosaic state at levels of 21% (*PIAS1*), 22% (*HIVEP2*), and 20% (*KANSL2*) in the patients. In a systematic attempt to study the role of de novo noncoding mutations in ID, 43 de novo mutations located either within the promoter regions, introns, or untranslated regions of all known ID genes were confirmed, but annotation of these mutations did not reveal a potential pathogenic role for these noncoding mutations.

Jiang et al. performed WGS in 32 families with ASD using the Illumina Hiseq 2000 platform.[52] The average sequence depth was 38.4X. They found that the number of de novo mutations significantly correlated with paternal age. Of these 32 probands, 15 (47%) were found to carry at least one de novo deleterious mutation, which suggested that WGS is a useful tool for detecting genetic variants associated with ASD.

In the latest report about whole-exome sequencing in ASD, the authors conducted the largest sample to date to detect rare coding variations in 3871 autism cases and 9937 ancestry-matched or parental controls.[53] Thirty-three autosomal genes with a false discovery rate (FDR) less than 0.1 and 107 with an FDR less than 0.3 were indicated to be associated with ASD. Of the 33 genes, 15 (45.5%) are known ASD risk genes; 11 have been reported previously with mutations in ASD patients (*SUV420H1, ADNP, BCL11A, CACNA2D3, CTTNBP2, GABRB3, CDC42BPB, APH1A, NR3C2, SETD5,* and *TRIO*) and seven are completely novel (*ASH1L, MLL3, ETFB, NAA15, MYO9B, MIB1,* and *VIL1*). They found significant enrichment for genes encoding messenger ribonucleic acids (RNAs) targeted by two neuronal RNA-binding proteins: *FMRP* and *RBFOX*. These two pathways expand the complexity of ASD neurobiology to posttranscriptional events, including splicing and translation. Protein—protein interaction network predicted genes form four natural clusters on the basis of network connectivity. The enriched pathways and biological functions for each of the four clusters are cell communication and synaptic transmission, transcriptional and chromatin regulation, cell junction and transforming growth factor-β pathway, and neurodegeneration.

Exome Sequencing in ID and ASD

The exome represents less than 2% of the human genome but it contains about 85% of known disease-causing variants, which makes exome sequencing a cost-effective and compelling approach for identifying disease genes. Exome sequencing combines NGS technology with the targeted capture and amplification of exons (approximately 40 Mbp of the genome). The efficacy of the capture depends on the percentage GC nucleotide composition of the targeted sequence (also known as GC capture bias). For exons with especially high GC content, exome sequencing can fail to produce enough coverage for accurate variant detection and calling.

Krumm et al. reviewed six family-based exome studies of ASD and ID and found that the genes involved in ASD and ID converge on three functional pathways: chromatin remodeling, Wnt signaling during development, and synaptic function.[54]

Hamdan et al. performed high-depth exome sequencing in 41 individuals with moderate or severe ID and their healthy parents.[55] De novo point mutations (DNMs) (including SNVs and small insertions/deletions) were assessed for the role in genetics of ID. Finally, 81 putative DNMs that affected the coding sequence or consensus splice sites (1.98 DNMs/proband) were identified and confirmed. The de novo SNV rate in the consensus coding sequences was 2.58×10^{-8} per base per generation in ID cases, which is significantly higher than the expected population rate of 1.65×10^{-8}. A significant excess of de novo nonsense and splice site mutations in the probands was observed compared with controls with no family history of ID, which suggests that at least a subset of them are pathogenic. Nine loss-of-function DNMs (nonsense, frameshift, and canonical splice variants) and three predicted damaging DNMs (an in-frame insertion and two missense mutations) were identified in genes previously associated with ID (*ARID1B*, *CHD2*, *FOXG1*, *GABRB3*, *GATAD2B*, *GRIN2B*, *MBD5*, *MED13L*, *SETBP1*, *TBR1*, *TCF4*, and *WDR45*), resulting in a diagnostic yield of 29%. Six predicted damaging DNMs were identified in genes (*SET*, *EGR1*, *PPP1CB*, *CHMP2A*, *PPP2R2B*, and *VPS4A*) that have biological functions relevant to ID. Enrichment for proteins implicated in glutamate receptor signaling pathways was observed using protein network analysis. The author concluded that DNMs represent a major cause of moderate or severe ID.

CONCLUSION

Genetic research tools are more powerful when used in combination. The Decipher Developmental Disorders Study group demonstrated a combinational approach using both exome sequencing and array-based detection of chromosomal rearrangement. The combined data led to the identification of 12 novel genes associated with developmental disorders.[56] Coe et al. combined 70 significant CNVs data detected from 29,085 children with developmental delay and candidate gene resequencing among 4716 additional cases with developmental delay or ASD. This integrated analysis of CNV and sequence variants pinpointed 10 genes enriched for putative loss of function.[57] We anticipate that the pace of gene discovery for ID and ASD will continue to grow using the combination of approaches discussed here. We hope and believe that a better understanding of the genetic underpinning will lead to better diagnosis, management, and treatment for patients with ID and ASD.

References

1. Chiurazzi P, Schwartz CE, Gecz J, Neri G. XLMR genes: update 2007. *Eur J Hum Genet* 2008;**16**(4):422−34.
2. Ropers HH, Hamel BC. X-linked mental retardation. *Nat Rev Genet* 2005;**6**(1):46−57.
3. Kleefstra T, Hamel BC. X-linked mental retardation: further lumping, splitting and emerging phenotypes. *Clin Genet* 2005;**67**(6): 451−67.
4. Mandel JL, Chelly J. Monogenic X-linked mental retardation: is it as frequent as currently estimated? The paradox of the ARX (Aristaless X) mutations. *Eur J Hum Genet* 2004;**12**(9):689−93.
5. Lubs HA, Stevenson RE, Schwartz CE. Fragile X and X-linked intellectual disability: four decades of discovery. *Am J Hum Genet* 2012; **90**(4):579−90.
6. Gilfillan GD, Selmer KK, Roxrud I, et al. SLC9A6 mutations cause X-linked mental retardation, microcephaly, epilepsy, and ataxia, a phenotype mimicking Angelman syndrome. *Am J Hum Genet* 2008;**82**(4):1003−10.
7. Nolan DK, Chen P, Das S, Ober C, Waggoner D. Fine mapping of a locus for nonsyndromic mental retardation on chromosome 19p13. *Am J Med Genet A* 2008;**146A**(11):1414−22.
8. Caliskan M, Chong JX, Uricchio L, et al. Exome sequencing reveals a novel mutation for autosomal recessive non-syndromic mental retardation in the TECR gene on chromosome 19p13. *Hum Mol Genet* 2011;**20**(7):1285−9.
9. Weiss LA, Arking DE, Gene Discovery Project of Johns H, the Autism C, Daly MJ, Chakravarti A. A genome-wide linkage and association scan reveals novel loci for autism. *Nature* 2009; **461**(7265):802−8.
10. Allen-Brady K, Robison R, Cannon D, et al. Genome-wide linkage in Utah autism pedigrees. *Mol psychiatry* 2010;**15**(10):1006−15.
11. A full genome screen for autism with evidence for linkage to a region on chromosome 7q. International Molecular Genetic Study of Autism Consortium. *Hum Mol Genet* 1998;**7**(3):571−8.
12. Autism Genome Project Consortium, Szatmari P, Paterson AD, et al. Mapping autism risk loci using genetic linkage and chromosomal rearrangements. *Nat Genet* 2007;**39**(3):319−28.
13. International Molecular Genetic Study of Autism C. A genomewide screen for autism: strong evidence for linkage to chromosomes 2q, 7q, and 16p. *Am J Hum Genet* 2001;**69**(3):570−81.
14. Lamb JA, Barnby G, Bonora E, et al. Analysis of IMGSAC autism susceptibility loci: evidence for sex limited and parent of origin specific effects. *J Med Genet* 2005;**42**(2):132−7.
15. Liu XQ, Paterson AD, Szatmari P, Autism Genome Project C. Genome-wide linkage analyses of quantitative and categorical autism subphenotypes. *Biol psychiatry* 2008;**64**(7):561−70.
16. Schellenberg GD, Dawson G, Sung YJ, et al. Evidence for multiple loci from a genome scan of autism kindreds. *Mol psychiatry* 2006; **11**(11):1049−60. 1979.
17. Freitag CM, Staal W, Klauck SM, Duketis E, Waltes R. Genetics of autistic disorders: review and clinical implications. *Eur child Adolesc psychiatry* 2010;**19**(3):169−78.
18. Trikalinos TA, Karvouni A, Zintzaras E, et al. A heterogeneity-based genome search meta-analysis for autism-spectrum disorders. *Mol psychiatry* 2006;**11**(1):29−36.
19. Talkowski ME, Rosenfeld JA, Blumenthal I, et al. Sequencing chromosomal abnormalities reveals neurodevelopmental loci that confer risk across diagnostic boundaries. *Cell* 2012;**149**(3):525−37.
20. Talkowski ME, Ernst C, Heilbut A, et al. Next-generation sequencing strategies enable routine detection of balanced chromosome rearrangements for clinical diagnostics and genetic research. *Am J Hum Genet* 2011;**88**(4):469−81.
21. Ropers HH. Genetics of intellectual disability. *Curr Opin Genet Dev* 2008;**18**(3):241−50.
22. Lander ES, Botstein D. Homozygosity mapping: a way to map human recessive traits with the DNA of inbred children. *Science* 1987; **236**(4808):1567−70.
23. Alkuraya FS. Discovery of rare homozygous mutations from studies of consanguineous pedigrees. In: Haines JL, Korf BR, editors. *Current protocols in human genetics*. John Wiley & Son; 2012 [Chapter 6: Unit 6.12].
24. Seelow D, Schuelke M, Hildebrandt F, Nurnberg P. Homozygosity-Mapper−an interactive approach to homozygosity mapping. *Nucleic Acids Res* 2009;**37**(Web Server issue):W593−9.
25. Carr IM, Flintoff KJ, Taylor GR, Markham AF, Bonthron DT. Interactive visual analysis of SNP data for rapid autozygosity mapping in consanguineous families. *Hum Mutat* 2006;**27**(10):1041−6.

26. Carr IM, Sheridan E, Hayward BE, Markham AF, Bonthron DT. IBDfinder and SNPsetter: tools for pedigree-independent identification of autozygous regions in individuals with recessive inherited disease. *Hum Mutat* 2009;**30**(6):960—7.

27. Morrow EM, Yoo SY, Flavell SW, et al. Identifying autism loci and genes by tracing recent shared ancestry. *Science* 2008;**321**(5886): 218—23.

28. Alkuraya FS. The application of next-generation sequencing in the autozygosity mapping of human recessive diseases. *Hum Genet* 2013;**132**(11):1197—211.

29. Carr IM, Morgan J, Watson C, et al. Simple and efficient identification of rare recessive pathologically important sequence variants from next generation exome sequence data. *Hum Mutat* 2013; **34**(7):945—52.

30. Carr IM, Bhaskar S, O'Sullivan J, et al. Autozygosity mapping with exome sequence data. *Hum Mutat* 2013;**34**(1):50—6.

31. Casey JP, Magalhaes T, Conroy JM, et al. A novel approach of homozygous haplotype sharing identifies candidate genes in autism spectrum disorder. *Hum Genet* 2012;**131**(4):565—79.

32. Sim NL, Kumar P, Hu J, Henikoff S, Schneider G, Ng PC. SIFT web server: predicting effects of amino acid substitutions on proteins. *Nucleic Acids Res* 2012;**40**(Web Server issue):W452—7.

33. Adzhubei IA, Schmidt S, Peshkin L, et al. A method and server for predicting damaging missense mutations. *Nat methods* 2010;**7**(4): 248—9.

34. Ferrer-Costa C, Orozco M, de la Cruz X. Sequence-based prediction of pathological mutations. *Proteins* 2004;**57**(4):811—9.

35. Tarpey PS, Smith R, Pleasance E, et al. A systematic, large-scale resequencing screen of X-chromosome coding exons in mental retardation. *Nat Genet* 2009;**41**(5):535—43.

36. Kenny EM, Cormican P, Furlong S, et al. Excess of rare novel loss-of-function variants in synaptic genes in schizophrenia and autism spectrum disorders. *Mol psychiatry* 2014;**19**(8):872—9.

37. Homer N, Merriman B, Nelson SF. BFAST: an alignment tool for large scale genome resequencing. *PloS One* 2009;**4**(11):e7767.

38. Koboldt DC, Larson DE, Chen K, Ding L, Wilson RK. Massively parallel sequencing approaches for characterization of structural variation. *Methods Mol Biol* 2012;**838**:369—84.

39. Li H, Durbin R. Fast and accurate short read alignment with Burrows-Wheeler transform. *Bioinformatics* 2009;**25**(14):1754—60.

40. Li H, Durbin R. Fast and accurate long-read alignment with Burrows-Wheeler transform. *Bioinformatics* 2010;**26**(5):589—95.

41. Li H, Ruan J, Durbin R. Mapping short DNA sequencing reads and calling variants using mapping quality scores. *Genome Res* 2008; **18**(11):1851—8.

42. Ning Z, Cox AJ, Mullikin JC. SSAHA: a fast search method for large DNA databases. *Genome Res* 2001;**11**(10):1725—9.

43. Rumble SM, Lacroute P, Dalca AV, Fiume M, Sidow A, Brudno M. SHRiMP: accurate mapping of short color-space reads. *PLoS Comput Biol* 2009;**5**(5):e1000386.

44. Zhao M, Wang Q, Wang Q, Jia P, Zhao Z. Computational tools for copy number variation (CNV) detection using next-generation sequencing data: features and perspectives. *BMC Bioinforma* 2013; **14**(Suppl. 11):S1.

45. Miller DT, Adam MP, Aradhya S, et al. Consensus statement: chromosomal microarray is a first-tier clinical diagnostic test for individuals with developmental disabilities or congenital anomalies. *Am J Hum Genet* 2010;**86**(5):749—64.

46. Liu L, Li Y, Li S, et al. Comparison of next-generation sequencing systems. *J Biomed Biotechnol* 2012;**2012**:251364.

47. Metzker ML. Sequencing technologies — the next generation. *Nat Rev Genet* 2010;**11**(1):31—46.

48. Schuster SC. Next-generation sequencing transforms today's biology. *Nat methods* 2008;**5**(1):16—8.

49. Shendure J, Ji H. Next-generation DNA sequencing. *Nat Biotechnol* 2008;**26**(10):1135—45.

50. Xi R, Kim TM, Park PJ. Detecting structural variations in the human genome using next generation sequencing. *Briefings Funct genomics* 2010;**9**(5—6):405—15.

51. Gilissen C, Hehir-Kwa JY, Thung DT, et al. Genome sequencing identifies major causes of severe intellectual disability. *Nature* 2014;**511**(7509):344—7.

52. Jiang YH, Yuen RK, Jin X, et al. Detection of clinically relevant genetic variants in autism spectrum disorder by whole-genome sequencing. *Am J Hum Genet* 2013;**93**(2):249—63.

53. De Rubeis S, He X, Goldberg AP, et al. Synaptic, transcriptional and chromatin genes disrupted in autism. *Nature* 2014;**515**(7526): 209—15.

54. Krumm N, O'Roak BJ, Shendure J, Eichler EE. A de novo convergence of autism genetics and molecular neuroscience. *Trends Neurosci* 2014;**37**(2):95—105.

55. Hamdan FF, Srour M, Capo-Chichi JM, et al. De novo mutations in moderate or severe intellectual disability. *PLoS Genet* 2014;**10**(10): e1004772.

56. The Deciphering Developmental Disorders Study. Large-scale discovery of novel genetic causes of developmental disorders. *Nature* 2014;**519**(7542):223—8.

57. Coe BP, Witherspoon K, Rosenfeld JA, et al. Refining analyses of copy number variation identifies specific genes associated with developmental delay. *Nat Genet* 2014;**46**(10):1063—71.

2

Genetic Causes of Autism Spectrum Disorders

Guillaume Huguet[1,2,3], Thomas Bourgeron[1,2,3,4,5]

[1]Institut Pasteur, Human Genetics and Cognitive Functions Unit, Paris, France; [2]CNRS UMR3571 Genes, Synapses and Cognition, Institut Pasteur, Paris, France; [3]University Paris Diderot, Sorbonne Paris Cité, Human Genetics and Cognitive Functions, Paris, France; [4]FondaMental Foundation, Créteil, France; [5]Gillberg Neuropsychiatry Centre, Sahlgrenska Academy, University of Gothenburg, Gothenburg, Sweden

INTRODUCTION

Autism spectrum disorders (ASDs) are a group of neuropsychiatric disorders characterized by problems with social communication as well as the presence of restricted interests and stereotyped and repetitive behaviors.[1-3] Epidemiological studies estimate that more than 1% of the population could receive a diagnosis of ASD.[4,5] Individuals with ASD can also have other psychiatric and medical conditions including intellectual disability (ID), epilepsy, motor control difficulties, attention-deficit hyperactivity disorder (ADHD), tics, anxiety, sleep disorders, depression, and gastrointestinal problems.[6,7] The term "ESSENCE" (early symptomatic syndromes eliciting neurodevelopmental clinical examinations) was coined by Christopher Gillberg to take into account this clinical heterogeneity and syndrome overlap.[6] There are four to eight times more males than females with ASD[5] but the sex ratio is more balanced in patients with ID and/or

dysmorphic features.[8] Autism can be studied as a category (affected versus unaffected) or as a quantitative trait using auto- or heteroquestionnaires such as the Social Responsiveness Scale or the Autism Quotient.[9-11] Using these tools, autistic traits seem to be normally distributed in clinical cases as well as in the general population.[9-11]

The causes of autism remain largely unknown, but twin studies have constantly shown a high genetic contribution to ASD. Molecular genetics studies have identified more than 100 ASD-risk genes carrying rare and penetrant deleterious mutations in approximately 10–25% of patients.[12,13] In addition, quantitative genetics studies have shown that common genetic variants could capture almost all of the heritability of ASD.[12,13] The genetic landscape of ASD is shaped by a complex interplay between common and rare variants and is most likely different from one individual to another.[14,15] Remarkably, the susceptibility genes seem[12] to converge in a limited number of biological pathways including chromatin remodeling,

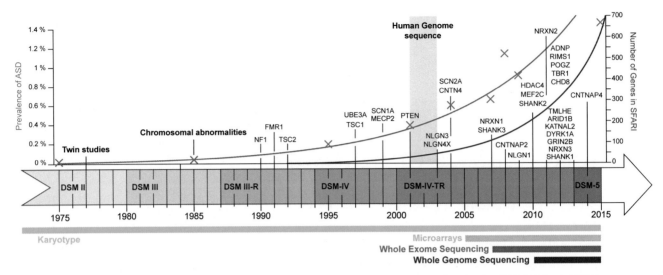

FIGURE 1   **History of the genetics of autism, from 1975 to 2015.** Increase in genes associated with ASD (SFARI, March 2015) is represented, together with the prevalence of ASD (data taken from the Centers for Disease Control and Prevention), the different versions of the *Diagnostic Statistical Manual* (from DSM II to DSM 5.0), and advances in genetics technology.

protein translation, actin dynamics, and synaptic functions.[12,16,17]

In this chapter, we will detail the advances of the genetics of ASD in the past four decades starting from twin studies, following with molecular genetics studies and ending with an investigation of the biological pathways associated with ASD[12,16–19] (Figure 1).

TWIN AND FAMILY STUDIES IN ASD

Based on more than 13 twin studies published between 1977 and 2015, researchers have estimated the genetic and environmental contribution to ASD (Figure 2). In 1977, the first twin study of autism by Folstein and Rutter[20] reported a cohort of 11 monozygotic (MZ) twins and 10 dizygotic (DZ) twins. This study showed that MZ twins were more concordant for autism in 36% (four of 11) compared with 0% (0 of 10) for DZ twins. When a broader autism phenotype was used, the concordance increased to 92% for MZ twins and 10% for DZ twins.[21] Since this first small-scale study, twin studies have constantly reported higher concordance for ASD in MZ compared with DZ.[21–24] Between 2005 and 2009, three twin studies with relatively large groups of twins (285–3419) have reported high concordances for ASD in MZ twins (77–95%) compared with DZ twins (31%).[25–27] Notably, MZ concordances were similar to those reported in the previous studies, but DZ concordances were higher. In 2010, Lichtenstein et al. reported a relatively low concordance for ASD in 39% of MZ twins compared with other studies (the concordance for DZ twins in that study was 15%).[28] However, as

previously indicated by studies using the broader autism phenotype, all discordant MZ twins of that cohort had symptoms of ESSENCE (e.g., ID, ADHD, language delay). A significant proportion of the genetic contribution to ASD was shown to be shared with other neurodevelopmental disorders such as ADHD (>50%) and learning disability (>40%).[28–31] In summary, when all twin studies are taken into account, concordance for ASD is roughly 45% for MZ twins and 16% for DZ twins.[21–24]

Family studies also showed that the recurrence of having a child with ASD increases with the proportion of the genome that the individual shares with one affected sibling or parent.[32–34] In a population-based sample of 14516 children diagnosed with ASD,[32] the relative risk for ASD (compared with the general population) was estimated to be 153.0 (95% confidence interval [CI], 56.7–412.8) for MZ twins, 8.2 (3.7–18.1) for DZ twins, 10.3 (9.4–11.3) for full siblings, 3.3 (95% CI, 2.6–4.2) for maternal half siblings, 2.9 (95% CI, 2.2–3.7) for paternal half siblings, and 2.0 (95% CI, 1.8–2.2) for cousins.

Heritability is the proportion of the phenotypic variation in a trait of interest, measured in a given studied population and in a given environment that is co-varying with genetic differences among individuals in the same population. In 1995, based on a twin study, Bailey et al. estimated the heritability of autism to be 91–93%.[21] Since then, the estimation of heritability has differed from one study to another, but the genetic variance has accounted for at least 38% and up to 90% of the phenotypic variance.[15,29,32] Using a large cohort of 14,516 children diagnosed with ASD,[32] the heritability was estimated to be 0.50 (95% CI, 0.45–0.56) and the

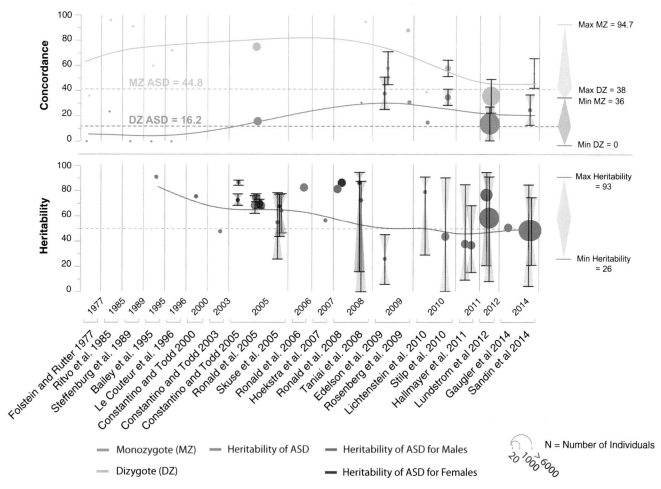

FIGURE 2 **The main twin studies in ASD.** A total of 13 twin studies and 17 heritability studies are depicted. Means of concordance and heritability weighted by sample size are presented on the right of the figure.

nonshared environmental influence was also 0.50 (95% CI, 0.44−0.55). Surprisingly, only the additive genetic component and the nonshared environment seemed to account for the risk of developing ASD.[32]

In summary, epidemiological studies provide crucial information on the heritability of ASD. However, they do not inform us about the genes involved or the number and frequency of their variants. In the past 15 years, candidate genes and whole-genome analyses have been performed to address these questions.

FROM CHROMOSOMAL REARRANGEMENTS TO COPY NUMBER VARIANTS IN ASD

The first genetic studies that associated genetic variants with autism used observations from cytogenetics studies.[35] However, because of the low resolution of the karyotypes (several megabytes), it was almost impossible to associate a specific gene with ASD using this approach. The prevalence of large chromosomal abnormalities is estimated to be <2%.[36] Because of progress in molecular technologies such as comparative genomic hybridization and single nucleotide polymorphism (SNP) arrays, the resolution of detection of genomic imbalances has dramatically increased. Depending on the platforms, copy number variants (CNVs) of more than 50 kb are now robustly detected.[37] Since the first articles published in 2006, a very large number of studies have investigated the contribution of CNVs in ASD.[38,39] Several studies using the Simons Simplex Collection could even provide an estimation of the frequency of the de novo CNVs in patients with ASD compared with their unaffected siblings.[40] Altogether, de novo CNVs are present in 4−7% of patients with ASD compared with 1−2% in unaffected siblings and controls.[40−42] The studies have also indicated that de novo CNVs identified in patients are most likely altering genes and most especially genes associated with synaptic functions and/or regulated by FMRP, the protein responsible for fragile X syndrome.[42,43] Beyond ASD, large CNVs (>400 kb) affecting exons are present in 15% of patients with developmental delay or ID.[44] Most of the CNVs are private to each individual, but some are recurrently observed in independent patients. For example, three loci on chromosomal regions 7q11, 15q11.2−13.3, and 16p11.2 have been strongly associated with ASD.[40,45−49]

In summary, large chromosomal rearrangements and CNVs increase the risk of having ASD in 5−10% of individuals[36,42,43]. To identify ASD-risk genes further, candidate genes and whole exome/genome studies were performed.

FROM CANDIDATE GENES TO WHOLE EXOME/GENOME SEQUENCING STUDIES IN ASD

The first approach to associating a gene with ASD was to select specific candidate genes based on data from functional or genetic studies, or a combination of both. This approach was successful in identifying several synaptic genes associated with ASD, such as NLGN3, NLGN4X, SHANK3, and NRXN1.[50−52] Because of advances in next-generation sequencing, we can now interrogate all genes of the genome in an unbiased manner using whole exome sequencing (WES) and whole genome sequencing (WGS).

To date, more than 18 WES studies of sporadic cases of ASD[53−70] have been performed, altogether comprising >4000 families (Table 1). In almost all of these studies, the authors have especially focused their analysis on the contribution of de novo SNVs in ASD. The average number of de novo coding SNVs per individual (including missense, splicing, frameshift, and stop-gain variants) is estimated to be approximately 0.86 in female patients, 0.73 in male patients, and 0.60 in unaffected male and female siblings.[71,72] Interestingly, de novo SNVs were three times more likely to be on the paternal chromosome than on the maternal one,[54,73] with an increase of almost two de novo mutations per year and doubling every 16.5 years.[73]

Based on these studies,[54−57] 3.6−8.8% of patients were shown to carry a de novo causative mutation,[57] with a twofold increase of deleterious mutations in patients compared with their unaffected siblings. In a meta-analysis using more than 2500 families, Iossifov et al.[66] found that de novo likely gene disrupting (LGD) mutations (frameshift, nonsense, and splice site) were more frequent in patients with ASD compared with unaffected siblings ($P = 5 \times 10^{-7}$). Carriers of these de novo LGD mutations were more likely diagnosed with a low nonverbal intelligence quotient. The de novo LGD mutations are significantly enriched in genes

involved in chromatin modeling factors ($P = 4 \times 10^{-6}$) and in genes regulated by the FMRP complex ($P = 4 \times 10^{-7}$). After these whole exome studies, targeted resequencing studies of the most compelling candidate genes were performed.[74] Ten genes carrying de novo mutations were significantly associated with ASD: CHD8, DYRK1A, GRIN2B, KATNAL2, RIMS1, SCN2A, POGZ, ADNP, ARID1B, and TBR1.

Only a few studies have analyzed the contribution of inherited SNVs in ASD. In 2013, Lim et al. (2013) analyzed WES of 933 patients (ASD) and 869 controls for the presence of rare complete human knockouts (KO) with homozygous or compound heterozygous loss-of-function variants (≤5% frequency).[60] They observed a significant twofold increase in complete KO in patients with ASD compared with controls and estimated that such complete KO mutations could account for 3% of patients with ASD. For the X chromosome, there was a significant 1.5-fold increase in complete KO in affected males compared with unaffected males, which could account for 2% of males with ASD.[60] The same year, Yu et al. analyzed 104 consanguineous families including 79 families with a single child with ASD (simplex families) and 25 families with more than one affected individual (multiplex families), collected by the Homozygosity Mapping Collaborative for Autism.[59] The researchers identified biallelic mutations in AMT, PEX7, SYNE1, VPS13B, PAH, and POMGNT1. Finally, a study by Krumm et al. ascertained the relative impact of inherited and de novo variants (CNVs or SNVs) on ASD risk in 2377 families.[70] Inherited truncating variants are enriched in probands (for SNV odds ratio = 1.14, $P = 0.0002$; for CNV odds ratio = 1.23, $P = 0.001$) compared with unaffected siblings.[70] Interestingly, they also observed a significant maternal transmission bias of inherited LGD to sons.[70] New ASD-risk genes were also identified, such as RIMS1, CUL7, and LZTR1.

To date, few WGS studies have been published in ASD (Table 1). Michaelson et al. analyzed 40 whole genome sequences of MZ twins concordant for ASD and their parents.[75] They proposed that ASD-risk genes could be hot spots of mutation in the genome and confirmed the association between ASD and de novo mutations in GPR98, KIRREL3, and TCF4. Shi et al. analyzed a large pedigree with two sons affected with ASD and six unaffected siblings, focusing on inherited mutations.[76] They identified ANK3 as the most likely candidate gene. In 2015, Yuen et al. analyzed 85 families with two children affected with ASD. That study represents the largest published WGS data set in ASD.[77] They identified 46 ASD-relevant mutations present in 36 of 85 families (42.4%). Only 16 ASD-relevant mutations of 46 identified (35%) were de novo. Interestingly, for more than half of the families (69.4%; 25 of 36), the two

TABLE 1 Summary of the Main Whole Exome/Genome Sequencing (WES/WGS) Studies in ASDs

Studies	Tech	No. ASD Analyzed in the Study	No. ASD Specific to This Study	No. ASD Coming from Other Studies	No. Controls	No. Unaffected Siblings	No. Parents	Analysis of De Novo Variants	Analysis of Inherited Variants
O'Roak et al.[53]	WES	20	20	–	–	20	38	X	–
O'Roak et al.[54]	WES	229	209	20[53]	–	50	418	X	–
Neale et al.[55]	WES	175	175	–	–	–	350	X	–
Sanders et al.[56]	WES	238	238	–	–	200	476	X	–
Iossifov et al.[57]	WES	343	343	–	–	343	686	X	X
Chahrour et al.[58]	WES	16	16	–	–	–	–	–	X
Yu et al.[59]	WES	401	163	238[55–57]	–	114	326	X	X
Lim et al.[60]	WES	1496	1004	492[56]	5474	–	–	X	X
Liu et al.[61]	WES	1039	–	1039[53–57,61]	869	–	–	–	X
He et al.[62]	WES	1867	–	1867[53–57,61]	870	593	1870	X	X
Willsey et al.[63]	WES	1099	56	1043[53–57,61]	–	56	112	X	X
Liu et al.[64]	WES	1967	–	1967[53–57,61,63,73]	870	593	2070	X	X
Samocha et al.[65]	WES	1078	–	1078[2–6,9]	–	343	2156	X	–
Iossifov et al.[66]	WES	2	1576	932[53–57,61]	–	1911	5016	X	–
An et al.[67]	WES	40	40	–	–	8	80	X	X
De Rubeis et al.[68]	WES	2270	–	2270[53–57,66]	5397	–	4540	X	X
Chang et al.[69]	WES	932	–	932[53,54,56,57,125]	–	593	1580	X	X
Krumm et al.[70]	WES	2377	–	2377[53–57,66]	–	1786	4754	X	X
Kong et al.[73]	WGS	40	44	–	–	7	136	X	–
Michaelson et al.[75]	WGS	20	20	–	–	–	–	X	–
Shi et al.[76]	WGS	1	1	–	–	6	2	X	X
Jiang et al.[126]	WGS	32	32	–	–	–	64	X	X
Yuen et al.[77]	WGS	85	85	32[126]	–	–	170	X	X
Nemirovsky et al.[78]	WGS	1	–	–	–	–	–	–	X

affected siblings did not share the same rare penetrant ASD-risk variant(s).

Whole genome sequencing is also efficient for identifying mutations in regions of the human genome that are wrongly annotated and regions that are highly GC-rich. For example, mutations on the *SHANK3* gene were rarely identified using WGS because of its high GC content.[49] In contrast, WGS could successfully identify *SHANK3* mutations.[77,78]

COMMON VARIANTS IN ASD

In the general population, one individual carries on average three million genetic variants compared with the reference human genome sequence.[79–81] The vast majority of variants (>95%) are so-called common variants shared with more than 5% of the human population.[79–81] Although there is not a clear border between common and rare variants, it is nevertheless interesting to estimate the role of the genetic variants found in the general population in the susceptibility to ASD.

Using quantitative genetics, Klei et al. estimated that common variants contributed to a high proportion of the liability of ASD: 40% in simplex families and 60% in multiplex one.[82] In 2014, the study of Gaugler et al. used the same methodology[83] and provided an estimation of the heritability (52.4%) that is almost exclusively caused by common variation, leaving only 2.6% of the liability to rare variants.[13] The contribution of common variants is therefore important, but unfortunately the causative SNPs remain unknown because they are numerous (>1000) and each is associated with a low risk. To date, the largest genome-wide association studies (GWAS) performed on <5000 families with ASD were underpowered to identify a single SNP with genome-wide significance.[84,85]

The recruitment of larger cohorts of patients with dimensional phenotypes is therefore warranted to better ascertain the heritability of ASD and identify genetic variants that explain most of the genetic variance.

THE GENETIC ARCHITECTURE OF ASD

Based on the results obtained from epidemiological and molecular studies, it is now accepted that the genetic susceptibility to ASD can be different from one individual to another with a combination of rare deleterious variants (R) and a myriad of low-risk alleles (also defined as the genetic background [B]). Most of the inherited part of ASD seems to result from common variants observed in the general population, with only a small contribution from rare variants (Figure 3). Importantly, whereas the de novo mutations are considered per se to be genetic factors, they do not contribute

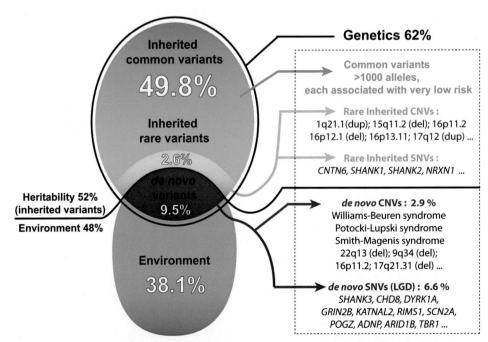

FIGURE 3   **Relative contributions of genetics and environment in ASD.** Based on twin and familial studies, it is estimated that the genetic and environmental contributions to ASD are approximately 50–50%. Most of the inheritable part seems to be due to common variants observed in the general population, with a small contribution from rare variants. Importantly, de novo mutations are genetic causes of ASD, but they do not contribute to heritability because they are present only in the patient. These de novo events are therefore considered environmental causes of ASD, but act on the deoxyribonucleic acid molecule.

to the heritability because they are present only in the patient (with the relatively rare exception of germinal mosaicisms present in one of the parental germ line and transmitted to multiple children). These de novo events could therefore be considered environmental causes of ASD, but acting on the deoxyribonucleic acid molecule. It is currently estimated that more than 500–1000 genes could account for these monogenic forms of ASD,[56,57] which confirms the high degree of genetic heterogeneity.

The interplay between the rare or de novo variants R and the background B will also influence the phenotypic diversity observed in patients carrying rare deleterious mutations. In some individuals, a genetic background B will be able to buffer or compensate for the impact of the rare genetic variations, R. In contrast, in some individuals the buffering capacity of B will not be sufficient to compensate the impact of R and they will develop ASD.[86,87] In the R and B model, ASD can be regarded as a collection of many genetic forms of autisms, each with a different etiology ranging from monogenic to polygenic models.

The presence of multiple hits of rare CNVs, SNVs or indels in a single individual also illustrates the complexity of the genetic landscape of ASD.[88–90] In addition, an analysis of the WGS of multiplex families indicates that clinically relevant mutations can be different from one affected sibling to another even in a single family.[77] It is therefore still difficult to ascertain robust genotype–phenotype relationships based on our current knowledge.

Fortunately, although the ASD-risk genes are numerous, they seem to converge in a limited number of biological pathways that are currently being scrutinized by many researchers.

BIOLOGICAL PATHWAYS ASSOCIATED WITH ASD

Unbiased pathway analyses indicated that ASD-risk genes seem to be enriched in groups of proteins with specific functions.[68,72,91–93] Pinto et al. analyzed the burden of CNVs in 2446 individuals with ASD and 2640 controls and found an enrichment in genes coding postsynaptic density proteins and FMRP targets.[42] Ronemus et al. reviewed the results of four WES studies and showed an enrichment of mutated genes in chromatin modifier genes ($P = 4 \times 10^{-6}$) and FMRP targets ($P = 7 \times 10^{-6}$).[72] Protein–protein interactions (PPI) analyses of genes carrying LGD mutations also showed enrichment in proteins involved in neuronal development and axon guidance, signaling pathways, and chromatin and transcription regulation. De Rubeis et al. also used PPI networks and showed enrichment in clusters of proteins involved in cell junction transforming growth factor-β pathway, cell communication and synaptic transmission, neurodegeneration, and transcriptional regulation.[68]

In parallel to the genetic studies, several transcriptomic analyses were performed using postmortem brains of individuals with ASD.[91,94] Several genes were differentially expressed or correlated between brain regions. Two network modules were identified. The first module was related to interneurons and to genes involved in synaptic function (downregulated in brains from ASD patients compared with controls). The second module was related to immunity and microglia activation (upregulated in brains from ASD patients compared with controls).

Based on these results, neurobiological studies using cellular and animal models have been performed to identify the main mechanisms leading to ASD. Remarkably, several studies showed that neuronal activity seems to regulate the function of many of the ASD-risk genes. This has led to the hypothesis that abnormal synaptic plasticity and failure of neuronal/synaptic homeostasis could have a key role in the susceptibility to ASD.[16,95,96] Here, we will depict only four main biological pathways associated with ASD: chromatin remodeling, protein synthesis, protein degradation, and synaptic function (Figure 4).

Chromatin remodeling: Mutations in genes encoding key regulators of chromatin remodeling and gene transcription (e.g., MECP2, MEF2C, HDAC4, CHD8, and CTNNB1) have been reported in individuals with ASD (Figure 4). Remarkably, a subset of these genes is regulated by neuronal activity and influences neuronal connectivity and synaptic plasticity.[97–99]

Protein synthesis: The level of synaptic proteins can be influenced by neuronal activity through global and local synaptic messenger ribonucleic acid (mRNA) translation.[100] Several genes involved in such activity-driven regulation of synaptic proteins have been found to be mutated in individuals with ASD.[101] For example, the mTOR pathway controls global mRNA translation and its deregulation causes diseases associated with increased cell proliferation and loss of autophagy, including cancer,[100] but it also increases the risk for ASD. Mutations in the repressor of the mTOR pathway, such as NF1, PTEN, and SynGAP1, cause an increase in translation in neurons and at the synapse.[95] Mutations of the FMRP–EIF4E–CYFIP1 complex cause fragile X syndrome and increase the risk of ASD.[102] This protein complex controls local translation of mRNA at the synapse and acts downstream of the Ras-ERK signaling pathway. This complex regulates the translation of more than 1000 specific genes, many of which are ASD-risk genes.[103–106] Alteration of this FMRP–EIF4E–CYFIP1 complex should therefore create an imbalance

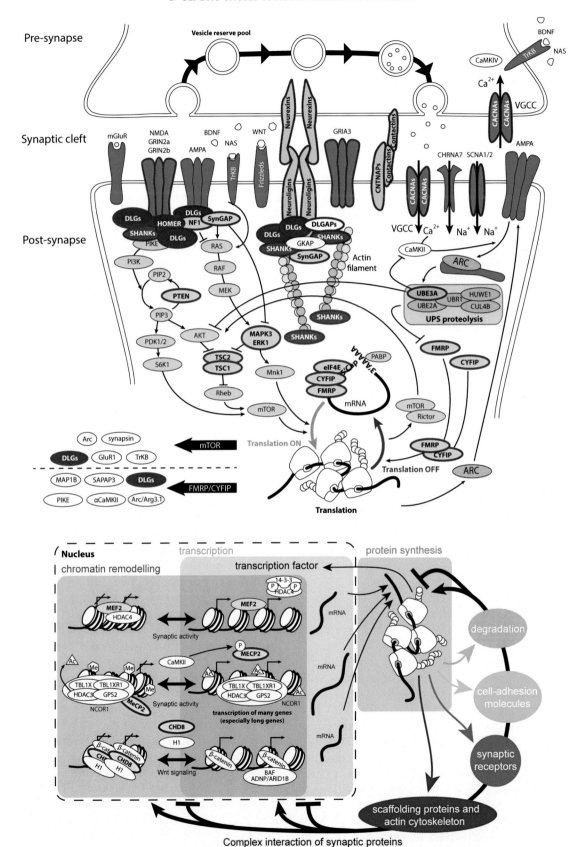

FIGURE 4 **Examples of biological pathways associated with ASD.** The ASD-risk genes code for proteins involved in chromatin remodeling, transcription, protein synthesis and degradation, cytoskeleton dynamics, and synaptic functions. Proteins associated with ASD are circled in red.

in the level of many synaptic proteins that are associated with ASD.

Protein degradation: The ubiquitin–proteasome system is central to degradation of the proteins and, consequently, for the regulation of synapse composition, assembly, and elimination.[107] The *UBE3A* gene encodes an ubiquitin ligase, is mutated in patients with Angelman syndrome, and is duplicated on the maternal chromosome 15q11 in individuals with ASD. Neuronal activity increases *UBE3A* transcription through the MEF2 complex and regulates excitatory synapse development by controlling the degradation of ARC, a synaptic protein that decreases long-term potentiation by promoting the internalization of α-amino-3-hydroxy-5-methyl-4-isoxazolepropionic acid receptors.[108]

Synaptic functions: Many proteins encoded by ASD-risk genes participate in different aspects of neuronal connectivity, such as glutamatergic (e.g., GRIN2B), GABAergic (e.g., GABRA3 and GABRB3), and glycinergic (e.g., GLRA2) neurotransmission, neuritogenesis (e.g., CNTN), the establishment of synaptic identity (e.g., cadherins and protocadherins), neuronal conduction (CNTNAP2), and permeability to ions (CACNA1, CACNA2D3, and SCN1A). Some of these proteins are directly involved in activity-driven synapse formation, such as the neurexins (NRXNs) and neuroligins (NLGNs). Some are scaffolding proteins involved in the positioning of cell-adhesion molecules and neurotransmitter receptors at the synapse.[109,110] For example, deletions, duplications, and coding mutations in the three *SHANK* genes (*SHANK1*, *SHANK2*, and *SHANK3*) have been recurrently reported in individuals with ASD[49] (see also Chapter 10). SHANK proteins assemble into large molecular platforms in interaction with glutamate receptors and actin-associated proteins.[111] In vitro, SHANK3 mutations identified in individuals with ASD reduce actin accumulation in spines, affecting the development and morphology of dendrites as well as axonal growth cone motility.[112] In mice, mutations in *SHANK3* decrease spine density in the hippocampus, but they also increase dendritic arborizations in striatal neurons.[113] Mice mutated in SHANK present with behavior resembling autistic features in humans. *Shank1* KO mice display increased anxiety, decreased vocal communication, decreased locomotion, and enhanced working memory, but decreased long-term memory.[114–116] *Shank2* KO mice present with hyperactivity, increased anxiety, repetitive grooming, and abnormalities in vocal and social behaviors.[117,118] *Shank3* KO mice show self-injurious repetitive grooming and deficits in social interaction and communication.[113,119–121]

PERSPECTIVES

In the past 30 years, significant progress has been made in the genetics of ASD. We now have better knowledge about the genetic architecture of this heterogeneous syndrome, and some of the biological pathways are being investigated using different approaches such as cellular and animal models. However, there are many aspects of the genetics of ASD that remain largely unknown.

The first challenge concerns the role of the common variants. These variants most likely have a key role in susceptibility to ASD and the severity of the symptoms. But because the impact of each single SNP is low, it is currently impossible to identify the risk alleles using conventional GWAS. In human quantitative traits such as height, neuroanatomical diversity, or intelligent quotient, very large cohorts of many thousands of individuals are necessary to identify the main causative SNPs.[122–124]

The second challenge concerns the stratification of patients and the role of ASD-risk genes during brain development and function. Based on our current knowledge, the genetic architecture of ASD seems to be different from one individual to another, with possibly contrasting impact on when and where neuronal connectivity could be atypical compared with the general population. For example, in animal models, several mutations lead to higher connectivity, whereas other mutations alter synaptic density. It is therefore crucial to increase our knowledge from a basic research perspective on the biological roles of the ASD-risk genes and their partners.

Finally, although we all agree that biological research is necessary to improve the quality of life for patients and their families, progress should also be made for better recognition and inclusion of people with neuropsychiatric conditions in our society (no mind left behind). It is hoped that increasing knowledge in genetics, neurology, and psychology will allow for better diagnosis, care, and integration of individuals with autism.

Acknowledgments

We thank Roberto Toro for critical reading of the manuscript. This work was funded by Institut Pasteur, the Bettencourt-Schueller foundation, Center National de la Recherche Scientifique, University Paris Diderot, Agence Nationale de la Recherche (SynDiv-ASD), the Conny-Maeva Charitable Foundation, the Cognacq Jay Foundation, the Orange Foundation, and the FondaMental Foundation.

References

1. Kanner L. Autistic disturbances of affective contact. *Nerv Child* 1943;**2**:217−50.

2. Asperger H. Die "Autistischen Psychopathen" im Kindesalter. *Arch Psychiatr Nervenkr* 1944;**177**:76−137.

3. Coleman M, Gillberg C. *The autisms*. Oxford University Press; 2012.

4. Developmental Disabilities Monitoring Network Surveillance Year Principal I. Prevalence of autism spectrum disorder among children aged 8 years − autism and developmental disabilities monitoring network, 11 sites, United States, 2010. *MMWR Surveill Summ* March 28, 2014;**63**(Suppl. 2):1−21.

5. Elsabbagh M, Divan G, Koh YJ, et al. Global prevalence of autism and other pervasive developmental disorders. *Autism Res* June 2012;**5**(3):160−79.

6. Gillberg C. The ESSENCE in child psychiatry: Early Symptomatic Syndromes Eliciting Neurodevelopmental Clinical Examinations. *Res Dev Disabil* November−December 2010;**31**(6):1543−51.

7. Moreno-De-Luca A, Myers SM, Challman TD, Moreno-De-Luca D, Evans DW, Ledbetter DH. Developmental brain dysfunction: revival and expansion of old concepts based on new genetic evidence. *Lancet Neurol* April 2013;**12**(4):406−14.

8. Miles JH, Takahashi TN, Bagby S, et al. Essential versus complex autism: definition of fundamental prognostic subtypes. *Am J Med Genet A* June 1, 2005;**135**(2):171−80.

9. Constantino JN. The quantitative nature of autistic social impairment. *Pediatr Res* May 2011;**69**(5 Pt 2):55R−62R.

10. Skuse DH, Mandy W, Steer C, et al. Social communication competence and functional adaptation in a general population of children: preliminary evidence for sex-by-verbal IQ differential risk. *J Am Acad Child Adolesc Psychiatry* February 2009;**48**(2):128−37.

11. Ronald A, Happe F, Price TS, Baron-Cohen S, Plomin R. Phenotypic and genetic overlap between autistic traits at the extremes of the general population. *J Am Acad Child Adolesc Psychiatry* October 2006;**45**(10):1206−14.

12. Huguet G, Ey E, Bourgeron T. The Genetic Landscapes of Autism Spectrum Disorders. *Annu Rev Genomics Hum Genet* 2013;**14**:191−213.

13. Gaugler T, Klei L, Sanders SJ, et al. Most genetic risk for autism resides with common variation. *Nat Genet* August 2014;**46**(8):881−5.

14. Gardener H, Spiegelman D, Buka SL. Perinatal and neonatal risk factors for autism: a comprehensive meta-analysis. *Pediatrics* August 2011;**128**(2):344−55.

15. Hallmayer J, Cleveland S, Torres A, et al. Genetic heritability and shared environmental factors among twin pairs with autism. *Arch Gen Psychiatry* November 2011;**68**(11):1095−102.

16. Toro R, Konyukh M, Delorme R, et al. Key role for gene dosage and synaptic homeostasis in autism spectrum disorders. *Trends Genet* August 2010;**26**(8):363−72.

17. Bourgeron T. A synaptic trek to autism. *Curr Opin Neurobiol* April 2009;**19**(2):231−4.

18. Abrahams BS, Geschwind DH. Advances in autism genetics: on the threshold of a new neurobiology. *Nat Rev Genet* May 2008;**9**(5):341−55.

19. Devlin B, Scherer SW. Genetic architecture in autism spectrum disorder. *Curr Opin Genet Dev* June 2012;**22**(3):229−37.

20. Folstein S, Rutter M. Genetic influences and infantile autism. *Nature* February 02, 1977;**265**(5596):726−8.

21. Bailey A, Le Couteur A, Gottesman I, et al. Autism as a strongly genetic disorder: evidence from a British twin study. *Psychol Med* 1995;**25**(1):63−77.

22. Ritvo ER, Freeman BJ, Mason-Brothers A, Mo A, Ritvo AM. Concordance for the syndrome of autism in 40 pairs of afflicted twins. *Am J Psychiatry* 1985;**142**(1):74−7.

23. Steffenburg S, Gillberg C, Hellgren L, et al. A twin study of autism in Denmark, Finland, Iceland, Norway and Sweden. *J Child Psychol Psychiatry Allied Discip* 1989;**30**(3):405−16.

24. Le Couteur A, Bailey A, Goode S, et al. A Broader Phenotype of Autism: The Clinical Spectrum in Twins. *J Child Psychol Psychiatry* 1996;**37**(7):785−801.

25. Ronald A, Happe F, Plomin R. The genetic relationship between individual differences in social and nonsocial behaviours characteristic of autism. *Dev Sci* September 2005;**8**(5):444−58.

26. Taniai H, Nishiyama T, Miyachi T, Imaeda M, Sumi S. Genetic influences on the broad spectrum of autism: study of proband-ascertained twins. *Am J Med Genet B Neuropsychiatr Genet* September 5, 2008;**147B**(6):844−9.

27. Rosenberg RE, Law JK, Yenokyan G, McGready J, Kaufmann WE, Law PA. Characteristics and concordance of autism spectrum disorders among 277 twin pairs. *Arch Pediatr Adolesc Med* October 2009;**163**(10):907−14.

28. Lichtenstein P, Carlstrom E, Rastam M, Gillberg C, Anckarsater H. The Genetics of Autism Spectrum Disorders and Related Neuropsychiatric Disorders in Childhood. *Am J Psychiatry* August 4, 2010;**167**. AiA:1−7.

29. Ronald A, Hoekstra RA. Autism spectrum disorders and autistic traits: a decade of new twin studies. *Am J Med Genet B Neuropsychiatr Genet* April 2011;**156B**(3):255−74.

30. Ronald A, Larsson H, Anckarsater H, Lichtenstein P. A twin study of autism symptoms in Sweden. *Mol Psychiatry* October 2010;**16**(10):1039−47.

31. Lundstrom S, Chang Z, Kerekes N, et al. Autistic-like traits and their association with mental health problems in two nationwide twin cohorts of children and adults. *Psychol Med* November 2011;**41**(11):2423−33.

32. Sandin S, Lichtenstein P, Kuja-Halkola R, Larsson H, Hultman CM, Reichenberg A. The familial risk of autism. *JAMA* May 7, 2014;**311**(17):1770−7.

33. Constantino JN, Zhang Y, Frazier T, Abbacchi AM, Law P. Sibling recurrence and the genetic epidemiology of autism. *Am J Psychiatry* November 2010;**167**(11):1349−56.

34. Risch N, Hoffmann TJ, Anderson M, Croen LA, Grether JK, Windham GC. Familial Recurrence of Autism Spectrum Disorder: Evaluating Genetic and Environmental Contributions. *Am J Psychiatry* June 27, 2014;**171**.

35. Gillberg C, Wahlstrom J. Chromosome abnormalities in infantile autism and other childhood psychoses: a population study of 66 cases. *Dev Med Child Neurol* June 1985;**27**(3):293−304.

36. Vorstman JA, Staal WG, van Daalen E, van Engeland H, Hochstenbach PF, Franke L. Identification of novel autism candidate regions through analysis of reported cytogenetic abnormalities associated with autism. *Mol Psychiatry* January 2006;**11**(1):18−28.

37. Pinto D, Darvishi K, Shi X, et al. Comprehensive assessment of array-based platforms and calling algorithms for detection of copy number variants. *Nat Biotechnol* June 2011;**29**(6):512−20.

38. Jacquemont ML, Sanlaville D, Redon R, et al. Array-based comparative genomic hybridisation identifies high frequency of cryptic chromosomal rearrangements in patients with syndromic autism spectrum disorders. *J Med Genet* November 2006;**43**(11):843−9.

39. Sebat J, Lakshmi B, Malhotra D, et al. Strong association of de novo copy number mutations with autism. *Science* April 20, 2007;**316**(5823):445−9.

40. Sanders SJ, Ercan-Sencicek AG, Hus V, et al. Multiple recurrent de novo CNVs, including duplications of the 7q11.23 Williams syndrome region, are strongly associated with autism. *Neuron* June 9, 2011;**70**(5):863−85.

41. Glessner JT, Wang K, Cai G, et al. Autism genome-wide copy number variation reveals ubiquitin and neuronal genes. *Nature* May 28, 2009;**459**(7246):569—73.

42. Pinto D, Delaby E, Merico D, et al. Convergence of genes and cellular pathways dysregulated in autism spectrum disorders. *Am J Hum Genet* May 1, 2014;**94**(5):677—94.

43. Pinto D, Pagnamenta AT, Klei L, et al. Functional impact of global rare copy number variation in autism spectrum disorders. *Nature* July 15, 2010;**466**(7304):368—72.

44. Cooper GM, Coe BP, Girirajan S, et al. A copy number variation morbidity map of developmental delay. *Nat Genet* September 2011;**43**(9):838—46.

45. Ballif BC, Hornor SA, Jenkins E, et al. Discovery of a previously unrecognized microdeletion syndrome of 16p11.2-p12.2. *Nat Genet* September 2007;**39**(9):1071—3.

46. Kumar RA, KaraMohamed S, Sudi J, et al. Recurrent 16p11.2 microdeletions in autism. *Hum Mol Genet* February 15, 2008; **17**(4):628—38.

47. Szafranski P, Schaaf CP, Person RE, et al. Structures and molecular mechanisms for common 15q13.3 microduplications involving CHRNA7: benign or pathological? *Hum Mutat* July 2010;**31**(7): 840—50.

48. Weiss LA, Shen Y, Korn JM, et al. Association between microdeletion and microduplication at 16p11.2 and autism. *N Engl J Med* February 14, 2008;**358**(7):667—75.

49. Leblond CS, Nava C, Polge A, et al. Meta-analysis of SHANK Mutations in Autism Spectrum Disorders: a gradient of severity in cognitive impairments. *PLoS Genet* September 2014;**10**(9): e1004580.

50. Jamain S, Quach H, Betancur C, et al. Mutations of the X-linked genes encoding neuroligins NLGN3 and NLGN4 are associated with autism. *Nat Genet* May 2003;**34**(1):27—9.

51. Durand CM, Betancur C, Boeckers TM, et al. Mutations in the gene encoding the synaptic scaffolding protein SHANK3 are associated with autism spectrum disorders. *Nat Genet* January 2007; **39**(1):25—7.

52. Szatmari P, Paterson AD, Zwaigenbaum L, et al. Mapping autism risk loci using genetic linkage and chromosomal rearrangements. *Nat Genet* March 2007;**39**(3):319—28.

53. O'Roak BJ, Deriziotis P, Lee C, et al. Exome sequencing in sporadic autism spectrum disorders identifies severe de novo mutations. *Nat Genet* June 2011;**43**(6):585—9.

54. O'Roak BJ, Vives L, Girirajan S, et al. Sporadic autism exomes reveal a highly interconnected protein network of de novo mutations. *Nature* May 10, 2012;**485**(7397):246—50.

55. Neale BM, Kou Y, Liu L, et al. Patterns and rates of exonic de novo mutations in autism spectrum disorders. *Nature* May 10, 2012; **485**(7397):242—5.

56. Sanders SJ, Murtha MT, Gupta AR, et al. De novo mutations revealed by whole-exome sequencing are strongly associated with autism. *Nature* April 4, 2012;**485**:237—41.

57. Iossifov I, Ronemus M, Levy D, et al. De novo gene disruptions in children on the autistic spectrum. *Neuron* April 26, 2012;**74**(2): 285—99.

58. Chahrour MH, Yu TW, Lim ET, et al. Whole-exome sequencing and homozygosity analysis implicate depolarization-regulated neuronal genes in autism. *PLoS Genet* 2012;**8**(4):e1002635.

59. Yu TW, Chahrour MH, Coulter ME, et al. Using whole-exome sequencing to identify inherited causes of autism. *Neuron* January 23, 2013;**77**(2):259—73.

60. Lim ET, Raychaudhuri S, Sanders SJ, et al. Rare complete knockouts in humans: population distribution and significant role in autism spectrum disorders. *Neuron* January 23, 2013;**77**(2):235—42.

61. Liu L, Sabo A, Neale BM, et al. Analysis of rare, exonic variation amongst subjects with autism spectrum disorders and population controls. *PLoS Genet* April 2013;**9**(4):e1003443.

62. He X, Sanders SJ, Liu L, et al. Integrated model of de novo and inherited genetic variants yields greater power to identify risk genes. *PLoS Genet* 2013;**9**(8):e1003671.

63. Willsey AJ, Sanders SJ, Li M, et al. Coexpression networks implicate human midfetal deep cortical projection neurons in the pathogenesis of autism. *Cell* November 21, 2013;**155**(5):997—1007.

64. Liu L, Lei J, Sanders SJ, et al. DAWN: a framework to identify autism genes and subnetworks using gene expression and genetics. *Mol Autism* 2014;**5**(1):22.

65. Samocha KE, Robinson EB, Sanders SJ, et al. A framework for the interpretation of de novo mutation in human disease. *Nat Genet* August 3, 2014;**46**.

66. Iossifov I, O'Roak BJ, Sanders SJ, et al. The contribution of de novo coding mutations to autism spectrum disorder. *Nature* November 13, 2014;**515**(7526):216—21.

67. An JY, Cristino AS, Zhao Q, et al. Towards a molecular characterization of autism spectrum disorders: an exome sequencing and systems approach. *Transl Psychiatry* 2014;**4**:e394.

68. De Rubeis S, He X, Goldberg AP, et al. Synaptic, transcriptional and chromatin genes disrupted in autism. *Nature* November 13, 2014;**515**(7526):209—15.

69. Chang J, Gilman SR, Chiang AH, Sanders SJ, Vitkup D. Genotype to phenotype relationships in autism spectrum disorders. *Nat Neurosci* February 2015;**18**(2):191—8.

70. Krumm N, Turner TN, Baker C, et al. Excess of rare, inherited truncating mutations in autism. *Nat Genet* June 2015;**47**(6):582—8.

71. Krumm N, O'Roak BJ, Shendure J, Eichler EE. A de novo convergence of autism genetics and molecular neuroscience. *Trends Neurosci* February 2014;**37**(2):95—105.

72. Ronemus M, Iossifov I, Levy D, Wigler M. The role of de novo mutations in the genetics of autism spectrum disorders. *Nat Rev Genet* February 2014;**15**(2):133—41.

73. Kong A, Frigge ML, Masson G, et al. Rate of de novo mutations and the importance of father's age to disease risk. *Nature* August 23, 2012;**488**(7412):471—5.

74. O'Roak BJ, Vives L, Fu W, et al. Multiplex targeted sequencing identifies recurrently mutated genes in autism spectrum disorders. *Science* December 21, 2012;**338**(6114):1619—22.

75. Michaelson JJ, Shi Y, Gujral M, et al. Whole-genome sequencing in autism identifies hot spots for de novo germline mutation. *Cell* December 21, 2012;**151**(7):1431—42.

76. Shi L, Zhang X, Golhar R, et al. Whole-genome sequencing in an autism multiplex family. *Mol Autism* 2013;**4**(1):8.

77. Yuen RK, Thiruvahindrapuram B, Merico D, et al. Whole-genome sequencing of quartet families with autism spectrum disorder. *Nat Med* February 2015;**21**(2):185—91.

78. Nemirovsky SI, Cordoba M, Zaiat JJ, et al. Whole genome sequencing reveals a de novo SHANK3 mutation in familial autism spectrum disorder. *PLoS One* 2015;**10**(2):e0116358.

79. Xue Y, Chen Y, Ayub Q, et al. Deleterious- and disease-allele prevalence in healthy individuals: insights from current predictions, mutation databases, and population-scale resequencing. *Am J Hum Genet* December 7, 2012;**91**(6):1022—32.

80. Fu W, O'Connor TD, Jun G, et al. Analysis of 6515 exomes reveals the recent origin of most human protein-coding variants. *Nature* January 10, 2013;**493**(7431):216—20.

81. Genome of the Netherlands C. Genome of the Netherlands C. Whole-genome sequence variation, population structure and demographic history of the Dutch population. *Nat Genet* August 2014;**46**(8):818—25.

82. Klei L, Sanders SJ, Murtha MT, et al. Common genetic variants, acting additively, are a major source of risk for autism. *Mol Autism* October 15, 2012;**3**(1):9.

83. Yang J, Lee SH, Goddard ME, Visscher PM. GCTA: a tool for genome-wide complex trait analysis. *Am J Hum Genet* January 7, 2011;**88**(1):76—82.

84. Anney R, Klei L, Pinto D, et al. Individual common variants exert weak effects on the risk for autism spectrum disorderspi. *Hum Mol Genet* November 1, 2012;**21**(21):4781−92.

85. Cross-Disorder Group of the Psychiatric Genomics C. Identification of risk loci with shared effects on five major psychiatric disorders: a genome-wide analysis. *Lancet* April 20, 2013;**381**(9875): 1371−9.

86. Rutherford SL. From genotype to phenotype: buffering mechanisms and the storage of genetic information. *Bioessays* December 2000;**22**(12):1095−105.

87. Hartman JL, Garvik B, Hartwell L. Principles for the buffering of genetic variation. *Science* February 9, 2001;**291**(5506):1001−4.

88. Leblond CS, Heinrich J, Delorme R, et al. Genetic and functional analyses of SHANK2 mutations suggest a multiple hit model of autism spectrum disorders. *PLoS Genet* February 2012;**8**(2): e1002521.

89. Girirajan S, Rosenfeld JA, Coe BP, et al. Phenotypic heterogeneity of genomic disorders and rare copy-number variants. *N Engl J Med* October 4, 2012;**367**(14):1321−31.

90. Girirajan S, Rosenfeld JA, Cooper GM, et al. A recurrent 16p12.1 microdeletion supports a two-hit model for severe developmental delay. *Nat Genet* March 2010;**42**(3):203−9.

91. Voineagu I, Wang X, Johnston P, et al. Transcriptomic analysis of autistic brain reveals convergent molecular pathology. *Nature* June 16, 2011;**474**(7351):380−4.

92. Uddin M, Tammimies K, Pellecchia G, et al. Brain-expressed exons under purifying selection are enriched for de novo mutations in autism spectrum disorder. *Nat Genet* July 2014;**46**(7): 742−7.

93. Hormozdiari F, Penn O, Borenstein E, Eichler EE. The discovery of integrated gene networks for autism and related disorders. *Genome Res* January 2015;**25**(1):142−54.

94. Gupta S, Ellis SE, Ashar FN, et al. Transcriptome analysis reveals dysregulation of innate immune response genes and neuronal activity-dependent genes in autism. *Nat Commun* 2014;**5**:5748.

95. Auerbach BD, Osterweil EK, Bear MF. Mutations causing syndromic autism define an axis of synaptic pathophysiology. *Nature* December 1, 2011;**480**(7375):63−8.

96. Belmonte MK, Bourgeron T. Fragile X syndrome and autism at the intersection of genetic and neural networks. *Nat Neurosci* October 2006;**9**(10):1221−5.

97. Cohen S, Gabel HW, Hemberg M, et al. Genome-wide activity-dependent MeCP2 phosphorylation regulates nervous system development and function. *Neuron* October 6, 2011;**72**(1): 72−85.

98. Ebert DH, Gabel HW, Robinson ND, et al. Activity-dependent phosphorylation of MeCP2 threonine 308 regulates interaction with NCoR. *Nature* July 18, 2013;**499**(7458):341−5.

99. Sando 3rd R, Gounko N, Pieraut S, Liao L, Yates 3rd J, Maximov A. HDAC4 governs a transcriptional program essential for synaptic plasticity and memory. *Cell* November 9, 2012;**151**(4):821−34.

100. Ma XM, Blenis J. Molecular mechanisms of mTOR-mediated translational control. *Nat Rev Mol Cell Biol* May 2009;**10**(5):307−18.

101. Kelleher 3rd RJ, Bear MF. The autistic neuron: troubled translation? *Cell* October 31, 2008;**135**(3):401−6.

102. Budimirovic DB, Kaufmann WE. What can we learn about autism from studying fragile X syndrome? *Dev Neurosci* 2011;**33**(5):379−94.

103. Fernandez E, Rajan N, Bagni C. The FMRP regulon: from targets to disease convergence. *Front Neurosci* 2013;**7**:191.

104. De Rubeis S, Pasciuto E, Li KW, et al. CYFIP1 coordinates mRNA translation and cytoskeleton remodeling to ensure proper dendritic spine formation. *Neuron* September 18, 2013;**79**(6):1169−82.

105. Santini E, Huynh TN, MacAskill AF, et al. Exaggerated translation causes synaptic and behavioural aberrations associated with autism. *Nature* January 17, 2013;**493**(7432):411−5.

106. Gkogkas CG, Khoutorsky A, Ran I, et al. Autism-related deficits via dysregulated eIF4E-dependent translational control. *Nature* January 17, 2013;**493**(7432):371−7.

107. Mabb AM, Ehlers MD. Ubiquitination in postsynaptic function and plasticity. *Annu Rev Cell Dev Biol* 2010;**26**:179−210.

108. Greer PL, Hanayama R, Bloodgood BL, et al. The Angelman Syndrome Protein Ube3A Regulates Synapse Development by Ubiquitinating Arc. *Cell* March 5, 2010;**140**(5):704−16.

109. Sheng M, Kim E. The postsynaptic organization of synapses. *Cold Spring Harb Perspect Biol* December 2011;**3**(12).

110. Choquet D, Triller A. The dynamic synapse. *Neuron* October 30, 2013;**80**(3):691−703.

111. Grabrucker AM, Schmeisser MJ, Schoen M, Boeckers TM. Postsynaptic ProSAP/Shank scaffolds in the cross-hair of synaptopathies. *Trends Cell Biol* October 2011;**21**(10):594−603.

112. Durand CM, Perroy J, Loll F, et al. SHANK3 mutations identified in autism lead to modification of dendritic spine morphology via an actin-dependent mechanism. *Molecular Psychiatry* January 2012;**17**(1):71−84.

113. Peca J, Feliciano C, Ting JT, et al. Shank3 mutant mice display autistic-like behaviours and striatal dysfunction. *Nature* April 28, 2011;**472**(7344):437−42.

114. Hung AY, Futai K, Sala C, et al. Smaller dendritic spines, weaker synaptic transmission, but enhanced spatial learning in mice lacking Shank1. *J Neurosci* February 13, 2008;**28**(7):1697−708.

115. Silverman JL, Turner SM, Barkan CL, et al. Sociability and motor functions in Shank1 mutant mice. *Brain Res* March 22, 2011;**1380**: 120−37.

116. Wohr M, Roullet FI, Hung AY, Sheng M, Crawley JN. Communication impairments in mice lacking Shank1: reduced levels of ultrasonic vocalizations and scent marking behavior. *PLoS One* 2011; **6**(6):e20631.

117. Schmeisser MJ, Ey E, Wegener S, et al. Autistic-like behaviours and hyperactivity in mice lacking ProSAP1/Shank2. *Nature* June 14, 2012;**486**(7402):256−60.

118. Won H, Lee H-R, Gee HY, et al. Autistic-like social behaviour in Shank2-mutant mice improved by restoring NMDA receptor function. *Nature* June 14, 2012;**486**(7402):261−5.

119. Bozdagi O, Sakurai T, Papapetrou D, et al. Haploinsufficiency of the autism-associated Shank3 gene leads to deficits in synaptic function, social interaction, and social communication. *Mol Autism* 2010;**1**(1):15.

120. Wang X, McCoy PA, Rodriguiz RM, et al. Synaptic dysfunction and abnormal behaviors in mice lacking major isoforms of Shank3. *Hum Mol Genet* August 1, 2011;**20**(15):3093−108.

121. Yang M, Bozdagi O, Scattoni ML, et al. Reduced Excitatory Neurotransmission and Mild Autism-Relevant Phenotypes in Adolescent Shank3 Null Mutant Mice. *J Neurosci* May 9, 2012; **32**(19):6525−41.

122. Toro R, Poline JB, Huguet G, et al. Genomic architecture of human neuroanatomical diversity. *Mol Psychiatry* September 16, 2014;**20**.

123. Yang J, Benyamin B, McEvoy BP, et al. Common SNPs explain a large proportion of the heritability for human height. *Nat Genet* July 2010;**42**(7):565−9.

124. Deary IJ, Yang J, Davies G, et al. Genetic contributions to stability and change in intelligence from childhood to old age. *Nature* February 9, 2012;**482**(7384):212−5.

125. Levy D, Ronemus M, Yamrom B, et al. Rare de novo and transmitted copy-number variation in autistic spectrum disorders. *Neuron* June 9, 2011;**70**(5):886−97.

126. Jiang YH, Yuen RK, Jin X, et al. Detection of clinically relevant genetic variants in autism spectrum disorder by whole-genome sequencing. *Am J Hum Genet* August 8, 2013;**93**(2):249−63.

3

Genetics of X-Linked Intellectual Disability

Charles E. Schwartz, Luigi Boccuto

JC Self Research Institute Greenwood Genetic Center, Greenwood, SC, USA

INTRODUCTION

Intellectual disability (ID) is characterized by significant limitations in both intellectual functioning and adaptive behavior.[1,2] Intellectual functioning refers to general mental capability and involves the ability to reason, plan, solve problems, think abstractly, comprehend complex ideas, learn quickly, and learn from experience. One way to measure intellectual functioning is the intellectual quotient, which in individuals affected with ID is usually below 70. Adaptive behavior is the collection of conceptual, social, and practical skills that are learned and performed by people in their everyday lives.

Because ID is generated by aberrations in the development of the central nervous system, symptoms occur during the developmental period and generally before age 18 years. Knowledge of the age of onset is important to differentiate ID from other conditions that can also affect mental and behavioral skills but are acquired later in life as a consequence of external factors, such as trauma or infections. The disorder is considered chronic and often co-occurs with other mental conditions such as depression, attention-deficit hyperactivity disorder, and autism spectrum disorder (ASD).[1] ID is a relatively common disorder with a prevalence of 2–3% of the general population.[3]

Several studies have consistently shown that affected males outnumber females by about 30%.[2,4–6] The biological inequity between males and females conferred by the presence of a single X chromosome in males has been considered to be primarily responsible for such a significant gender bias, suggesting a primary role for genes on the X chromosome in the causation of ID. However, this genetic imbalance is partially compensated for by the random inactivation of one of the two X chromosomes in female cells (the Lyon hypothesis[7]). As a result, any alteration in an X-linked gene will fully express itself in a male, whereas X-inactivation will mitigate the effect in females. Some have argued that the vulnerability of males to X-linked gene alterations provides a means for evolution to select for positive contributions of genes involved in brain development and cognitive function.[8,9] The number of ID genes on the X exceeds that expected based on its DNA amount relative to the whole genome. This evolutionary role may explain why the X appears to contain an exceptional number of genes involved in cognitive and brain development.[10]

The prevalence of X-linked ID (XLID) in the male population has been estimated at 1.7 cases in 1000 births, with a range of 0.5−3/1000 births.[2,8,11,12] XLID thus competes with aberrations of the autosomal chromosomes as the most frequent cause of ID.

HISTORY OF XLID

Before the identification of the first causative genes, the study of XLID was predominantly based on clinical evaluation, linkage analysis, and exploration of chromosome rearrangements. However, many conditions shared numerous common features, and without a molecular test the differential diagnosis was problematic.

As is evident from Table 1, the identification of genes responsible for XLID was limited in the first decade of exploration (1981−1990) by the available methodologies. Apart from cytogenetic analysis, the strategy was limited to searching for genes responsible for enzymes known to be involved (HPRT, PGK1, OTC, and PHDA1) or in the single case of the PLP1 gene, where the molecular pathway was known. The use of chromosomal rearrangements and the application of linkage analysis led to a drastic increase in known XLID genes, from 7 (1981−1990) to 29 (1991−2000) (Table 1). This number more than doubled in the next decade (2001−2010) as sequencing of genes became easier, allowing for high-throughput screening of a large number of samples for a small number of candidate genes or for all of the genes on the X chromosome. The pace of gene discovery has slowed since then, not because of limitations in methodology

but because of a decrease in the number of clearly defined families with XLID available for analysis. It is also likely that most alterations in the coding regions have been identified and the remaining males with XLID have pathogenic changes which alter noncoding regulatory elements.

Genetic tests allowed for a better estimate of the prevalence of XLID conditions. For example, Fragile X syndrome, caused by mutations in the FMR1 gene (Xq27.3), is the most commonly diagnosed XLID syndrome, with a prevalence of 1 in 4000 in the male population.[2,13,14] This condition alone accounts for about 2% of males and about 0.3% of females with ID.[2] Among families suspected to have XLID, 40−50% of responsible mutations can now be identified; the most commonly affected genes, besides FMR1, are ARX (5−6%) and MECP2, OPHN1, PQBP1, and KDM5C (1−4% each).[2,14] The detection rate of mutations in XLID genes is much lower in sporadic males, which suggests the importance of the inheritance pattern to distinguish X-linked from autosomal forms of ID.

CLASSIFICATION OF XLID

In the 1970s, for example, the term "Renpenning syndrome" was used as a generic reference for XLID.[15−18] This broad usage was applied to both nonsyndromal and syndromal XLID, including well-characterized disorders such as the Fragile X syndrome. Turner et al.[19−21] argued that this designation should be used only for nonsyndromal XLID, specifically cases lacking macrocephaly or microcephaly, epilepsy, major malformations or more than one minor malformation, and neurological signs. In the early 1990s, this idea of distinguishing XLID based on the presence or absence of distinct clinical findings was embraced by both clinicians and researchers. XLID disorders are now broken out into two broad categories: syndromal and nonsyndromal. The first group includes conditions in which the cognitive impairment occurs in the presence of other clinical findings which set the affected individual apart from a normal sib or another normal male. Thus, currently, Renpenning syndrome identifies a condition characterized by cognitive impairment, microcephaly, and a tendency toward short stature and small testes, caused by mutations in the PQBP1 gene.[22] Although better defined both clinically and genetically, this syndrome still encompasses several allelic conditions such as Sutherland−Haan, Porteous, Golabi−Ito−Hall, and Hamel cerebropalatocardiac syndromes.[23−26] Mutations in 103 genes are responsible for 125 of the known 160 XLID syndromes (Figure 1).

TABLE 1　Tabulation of Identification of XLIDs by Decade and Methodology

Decade	# XLID Genes	Methodology						
		Met-Fu	Rea	Can	Mol-Fu	Seq	MCGH	Exp
1981−1990	7	5	1		1			
1991−2000	29	1	12	16				
2001−2010	65	1	18	27	4	13	1	1
2011−2015	29		1			27	1	

Met-Fu, follow-up of a known metabolic pathway; Rea, use of a chromosomal rearrangement; Can, candidate gene screening within a linkage interval; Mol-Fu, follow-up of a known molecular pathway; Seq, sequencing, either X-exome or whole exome; MCGH, genomic microarray; Exp, gene expression analysis.

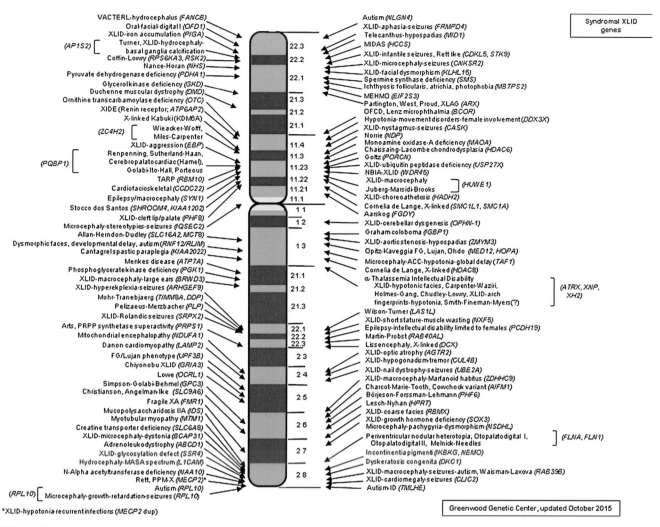

FIGURE 1 **Ideogram of the X chromosome showing X-linked intellectual disability (XLID) syndromes.** *Arrows,* locations of the syndromal XLID genes which have been cloned and carry pathogenic mutations; *parentheses,* genes for each syndrome. *Used with permission of the Greenwood Genetic Center.*

Syndromal XLID

Abnormal head circumference, either reduced or increased, has often been reported in syndromal XLID. Microcephaly is a feature present in 40 XLID syndromes.[2] For some syndromes, such as Renpenning,[22–27] Borjeson—Forssman—Lehman,[28–30] Coffin—Lowry (CLS),[31–33] and Rett,[34,35] it can be regarded as a significant clinical finding although it is less frequent in *ARX*-associated XLID,[36–38] Abidi syndrome,[39] and ornithine transcarbamoylase deficiency.[40–42] On the other hand, macrocephaly occurs in only 11 syndromes[2]; it is usually present in Fragile X,[43–45] Lujan,[46–48] Clark—Baraitser,[49–52] and FG syndromes,[53–55] less commonly in Simpson—Golabi—Behmel[56–58] and Snyder—Robinson syndromes.[59,60] In some disorders, an increased head circumference results from hydrocephaly: Pettigrew syndrome,[61,62]

APIS2-associated XLID,[62,63] and the hydrocephaly—MASA spectrum.[64–66]

Of the various neurological problems that are often reported in syndromal XLID, seizures occur most frequently; they are usually present in 47 XLID syndromes[2] such as Aicardi,[67–69] Cantu,[70] Christianson,[71] Fragile X,[43–45] Rett,[34,35] Pettigrew,[61,62] Menkes,[72,73] and Smith—Fineman—Myers syndromes,[74] as well as ornithine transcarbamoylase[40,41] and creatine transporter deficiency[75–77] and *ARX*-associated[36–38] and *FLNA*-associated XLIDs,[78,79] to mention a few. Seizures are observed in another 24 syndromes.[2] However, in these, they are present in fewer than half of patients and thus cannot be considered a hallmark feature. Spastic paraplegia is present in 43 syndromes and unsurprisingly is found in syndromes which also have seizures as a clinical finding, such as those mentioned previously.[2] However, it can be observed as a major feature without seizures, as is the case for Goldblatt spastic paraplegia, XLID—spastic paraplegia type 7, and XLID—spastic paraplegia-athetosis.[2] Surprisingly, results of disruption of neuronal migration, such as lissencephaly, polymicrogyria, and subcortical heterotopias, are a hallmark feature noted in only seven XLID syndromes: Aicardi,[67–69] X-linked lissencephaly,[80,81] CK syndromes,[82,83] ARX-associated[36–38] and FLNA-associated XLIDs.[78,79] Thus observing any of these features in males with ID, especially if there is a family history, can greatly assist one in making a clinical diagnosis and therefore suggesting proper gene testing.

Sensory problems which can be assumed to reflect some neurological problem are common. In fact, ocular anomalies are noted in 55 XLID syndromes, which make the organ system the most frequently affected in XLID syndromes. Ocular findings range from anophthalmia/microphthalmia (Aicardi syndrome[67–69]) to coloboma (Renpenning syndrome[22–27]), and retinopathy (cerebro-oculo-genital syndrome[84,85]) and to optic atrophy (Goltz syndrome[86,87]), nystagmus (Pelizaeus—Merzbacher syndrome[88,89]) and corneal clouding (MIDAS syndrome[90,91]). On the other hand, hearing loss is observed in 13 XLID syndromes such as Gustavson, X-linked ataxia—deafness—dementia, Mohr—Tranebjaerg, and Juberg—Marsidi—Brooks syndromes.[2] As with the presence of neuronal migration problems, the clinician can use deafness to focus on the most likely XLID conditions in a differential diagnosis list of disorders.

Other organ systems are affected in males with syndromal XLID. Abnormalities in the urogenital track are observed in 43 XLID syndromes,[2] and in some cases the presence of the abnormality can be extremely helpful in making the diagnosis, such as Aarskog syndrome,[92,93] cerebro-oculo-genital,[84,85] lissencephaly and abnormal genitalia, X-linked,[94,95] and Simpson—Golabi—Behmel[56–58] syndromes, to mention a few. Cardiac malformations occur at a low frequency; only six XLID syndromes (MIDAS, cerebro-palato-cardiac, TARP, craniofacioskeletal (males only), myotubular myopathy, and Bergia cardiomyopathy) have this as a major finding.[2] Thus, the presence of this clinical finding should be extremely useful to the clinician. However, it can be present in some patients in 10 other XLID syndromes.[2] Since these latter syndromes have other findings, heart defects in conjunction with the clinical findings should also prove useful in making a proper clinical diagnosis.

Nonsyndromal XLID

The nonsyndromal XLID category is composed of conditions with ID as the only clinical finding which clearly distinguishes an affected male from a normal one. As shown in Figure 2, mutations in 48 genes are responsible for 53 of over 99 families with nonsyndromal XLID. The figure also highlights the overlap between the syndromal and nonsyndromal groups. On the right side of the ideogram are the 21 genes which have been associated with both syndromal and nonsyndromal XLID. The phenotype associated with alterations of those genes depends on the mutation. In some cases, such as those with OPHN1 and ARX mutations, clinical reexamination has found syndromal manifestations in families previously considered to have nonsyndromal XLID.[96–98]

In the case of the creatine transporter deficiency syndrome, the very classification changed from nonsyndromal to syndromal when the causative gene, SLC6A8, was discovered. Mutations in this gene affect a creatine transporter, ultimately leading to increased creatine serum levels and providing a biochemical means by which an affected male could be distinguished from a normal sib. Therefore, the addition of this biochemical abnormality to the mental impairment constitutes a syndromal status.[10] When evaluating a male with apparent nonsyndromal XLID, it is no longer possible to exclude from consideration a gene associated with an XLID syndrome.

The far right part of Figure 2 indicates the 44 nonsyndromal XLID families that have been mapped for which no gene has yet been identified. Because many of the 44 families have tested negative for the XLID genes within their linkage intervals (the bar), many X-linked genes or other genetic events must still exist which result in XLID. Because at least 36 XLID syndromes have no genetic cause, either,[99] the number of potential XLID genes will likely exceed 150, as previously predicted.[100]

Genotype—Phenotype Correlation: Redefining XLID

Identification of X-linked genes causing ID raised some questions about the diagnosis and definition of XLID conditions. Clinical reevaluation of families with XLID previously reported, the observation of new features in most recently ascertained families, and the incorporation of molecular technologies in diagnosis resulted in lumping, splitting, and reclassification of a number of XLID disorders. With the variability and imprecision with which clinical evaluations are carried out, it is inevitable that some individuals with XLID will be incorrectly included in existing diagnostic categories whereas others will be incorrectly excluded. The extent to which individuals and families can be evaluated depends on the setting, access to historical

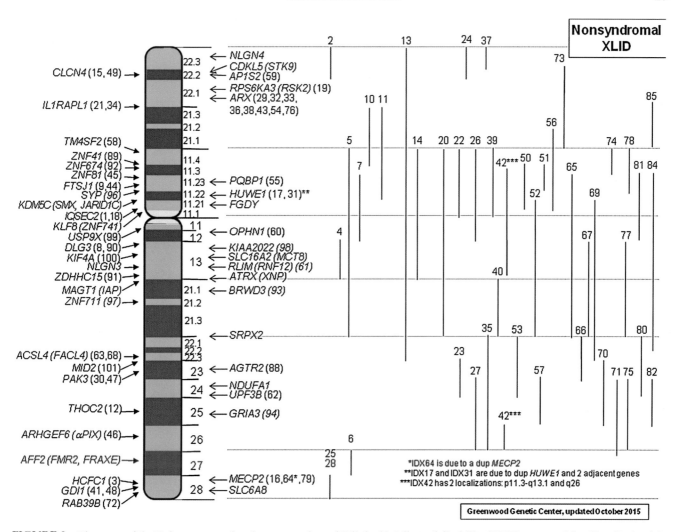

FIGURE 2 **Ideogram of the X chromosome showing nonsyndromal X-linked intellectual disability (XLID) genes and families.** On the right side of the figure are the linkage limits for XLID families which have been mapped (lod score > 2) but the genes are not yet cloned. *Solid arrows on left*, locations of nonsyndromal XLID genes which have been cloned; *open arrows on right*, genes that cause both syndromal and nonsyndromal XLID. *Used with permission of the Greenwood Genetic Center.*

information, availability and ages of affected and unaffected family members, and the experience and expertise of the observers.

The previous section discussed how mutations in the same gene can cause both syndromal and nonsyndromal XLID. Further studies proved that the phenotype variability associated with some X-linked genes can encompass entirely different conditions, such as was reported for the *PQBP1* gene.[22–25] Differences in phenotype can result from mutations in different domains of a gene and from contributions from the genetic background. On the other hand, some individuals with the same clinical diagnosis have been found to carry pathogenic mutations in different XLID genes, which indicates significant genotype variability and highlights the importance of combining clinical and molecular investigations.

A typical example of phenotype heterogeneity is provided by the *ARX* gene, located in Xp22.11 and responsible for a relatively large percentage (1–2%) of XLID conditions, often designated *ARX*-associated XLID. Alterations of this gene were found in a number of nonsyndromal families (listed in Figure 2 as numbers 29, 32, 33, 36, 38, 43, 54, and 76), an X-linked dystonia (Partington syndrome), X-linked infantile spasms (West syndrome), X-linked lissencephaly with abnormal genitalia, hydranencephaly and abnormal genitalia, and Proud syndrome (Figure 1).[37,96,101–106]

Another gene associated with multiple phenotypes is *ATRX* (Xq21.1). Initially the phenotype caused by *ATRX* mutations was confused with CLS, especially in young males. However, once both *ATRX*[107] and the gene for CLS, *RPS6KA3* (*RSK2*),[31] were identified, genetic testing assisted clinicians in distinguishing between these two XLID syndromes. Mutations in the *ATRX* gene were thought to cause alpha-thalassemia with ID (ATRX syndrome) but once a genetic test was used to screen a large number of males with hypotonic facies, ID, and other features of ATRX, causative alterations in other disorders were identified.[107,108] Currently, as shown in Figure 1, four other named XLID syndromes (Carpenter—Waziri, Holmes—Gang, Chudley—Lowry, and XLID—arch fingerprints-hypotonia) have been found to be allelic variants of ATRX syndrome, as have certain families with spastic paraplegia and nonsyndromal XLID (Figures 1 and 2).[39,109–113] One family clinically diagnosed as having Smith—Fineman—Myers syndrome was also found to harbor an *ATRX* mutation, although the gene has not been analyzed in the original family.[114] In addition, a family clinically diagnosed as having Juberg—Marsidi syndrome (JMS)[115] was found to have a mutation in *ATRX*.[116] However, a molecular analysis of a surviving male from the family originally reported by Juberg and Marsidi[117] identified a mutation in the *HUWE1* gene at Xp11.2.[118] The same mutation, p.Gly4310Arg, was found in a family reported by Brooks et al.[119] Upon evaluation, both JMS and Brooks syndrome are similar clinically.[120] This clinical presentation is different from that associated with *ATRX*-related XLID syndromes. Thus, although the literature states JMS results from an *ATRX* mutation, this is clearly not the situation. The family described by Mattei et al.[115] does not have JMS; rather it likely has ATRX.

These examples provide an idea of syndrome lumping caused by phenotype heterogeneity in XLID conditions. Perhaps even more challenging is syndrome splitting owing to genotype heterogeneity, in which different genes can cause the same condition. FG (or Opitz—FG) syndrome provides one of the best examples of syndrome splitting. This condition, first described by Opitz and Kaveggia,[53] presents with macrocephaly, downslanting palpebral fissures, imperforate anus or severe constipation, broad and flat thumbs and large toes, hypotonia, and ID. After the original family, several reports contributed to broaden the clinical manifestations attributed to this syndrome, but no single trait was pathognomonic or required for the diagnosis.[121–126] As a result, multiple localizations on the X chromosome were proposed for different FG families.[124–130] A recurring mutation, p.Arg961Trp in the *MED12* gene (Xq13.1), was detected in six families with the clinical diagnosis of FG, including the original family described by Opitz and Kaveggia.[131] In addition to the manifestations listed previously, two findings were consistently noted: small ears and friendly behavior. Clinical reevaluation and genetic sequencing of *MED12* were performed on several individuals who carried the FG diagnosis. The results showed that although most of these patients had one or more findings overlapping with the FG phenotype, none had the p.Arg961Trp substitution or other *MED12* mutations.[55,132] Instead, mutations in other XLID genes (*FMR1*, *FLNA*, *ATRX*, *CASK*, and *MECP2*) were found, along with duplications or deletions of the autosomes.[55,132] Considering the degree of heterogeneity within FG syndrome, it has been suggested that the vast majority of individuals so designated should best be considered to have ID of undetermined cause, especially if proven to carry no *MED12* mutations.[2,10]

The frequency with which the process of lumping and splitting has occurred in the history of XLID has been extremely instructive for both clinical and molecular investigators. Moreover, the process of reclassifying and refining the XLID conditions owing to gene identifications has been one of the most important contributions by geneticists to clinical medicine.[10] The underlying mechanisms or pathways by which mutations in different genes result in similar phenotypes and different mutations in a single gene result in disparate phenotypes, although not yet fully elucidated, will provide valuable insight into the era of translational medicine.

DISEASE MECHANISMS

Analysis of the greater than 130 known genes involved in XLID has provided valuable insight into many disease mechanisms involved in cognitive impairment and brain development (see also Chapter 9). Three major functions are represented by proteins encoded for by XLID genes: 31.5% are involved in binding, 26.6% have catalytic activity, and 10.5% have transcription regulatory activity. Another two functions, transporter activity and receptor activity, contribute equally at about 7.5%.[10] As for the proteins' localization within the cell, the four major subcellular fractions account for 30% in the nucleus, 28% in the cytoplasm, 18% in the membranes, and 16% in cellular organelles.[133]

Proteins involved with XLID fall into four generalized biological functions thought to be critical for neuronal morphology and integrity: presynaptic vesicle cycling and transport; cytoskeleton dynamics; cell adhesion and trans-synaptic signaling; and translation regulation.[10] It is interesting that about the same number of genes (five to seven) fall within each of the four biological functions. These genes can be grouped in another way which might provide some additional insights (Table 2). It is intriguing that although proteins associated with both syndromal and nonsyndromal

TABLE 2 X-Linked Intellectual Disability (XLID) Genes Involved in Neuronal Morphology and Function Grouped by Association with Type of XLID

Classification	Syndromal XLID	Nonsyndromal XLID	Both
Presynaptic vesicle cycling and transport	2	3	2
Cytoskeletal dynamics	2	3	2
Cell adhesion and transsynaptic signaling	1	2	
Translational regulation	4		2

XLID are involved in the first and second classifications, those found to be involved with syndromal forms of XLID are also classified as being involved in translational regulation. It is impossible at this time to assign significance to this observation, but it certainly warrants more exploration.

Presynaptic Vesicle Cycling and Transport

The synapse is a remarkably specialized environment allowing translation from an electrophysiological message to a chemical one on the presynaptic side and an opposite conversion on the postsynaptic site. Presynaptic and postsynaptic specializations form in precise opposition to each other at sites where axons contact specific target cells. Neurotransmitters such as glutamate or γ-aminobutyric acid (GABA) are synthesized by the presynaptic neurons and stored in synaptic vesicles (SVs) at presynaptic terminals. A critical step in presynaptic differentiation is the clustering of SVs near neurotransmitters release sites, the active zone, where vesicle fusion and exocytosis of neurotransmitters occur.[134] Several presynaptic molecules involved in the regulation of synaptic vesicle release, that involves a multistep process including vesicle endocytosis (transport/mobilization), docking, priming, fusion, and recycling, have been identified and are found to be defective in XLID.

The synapsins (Syns) are a family of neuron specific phosphoproteins which localize in the presynaptic compartments and interact with each other, actin, and the cytosolic surface of SVs (reviewed in Cesca et al.[135]) They help maintain a reserve pool of vesicles by tethering SVs to each other and to actin to regulate the availability of SVs for release through their phosphorylation-dependent dissociation from SVs and actin and have a role in the postdocking step of exocytosis.[136-139] SYN1 mutations are associated with a syndromal XLID characterized by epilepsy, macrocephaly, and/or autism[140,141] (Figure 1). Neurons from single or multiple Syn knockout mice show impairment in inhibitory neurotransmission and enhancement in excitatory transmission, accompanied by alteration in synaptic plasticity. A selective decrease in the density of SVs is noted in presynaptic compartments. In the absence of Syns, SVs show higher mobility and become dispersed along axons.[142,143] Lack of Syn1 and/or Syn11 triggers a strong epileptic phenotype in mice associated with cognitive impairments.[144]

Guanosine diphosphate (GDP) dissociation inhibitor (αGDI), a protein encoded by the XLID *GDI1* gene, controls the cycling of RAB guanosine triphosphate (GTP)ases that act as molecular switches between the active GTP-bound and inactive GDP-bound state and are involved in intracellular vesicle trafficking.[145] GDI1 knockout mice exhibit a large decrease in the reserve pool of SVs and short-term memory deficit.[146,147] Mutations in another small GTPase gene, RAB39B, cause a syndromal XLID associated with autism, epilepsy, and macrocephaly.[148] Its downregulation leads to an alteration in the number and morphology of neurite growth cones and a significant reduction in presynaptic compartments and supports the importance of the intracellular trafficking mediated by the αGDI−RAB pathway in cognitive and behavioral function.

Defects in *IL1RAPL1* have been associated with XLID and autism[149−152] (Figure 2) (see also Chapter 11). IL1RAPL1 belongs to the Toll/IL-1 receptor family and interacts with neuronal calcium sensor-1 and inhibits calcium-dependent exocytosis, neurotransmitter release, and nerve growth factor−induced neurite elongation.[153,154] Pavlowsky and coworkers identified PSD-95 as a novel partner of IL1RAPL1 and showed that it regulates dendritic spine number and PSD-95 localization to excitatory synapses by controlling c-jun terminal kinase activity and PSD-95 phosphorylation.[155,156] Through transsynaptic interaction with presynaptic protein phosphatase-δ, IL1RAPL1 has been found to mediate synapse formation.[157] IL1RAPL1 has been shown to interact with Mcf2-like (Mcf2l), a Rho guanine exchange factor, through the cytoplasmic Toll/IL-1 receptor domain and regulates the formation and stabilization of glutamatergic excitatory synapses of cortical neurons through RhoA signaling.[158]

The *SYP* gene encodes synaptophysin, an integral membrane protein found in transport vesicle and interacting with synaptobrevin. Synaptophysin represents an essential component of the SNARE (soluble N-ethylmaleimide−sensitive factor attachment protein receptor) complex, which mediates the SV fusion with the presynaptic membrane, allowing vesicle exocytosis and release of the neurotransmitter into the synaptic cleft. *SYP* mutations have been detected in cases with nonsyndromal XLID and XLID with epilepsy[159] (Figure 2). At the presynaptic site, reduced or defective OPHN1 signaling has been shown to impair SV cycling at hippocampal synapses. It forms a complex with endophilin A1, a protein implicated in membrane curvature generation during SV endocytosis.[160]

The *CASK* gene, located at Xp11.4, encodes a calcium/calmodulin-dependent serine protein kinase that is a member of the membrane-associated guanyl kinase family of scaffolding proteins.[161–163] CASK binds to the cytoplasmic tails of the presynaptic cell adhesion molecule β-neurexin.[164] Mutations in this gene have been described in patients with an FG phenotype,[129] XLID and microcephaly with pontine and cerebellar hypoplasia,[163] and XLID with or without nystagmus[159] (Figure 1).

Cytoskeletal Dynamics

The cytoskeleton is critical for cell structure, polarization and migration, and, more specifically, for neuronal cells; it has a pivotal role in regulating the structure and dynamics of dendrites and spines, axon outgrowth, and synapse formation. Once synapses have been formed, the neuronal cytoskeleton supports their maintenance and maturation and thus the synaptic cytoskeleton is essential for stabilization and remodeling of synaptic connections.[165] Actin filaments are the predominant cytoskeletal element in dendritic spines whereas actin and microtubules constitute the cytoskeleton of dendrites.[166–168] Both the formation and reorganization of spines are accompanied by dynamic rearrangements of actin filaments.[169,170] Inhibition of actin polymerization attenuates long-term potentiation maintenance, whereas long-term depotentiation (LTD) is associated with actin filament disassembly.[172] Signaling molecules and pathways that regulate actin-cytoskeleton organization have a major impact on the structure and function of dendrites and spines. Key molecules mediating changes in these structures are actin-binding proteins and members of the family of small Rho GTPases such as, RhoA, Rac, and Cdc42.[171]

Rho GTPases function as molecular switches, cycling between an inactive GDP-bound state and an active GTP-bound state. The activity is regulated by positive regulators (guanine nucleotide exchange factors (GEFs)), negative regulators (GTPase activating proteins (GAPs)), and GDIs.[172,173]

The XLID gene *OPHN1* (Xq12) encodes oligophrenin 1, a Rho GTPase-activating protein (Rho-GAP), expressed both presynaptically and postsynaptically in axons, dendrites, and spines, that has an important role in the activity-dependent maturation and plasticity of excitatory synapses by regulating their structural and functional stability[174] (Figures 1 and 2). Oligophrenin 1 was found to regulate RhoA negatively and interact

with the postsynaptic protein Homer; knockdown of oligophrenin-1 levels in CA1 neurons in rat hippocampal slices resulted in significantly decrease spine length.[173] Synaptic activity through N-methyl-D-aspartate receptor activation drives OPHN1 into dendritic spines, where it forms a complex with α-amino-3-hydroxy-5-methyl-4-isoxazolepropionic acid (AMPA) receptors and selectively enhances AMPA receptor–mediated synaptic transmission and spine size by stabilizing synaptic AMPA receptor, which suggests that normal activity-driven glutamatergic synapse development is impaired by perturbation of OPHN1 function.[174]

PAK3, an XLID protein encoded by the homonymous gene (Xq23), is a member of the large family of p21-activating kinases (PAKs), which are downstream effectors for Rac and Cdc42.[175–177] Mutations of the *PAK3* gene have been reported in families with nonsyndromal XLID.[178,179] Activation of PAK by Rac1 or Cdc42 leads to the activation of LIMK1, which in turn phosphorylates and inactivates cofilin, a crucial modulator of actin dynamics.[180,181] Downregulation of PAK3 results in morphological spine abnormalities, including an increased proportion of abnormally elongated, thin and immature spines, and variable defects in synaptic plasticity.[182–184] Studies showed that PAK3 is specifically recruited in the spine head of activated spines. In addition, researchers found a small reduction of PAK3 in the nearby dendrite as opposed to more distal parts of the dendrite. This result suggests that the redistribution of PAK3 relieves its negative action on spine growth in the nearby dendrite and thereby promotes a local formation of new spines, as seen with PAK3 inhibition.[183]

Other XLID proteins, FGD1, ARHGEF9 (collybistin), and ARHGEF6 (αPIX), are GEFs. ARHGEF9 and FGD1 are specific for Cdc42, whereas ARHGEF6 activates both Rac1 and Cdc42. *ARHGEF9*, which encodes a Cdc42 GEF protein, collybistin, is specifically enriched in neuronal dendrites and involved in the formation of inhibitory synapses.[185–188] Collybistin is essential for the clustering of the postsynaptic scaffold protein gephyrin, and along with Cdc42 regulates GABAergic postsynaptic densities.[188,189] ARHGEF6, which was initially isolated as a PAK interacting protein, localizes specifically at the postsynaptic compartment of excitatory synapses.[190] Knockdown of the rat Arhgef6 in cultured hippocampal neurons resulted in abnormalities in spine morphology similar to those reported with knockdown of PAK3. This phenotype could be rescued by a constitutively active form of PAK3.[190] *Arhgef6* knockout mice exhibited an increase in both dendritic length and spine density, accompanied by an overall loss in spine synapses and showed a dramatic reduction in levels of the active Rac1 and Cdc42 in the hippocampus.[191]

The *IQSEC2* gene (Xp11.22) encodes a guanine nucleotide exchange factor for the small GTPase, ADP-ribosylation factor 6 (ARF6), which localizes to the postsynaptic density of excitatory synapses.[192,193] ARF6 is known to regulate endosomal trafficking and actin dynamics.[194,195]

Cell-Adhesion and Transsynaptic Signaling

Cell-adhesion molecules (CAMs) have critical roles in brain development and are crucial for the initial contact between presynaptic and postsynaptic compartments and functional maturation and maintenance of synapses.[196,197] Neuronal CAMs provide anchors for scaffolding proteins.[197,198] Most CAMs at synaptic clefts are members of the cadherin family, immunoglobulin superfamilies, integrin family, and neurexins and their binding partners, the neuroligins. Mutations in several of these neuronal CAMs are associated with ID and ASD or ASD susceptibility. The finding of many independent, individually rare genetic variants in synaptic CAMs such as *CDH9*, *CDH10*, *CDH15*, *PTCHD1*, *PCDH9*, *PCDH10*, *PCDH19*, *CNTN4*, *CNTNAP2*, *KIRREL3*, *NLGN3*, *NLGN4X*, and *NRXN1* implies that synaptic cell-adhesion pathways have a significant role in cognitive and behavioral function[199–211] (see also Chapter 11). However, clinical heterogeneity has been reported in several individuals with mutations in synaptic CAMs, which suggests the existence of a compensatory mechanism or concomitance of other unknown genetic or nongenetic factors. Also, studies suggest that synaptic adhesion molecules might have overlapping functions or act together at synaptic sites because no single pair of synaptic adhesion molecules seems to be sufficient to accomplish all aspects of synaptic development.[212]

An important family of synaptic CAMs is composed of the neurexin and neuroligin proteins. Interactions between presynaptic neurexins and postsynaptic neuroligins, which act as calcium-dependent CAMS in both excitatory and inhibitory synapse formation, have been studied extensively. Neurexins encode two major isoforms, α (long) and β (short), differing in their extracellular domains. Binding of neurexins to neuroligins is mediated by the sixth laminin, neurexin, sex hormone–binding globulin (LNS) domain of α-neurexin, and the single LNS domain of β-neurexin.[213] Both neuroligins and neuroxin exhibit synaptogenic activity in cell culture assays.[214–217] However, double or triple α-neurexin knockout mice exhibit a synaptic transmission defect with no impairment in synapse formation.[218] Similarly, mice deficient in one or more neuroligin genes show normal synapse numbers but alterations in the recruitment of postsynaptic receptors to glutamatergic, GABAergic, and glycinergic synapses.[219,220] Chubykin and coworkers reported that different neuroligins act on distinct types of synapses via activity-dependent mechanisms.[221] Mutations in the *NLGN4* gene have been reported in all affected members of a large French family with XLID, with or without autism or pervasive developmental disorder.[222]

Translational Regulation, Protein Degradation, and Turnover

The balance between protein synthesis and degradation is crucial for the proper function of synapses. It has been proven that both de novo protein synthesis[223] and the ubiquitin proteasome system (UPS)[224–226] have an important function in synaptic transmission and plasticity. These observations suggest that changes in synaptic transmission involve extensive regulation of the synaptic proteome.

The synaptic proteome is also affected by the nonsense-mediated mRNA decay (NMD) pathway that provides a translation-coupled quality control system. The NMD functions not only in degrading aberrant mRNAs with a premature termination codon but also in regulating the transcriptome (reviewed in Nguyen et al.[227]). Mutations in the NMD-associated gene, *UPF3B*, located at Xq24 (Figure 1), have been found in both syndromal and nonsyndromal XLID.[124]

The UPS comprises a group of enzymes, an ubiquitin-activating enzyme (E1), an ubiquitin-conjugating enzyme (E2), and an ubiquitin ligase (E3), that activates and then attaches a 76–amino acid protein ubiquitin to lysine residues of specific substrates. Thus, ubiquitination posttranslationally modifies protein function and triggers the subsequent degradation of ubiquitinated proteins by the 26S proteasome. Various components of the multicomplex UPS are necessary for proper development of the brain, axon outgrowth and guidance, synapse development, and plasticity. It has been shown that protein degradation through the UPS controls proper synaptic balance by maintaining optimal protein levels, thus promoting functional equilibrium.[223,224,229]

Deficiency of the XLID gene *UBE2A* (Xq24), which encodes an ubiquitin-conjugating enzyme (E2) (RAD6A), has been shown to cause defective synaptic function as a consequence of mitochondrial failure in *Drosophila*.[230] Using both in vitro and in vivo ubiquitination assays, RAD6A in conjugation with an E3 ubiquitin ligase such as Parkin ubiquitinates mitochondrial proteins to facilitate the clearance of dysfunctional mitochondria in cells.[230] The XLID gene *MID1* (Xp22.2) encodes a microtubule-associated ubiquitin E3 ligase and is responsible for the Thelecanthus–hypospadias syndrome (or Opitz–GBBB type I syndrome)

(Figure 1).[231] This protein facilitates MID1-dependent regulation of protein phosphatase 2A (PP2A). It has been shown to catalyze the polyubiquitination of alpha 4, a key regulator of PP2A and mTOR.[232]

The *CUL4B* gene (Xq23) produces a member of the cullin family of E3 ligase complexes that acts as scaffold proteins and recruits specific substrates for ubiquitination and subsequent degradation.[233–235] Lack of Cul4b in mice leads to embryonic lethality.[236,237] Some dendritic features, including the complexity, diameter, and spine density in the hippocampal neurons, were affected by Cul4b deletion.[236] CUL4B has been implicated in degradation of Cdt1 (chromatin licensing and DNA replication factor 1) and camptothecin (CPT)-induced topoisomerase I (Topo I).[238] Patients harboring *CUL4B* mutation-derived cells show impaired CPT-induced Topo I degradation and increased Topo I–mediated DNA breakage.[237] CUL4B positively regulates the CDK2–CDC6 cascade, promoting DNA replication licensing.[239] Interestingly, the authors found that the upregulation of CDK2 by CUL4B is through the transcription repression of miR-372/373.[239] CUL4B has also been shown to target WDR5, a core subunit of histone H3 lysin 4 methyl transferase complexes for ubiquitination and degradation.[240] *CUL4B* mutations are defective in promoting TSC2 and cyclin E degradation and positively regulating mTOR signaling in neocortical neurons.[241] Activation of the mTOR pathway increases dendritic complexity[242,243] and has been observed in mouse models of Fragile X and tuberous sclerosis, two important causes of ID.[244,245]

FUTURE CHALLENGES AND THERAPEUTIC APPROACHES

Study of the pathogenetic mechanisms indicates how XLID genes are involved in various physiological processes; many of these genes converge on distinct and common pathways altering neuronal functions.[246] A growing understanding of genes, pathways, and associated molecular and cellular mechanisms in many cases of ID provides a means for exploring therapeutic approaches.

Two examples of such approaches involve XLID syndromes caused by mutations in transporter genes: Allan–Herndon–Dudley syndrome (*MCT8*, thyroid hormone transporter, Xq13.2), and creatine transporter deficiency syndrome (*SLC6A8*, Xq28). In both cases the strategy was based on supplementation of analogues of the missing compounds. Trials are currently under investigation within multiple laboratories.[10,247,248] Another condition, Snyder–Robinson syndrome, caused by mutations in the *SMS* gene (spermine synthase, Xp22.11), has been treated with supplementation by spermine. Although as yet unsuccessful, the approach has provided valuable information about the transport of spermine into the brain which will prove useful for future studies.[10]

Aside from enzyme replacement models, several studies suggest that neurological disorders such as Rett syndrome and Fragile X syndrome are not permanent, and hint at the possibility of rescuing, reversing, or ameliorating neurological deficits.[249–251]

However, a paper by Auerbach et al.[252] highlighted at least one potential problem with the assumption that knowledge of pathways may have universal therapeutic benefits. Auerbach and coworkers showed that even though mutations in the *Tsc2* gene and the *Fmr1* gene in mice resulted in LTD, *Tsc2* mutations caused diminished protein synthesis whereas *Fmr1* mutations caused excessive protein synthesis. As a result, each required different treatments to arrive at the same end point. Therefore, extrapolating to humans, a therapy designed for ID is not likely to be helpful in all cases (which is already known); in fact, it might even be deleterious for some individuals. Therefore, in-depth knowledge of the pathway may be necessary for each patient as therapies are developed using information gleamed from this systems approach.

References

1. American Psychiatric Association. *Diagnostic and statistical manual of mental disorders*. 5th ed. Arlington (VA): American Psychiatric Publishing; 2013.
2. Stevenson R, Schwartz C, Rogers C. *Atlas of X-linked intellectual disability syndromes*. New York: Oxford Press; 2012.
3. Perou R, Bitsko RH, Blumberg SJ, Pastor P, Ghandour RM, Gfroerer JC, et al. Mental health surveillance among children—United States 2005—2011. *Morb Mortal Wkly Rep Surveill Summ* 2013;**62**:1—35. Washington (DC).
4. Penrose LS. *A clinical and genetic study on 1280 cases of mental defect*. Special report series. Medical research council, No. 229. London: Her Majesty's Stationery Office; 1938.
5. Lehrke RG. X-linked mental retardation and verbal disability. *Birth Defects Orig Artic Ser* 1974;**X**(1):1—100.
6. Herbst DS, Miller JR. Non-specific X-linked mental retardation II: the frequency in British Columbia. *Am J Med Genet* 1980;**7**:461.
7. Lyon MF. Gene action in the X-chromosome of the mouse (*Mus musculus* L.). *Nature* 1961;**190**:372—3.
8. Turner G. Finding genes on the X chromosome by which homo may have become sapiens. *Am J Hum Genet* 1996;**58**:1109—10.
9. Turner G. Intelligence and the X chromosome. *Lancet* 1996;**347**:1814—5.
10. Schwartz CE. X-linked intellectual disability genetics. In: *eLS*. Chichester: John Wiley & Sons, Ltd; 2015.
11. Roper HH, Hamel BC. X-linked mental retardation. *Nat Rev Genet* 2005;**6**:46—57.
12. Chelly J, Khefaoui M, Francis F, Cherif B, Bienvenu T. Genetics and pathophysiology of mental retardation. *Eur J Hum Genet* 2006;**14**:701—13.
13. Oberlé I, Rousseau F, Heitz D, Kretz C, Devys D, Hanauer A, et al. Instability of a 550-base pair DNA segment and abnormal methylation in fragile X syndrome. *Science* 1991;**252**:1097—102.

14. Chiurazzi P, Schwartz CE, Gecz J, Neri G. XLMR genes: update 2007. *Eur J Hum Genet* 2008;**16**:422−34.

15. Steele MW, Chorazy AL. Renpenning's syndrome. *Lancet* 1974; **2**:752.

16. Howard-Peebles PN, Stoddard GR, Mims MG. Familial X-linked mental retardation, verbal disability, and marker X chromosomes. *Am J Hum Genet* 1979;**31**:214.

17. Jennings M, Hall JG, Hoehn H. Significance of phenotypic and chromosomal abnormalities in X-linked mental retardation (Martin-Bell or Renpenning syndrome). *Am J Med Genet* 1980;**7**:417.

18. Proops R, Webb T. The 'fragile' X chromosome in the Martin-Bell-Renpenning syndrome and in males with other forms of familial mental retardation. *J Med Genet* 1981;**18**:366.

19. Turner G, Turner B, Collins E. Renpenning's syndrome − X-linked mental retardation. *Lancet* 1970;**2**:365.

20. Turner G, Turner B, Collins E. X-linked mental retardation without physical abnormality: Renpenning's syndrome. *Dev Med Child Neurol* 1971;**13**:71.

21. Turner G, Engisch B, Lindsay DG, Turner B. X-linked mental retardation without physical abnormality (Renpenning's syndrome) in sibs in an institution. *J Med Genet* 1972;**9**:324−30.

22. Lenski C, Abidi F, Meindl A, Gibson A, Platzer M, Frank Kooy R, et al. Novel truncating mutations in the polyglutamine tract binding protein 1 gene (PQBP1) cause Renpenning syndrome and X-linked mental retardation in another family with microcephaly. *Am J Hum Genet* 2004;**74**:777−80.

23. Kalscheuer VM, Freude K, Musante L, Jensen LR, Yntema HG, Gécz J, et al. Mutations in the polyglutamine binding protein 1 gene cause X-linked mental retardation. *Nat Genet* 2003;**35**: 313−5.

24. Stevenson RE, Bennett CW, Abidi F, Kleefstra T, Porteous M, Simensen RJ, et al. Renpenning syndrome comes into focus. *Am J Med Genet A* 2005;**134**:415−21.

25. Lubs H, Abidi FE, Echeverri R, Holloway L, Meindl A, Stevenson RE, et al. Golabi-Ito-Hall syndrome results from a missense mutation in the WW domain of the PQBP1 gene. *J Med Genet* 2006;**43**:e30.

26. Schwartz CE, Gurrieri F, Neri G. Intellectual disability syndromes. In: Charney DS, Buxbaum JD, Sklar P, Nestler EJ, editors. *Neurobiology of mental illness.* New York: Oxford Press; 2013. p. 1010−21.

27. Germanaud D, Rossi M, Bussy G, Gérard D, Hertz-Pannier L, Blanchet P, et al. The Renpenning syndrome spectrum: new clinical insights supported by 13 new *PQBP1*-mutated males. *Clin Genet* 2011;**79**:225−35.

28. Borjeson M, Forssman H, Lehmann O. An X-linked recessively inherited syndrome characterized by grave mental deficiency epilepsy and endocrine disorder. *Acta Med Scand* 1962;**171**:13−21.

29. Turner G, Gedeon A, Mulley J, Sutherland G, Rae J, Power K, et al. Borjeson-Forssman-Lehmann syndrome: clinical manifestations and gene localization to Xq26-27. *Am J Med Genet* 1989;**34**:463−9.

30. Turner G, Lower KM, White SM, Delatycki M, Lampe AK, Wright M, et al. The clinical picture of the Borjeson-Forssman-Lehmann syndrome in males and heterozygous females with *PHF6* mutations. *Clin Genet* 2004;**65**:226−32.

31. Trivier E, De Cesare D, Jacquot S, Pannetier S, Zackai E, Young I, et al. Mutations in the kinase *Rsk-2* associated with Coffin-Lowry syndrome. *Nature* 1996;**384**:567−70.

32. Hunter AGW. Coffin-Lowry syndrome: a 20-year follow-up and review of long-term outcomes. *Am J Med Genet* 2002;**111**:345−55.

33. Marques Pereira P, Schneider A, Pannetier S, Heron D, Hanauer A. Coffin-lowry syndrome. *Eur J Hum Genet* 2010;**18**:627−33.

34. Hagberg B, Aicardi J, Dias K, Ramos O. A progressive syndrome of autism, dementia, ataxia, and loss of purposeful hand use in girls: Rett's syndrome: report of 35 cases. *Ann Neurol* 1983;**14**: 471−9.

35. Neul JL, Kaufmann WE, Glaze DG, Christodoulou J, Clarke AJ, Bahi-Buisson N, et al. Rett syndrome: revised diagnostic criteria and nomenclature. *Ann Neurol* 2010;**68**:944−50.

36. VK P, Levine C, Carpenter NJ. New X-linked syndrome with seizures, acquired microcephaly, and agenesis of the corpus callosum. *Am J Med Genet* 1992;**43**:458−66.

37. Kato M, Das S, Petras K, Kitamura K, Morohashi K, Abuelo DN, et al. Mutations of ARX are associated with striking pleiotropy and consistent genotype-phenotype correlation. *Hum Mutat* 2004;**23**:147−59.

38. Shoubridge C, Fullston T, Gécz J. ARX spectrum disorders: making inroads into the molecular pathology. *Hum Mutat* 2010;**31**: 889−900.

39. Abidi F, Hall BD, Cadle RG, Feldman GL, Lubs HA, Ouzts LV, et al. X-linked mental retardation with variable stature, head circumference, and testicular volume linked to Xq12-q21. *Am J Med Genet* 1999;**85**:223−9.

40. Bachmann C. Ornithine carbamoyl transferase deficiency: findings, models and problems. *J Inherit Metab Dis* 1992;**15**:578−91.

41. Matsuda I, Matsuura T, Nishiyori A, Komaki S, Hoshide R, Matsumoto T, et al. Phenotypic variability in male patients carrying the mutant ornithine transcarbamylase (OTC) allele, Arg40His, ranging from a child with an unfavourable prognosis to an asymptomatic older adult. *J Med Genet* 1996;**33**:645−8.

42. Genet S, Cranston T, Middleton-Price HR. Mutation detection in 65 families with a possible diagnosis of ornithine carbamoyltransferase deficiency including 14 novel mutations. *J Inherit Metab Dis* 2000;**23**:669−76.

43. de Vries BB, Halley DJ, Oostra BA, Niermeijer MF. The fragile X syndrome. *J Med Genet* 1998;**35**:579−89.

44. Terracciano A, Chiurazzi P, Neri G. Fragile X syndrome. *Am J Med Genet C Semin Med Genet* 2005;**137C**:32−7.

45. Lubs HA, Stevenson RE, Schwartz CE. Fragile X and X-linked intellectual disability: four decades of discovery. *Am J Hum Genet* 2012;**90**:579−90.

46. Lujan JE, Carlis ME, Lubs HA. A form of X-linked mental retardation with marfanoid habitus. *Am J Med Genet* 1984;**17**: 311−22.

47. Fryns JP, Buttiens M. X-linked mental retardation with marfanoid habitus. *Am J Med Genet* 1987;**28**:267−74.

48. Lalatta F, Livini E, Selicorni A, Briscioli V, Vita A, Lugo F, et al. X-linked mental retardation with marfanoid habitus: first report of four Italian patients. *Am J Med Genet* 1991;**38**:228−32.

49. Atkin JF, Flaitz K, Patil S, Smith W. A new X-linked mental retardation syndrome. *Am J Med Genet* 1985;**21**:697−705.

50. Clark RD, Baraitser M. A new X-linked mental retardation syndrome. *Am J Med Genet* 1987;**26**:13−5.

51. Baraitser M, Reardon W, Vijeratnam S. Nonspecific X-linked mental retardation with macrocephaly and obesity: a further family. *Am J Med Genet* 1995;**57**:380−4.

52. Mendicino A, Sabbadini G, Pergola MS. Clark-Baraitser syndrome: report of a new case and review of the literature. *Clin Dysmorph* 2005;**14**:133−5.

53. Opitz JM, Kaveggia EG. The FG syndrome: an X-linked recessive syndrome of multiple congenital anomalies and mental retardation. *Z Kinderheilk* 1974;**117**:1−18.

54. Graham Jr JM, Superneau D, Rogers RC, Corning K, Schwartz CE, Dykens EM. Clinical and behavioral characteristics in FG syndrome. *Am J Med Genet* 1999;**85**:470−5.

55. Clark RD, Graham Jr JM, Friez MJ, Hoo JJ, Jones KL, McKeown C, et al. FG syndrome, an X-linked multiple congenital anomaly syndrome: the clinical phenotype and an algorithm for diagnostic testing. *Genet Med* 2009;**11**:769−75.

56. Simpson JL, Landey S, New M, German J. A previously unrecognized X-linked syndrome of dysmorphia. *Birth Defects Orig Art Ser* 1975;**XI**:18−24.

57. Gurrieri F, Cappa M, Neri G. Further delineation of the Simpson-Golabi-Behmel (SGB) syndrome. *Am J Med Genet* 1992; **44**:136–7.

58. Neri G, Gurrieri F, Zanni G, Lin A. Clinical and molecular aspects of the Simpson-Golabi-Behmel syndrome. *Am J Med Genet* 1998; **79**:279–83.

59. Snyder RD, Robinson A. Recessive sex-linked mental retardation in the absence of other recognizable abnormalities: report of a family. *Clin Pediat* 1969;**8**:669–74.

60. Arena JF, Schwartz C, Ouzts L, Stevenson R, Miller M, Garza J, et al. X-linked mental retardation with thin habitus, osteoporosis, and kyphoscoliosis: linkage to Xp21.3-p22.12. *Am J Med Genet* 1996;**64**:50–8.

61. Pettigrew AL, Jackson LG, Ledbetter DH. New X-linked mental retardation disorder with Dandy-Walker malformation, basal ganglia disease, and seizures. *Am J Med Genet* 1991;**38**:200–7.

62. Turner G, Gedeon A, Kerr B, Bennett R, Mulley J, Partington M. Syndromic form of X-linked mental retardation with marked hypotonia in early life, severe mental handicap, and difficult adult behavior maps to Xp22. *Am J Med Genet A* 2003;**117A**:245–50.

63. Saillour Y, Zanni G, Des Portes V, Heron D, Guibaud L, Iba-Zizen MT, et al. Mutations in the *AP1S2* gene encoding the sigma 2 subunit of the adaptor protein 1 complex are associated with syndromic X-linked mental retardation with hydrocephalus and calcifications in basal ganglia. *J Med Genet* 2007;**44**:739–44.

64. Bianchine JW, Lewis Jr RC. The MASA syndrome: a new heritable mental retardation syndrome. *Clin Genet* 1974;**5**:298–306.

65. Schrander-Stumpel C, Howeler C, Jones M, Sommer A, Stevens C, Tinschert S, et al. Spectrum of X-linked hydrocephalus (HSAS), MASA syndrome, and complicated spastic paraplegia (SPG1): clinical review with six additional families. *Am J Med Genet* 1995;**57**:107–16.

66. Vos YJ, de Walle HE, Bos KK, Stegeman JA, Ten Berge AM, Bruining M, et al. Genotype-phenotype correlations in L1 syndrome: a guide for genetic counselling and mutation analysis. *J Med Genet* 2010;**47**:169–75.

67. Aicardi J, Chevrie JJ, Rousselie F. Le syndrome spasmes en flexion, agenesic calleuse, anomalies chorio-retiniennes. *Arch Franc Pediat* 1969;**26**:1103–20.

68. Donnenfeld AE, Packer RJ, Zackai EH, Chee CM, Sellinger B, Emanuel BS. Clinical, cytogenetic, and pedigree findings in 18 cases of Aicardi syndrome. *Am J Med Genet* 1989;**32**:461–7.

69. Sutton VR, Hopkins BJ, Eble TN, Gambhir N, Lewis RA, Van den Veyver IB. Facial and physical features of Aicardi syndrome: infants to teenagers. *Am J Med Genet* 2005;**138**:254–8.

70. Cantu JM, Hernandez A, Larracilla J, Trejo A, Macotela-Ruiz E. A new X-linked recessive disorder with dwarfism, cerebral atrophy, and generalized keratosis follicularis. *J Pediatr* 1974;**84**:564–7.

71. Christianson AL, Stevenson RE, van der Meyden CH, Pelser J, Theron FW, van Rensburg PL, et al. X linked severe mental retardation, craniofacial dysmorphology, epilepsy, ophthalmoplegia, and cerebellar atrophy in a large South African kindred is localised to Xq24-q27. *J Med Genet* 1999;**36**:759–66.

72. Menkes JH, Alter M, Steigleder GK, Weakley DR, Sung JH. A sex-linked recessive disorder with retardation of growth, peculiar hair and focal cerebral and cerebellar degeneration. *Pediatrics* 1962;**29**:764–79.

73. Barnard RO, Best PV, Erdohazi M. Neuropathology of Menkes' disease. *Dev Med Child Neurol* 1978;**20**:586–97.

74. Smith RD, Fineman RM, Myers GG. Short stature, psychomotor retardation, and unusual facial appearance in two brothers. *Am J Med Genet* 1980;**7**:5–9.

75. Salomons GS, van Dooren SJM, Verhoeven NM, Cecil KM, Ball WS, Degrauw TJ, et al. X-linked creatine-transporter gene (*SLC6A8*) defect: a new creatine-deficiency syndrome. *Am J Hum Genet* 2001;**68**:1497–500.

76. Hahn KA, Salomons GS, Tackels-Horne D, Wood TC, Taylor HA, Schroer RJ, et al. X-linked mental retardation with seizures and carrier manifestations is caused by a mutation in the creatine-transporter gene (*SLC6A8*) located in Xq28. *Am J Hum Genet* 2002; **70**:1349–56.

77. van de Kamp JM, Betsalel OT, Mercimek-Mahmutoglu S, Abulhoul L, Grunewald S, Anselm I, et al. Phenotype and genotype in 101 males with X-linked creatine transporter deficiency. *J Med Genet* 2013;**50**:463–72.

78. Fox JW, Lamperti ED, Eksioğlu YZ, Hong SE, Feng Y, Graham DA, et al. Mutations in *filamin 1* prevent migration of cerebral cortical neurons in human periventricular heterotopia. *Neuron* 1998;**21**:1315–25.

79. Robertson SP. Filamin A: phenotypic diversity. *Curr Opin Genet Dev* 2005;**15**:301–7.

80. Dobyns WB, Elias ER, Newlin AC, Pagon RA, Ledbetter DH. Causal heterogeneity in isolated lissencephaly. *Neurology* 1992; **42**:1375–88.

81. Matsumoto N, Leventer RJ, Kuc JA, Mewborn SK, Dudlicek LL, Ramocki MB, et al. Mutation analysis of the *DCX* gene and genotype/phenotype correlation in subcortical band heterotopia. *Eur J Hum Genet* 2001;**9**:5–12.

82. du Souich C, Chou A, Yin J, Oh T, Nelson TN, Hurlburt J, et al. Characterization of a new X-linked mental retardation syndrome with microcephaly, cortical malformation, and thin habitus. *Am J Med Genet A* 2009;**149A**:2469–78.

83. McLarren KW, Severson TM, du Souich C, Stockton DW, Kratz LE, Cunningham D, et al. Hypomorphic temperature-sensitive alleles of *NSDHL* cause CK syndrome. *Am J Hum Genet* 2010;**87**:905–14.

84. Siber M. X-linked recessive microcephaly, microphthalmia with corneal opacities, spastic quadriplegia, hypospadias and cryptorchidism. *Clin Genet* 1984;**26**:453–6.

85. Duker JS, Weiss JS, Siber M, Bieber FR, Albert DM. Ocular findings in a new heritable syndrome of brain, eye, and urogenital abnormalities. *Am J Ophthalmol* 1985;**15**(99):51–5.

86. Goltz RW, Peterson Jr WC, Gorlin RJ, Ravits HG. Focal dermal hypoplasia. *Arch Derm* 1962;**86**:708–17.

87. Maas SM, Lombardi MP, van Essen AJ, Wakeling EL, Castle B, Temple IK, et al. Phenotype and genotype in 17 patients with Goltz-Gorlin syndrome. *J Med Genet* 2009;**46**:716–20.

88. Gencic S, Abuelo D, Ambler M, Hudson LD. Pelizaeus-Merzbacher disease: an X-linked neurologic disorder of myelin metabolism with a novel mutation in the gene encoding proteolipid protein. *Am J Hum Genet* 1989;**45**:435–42.

89. Arena JF, Schwartz C, Stevenson R, Lawrence L, Carpenter A, Duara R, et al. Spastic paraplegia with iron deposits in the basal ganglia: a new X-linked mental retardation syndrome. *Am J Med Genet* 1992;**43**:479–90.

90. al-Gazali LI, Mueller RF, Caine A, Antoniou A, McCartney A, Fitchett M, et al. Two 46,XX,t(X;Y) females with linear skin defects and congenital microphthalmia: a new syndrome at Xp22.3. *J Med Genet* 1990;**27**:59–63.

91. Bird LM, Krous HF, Eichenfield LF, Swalwell CI, Jones MC. Female infant with oncocytic cardiomyopathy and microphthalmia with linear skin defects (MLS): a clue to the pathogenesis of oncocytic cardiomyopathy? *Am J Med Genet* 1994;**53**:141–8.

92. Aarskog D. A familial syndrome of short stature associated with facial dysplasia and genital anomalies. *J Pediatr* 1970;**77**:856–61.

93. Orrico A, Galli L, Cavaliere ML, Garavelli L, Fryns JP, Crushell E, et al. Phenotypic and molecular characterisation of the Aarskog-Scott syndrome: a survey of the clinical variability in light of *FGD1* mutation analysis in 46 patients. *Eur J Hum Genet* 2004;**12**:16–23.

94. Bonneau D, Toutain A, Laquerrière A, Marret S, Saugier-Veber P, Barthez MA, et al. X-linked lissencephaly with absent corpus callosum and ambiguous genitalia (XLAG): clinical, magnetic resonance imaging, and neuropathological findings. *Ann Neurol* 2002;**51**:340−9.

95. Bhat SS, Rogers RC, Holden KR, Srivastava AK. A novel in-frame deletion in *ARX* is associated with lissencephaly with absent corpus callosum and hypoplastic genitalia. *Am J Med Genet A* 2005;**138**:70−2.

96. Frints SG, Froyen G, Marynen P, Willekens D, Legius E, Fryns JP. Re-evaluation of MRX36 family after discovery of an *ARX* gene mutation reveals mild neurological features of Partington syndrome. *Am J Med Genet* 2002;**112**:427−8.

97. Bergmann C, Zerres K, Senderek J, Rudnik-Schoneborn S, Eggermann T, Häusler M, et al. Oligophrenin 1 (*OPHN1*) gene mutation causes syndromic X-linked mental retardation with epilepsy, rostral ventricular enlargement and cerebellar hypoplasia. *Brain* 2003;**126**(Pt 7):1537−44.

98. Philip N, Chabrol B, Lossi AM, Cardoso C, Guerrini R, Dobyns WB, et al. Mutations in the oligophrenin-1 gene (OPHN1) cause X linked congenital cerebellar hypoplasia. *J Med Genet* 2003;**40**:441−6.

99. Greenwood genetic center website: www.ggc.org.

100. Stevenson RE, Schwartz CE. Clinical and molecular contributions to the understanding of X-linked mental retardation. *Cytogenet Genome Res* 2002;**99**:265−75.

101. Strømme P, Mangelsdorf ME, Scheffer IE, Gécz J. Infantile spasms, dystonia, and other X-linked phenotypes caused by mutations in Aristaless related homeobox gene. *Arx Brain Dev* 2002;**24**:266−8.

102. Strømme P, Mangelsdorf ME, Shaw MA, Lower KM, Lewis SM, Bruyere H, et al. Mutations in the human ortholog of Aristaless cause X-linked mental retardation and epilepsy. *Nat Genet* 2002;**30**:441−5.

103. Bienvenu T, Poirier K, Friocourt G, Bahi N, Beaumont D, Fauchereau F, et al. *ARX*, a novel Prd-class-homeobox gene highly expressed in the telencephalon, is mutated in X-linked mental retardation. *Hum Mol Genet* 2002;**11**:981−91.

104. Kitamura K, Yanazawa M, Sugiyama N, Miura H, Iizuka-Kogo A, Kusaka M, et al. Mutation of *ARX* causes abnormal development of forebrain and testes in mice and X-linked lissencephaly with abnormal genitalia in humans. *Nat Genet* 2002;**32**:359−69.

105. Uyanik G, Aigner L, Martin P, Gross C, Neumann D, Marschner-Schäfer H, et al. *ARX* mutations in X-linked lissencephaly with abnormal genitalia. *Neurology* 2003;**61**:232−5.

106. Stepp ML, Cason AL, Finnis M, Mangelsdorf M, Holinski-Feder E, Macgregor D, et al. XLMR in MRX families 29, 32, 33 and 38 results from the dup24 mutation in the *ARX* (Aristaless related homeobox) gene. *BMC Med Genet* 2005;**6**:16.

107. Gibbons RJ, Picketts DJ, Villard L, Higgs DR. Mutations in a putative global transcriptional regulator cause X-linked mental retardation with alpha-thalassemia (ATR-X syndrome). *Cell* 1995;**80**:837−45.

108. Villard L, Fontes M. Alpha-thalassemia/mental retardation syndrome, X-Linked (ATR-X, MIM #301040, *ATR-X/XNP/XH2* gene MIM #300032). *Eur J Hum Genet* 2002;**10**:223−5.

109. Lossi AM, Millán JM, Villard L, Orellana C, Cardoso C, Prieto F, et al. Mutation of the *XNP/ATR-X* gene in a family with severe mental retardation, spastic paraplegia and skewed pattern of X inactivation: demonstration that the mutation is involved in the inactivation bias. *Am J Hum Genet* 1999;**65**:558−62.

110. Stevenson RE, Abidi F, Schwartz CE, Lubs HA, Holmes LB. Holmes-Gang syndrome is allelic with XLMR-hypotonic face syndrome. *Am J Med Genet* 2000;**94**:383−5.

111. Guerrini R, Shanahan JL, Carrozzo R, Bonanni P, Higgs DR, Gibbons RJ. A nonsense mutation of the *ATRX* gene causing mild mental retardation and epilepsy. *Ann Neurol* 2000;**47**:117−21.

112. Yntema HG, Poppelaars FA, Derksen E, Oudakker AR, van Roosmalen T, Jacobs A, et al. Expanding phenotype of *XNP* mutations: mild to moderate mental retardation. *Am J Med Genet* 2002;**110**:243−7.

113. Abidi FE, Cardoso C, Lossi AM, Lowry RB, Depetris D, Mattéi MG, et al. Mutation in the 5′ alternatively spliced region of the *XNP/ATR-X* gene causes Chudley-Lowry syndrome. *Eur J Hum Genet* 2005;**13**:176−83.

114. Villard L, Fontès M, Adès LC, Gecz J. Identification of a mutation in the *XNP/ATR-X* gene in a family reported as Smith-Fineman-Myers syndrome. *Am J Med Genet* 2000;**91**:83−5.

115. Mattei JF, Collignon P, Ayme S, Giraud F. X-linked mental retardation, growth retardation, deafness and microgenitalism. A second familial report. *Clin Genet* 1983;**23**:70−4.

116. Villard L, Gecz J, Mattéi JF, Fontés M, Saugier-Veber P, Munnich A, et al. *XNP* mutation in a large family with Juberg-Marsidi syndrome. *Nat Genet* 1996;**12**:359−60.

117. Juberg RC, Marsidi I. A new form of X-linked mental retardation with growth retardation, deafness, and microgenitalism. *Am J Hum Genet* 1980;**32**:714−22.

118. Friez MJ, Brooks SS, Abidi F, Schwartz CE, Stevenson RE. Juberg-Marsidi syndrome and Brooks syndrome are allelic X-linked intellectual disability syndromes due to a *HUWE1* mutation. In: *15th international workshop on fragile X and early-onset cognitive disorders*; September 5, 2011. Berlin (Germany).

119. Brooks SS, Wisniewski K, Brown WT. New X-linked mental retardation (XLMR) syndrome with distinct facial appearance and growth retardation. *Am J Med Genet* 1994;**51**:586−90.

120. Friez MJ, Brooks SS, Stevenson RE, Seabold C, McGee S, Saxon S, et al. Juberg-Marsidi syndrome and Brooks syndrome are allelic X-linked intellectual disability syndromes due to a single mutation (p.G4310R) in HUWE1. *Clin Genet* 2015 [submitted for publication].

121. Opitz JM, Richieri-da Costa A, Aase JM, Benke PJ. FG syndrome update 1988: note of 5 new patients and bibliography. *Am J Med Genet* 1988;**30**:309−28.

122. Romano C, Baraitser M, Thompson E. A clinical follow-up of British patients with FG syndrome. *Clin Dysmorphol* 1994;**3**:104−14.

123. Ozonoff S, Williams BJ, Rauch AM, Opitz JO. Behavior phenotype of FG syndrome: cognition, personality, and behavior in eleven affected boys. *Am J Med Genet* 2000;**97**:112−8.

124. Jehee FS, Rosenberg C, Krepischi-Santos AC, Kok F, Knijnenburg J, Froyen G, et al. An Xq22.3 duplication detected by comparative genomic hybridization microarray (Array-CGH) defines a new locus (*FGS5*) for FG syndrome. *Am J Med Genet A* 2005;**139**:221−6.

125. Tarpey PS, Raymond FL, Nguyen LS, Rodriguez J, Hackett A, Vandeleur L, et al. Mutations in *UPF3B*, a member of the nonsense-mediated mRNA decay complex, cause syndromic and nonsyndromic mental retardation. *Nat Genet* 2007;**39**:1127−33.

126. Unger S, Mainberger A, Spitz C, Bähr A, Zeschnigk C, Zabel B, et al. *Filamin A* mutation is one cause of FG syndrome. *Am J Med Genet A* 2007;**143A**:1876−9.

127. Briault S, Hill R, Shrimpton A, Zhu D, Till M, Ronce N, et al. A gene for FG syndrome maps in the Xq12-q21.31 region. *Am J Med Genet* 1997;**73**:87−90.

128. Briault S, Villard L, Rogner U, Coy J, Odent S, Lucas J, et al. Mapping of X chromosome inversion breakpoints [inv(X)(q11q28)] associated with FG syndrome: a second FG locus [*FGS2*]? *Am J Med Genet* 2000;**95**:178−81.

129. Piluso G, D'Amico F, Saccone V, Bismuto E, Rotundo IL, Di Domenico M, et al. A missense mutation in *CASK* causes FG syndrome in an Italian family. *Am J Hum Genet* 2009;**84**:162−77.

130. Dessay S, Moizard MP, Gilardi JL, Opitz JM, Middleton-Price H, Pembrey M, et al. FG syndrome: linkage analysis in two families supporting a new gene localization at Xp22.3 [FGS3]. *Am J Med Genet* 2002;**112**:6–11.

131. Risheg H, Graham Jr JM, Clark RD, Rogers RC, Opitz JM, Moeschler JB, et al. A recurrent mutation in *MED12* leading to R961W causes Opitz-Kaveggia syndrome. *Nat Genet* 2007;**39**: 451–3.

132. Lyons MJ, Graham Jr JM, Neri G, Hunter AG, Clark RD, Rogers RC, et al. Clinical experience in the evaluation of 30 patients with a prior diagnosis of FG syndrome. *J Med Genet* 2009;**46**:9–13.

133. Ropers HH. Genetics of intellectual disability. *Curr Opin Genet Dev* 2008;**18**:241–50.

134. Sudhof TC. The synaptic vesicle cycle. *Annu Rev Neurosci* 2004;**27**: 509–47.

135. Cesca F, Baldelli P, Valtorta F, Benfenati F. The synapsins: key actors of synapse function and plasticity. *Prog Neurobiol* 2010;**91**: 313–48.

136. Baldelli P, Fassio A, Valtorta F, Benfenati F. Lack of synapsin I reduces the readily releasable pool of synaptic vesicles at central inhibitory synapses. *J Neurosci* 2007;**27**:13520–31.

137. Chi P, Greengard P, Ryan TA. Synapsin dispersion and reclustering during synaptic activity. *Nat Neurosci* 2001;**4**:1187–93.

138. Chi P, Greengard P, Ryan TA. Synaptic vesicle mobilization is regulated by distinct synapsin I phosphorylation pathways at different frequencies. *Neuron* 2003;**38**:69–78.

139. Chiappalone M, Casagrande S, Tedesco M, Valtorta F, Baldelli P, Martinoia S, et al. Opposite changes in glutamatergic and GABAergic transmission underlie the diffuse hyperexcitability of synapsin I-deficient cortical networks. *Cereb Cortex* 2009;**19**: 1422–39.

140. Fassio A, Patry L, Congia S, Onofri F, Piton A, Gauthier J, et al. SYN1 loss-of-function mutations in autism and partial epilepsy cause impaired synaptic function. *Hum Mol Genet* 2011;**20**: 2297–307.

141. Giannandrea M, Guarnieri FC, Gehring NH, Monzani E, Benfenati F, Kulozik AE, et al. Nonsense-mediated mRNA decay and loss-of-function of the protein underlie the X-linked epilepsy associated with the W356x mutation in synapsin I. *PLoS One* 2013; **8**:e67724.

142. Fornasiero EF, Raimondi A, Guarnieri FC, Orlando M, Fesce R, Benfenati F, et al. Synapsins contribute to the dynamic spatial organization of synaptic vesicles in an activity-dependent manner. *J Neurosci* 2012;**32**:12214–27.

143. Orenbuch A, Shalev L, Marra V, Sinai I, Lavy Y, Kahn J, et al. Synapsin selectively controls the mobility of resting pool vesicles at hippocampal terminals. *J Neurosci* 2012;**32**:3969–80.

144. Greco B, Manago F, Tucci V, Kao HT, Valtorta F, Benfenati F. Autism-related behavioral abnormalities in synapsin knockout mice. *Behav Brain Res* 2013;**251**:65–74.

145. Takai Y, Sasaki T, Matozaki T. Small GTP-binding proteins. *Physiol Rev* 2001;**81**:153–208.

146. Bianchi V, Farisello P, Baldelli P, Meskenaite V, Milanese M, Vecellio M, et al. Cognitive impairment in GDI1-deficient mice is associated with altered synaptic vesicle pools and short-term synaptic plasticity, and can be corrected by appropriate learning training. *Hum Mol Genet* 2009;**18**:105–17.

147. Bianchi V, Gambino F, Muzio L, Toniolo D, Humeau Y, D'Adamo P. Forebrain deletion of αGDI in adult mice worsens the pre-synaptic deficit at cortico-lateral amygdala synaptic connections. *PLoS One* 2012;**7**:e29763.

148. Giannandrea M, Bianchi V, Mignogna ML, Sirri A, Carrabino S, D'Elia E, et al. Mutations in the small GTPase gene RAB39B are responsible for X-linked mental retardation associated with autism, epilepsy, and macrocephaly. *Am J Hum Genet* 2010;**86**:185–95.

149. Carrie A, Jun L, Bienvenu T, Vinet MC, McDonell N, Couvert P, et al. A new member of the IL-1 receptor family highly expressed in hippocampus and involved in X-linked mental retardation. *Nat Genet* 1999;**23**:25–31.

150. Bhat SS, Ladd S, Grass F, Spence JE, Brasington CK, Simensen RJ, et al. Disruption of the IL1RAPL1 gene associated with a pericentromeric inversion of the X chromosome in a patient with mental retardation and autism. *Clin Genet* 2008;**73**:94–6.

151. Piton A, Michaud JL, Peng H, Aradhya S, Gauthier J, Mottron L, et al. Mutations in the calcium-related gene IL1RAPL1 are associated with autism. *Hum Mol Genet* 2008;**17**:3965–74.

152. Piton A, Gauthier J, Hamdan FF, Lafreniere RG, Yang Y, Henrion E, et al. Systematic resequencing of X-chromosome synaptic genes in autism spectrum disorder and schizophrenia. *Mol Psychiatry* 2011;**16**:867–80.

153. Bahi N, Friocourt G, Carrie A, Graham ME, Weiss JL, Chafey P, et al. IL1 receptor accessory protein like, a protein involved in X-linked mental retardation, interacts with neuronal calcium sensor-1 and regulates exocytosis. *Hum Mol Genet* 2003;**12**:1415–25.

154. Gambino F, Pavlowsky A, Begle A, Dupont JL, Bahi N, Courjaret R, et al. IL1-receptor accessory protein-like 1 (IL1RAPL1), a protein involved in cognitive functions, regulates N-type Ca^{2+}-channel and neurite elongation. *Proc Natl Acad Sci USA* 2007;**104**:9063–8.

155. Pavlowsky A, Gianfelice A, Pallotto M, Zanchi A, Vara H, Khelfaoui M, et al. A postsynaptic signaling pathway that may account for the cognitive defect due to IL1RAPL1 mutation. *Curr Biol* 2010;**20**:103–15.

156. Pavlowsky A, Zanchi A, Pallotto M, Giustetto M, Chelly J, Sala C, et al. Neuronal JNK pathway activation by IL-1 is mediated through IL1RAPL1, a protein required for development of cognitive functions. *Commun Integr Biol* 2010;**3**:245–7.

157. Yoshida T, Yasumura M, Uemura T, Lee SJ, Ra M, Taguchi R, et al. IL-1 receptor accessory protein-like 1 associated with mental retardation and autism mediates synapse formation by trans-synaptic interaction with protein tyrosine phosphatase delta. *J Neurosci* 2011;**31**:13485–99.

158. Hayashi T, Yoshida T, Ra M, Taguchi R, Mishina M. IL1RAPL1 associated with mental retardation and autism regulates the formation and stabilization of glutamatergic synapses of cortical neurons through RhoA signaling pathway. *PLoS One* 2013;**8**: e66254.

159. Tarpey PS, Smith R, Pleasance E, Whibley A, Edkins S, Hardy C, et al. A systematic, large-scale resequencing screen of X-chromosome coding exons in mental retardation. *Nat Genet* 2009;**41**:535–43.

160. Nakano-Kobayashi A, Kasri NN, Newey SE, Van Aelst L. The Rho-linked mental retardation protein OPHN1 controls synaptic vesicle endocytosis via endophilin A1. *Curr Biol* 2009;**19**:1133–9.

161. Hackett A, Tarpey PS, Licata A, Cox J, Whibley A, Boyle J, et al. CASK mutations are frequent in males and cause X-linked nystagmus and variable XLMR phenotypes. *Eur J Hum Genet* 2010;**18**:544–52.

162. Hsueh YP. The role of the MAGUK protein CASK in neural development and synaptic function. *Curr Med Chem* 2006;**13**:1915–27.

163. Najm J, Horn D, Wimplinger I, Golden JA, Chizhikov VV, Sudi J, et al. Mutations of CASK cause an X-linked brain malformation phenotype with microcephaly and hypoplasia of the brainstem and cerebellum. *Nat Genet* 2008;**40**:1065–7.

164. Sun M, Liu L, Zeng X, Xu M, Liu L, Fang M, et al. Genetic interaction between Neurexin and CAKI/CMG is important for synaptic function in Drosophila neuromuscular junction. *Neurosci Res* 2009;**64**:362–71.

165. Dent EW, Merriam EB, Hu X. The dynamic cytoskeleton: backbone of dendritic spine plasticity. *Curr Opin Neurobiol* 2011; **21**:175–81.

166. Fifkova E, Delay RJ. Cytoplasmic actin in neuronal processes as a possible mediator of synaptic plasticity. *J Cell Biol* 1982;**95**:345−50.

167. Hoogenraad CC, Bradke F. Control of neuronal polarity and plasticity—a renaissance for microtubules? *Trends Cell Biol* 2009; **19**:669−76.

168. Matus A, Ackermann M, Pehling G, Byers HR, Fujiwara K. High actin concentrations in brain dendritic spines and postsynaptic densities. *Proc Natl Acad Sci USA* 1982;**79**:7590−4.

169. Matus A. Actin-based plasticity in dendritic spines. *Science* 2000; **290**:754−8.

170. Rex CS, Gavin CF, Rubio MD, Kramar EA, Chen LY, Jia Y, et al. Myosin IIb regulates actin dynamics during synaptic plasticity and memory formation. *Neuron* 2010;**67**:603−17.

171. Hotulainen P, Hoogenraad CC. Actin in dendritic spines: connecting dynamics to function. *J Cell Biol* 2010;**189**:619−29.

172. Ba W, van der Raadt J, Nadif Kasri N. Rho GTPase signaling at the synapse: Implications for intellectual disability. *Exp Cell Res* 2013; **319**:2368−74.

173. Govek EE, Newey SE, Akerman CJ, Cross JR, Van der Veken L, Van Aelst L. The X-linked mental retardation protein oligophrenin-1 is required for dendritic spine morphogenesis. *Nat Neurosci* 2004;**7**:364−72.

174. Nadif Kasri N, Nakano-Kobayashi A, Malinow R, Li B, Van Aelst L. The Rho-linked mental retardation protein oligophrenin-1 controls synapse maturation and plasticity by stabilizing AMPA receptors. *Genes Dev* 2009;**23**:1289−302.

175. Allen KM, Gleeson JG, Bagrodia S, Partington MW, MacMillan JC, Cerione RA, et al. PAK3 mutation in nonsyndromic X-linked mental retardation. *Nat Genet* 1998;**20**:25−30.

176. Kreis P, Thevenot E, Rousseau V, Boda B, Muller D, Barnier JV. The p21-activated kinase 3 implicated in mental retardation regulates spine morphogenesis through a Cdc42-dependent pathway. *J Biol Chem* 2007;**282**:21497−506.

177. Rousseau V, Goupille O, Morin N, Barnier JV. A new constitutively active brain PAK3 isoform displays modified specificities toward Rac and Cdc42 GTPases. *J Biol Chem* 2003;**278**:3912−20.

178. Gedeon AK, Nelson J, Gecz J, Mulley JC. X-linked mild non-syndromic mental retardation with neuropsychiatric problems and the missense mutation A365E in PAK3. *Am J Med Genet* 2003;**120A**:509−17.

179. Peippo M, Koivisto AM, Sarkamo T, Sipponen M, von Koskull H, Ylisaukko-oja T, et al. PAK3 related mental disability: further characterization of the phenotype. *Am J Med Genet* 2007;**143A**:2406−16.

180. Arber S, Barbayannis FA, Hanser H, Schneider C, Stanyon CA, Bernard O, et al. Regulation of actin dynamics through phosphorylation of cofilin by LIM-kinase. *Nature* 1998;**393**:805−9.

181. Edwards DC, Sanders LC, Bokoch GM, Gill GN. Activation of LIM-kinase by Pak1 couples Rac/Cdc42 GTPase signalling to actin cytoskeletal dynamics. *Nat Cell Biol* 1999;**1**:253−9.

182. Boda B, Alberi S, Nikonenko I, Node-Langlois R, Jourdain P, Moosmayer M, et al. The mental retardation protein PAK3 contributes to synapse formation and plasticity in hippocampus. *J Neurosci* 2004;**24**:10816−25.

183. Dubos A, Combeau G, Bernardinelli Y, Barnier JV, Hartley O, Gaertner H, et al. Alteration of synaptic network dynamics by the intellectual disability protein PAK3. *J Neurosci* 2012;**32**:519−27.

184. Meng J, Meng Y, Hanna A, Janus C, Jia Z. Abnormal long-lasting synaptic plasticity and cognition in mice lacking the mental retardation gene PAK3. *J Neurosci* 2005;**25**:6641−50.

185. Kneussel M, Brandstatter JH, Gasnier B, Feng G, Sanes JR, Betz H. Gephyrin-independent clustering of postsynaptic GABA(A) receptor subtypes. *Mol Cell Neurosci* 2001;**17**:973−82.

186. Kneussel M, Engelkamp D, Betz H. Distribution of transcripts for the brain-specific GDP/GTP exchange factor collybistin in the developing mouse brain. *Eur J Neurosci* 2001;**13**:487−92.

187. Papadopoulos T, Korte M, Eulenburg V, Kubota H, Retiounskaia M, Harvey RJ, et al. Impaired GABAergic transmission and altered hippocampal synaptic plasticity in collybistin-deficient mice. *EMBO J* 2007;**26**:3888−99.

188. Tyagarajan SK, Ghosh H, Harvey K, Fritschy JM. Collybistin splice variants differentially interact with gephyrin and Cdc42 to regulate gephyrin clustering at GABAergic synapses. *J Cell Sci* 2011;**124**:2786−96.

189. Korber C, Richter A, Kaiser M, Schlicksupp A, Mukusch S, Kuner T, et al. Effects of distinct collybistin isoforms on the formation of GABAergic synapses in hippocampal neurons. *Mol Cell Neurosci* 2012;**50**:250−9.

190. Node-Langlois R, Muller D, Boda B. Sequential implication of the mental retardation proteins ARHGEF6 and PAK3 in spine morphogenesis. *J Cell Sci* 2006;**119**:4986−93.

191. Ramakers GJ, Wolfer D, Rosenberger G, Kuchenbecker K, Kreienkamp HJ, Prange-Kiel J, et al. Dysregulation of Rho GTPases in the alphaPix/Arhgef6 mouse model of X-linked intellectual disability is paralleled by impaired structural and synaptic plasticity and cognitive deficits. *Hum Mol Genet* 2012;**21**:268−86.

192. Shoubridge C, Tarpey PS, Abidi F, Ramsden SL, Rujirabanjerd S, Murphy JA, et al. Mutations in the guanine nucleotide exchange factor gene IQSEC2 cause nonsyndromic intellectual disability. *Nat Genet* 2010;**42**:486−8.

193. Shoubridge C, Walikonis RS, Gecz J, Harvey RJ. Subtle functional defects in the Arf-specific guanine nucleotide exchange factor IQSEC2 cause non-syndromic X-linked intellectual disability. *Small GTPases* 2010;**1**:98−103.

194. D'Souza-Schorey C, Chavrier P. ARF proteins: roles in membrane traffic and beyond. *Nature Reviews: Mol Cell Biol* 2006;**7**:347−58.

195. Grant BD, Donaldson JG. Pathways and mechanisms of endocytic recycling. *Nature Reviews: Mol Cell Biol* 2009;**10**:597−608.

196. Betancur C, Sakurai T, Buxbaum JD. The emerging role of synaptic cell-adhesion pathways in the pathogenesis of autism spectrum disorders. *Trends Neurosci* 2009;**32**:402−12.

197. Missler M, Sudhof TC, Biederer T. Synaptic cell adhesion. *Cold Spring Harb Perspect Biol* 2012;**4**:a005694.

198. Scheiffele P. Cell-cell signaling during synapse formation in the CNS. *Annu Rev Neurosci* 2003;**26**:485−508.

199. Bakkaloglu B, O'Roak BJ, Louvi A, Gupta AR, Abelson JF, Morgan TM, et al. Molecular cytogenetic analysis and resequencing of contactin associated protein-like 2 in autism spectrum disorders. *Am J Hum Genet* 2008;**82**:165−73.

200. Berkel S, Marshall CR, Weiss B, Howe J, Roeth R, Moog U, et al. Mutations in the SHANK2 synaptic scaffolding gene in autism spectrum disorder and mental retardation. *Nat Genet* 2010;**42**:489−91.

201. Bhalla K, Luo Y, Buchan T, Beachem MA, Guzauskas GF, Ladd S, et al. Alterations in CDH15 and KIRREL3 in patients with mild to severe intellectual disability. *Am J Hum Genet* 2008;**83**: 703−13.

202. Glessner JT, Wang K, Cai G, Korvatska O, Kim CE, Wood S, et al. Autism genome-wide copy number variation reveals ubiquitin and neuronal genes. *Nature* 2009;**459**:569−73.

203. Jiang YH, Yuen RK, Jin X, Wang M, Chen N, Wu X, et al. Detection of clinically relevant genetic variants in autism spectrum disorder by whole-genome sequencing. *Am J Hum Genet* 2013; **93**:249−63.

204. Morrow EM, Yoo SY, Flavell SW, Kim TK, Lin Y, Hill RS, et al. Identifying autism loci and genes by tracing recent shared ancestry. *Science* 2008;**321**:218−23.

205. Noor A, Whibley A, Marshall CR, Gianakopoulos PJ, Piton A, Carson AR, et al. Disruption at the PTCHD1 locus on Xp22.11 in autism spectrum disorder and intellectual disability. *Sci Transl Med* 2010;**2**:49−68.

206. O'Roak BJ, Vives L, Girirajan S, Karakoc E, Krumm N, Coe BP, et al. Sporadic autism exomes reveal a highly interconnected protein network of de novo mutations. *Nature* 2012;**485**:246−50.

207. Pagnamenta AT, Khan H, Walker S, Gerrelli D, Wing K, Bonaglia MC, et al. Rare familial 16q21 microdeletions under a linkage peak implicate cadherin 8 (CDH8) in susceptibility to autism and learning disability. *J Med Genet* 2011;**48**:48−54.

208. Pinto D, Pagnamenta AT, Klei L, Anney R, Merico D, Regan R, et al. Functional impact of global rare copy number variation in autism spectrum disorders. *Nature* 2010;**466**:368−72.

209. Sanders SJ, Ercan-Sencicek AG, Hus V, Luo R, Murtha MT, Moreno-De-Luca D, et al. Multiple recurrent de novo CNVs, including duplications of the 7q11.23 Williams syndrome region, are strongly associated with autism. *Neuron* 2011;**70**:863−85.

210. Vincent AK, Noor A, Janson A, Minassian BA, Ayub M, Vincent JB, et al. Identification of genomic deletions spanning the PCDH19 gene in two unrelated girls with intellectual disability and seizures. *Clin Genet* 2012;**82**:540−5.

211. Wang K, Zhang H, Ma D, Bucan M, Glessner JT, Abrahams BS, et al. Common genetic variants on 5p14.1 associate with autism spectrum disorders. *Nature* 2009;**459**:528−33.

212. Srivastava AK, Schwartz CE. Intellectual disability and autism spectrum disorders: causal genes and molecular mechanisms. *Neurosci Biobehav Rev* 2014;**46**(Pt 2):161−74.

213. Reissner C, Klose M, Fairless R, Missler M. Mutational analysis of the neurexin/neuroligin complex reveals essential and regulatory components. *Proc Natl Acad Sci USA* 2008;**105**:15124−9.

214. Chih B, Engelman H, Scheiffele P. Control of excitatory and inhibitory synapse formation by neuroligins. *Science* 2005;**307**:1324−8.

215. Graf ER, Zhang X, Jin SX, Linhoff MW, Craig AM. Neurexins induce differentiation of GABA and glutamate postsynaptic specializations via neuroligins. *Cell* 2004;**119**:1013−26.

216. Nam CI, Chen L. Postsynaptic assembly induced by neurexin-neuroligin interaction and neurotransmitter. *Proc Natl Acad Sci USA* 2005;**102**:6137−42.

217. Zhang C, Atasoy D, Arac D, Yang X, Fucillo MV, Robison AJ, et al. Neurexins physically and functionally interact with GABA(A) receptors. *Neuron* 2010;**66**:403−16.

218. Dudanova I, Tabuchi K, Rohlmann A, Sudhof TC, Missler M. Deletion of alpha-neurexins does not cause a major impairment of axonal pathfinding or synapse formation. *J Comp Neurol* 2007;**502**:261−74.

219. Missler M, Zhang W, Rohlmann A, Kattenstroth G, Hammer RE, Gottmann K, et al. Alpha-neurexins couple Ca^{2+} channels to synaptic vesicle exocytosis. *Nature* 2003;**423**:939−48.

220. Varoqueaux F, Aramuni G, Rawson RL, Mohrmann R, Missler M, Gottmann K, et al. Neuroligins determine synapse maturation and function. *Neuron* 2006;**51**:741−54.

221. Chubykin AA, Atasoy D, Etherton MR, Brose N, Kavalali ET, Gibson JR, et al. Activity-dependent validation of excitatory versus inhibitory synapses by neuroligin-1 versus neuroligin-2. *Neuron* 2007;**54**:919−31.

222. Laumonnier F, Bonnet-Brilhault F, Gomot M, Blanc R, David A, Moizard MP, et al. X-linked mental retardation and autism are associated with a mutation in the NLGN4 gene, a member of the neuroligin family. *Am J Hum Genet* 2004;**74**:552−7.

223. Cajigas IJ, Will T, Schuman EM. Protein homeostasis and synaptic plasticity. *EMBO J* 2010;**29**:2746−52.

224. Mabb AM, Ehlers MD. Ubiquitination in postsynaptic function and plasticity. *Annu Rev Cell Dev Biol* 2010;**26**:179−210.

225. Segref A, Hoppe T. Think locally: control of ubiquitin-dependent protein degradation in neurons. *EMBO Re* 2009;**10**:44−50.

226. Tai HC, Schuman EM. Ubiquitin, the proteasome and protein degradation in neuronal function and dysfunction. *Nat Rev Neurosci* 2008;**9**:826−38.

227. Nguyen LS, Wilkinson M, Gecz J. Nonsense-mediated mRNA decay: inter-individual variability and human disease. *Neurosci Biobehav Rev* 2013;**46**(Pt 2):175−86. S0149-7634(13)00270-4.

228. Bingol B, Schuman EM. Activity-dependent dynamics and sequestration of proteasomes in dendritic spines. *Nature* 2006;**441**:1144−8.

229. Ehlers MD. Activity level controls postsynaptic composition and signaling via the ubiquitin-proteasome system. *Nat Neurosci* 2003;**6**:231−42.

230. Haddad DM, Vilain S, Vos M, Esposito G, Matta S, Kalscheuer VM, et al. Mutations in the intellectual disability gene Ube2a cause neuronal dysfunction and impair parkin-dependent mitophagy. *Mol Cell* 2013;**50**:831−43.

231. Quaderi NA, Schweiger S, Gaudenz K, Franco B, Rugarli EI, Berger W, et al. Opitz G/BBB syndrome, a defect of midline development, is due to mutations in a new RING finger gene on Xp22. *Nat Genet* 1997;**17**:285−91.

232. Du H, Huang Y, Zaghlula M, Walters E, Cox TC, Massiah MA. The MID1 E3 ligase catalyzes the polyubiquitination of Alpha4 (alpha4), a regulatory subunit of protein phosphatase 2A (PP2A): novel insights into MID1-mediated regulation of PP2A. *J Biol Chem* 2013;**288**:21341−50.

233. Badura-Stronka M, Jamsheer A, Materna-Kiryluk A, Sowinska A, Kiryluk K, Budny B, et al. A novel nonsense mutation in CUL4B gene in three brothers with X-linked mental retardation syndrome. *Clin Genet* 2010;**77**:141−4.

234. Tarpey PS, Raymond FL, O'Meara S, Edkins S, Teague J, Butler A, et al. Mutations in CUL4B, which encodes a ubiquitin E3 ligase subunit, cause an X-linked mental retardation syndrome associated with aggressive outbursts, seizures, relative macrocephaly, central obesity, hypogonadism, pes cavus, and tremor. *Am J Hum Genet* 2007;**80**:345−52.

235. Zou Y, Liu Q, Chen B, Zhang X, Guo C, Zhou H, et al. Mutation in CUL4B, which encodes a member of cullin-RING ubiquitin ligase complex, causes X-linked mental retardation. *Am J Hum Genet* 2007;**80**:561−6.

236. Chen CY, Tsai MS, Lin CY, Yu IS, Chen YT, Lin SR, et al. Rescue of the genetically engineered Cul4b mutant mouse as a potential model for human X-linked mental retardation. *Hum Mol Genet* 2012;**21**:4270−85.

237. Jiang B, Zhao W, Yuan J, Qian Y, Sun W, Zou Y, et al. Lack of Cul4b, an E3 ubiquitin ligase component, leads to embryonic lethality and abnormal placental development. *PLoS One* 2012;**7**:e37070.

238. Kerzendorfer C, Whibley A, Carpenter G, Outwin E, Chiang SC, Turner G, et al. Mutations in cullin 4B result in a human syndrome associated with increased camptothecin-induced topoisomerase I-dependent DNA breaks. *Hum Mol Genet* 2010;**19**:1324−34.

239. Zhou P, Pang ZP, Yang X, Zhang Y, Rosenmund C, Bacaj T, et al. Syntaxin-1 N-peptide and Habc-domain perform distinct essential functions in synaptic vesicle fusion. *EMBO J* 2013;**32**:159−71.

240. Nakagawa T, Xiong Y. X-linked mental retardation gene CUL4B targets ubiquitylation of H3K4 methyltransferase component WDR5 and regulates neuronal gene expression. *Mol Cell* 2011;**43**:381−91.

241. Wang HL, Chang NC, Weng YH, Yeh TH. XLID CUL4B mutants are defective in promoting TSC2 degradation and positively regulating mTOR signaling in neocortical neurons. *Biochim Biophys Acta* 2013;**1832**:585−93.

242. Jaworski J, Spangler S, Seeburg DP, Hoogenraad CC, Sheng M. Control of dendritic arborization by the phosphoinositide-3'-kinase-Akt-mammalian target of rapamycin pathway. *J Neurosci* 2005;**25**:11300−12.

243. Kumar V, Zhang MX, Swank MW, Kunz J, Wu GY. Regulation of dendritic morphogenesis by Ras-PI3K-Akt-mTOR and Ras-MAPK signaling pathways. *J Neurosci* 2005;**25**:11288−99.

244. Ehninger D, Han S, Shilyansky C, Zhou Y, Li W, Kwiatkowski DJ, et al. Reversal of learning deficits in a Tsc2$^{+/-}$ mouse model of tuberous sclerosis. *Nat Med* 2008;**14**:843−8.

245. Sharma A, Hoeffer CA, Takayasu Y, Miyawaki T, McBride SM, Klann E, et al. Dysregulation of mTOR signaling in fragile X syndrome. *J Neurosci* 2010;**30**:694−702.

246. Delorme R, Ey E, Toro R, Leboyer M, Gillberg C, Bourgeron T. Progress toward treatments for synaptic defects in autism. *Nat Med* 2013;**19**:685−94.

247. Dunbar M, Jaggumantri S, Sargent M, Stockler-Ipsiroglu S, van Karnebeek CD. Treatment of X-linked creatine transporter (SLC6A8) deficiency: systematic review of the literature and three new cases. *Mol Genet Metab* 2014;**112**:259−74.

248. Kersseboom S, Horn S, Visser WE, Chen J, Friesema EC, Vaurs-Barrière C, et al. In vitro and mouse studies support therapeutic utility of triiodothyroacetic acid in MCT8 deficiency. *Mol Endocrinol* 2014;**28**(12).

249. Chang S, Bray SM, Li Z, Zarnescu DC, He C, Jin P, et al. Identification of small molecules rescuing fragile X syndrome phenotypes in *Drosophila*. *Nat Chem Biol* 2008;**4**:256−63.

250. Dölen G, Carpenter RL, Ocain TD, Bear MF. Mechanism-based approaches to treating fragile X. *Pharmacol Ther* 2010;**127**:78−93.

251. Guy J, Gan J, Selfridge J, Cobb S, Bird A. Reversal of neurological defects in a mouse model of Rett syndrome. *Science* 2007;**315**:1143−7.

252. Auerbach BD, Osterweil EK, Bear MF. Mutations causing syndromic autism define an axis of synaptic pathophysiology. *Nature* 2011;**480**:63−8.

4

Genetic Causes of Intellectual Disability: The Genes Controlling Cortical Development

Yoann Saillour[1,2], *Jamel Chelly*[3,4]

[1]Institut Cochin, Université Paris Descartes, CNRS (UMR 8104), Paris, France; [2]INSERM U1016, Paris, France; [3]IGBMC, Department of Translational Medicine and Neurogenetics, Inserm U964, CNRS UMR 7104, Université de Strasbourg, Illkirch Cedex, France; [4]Pôle de biologie, Hôpitaux Universitaires de Strasbourg, Strasbourg, France

INTRODUCTION

In vertebrates, the cerebral cortex is the outer layer of the gray matter that covers the cerebral hemispheres. It is responsible for higher functions of the nervous system and specific parts of the cortex control specific functions, including sensation, voluntary muscle movement, language, thought, reasoning, and memory. The large size and surface of the cerebral cortex in humans distinguish them from other animals. Whereas less evolved brains are lissencephalic, more evolved cortex brains are usually gyrencephalic (with gyrations) because they are shaped and modeled by grooves and folds called circumvolutions that drastically expand cortical surface.[1–3] At the cellular level, the cortex is characterized by a recognizable cytoarchitecture with six layers of neurons (I–VI). Cerebral corticogenesis is a highly dynamic process that includes progenitor proliferation, cell cycle exit, and neuronal migration and differentiation. Once differentiated and properly located in the nervous system, synapses and establishment of neuronal synaptic communication sustain the whole nervous system activity. A highly sophisticated molecular network has evolved to allow tight control of these processes of proliferation, polarization, migration, and differentiation, which are crucial for the proper development and organization of the cortex and its highly elaborated cytoarchitecture.

At first sight, the heterogeneity of developmental disorders affecting the cortex recapitulates its development, because impairments in the different steps are associated with specific features. For instance, early genetic assaults on proliferation and neuronal production might lead to microcephaly. Remarkably, most microcephaly-related genes encode proteins associated with centrosomes or centrosomal-related functions such as mitotic microtubule spindle structure, cilia function, and cell cycle checkpoint proficiency. After neurogenesis, the disruption of neuronal migration resulting from genetic mutations represents a major cause of cortical dysgeneses, traditionally called neuronal migration disorders, and encompasses a large variety of cortical malformations. Interestingly, many of these genes encode important effectors that modulate cytoskeletal dynamics during mitosis of progenitor proliferation, and/or the migration of neuronal cells. Structural cortical abnormalities characterizing neuronal migration disorders often are associated with dramatic cognitive impairment and epilepsy, and in many cases motor and neurological deficits. Finally, subtle deregulation of later developmental processes concerning neuronal differentiation, synaptogenesis, and neuronal connectivity and synaptic plasticity has emerged over the past few years as a major pathophysiological mechanism underlying neurodevelopmental disorders with no apparent brain malformations such as intellectual disability (ID), autism spectrum disorders, epilepsy, and psychiatric and behavioral conditions. As detailed in the other chapters, these groups of neurodevelopmental disorders have been shown to result from defects in genes encoding proteins enriched in synaptic compartments or transcription factor and chromatin remodeling factors regulating the expression of proteins enriched at the synaptic level.[4]

In the current chapter, we will briefly describe some of the major concepts and processes involved in cortex development, and discuss how the recent development in human genetics of malformation of cortical development disorders, consistently associated with ID, contributed to improve our understanding of the critical molecular actors regulating neuronal migration in the cerebral cortex. We will also discuss the emerging genetic overlaps between groups of ID with malformations of cortical development (MCD) and ID with no apparent MCD. Finally, we will highlight examples from the literature illustrating potential reversibility of cellular defects and phenotypes in experimental models mimicking neuronal migration disorders.

DEVELOPMENT OF THE MAMMALIAN BRAIN CORTEX

Basically, two main streams of work have contributed to a better understanding of developmental processes underlying cerebral cortex formation and organization. First, a fine and thorough description of the developing cortex in primates pioneered by Rakic and Caviness led to the emergence of strong principles and concepts such as: (1) the existence of both radial and tangential migrations of pyramidal neurons and interneurons, respectively; (2) correlation between the date of birth of postmitotic cells and their positions in the cortical plate; and (3) the concept of inside-out migration and organization[5–7] (Figure 1(A–C)). Further studies from different groups uncovered (1) symmetric and asymmetric cell division and the lineage of radial glial cells and their role as neuronal progenitors, (2) the concept of intermediate progenitor cells, and (3) the importance of postmitotic neuronal polarization and its role in the regulation of migration and early steps of differentiation[8–12] (Figure 1(B)). The second stream of work is based on data generated from human genetic investigations of neurodevelopmental disorders and analyses of mouse models. Indeed, over the past 2 decades, genetic approaches combined with the new generation technologies (NGS) for large-scale whole genome mapping and whole exome sequencing (WES) have led to considerable progress in identifying most genetic factors underlying malformations of the cerebral cortex, as well as significant improvement in knowledge of molecular and biological bases of cortical development.[13,14]

As illustrated in Figure 1 and reviewed by Jaglin and Chelly,[15] early cortical developmental phases include proliferation and neurogenesis required for the production of pyramidal neurons and interneurons populations. The onset of active neurogenesis, at approximately embryonic day (E)33 in the human dorsal telencephalon and E10 in mice, follows a period of proliferative symmetrical divisions and is marked by the first asymmetrical divisions of radial glial cells in the periventricular neuroepithelium.[12,16] This type of mitosis produces one daughter cell that remains a progenitor and one postmitotic cell that will give rise to a pyramidal neuron either directly or indirectly through an intermediate progenitor cell (IP)[11,12,17–20] (Figure 1(B)). The pool of IPs further contributes to the formation of the subventricular zone (SVZ) and the final population of neurons. Concomitantly, inhibitory interneurons are generated in the ganglionic eminences and migrate tangentially in direction of the cortex (Figure 1(A)).

As far as pyramidal neurons are concerned, overlapping with the period of neurogenesis, successive waves

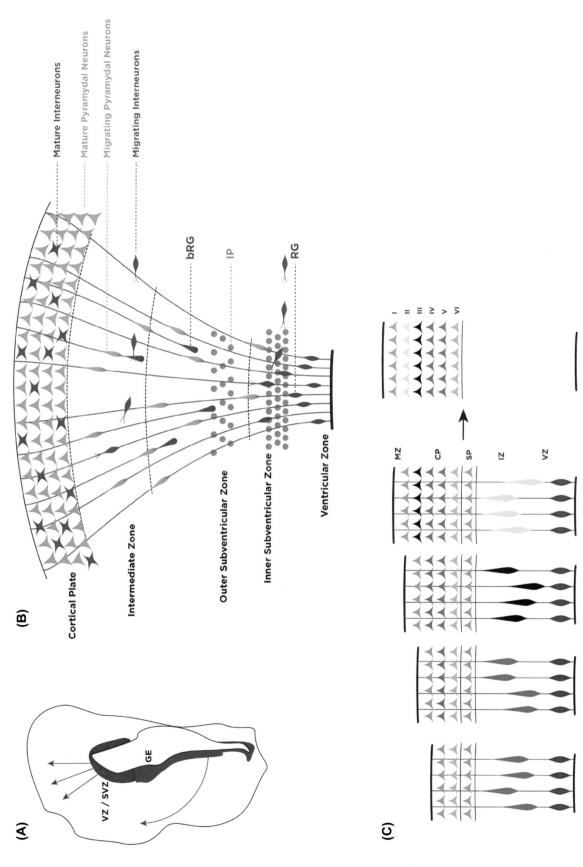

FIGURE 1 **Human cortical development.** (A) Schematic illustration of human forebrains at the peak of corticogenesis. The main source of interneurons is the ganglionic eminence (GE) of the ventral telencephalon, which migrates tangentially to the neocortex in the dorsal telencephalon. Pyramidal neurons are produced in the ventricular and the sub-ventricular zones (VZ/SVZ) and migrate radially to the cortical plate. (B) Radial glial (RG) cells most often generate IP cells that divide mainly in the inner subventricular zone to produce pairs of pyramidal neurons. These neurons use RG fibers to migrate toward the cortical plate, where they differentiate in mature excitatory neurons. Observations have also demonstrated the presence of outer subventricular zone radial glia-like (oRG) cells increasing the number of fibers used by the neurons to migrate. Interneurons generated in the ganglionic eminences migrate tangentially toward the cortex and finish their journey in the cortical plate. (C) Cortical layering. During embryonic stages, pyramidal neurons generated by radial glial cells in the ventricular zone (VZ) undertake a radial migration to the cortical plate in an inside-out manner. As a consequence, each wave of neurons migrates through the intermediate zone (IZ) and the subplate (SP) and finally passes its predecessors to settle underneath the marginal zone (MZ). As a result, and after developmental transition of the subplate and its disappearance, mature cortex is organized as a six layered structure.

of postmitotic neurons further migrate radially along radial glia fibers toward the surface of the cortex through the entire cortical plate and settle in superficial regions as soon as gestational weeks (GW)7−8 in human and nonhuman primates and E14 in mice. Migration process follows an inside-out order in which the younger neurons bypass deep-layers populated by early-born neurons and settle in the superficial layer underneath the marginal zone (Figure 1(C)).

Studies based on cellular live imaging techniques revealed that postmitotic neurons do not migrate directly to the cortical plate but instead undergo distinct phases of migration interspersed by phases of morphological changes and polarization.[11,21] Neurally committed cells are bipolar and delaminate from the ventricular surface to move radially to the SVZ. The second phase consists of a migratory arrest for several hours that comes together with morphological changes leading to multipolar morphology. The third phase, which concerns a significant fraction but not all neurons, consists of a retrograde move toward the ventricular zone with a switch back to bipolar morphology. Finally, neurons enter the fourth phase of migration during which they migrate toward the cortical plate along radial glia fibers. Once they reach their predestined final position in the cortical plate, neuronal cells detach from the radial glia fiber and switch to terminal translocation mode.[22]

During radial neuronal migration process, morphological changes and polarization (i.e., the transition from multipolar to bipolar stage) are a prerequisite for the initiation of radial migration and rely on the proper function of the signaling pathways (for review, see Ref. 23 as well as the proper downstream modulation of cytoskeleton dynamics). Indeed, it has been shown by different groups that the experimental disruption of various genes related to these processes often leads to disruption of the transition from a multipolar to a bipolar morphology.[24−26]

Modulation of cytoskeleton stability is involved not only in the early process of polarization but also in the plasticity and sustainability of the migrating neuron's morphology. For instance, the growth of the leading process requires a highly dynamic actin cytoskeleton and an elongating stable microtubule network, both of which are under the control of molecular complexes involved in the polarization homeostasis.[23,27]

Finally, a further aspect of corticogenesis is the development of cortical connectivity of projection neurons that requires proper axonal growth and guidance toward cortical or subcortical targets, located in structures including the thalamus, brain stem, or spinal cord.[28] In human and many other primates, these highly regulated developmental steps and processes lead to the formation of a brain surface characterized by a succession of infolding (gyri) separated by fissures or sulci and a cortex composed of six layers of neurons that integrate highly connected pyramidal and interneurons (Figure 1(C)).

GENETIC BASES OF CORTICAL MALFORMATIONS AND THEIR CONTRIBUTION TO BETTER UNDERSTANDING NORMAL CORTICAL DEVELOPMENT

Malformations of cortical development are characterized by abnormal organization and layering of the cerebral cortex resulting from mispositioning of neuronal cells. They are recognized as a major cause of disorders with neurodevelopmental delay, including severe conditions of the ID spectrum, drug-resistant epilepsy, and motor impairments. These pathologies can be classified according to various criteria, in particular clinical, radiological, or genetic features. However, so far, the widely used classification of MCD is the one that takes into account disrupted neurodevelopmental processes, developed and regularly updated by Barkovich and colleagues.[29,30] Using the criteria of which biological process is likely to be affected, the most recent classification proposes three major groups of MCDs: MCDs resulting from (1) abnormal neuronal progenitor proliferation or neuronal death, (2) defects of migration of postmitotic neuronal, or (3) postmigration developmental anomalies, including those affecting neuronal organization in the cortical layers.[31] For instance, in disorders related to proliferation defects (or of the balance between proliferation and apoptosis), the number of cells is significantly reduced, resulting in an abnormally small head (microcephaly). In disorders of migration, neurons do not reach their correct destination in the cortical plate, by remaining at the ventricular surface (periventricular nodular heterotopia [PNH]), arresting in the white matter (subcortical band heterotopia [SBH]), or forming a disordered, often thickened cortical plate. This thicker cortex affects the formation of normal gyration, leading to a reduced gyral pattern or a smooth appearance of the cortical surface (lissencephaly or classic or type I lissencephaly). Other types of lissencephaly (cobblestone lissencephaly or type II lissencephaly) are associated with overmigration of neurons to the pial surface.[13,32] The current classification, disorders of cortical organization or late migration, is composed mostly of polymicrogyria, a heterogeneous group of malformations with multiple small gyri and an abnormally thin or thick cortex, sometimes so severely affecting brain structure as to cause clefting between the ventricular and meningeal surface (schizencephaly).[31] Although this classification remains highly relevant for clinical and diagnostic purposes, genetic and functional data support the hypothesis that several types of MCD result from deregulation of multiple developmental processes, and that proliferation and migration are genetically and functionally interdependent.[15,33,34]

Although little is known about differentiation and behavioral and functional status of misplaced neuronal cells, as well as their consequences on the functioning of disorganized cortex that characterize MCDs, we can hypothesize that mispositioning of cortical neurons and layering disorganization of the cortex are associated with massive changes in synaptic activity, connectivity, and communication, therefore preventing proper neuronal functioning, including adapted integration of stimulus and information. These neuroanatomical and cytoarchitectural abnormalities and their functional consequences are likely neurobiological and cellular substrates for neurodevelopmental delay and neurological symptoms such as epilepsy consistently associated with MCD.

Here, for the sake of clarity, we propose an overview on genetic and neurodevelopmental characteristics underlying major groups of MCDs (see also Table 1).

Malformations Resulting From Abnormal Neurogenesis

Malformations within this group can further be subdivided into two subgroups: reduced proliferation or excess of apoptosis (microcephaly), and increased proliferation (or decreased apoptosis) (megalencephly and hemimegalencephaly). Because macrocephaly often represents a clinical feature of a large array of disorders, we will highlight the group of developmental disorders called microcephaly vera (Figure 2(C and D)). Microcephaly vera (true macrocephaly), also called autosomal recessive primary microcephaly (microcephaly primary hereditary [MCPH]), is a rare genetic disorder characterized by a reduction of head circumference at birth of at least 2 standard deviations below normal age- and sex-matched controls, associated with ID. These patients typically display no obvious cortical brain disorganization, although it has been shown that specific gene-related disorders such as WDR62-related disorders encompass a spectrum of phenotypes that include patients with microcephaly alone and those presenting microcephaly and severe cortical malformations.[35,36]

There were originally seven genetic loci mapped for MCPH that were associated with mutated genes: MCPH1, ASPM, CDK5RAP2, CENPJ, STIL, WDR62, and CEP152.[35-41] Recent genetic studies mainly of consanguineous Pakistani families revealed the implication of

additional genes such as CEP63,[42] CEP135,[43] CDK6,[44] PHC1,[45] ZNF335,[46] CASC5,[47] and HsSAS-6[48] (Table 1). Remarkably, most of these microcephaly genes encode the protein of centrosome or centrosomal-related processes that have critical roles in cell division and especially in mitotic spindle formation, and also in neuronal migration.

All MCPH loci except one were reported in Pakistani families and the number of Pakistani families tested for MCPH represents almost half of families analyzed worldwide. These statements can be correlated with a high rate of consanguinity (about 61%) and the large family size observed in this country.[49]

Microcephaly primary hereditary is thought to arise from alterations in the size of the neuronal progenitor pool. Indeed, MCPH gene (Mcph1, Aspm, Cdk5rap2, and Cenpj) disruption in mice results mainly in primary microcephaly, mimicking human MCPH symptoms, owing to abnormal proliferation of neuroprogenitors caused by imbalance of the symmetric–asymmetric division rate, premature exit of the cell cycle, and/or increased cell death. Compromised homologous recombination deoxyribonucleic acid (DNA) repair and increased genomic instability have been also observed in these models[50-55] (Table 1).

Although our understanding of the bases underlying ID remains poor, in particular in view of the striking intra- and interfamilial heterogeneity regarding the severity of ID, it is reasonable to think that impaired progenitor proliferation lead to a deficit of neurons in the brain and therefore to limited capability of connectivity and the outbreak of ID in patients. Therefore, these diseases can shed light on the pathophysiology of the heterogeneous group of ID with no major apparent cortical abnormalities.

It is also proposed that MCPH-related genes were targets of positive selection in primates and human ancestors, which suggesting potential roles in controlling neuron number and brain size in evolution[56,57]

Malformations Resulting From Neuronal Migration Defects

For cortical malformations associated with neuronal migration abnormalities, the common hallmark is that pools of neurons do not reach their correct destination in the cortical plate by remaining at the ventricular surface (PNH) (Figure 2(E)), arresting in the white matter (SBH) (Figure 2(F)), or forming a disordered, often thickened, cortical plate. This thicker cortex affects the formation of normal gyration, leading to a reduced gyral pattern or a smooth appearance of the cortical surface (classic lissencephaly or type I lissencephaly). Other types of lissencephaly

TABLE 1   Summary of Genetic Bases of Malformations of Cortical Development and Related Rodent Phenotypes in Constitutive or RNA Interference (RNAi) Knockdown Models

Malformation of Cortical Development	Gene	Protein Function	Anomalies of Central Nervous System (CNS) in Constitutive Models (KO/ENU/Spontaneous)	Anomalies of CNS in RNAi in Utero Models	References
Microcephaly					
Hereditary primary microcephaly	MCPH1	Chromosome condensation	Microcephaly Apoptosis Defaults in neuronal progenitor division	—	37[a] 155 50
	ASPM	Mitotic spindle-associated protein	Microcephaly Altered cleavage plan in radial glial cells	Decrease of progenitor's proliferation Altered cleavage plan of progenitors Stop of radial migration	38[a] 156 54 157
	CDK5RAP2	Centrosome-associated protein	Microcephaly Decrease in progenitor's population Premature exit of cell cycle and death of progenitors	Decrease in radial glial cells Increase in basal progenitors Decrease in progenitor's proliferation Premature neuronal differentiation	39[a] 53 158
	CENPJ	Centrosome-associated protein	Microcephaly Dysregulation of cleavage plan and death of progenitors	—	39[a] 55
	STIL	Centrosome-associated protein	Early embryonic death Neural tube defects	—	40[a]
	CEP152	Centrosome-associated protein	—	—	41[a]
	CASC5	Centrosome-associated protein	Embryonic death	—	47[a]
	CEP63	Centrosome associated protein	—	—	42[a]
	CEP135	Centrosome-associated protein	—	—	43[a]
	CDK6	Kinase	—	—	44[a]
	ZNF335	Zing finger protein	Reduction in cortical size	Altered progenitor cell proliferation and self-renewal Premature cell cycle exit Decreased cell size Abnormal dendritic shape and orientation	46[a]
	PHC1	Chromatin remodeling complex	—	—	45[a]
	HsSAS-6	Centrosome-associated protein	—	—	48[a]
Isolated microcephaly or associated with pachygyria/PMG and cerebellar hypoplasia	WDR62	Centrosome-associated protein	—	Decrease in progenitor's proliferation	35[a] 36[a] 159

Continued

Classic Lissencephaly (LisI)

Phenotype	Gene	Protein function	Description	Cellular defect	References
Agyria/pachygyria/ isolated SBH	PAFAH1B1 (LIS1)	Microtubule-associated protein	Disorganization of cortical plate; Decrease in branching of interneurons	Altered division of radial glial cells; Morphological abnormalities of multipolar neurons; Stop of radial migration	160[a]; 161; 162; 163
	DCX	Microtubule-associated protein	Alteration of nucleokinesis and branching in interneurons; Ectopic neuronal layer in hippocampus	Stop of radial migration	71[a]; 72[a]; 164; 165
	KIF2A	Microtubule depolymerase	Ventricular dilatation; Altered lamination of cortex and hippocampus; Axonogenesis default	—	86[a]; 166; 167
	TUBG1	Centrosome-associated protein	Embryonic death	Stop of radial migration	86[a]; 168
Agyria-pachygyria associated with hypoplasia of cerebellum and brain stem, basal ganglia dysmorphia, and microcephaly	TUBA1A	Microtubules unit	Cortical layer disruption; Ectopic neuronal layer in hippocampus	—	81[a]
Agyria-pachygyria associated with genital anomalies	ARX	Transcription factor	Delay in tangential migration; Interneuron loss; Decrease in progenitor's population; Reduction of superficial layers of cortex	Altered proliferation of progenitors; Morphological anomalies in multipolar neurons; Stop of radial migration	136[a]; 169; 170
Agyria-pachygyria with severe cerebellar hypoplasia	RELN	Secreted glycoprotein	Inversed cortical lamination	—	171[a]; 5
	VLDLR	Membrane receptor	Inverse cortical lamination	—	172[a]; 173

Subcortical band heterotopia (SBH)

Phenotype	Gene	Protein function	Description	Cellular defect	References
SBH	DCX	Microtubule-associated protein	Alteration of nucleokinesis and branching in interneurons; Ectopic neuronal layer in hippocampus	Stop of radial migration	72[a]
Giant SBH	EML1	Microtubule-associated protein	Giant laminar heterotopia; Proliferation defect	Proliferation defect	80[a]

Periventricular Nodular Heterotopia (PVNH)

Phenotype	Gene	Protein function	Description	Cellular defect	References
PVNH	FLNA	Actin-associated protein	Microcephaly; Thin cortex; Decreased population of progenitors	Altered radial glial cells; Morphological anomalies of multipolar neurons; Stop of radial migration	174[a]; 58; 175; 176; 177
PVNH associated with microcephaly	ARFGEF2	Vesicular trafficking	Periventricular heterotopia	—	60[a]; 178

TABLE 1   Summary of Genetic Bases of Malformations of Cortical Development and Related Rodent Phenotypes in Constitutive or RNA Interference (RNAi) Knockdown Models—cont'd

Malformation of Cortical Development	Gene	Protein Function	Anomalies of Central Nervous System (CNS) in Constitutive Models (KO/ENU/Spontaneous)	Anomalies of CNS in RNAi in Utero Models	References
Cobblestone Lissencephaly (LisII)					
Walker–Warburg syndrome/Muscle –eye–brain syndrome	POMT1	Extracellular matrix glycosylation	Early embryonic death Disruption of pial membrane		118[a] 179
	POMT2	Extracellular matrix glycosylation	Disruption of pial membrane Overmigration of pyramidal neurons Defect in migration of cerebellar neurons Anomalies of hippocampus morphology		119[a] 133
	POMGnT1	Extracellular matrix glycosylation	Disruption of pial membrane Anomalies of hippocampus morphology		120[a] 131
	LARGE	Extracellular matrix glycosylation	Disruption of pial membrane Anomalies of hippocampus morphology		121[a] 180
	B3GALNT2	Extracellular matrix glycosylation	—		124[a]
	B3GNT1	Extracellular matrix glycosylation	Disruption of pial membrane Defect in neuronal migration Anomalies of axonal guidance		125 181[a] 134
	GTDC2	Extracellular matrix glycosylation	—		126[a]
	ISPD	Extracellular matrix glycosylation	Disruption of pial membrane Defect in neuronal migration Anomalies of axonal guidance		129[a] 130[a] 117[a] 134
	TMEM5	Extracellular matrix glycosylation	—		117[a]
	LAMB1	Extracellular matrix glycosylation	Early embryonic death		128[a] 182
	POMK	Extracellular matrix glycosylation			127[a]
Walker–Warburg syndrome/Fukuyama syndrome	FKTN	Extracellular matrix glycosylation	Disruption of pial membrane Overmigration of pyramidal neurons Lamination defect of cortical and hippocampal cortices	—	122[a] 135
	FKRP	Extracellular matrix glycosylation	Ventricular dilatation Decreased number of cortical neurons Defects in cortical, cerebellar, and hippocampal organizations	—	123[a] 183

Polymicrogyria (PMG)

Phenotype	Gene	Function			References
Bilateral frontoparietal PMG / Cerebellar anomalies	GPR56	Transmembrane receptor	Disruption of pial membrane; Overmigration of pyramidal neurons	—	98[a]; 100,184
Frontal/bilateral perisylvian PMG	DYNC1H1	Intracellular transport	KO: Embryonic death; ENU: Motor neuron degeneration	Stop of radial migration; Disruption of nucleus and Centrosome coupling in migrating neurons	86[a]; 185; 186; 63
Diffuse PMG	KBP	Intracellular transport	—	—	187[a]
Multifocal bilateral PMG / Hypoplasia of cerebellum and brain stem	TUBB2B	Microtubules unit	Decreased of cortex thickness; Ventricular dilatation; Decrease in interneuron population	Stop of radial migration	81[a]; 188; 84
Dysmorphia of basal ganglia / Microcephaly	TUBB3	Microtubules unit	Anomalies of axonal guidance	Altered proliferation of intermediate progenitors; Morphological anomalies in multipolar neurons; Delay of radial migration	85[a]; 189
	TUBB5	Microtubules unit	—	Increased cell cycle length in radial glial cells; Slight delay in migration of pyramidal neurons	83[a]
Unilateral/diffuse PMG	PAX6	Transcription factor	Increased number of Reelin+ and Calretinin + neurons; Neuronal subcortical heterotopia	—	190[a]; 191; 192
Undetermined PMG	TBR2	Transcription factor	Microcephaly; Decreased number of intermediate progenitors; Altered differentiation of pyramidal neurons; No neurogenesis in hippocampus	—	89[a]; 193

Schizencephaly

Phenotype	Gene	Function			References
Schizencephaly	SHH	Morphogen	Decreased size of cortex; Altered cell cycle in progenitors; Apoptosis of progenitors; Defects in cortical lamination	—	110[a]; 194
	SIX3	Transcription factor	Abnormal morphology of cerebral commissures	—	110[a]; 195

[a]Article demonstrating gene implication in MCD.

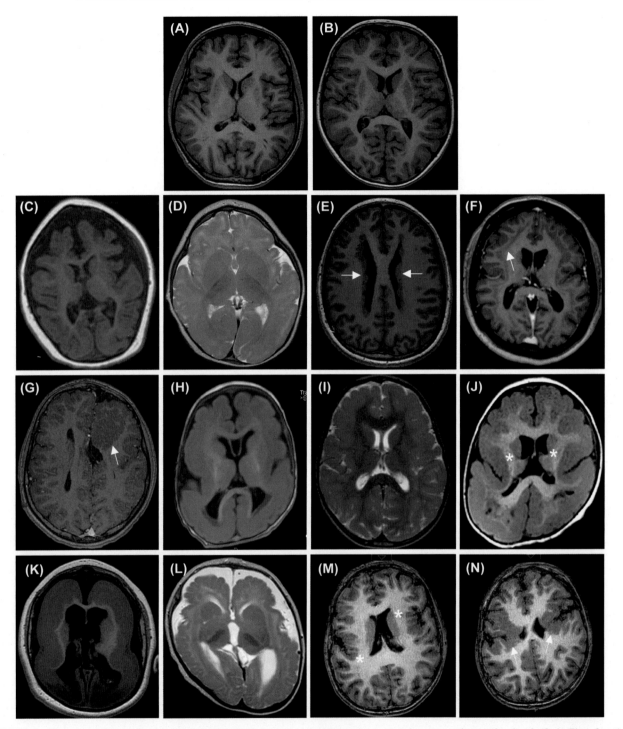

FIGURE 2 **Brain magnetic resonance imaging (MRI) of controls and MCD patients.** Axial sections of control individuals (A,B) and patients with primary microcephaly alone (C) or associated with simplified gyral pattern encompassing too few gyri and shallow sulci, normal myelination, and normal thickness of the cortex (D). Characteristic images of periventricular (E), laminar subcortical (F), and giant subcortical heterotopias (G) are highlight by white arrows. The lissencephaly spectrum encompasses Lis1-like pachygyria, with a posterior predominance of the malformation with only few sulci visible in frontal regions (H), Doublecortin-like pachygyria, presenting an anterior predominance of the malformation (I), tubulin-like pachygyria associating pachygyria with dysmorphia of basal ganglia (asterisk) (J), and complete agyria (K). Note that the pachygyric/agyric cortex appears to be thick. Polymicrogyria can be diffuse (L), restricted in an area (i.e., the perisylvian zone) (asterisks) (M), or surrounding schizencephalic clefts as in (N) (arrows). These cleft did not communicate with the lateral ventricle.

(cobblestone lissencephaly or type II lissencephaly) are associated with massive overmigration of neurons into the leptomeningeal space and beyond the pial surface because of the loss of glia limitans integrity.[13,32] Refinement of these malformations can further be obtained by taking into account developmental abnormalities of other brain structures such as, corpus callosum, cerebellum, brain stem, internal capsule, and basal ganglia.

Periventricular nodular heterotopia is the most frequent neuronal heterotopia. It is characterized by bilateral ectopic nodules along the lateral ventricles (Figure 2(E)). Mutations in the X-linked filamin A (*FLNA*) gene, encoding an actin binding protein that serves as scaffold for over 30 proteins,[58] account for about 50% of PNH cases, mostly females observed mainly for epilepsy and more less severe ID. Although *FLNA* mutations are generally lethal in male fetuses, a few living boys have been reported to carry mutations in this gene.[59] A second rare form of autosomal recessive PNH with microcephaly associated with mutations in *ARFGEF2* gene, encoding for the brefeldin A inhibited guanine-exchange factor 2, has been also described.[60]

Different types of PNH have also been described as linked to various deletions in 1p36, 7q11, and 5q14.3-q15 or duplications involving 5p15.[61,62]

Type I lissencephaly (classical lissencephaly), literally "smooth brain," is a rare disease characterized by impoverishment of the cortical gyration development associated with thickening of the cortex and disappearance of its normal six layered lamination that is replaced by four layers of immature neurons. These features reflect the incapacity of neurons to migrate correctly from the ventricular zone to reach their final destination in the proper cortical layer, and in particular to migrate across neuronal layers already positioned. In clinical practice, the term "lissencephaly" is used to designate the spectrum of malformations encompassing phenotypes with a decrease number of the cortical gyri, also called "pachygyria" (Figure 2(H, I, K)) and phenotypes with complete lack of cortical circumvolution called "agyria" (Figure 2(J)), as well as cortical band heterotopia (band of neuronal cells arrested in the white matter) (Figure 2(F)). These malformations are also sorted by the anteroposterior gradient of gyration anomaly. In many cases, it is indeed possible to distinguish anteroposterior (a > p) forms of lissencephaly, in which the malformation is more present in frontal zones of the brain (Figure 2(I)), from posteroanterior syndromes presenting a predominance of the malformation in parietal and occipital brain areas (Figure 2(H)). Although to date, the pathophysiological basis of this gradient remain poorly understood, this topographic difference

can be useful to orientate genetic explorations of classical lissencephaly.

Patients with classical lissencephaly have severe disabilities, hypotonia, and early drug-resistant epilepsy. However, with tremendous progress of fetal imaging, antenatal diagnosis has increased dramatically over the past few years. Accordingly, the frequency of classical lissencephaly diagnosed in postnatal stages decreased and pachygyria conditions are mainly observed.

When the lissencephaly is associated with an anomaly of the hindbrain or other malformative signs, such as genital anomalies, one speaks about the variant lissencephaly. Their genetic etiologies differ from those of the classical lissencephalies (Table 1).

Until recently, only four genes were associated with human type I lissencephaly: *LIS1* or PAFAH1B1, platelet-activating factor acetyl hydrolase (isoform Ib), *DCX* (Doublecortin), *ARX* (Aristaless-related homeobox), and *RELN* (Reelin) (reviewed in Ref. 13). Functional studies revealed that the LIS1 protein is involved in the regulation of the molecular motor complex formed by Dynein and Nudel proteins[63] and that Doublecortin is a microtubule-associated protein that both induces nucleation and stabilizes microtubules by linking adjacent tubulin protofilaments.[64,65] The genetic suppression in mice of Dcx or Lis1 is associated with neuronal migration defects.[66-68]

Mutations in *Lis1* and *DCX* account for about 85% of classical lissencephaly cases,[69] although most are linked to de novo mutations in the *LIS1* gene. Patients with *LIS1* mutations have a p > a gradient (more pronounced posterior pachygyria) whereas mutations in *DCX* lead to a > p lissencephalies.[70]

For X-linked lissencephaly associated with mutations in the *DCX* gene located in Xq22.3,[71,72] male patients hemizygous for *DCX* mutations develop a classical lissencephaly whereas transmitting females are less symptomatic and display subcortical laminar heterotopia, or even asymptomatic.[73] Subcortical band heterotopia, also called "double cortex," is considered a mild form of lissencephaly because of the common genetic bases and pathophysiological mechanisms. The bilateral ectopic band of neurons can be of different thicknesses with a normal or simplified cortex (Figure 2(F)). Patients with SBH have drug-resistant epilepsy associated with moderate ID in half of cases. Almost all cases of SBH are females with heterozygous mutation in the *DCX* gene. Mutations in *DCX* account for more than 90% of cases.[74,75] Rare male cases of SBH with either hemizygous missense mutations predicted to have mild consequences in protein function or somatic mutations were also reported.[76-78] Furthermore, few missense mutations in the *PAFAH1B1* gene have also been found.[79] Finally, in one study, homozygote or compound heterozygous mutations in *EML1* gene have been identified in two families with "giant" band heterotopia (Figure 2(G)). Indeed, magnetic resonance imaging (MRI) sections revealed huge subcortical masses that start at the ventricle and expand to the subcortical matter, associated with a polymicrogyric cortex facing the heterotopic lesions.[80]

As mentioned, *LIS1* and *DCX* genes both encode proteins involved in microtubule homeostasis. In line with these findings, the importance of the cytoskeleton in neuronal migration disorders was further reinforced by the characterization of patients with lissencephaly, pachygyria, band heterotopia, and polymicrogyria (PMG) carrying mutations in the α- and β-tubulin genes.

Tubulin alpha 1A (TUBA1A) was the first tubulin isoform shown through reverse genetic approach to be involved in human cortical malformations. Keays et al.[81] found lamination defects in the hippocampus and moderate disorganization of the cortex of a mutant mouse strain generated by random *N*-ethyl *N*-nitrosourea (ENU) mutagenesis. Further genetic investigations revealed that the mutant strain carries a heterozygous missense mutation (p.Ser140Gly) in the autosomal *Tuba1a* gene that encodes an α-tubulin subunit. Neuroanatomical similarities between the Tuba1a mutant and Dcx-deficient mice,[67] and the fact that Doublecortin is a microtubule-associated protein,[64] led the authors to analyze *TUBA1A* in patient with MCD and unknown genetic causes. Thus, de novo mutations in *TUBA1A* were also identified in type I lissencephaly patients.[81,82] The clinical features of *TUBA1A*-related cortical dysgeneses, which are commonly associated with a striking perisylvian or posterior predominant pachygyria, have been refined.[97]

However, in addition to microcephaly, rare occurrences of agyria and subcortical heterotopia demonstrate that *TUBA1A*-related lissencephaly could encompass a large spectrum of cortical abnormalities. This abnormal gyral pattern is combined with dysgenesis of the anterior limb of the internal capsule to give a dysmorphic aspect to the basal ganglia (Figure 2(K)). This combination constitutes specific features associated with *TUBA1A* mutations. Moreover, the analysis of several fetal cases, aged from 23 to 35 GW, have revealed cellular abnormalities suggesting that pyramidal neurons and interneurons might be equally affected, as well as neuronal axonal guidance and/or growth defects, in addition to early neuronal differentiation abnormalities likely to be involved in the pathogeny of *TUBA1A*-related cortical dysgeneses.[33]

In continuation of these findings and the hypothesis that tubulins and microtubule-related proteins are relevant candidates for MCD, Keays and associates

identified *TUBB5*,[83] and Chelly and coworkers used expression and WES-based approaches and showed the implications of *TUBB2B*,[84] *TUBB3*,[85] *DYNC1H1*, *KIF2A*, and *TUBG1* in a large spectrum of neuronal migration disorders[86] (Table 1). These data emphasize the association between microtubule-related cellular process and proper cortical development.

Malformations Thought to Be Related to Late Migration and/or Postmigrational Defects

Polymicrogyria. Disorders associated with PMG represent the most common type of cortical malformation and were first described in 1915 by Bielschowsky. The term "polymicrogyria" refers to abnormal development of the cortical layers and formation of multiple little gyri with an excess of shallow sulci.[87] At the histologic level, several types of cortex disorganization are described with disappearance of the six-layered normal cortical structure in all cases. With increased performance of brain MRI, several subtypes of PMG are recognized based on differences in extension and topography of gyral abnormalities. and focal, multifocal. and diffused PMG could be differentiated (Figure 2(L)). Multifocal PMG is unilateral, bilateral symmetric, or bilateral asymmetric. Most frequent PMG syndromes are bilateral perisylvian and frontoparietal polymicrogyria (Figure 2(M)). Clinical presentation of patients with PMG encompasses focal neurologic symptoms (hemiparesis or partial epilepsy) and severer developmental troubles including quadriparesis, drug-resistant epilepsy, and profound mental disability.

Polymicrogyria has multiple genetic and nongenetic etiologies. Although progress in deciphering genetic causes and genes involved is constant, the molecular basis of this heterogeneous group of malformation remains elusive. So far, with the exception of *GPR56* (G protein–coupled receptor 56) and *TUBB2B* (detailed below), patients (or family) have mainly private variations in a variety of genes that have been reported. For these latter genes, the association between mutations and PMG was reported in only a few cases: paired box gene 6 (*PAX6*) in PMG associated with aniridia,[88] *TBR2* (EOMES; eomesodermin homolog),[89] *KIAA1279*, and nonhomologous end-joining factor 1 in diffuse PMG[90,91] and RAB3 GTPase-activating protein in frontal PMG,[92] and *SRPX2* in which a missense mutation has been reported in BPP with epilepsy.[93] Genetic heterogeneity for PMG is even more complex if we include linkage data and copy number variations associated with heterogeneous syndromes in which PMG is not a constant feature. These include a 5.2-Mb interval in Xq28 identified owing to a linkage study in five different families with BPP,[94] a deletion in 22q11.2 not consistently associated with variable BPP,[95] and a set of chromosomic rearrangements in a cohort of 29 patients that highlighted numerous loci (1p36.3, 2p16.1-p23, 4q21.21-q22.1, 6q26-q27, 21q21.3-q22.1, 1q44, and 18p) that have to be take into account for future genetic studies.[96]

In some other cases of PMG, identified mutations reside in genes known to be involved in other forms of MCD (i.e., *TUBA1A*, *TUBB3*, and *DYNC1H1*).[86,97]

While keeping in mind this complex and evolving knowledge regarding genetics of PMG, consistent major genetic findings are GPR56 and tubulin genes and their implications in autosomal recessive bilateral frontoparietal PMG (BFPP) and sporadic cases of peculiar PMG, respectively. Patients with BFPP also have global development delay, epilepsy, ventricular dilatation, and anomalies of the cerebellum and brain stem. The molecular causes of this type of malformation are usually homozygous mutations in the *GRP56* gene encoding a transmembrane protein interacting with the extracellular matrix. These mutations are mainly missense mutations located in the extracellular domain.[98] Histopathological studies of the only reported fetal case demonstrated disruption of the basal membrane associated with overmigration of the neurons in the extracortical space, strongly reminiscent of what is seen in cobblestone lissencephaly.[99] These data suggest a physiopathological continuum between cobblestone lissencephaly and PMG. These features are also found in the knockout mice model of *Gpr56*, leading one to suppose that human mutations could act as loss-of-function mutations.[100]

For PMG resulting from mutations in tubulin genes, a study by Bahi-Buisson et al.[97] reviewed clinical and imaging data of 80 patients with malformations of cortical development related to de novo mutations in *TUBA1A*, *TUBB2B*, *TUBB3*, *TUBB5*, and *TUBG1* genes, collectively known as tubulinopathies. Six years after the discovery of TUBA1A, this study, together with data from the literature, showed that mutations in tubulin genes are responsible for a large spectrum of brain developmental defects, although mutations in each tubulin gene are responsible for a predominant phenotype.[97] This study also showed the presence of the key features defining the tubulinopathy spectrum. These include dysmorphic basal ganglia, hypoplasia or agenesis of the corpus callosum and brain stem, and cerebellar hypoplasia.

As far as PMG is concerned, the study confirmed that patients with malformations suggestive of PMG do not display all of the characteristics of typical PMG. These cases were therefore defined as PMG-like cortical dysplasia. Indeed, *TUBA1A*, *TUBB2B*, *TUBB3*, or *TUBB5*-related PMG more closely resemble coarse PMG with a thick cortex and irregular surfaces on both the pial and gray—white junction sides. Of note, one of the distinctive signs of atypical PMG is the absence of deep infolding that is usually highly suggestive of PMG.[31] These observations led Cushion et al.[101] to propose the concept of atypical PMG or PMG-like cortical dysplasia. This is further reinforced by neuropathological anomalies of a fetal case of *TUBB2B*-related PMG that we previously described.[15,84,101] Histological features were composed of disorganization of cortical layering, which is consistent with unlayered PMG, but also signs combining neuronal overmigration through breaches in the pial basement membrane and neuronal heterotopias reminiscent of cobblestone lissencephaly rather than classic PMG.[15,33,101] Moreover, this study and others found a significant number of patients with a milder neurological phenotype and only highly localized areas of irregular cortex, described as focal PMG. In these patients, main features reminiscent of a tubulinopathy are the abnormal basal ganglia, corpus callosum abnormalities, and cerebellar hypoplasia.[101] This group of malformations is mainly associated with *TUBB3* mutations but is also reported with *TUBB2B* and *TUBA1A* mutations.[101,102] These observations suggest that tubulinopathies may be responsible for a subset of intellectually disabled children with corpus callosum abnormalities, either hypogenesis or dysmorphic and cerebellar hypoplasia without obvious cortical malformations.

Schizencephaly. Schizencephaly is a rare congenital disorder defined by the presence of unilateral or bilateral transcortical cleft extending from the ventricular surface to the pial surface, lined with gray matter and filled with cerebrospinal fluid (Figure 2(N)). The clefts mostly involve the perisylvian regions and their walls can be widely separated or closed. The cortex around the cleft display PMG characteristics. Pathophysiological mechanisms underlying these abnormalities are poorly understood, although proliferation or abnormal cortical organization defects have been proposed. Patients can be almost normal or have microcephaly, seizures, and severe intellectual and motor delay, depending on the gravity and extent of the clefts.[103,104] Two initial reports of de novo heterozygous mutations in homeobox gene *EMX2* identified this gene as an important actor of schizencephaly etiology.[105,106] However, most of the described mutations are considered unconvincing and the knockout mouse model has no relevant phenotype.[107–109] Thus, the interest in EMX2 in our understanding of schizencephaly is decreasing. More recently, several heterozygous mutations in three other genes have been reported: *SHH* and *SIX3*, two genes also associated with holoprosencephaly, and *COL4A1* in association with porencephaly.[110–112] Finally, an association between mutations in *WDR62* (shown to be involved in a wide range of MCD) and schizencephaly was also reported.[35]

Malformations Resulting From Pial Basement Membrane Defects: Type II Lissencephaly (or Cobblestone Lissencephaly)

Although this group of malformations, called cobblestone lissencephaly or type II lissencephaly, exhibits neuronal migration abnormalities, it basically represents a peculiar brain malformation with characteristic brain imaging anomalies, defined as cortical dysplasia combined with dysmyelination, dysplastic cerebellum with cysts, and brain stem hypoplasia. Moreover, this group of cortical dysgeneses was shown to be associated with pial basement membrane defects and overmigration of neuronal cells into the meningeal space, creating an extra cortical layer that lead to an irregular cobblestone brain surface. The pial surface of the cortex is limited by a basement membrane, which is a specialized structure of extracellular matrix serving as an anchor for radial glial end feet.[113] The underlying mechanism for type II lissencephaly is disruption of the glia limitans in which breaches are formed. This further allows the migrating neurons to pass beyond the pial basement membrane and settle within the meningeal space.

Cobblestone lissencephaly is a characteristic feature found in different autosomal diseases syndromes: Walker–Warburg syndrome, muscle–eye–brain disease, and Fukuyama muscular dystrophy.[114–116] These three pathologies are now classified as muscular dystrophy-dystroglycanopathy with brain and eye anomalies (MDDGA) because of their association with autosomal recessive mutations in genes encoding posttranslational modification proteins of α-dystroglycan, a receptor for the extracellular matrix. Until now, 13 MDDGA-related genes have been identified and account for around 60% of patients: *POMT1*, *POMT2*, *POMGNT1*, *POMK*, *LARGE*, *FKTN*, *FKRP*, *B3GALNT2*, *B3GNT1*, *GTDC2*, *ISPD*, *TMEM5*, and *LAMB1*[117–130] (Table 1). All of these genes are known to encode proteins that ensure posttranslational modifications of transmembrane and extracellular matrix components.

Constitutive reduced expression of Pomt1, Pomt2, Pomgnt1, B3gnt1, Ispd, and Fktn in mice leads to a brain phenotype characterized by disruption of the pial basement membrane and overmigration of neurons in the extracortical region correlated with disorganization of underneath cortical layers.[131–135] Altogether, these data suggest that these proteins are involved in the development and maintenance of the basement membrane.

DISCUSSION

ID With Malformations of Cortical Development versus ID Without Apparent Malformations

This dichotomy is, of course, convenient for clinical and diagnostic purposes. However, when investigating genetic disorders, one should keep in mind that even the same mutation in a single gene can produce a remarkably wide range of associated clinical phenotypes. It is therefore reasonable to expect that mutations in some MCD-related genes might lead to clinical phenotypes limited to ID (with no apparent MCD). Whereas this issue of phenotypic heterogeneity is well known and might appear as the rule in human genetics, molecular and biological pathomechanisms are rarely understood. For the few genetic disorders in which clear genotype–phenotype correlations and/or mutations-related functional consequences correlate with specific phenotypes, such robust basic observations could be used as an entry point to dissect and understand these correlations further. In the field of MCD, there is the intriguing example of *ARX*, in which where loss-of-function mutations are associated with XLAG syndrome characterized by severe lissencephaly and ambiguous genitalia development,[136] whereas the polyalanine expansion mutation is associated with a striking large spectrum of ID (expanding from West syndrome to mild ID) without gross MCD. This example roughly illustrates the idea that mutation-related protein functional differences underlie the occurrence or not of MCD, but it also perfectly illustrates the poorly understood issue of phenotypic heterogeneity and variability of ID severity. Indeed, the most frequent *ARX* mutations corresponding to polyalanine expansion mutations owing to either a c.304ins(GCG)7 (16 increasing to 23 alanines) or a c.428_451dup (12 increasing to 20 alanines) account for a considerable proportion (about 45%) of *ARX* mutations that are related to at least seven well-defined clinical entities that have been described. The spectrum covers severe encephalopathy with profound ID (West syndrome) and clinical phenotypes characterized by neurodevelopmental delay and mild ID, and includes Ohtahara, Partington, and Proud syndromes, X-linked infantile spasms, X-linked myoclonic epilepsy, and nonsyndromic ID.[137] The usually proposed hypothesis that awaits convincing demonstration suggests modulatory effects of the individual genetic background and its considerable scope on variability in gene and protein expression. This implies that one might expect to see considerable variation in the effect of mutations in the same gene, and even of identical mutations, from one affected individual to another.

With the unprecedented power of NGS technologies, complete mono-dimension information based on DNA analysis and extensive genotyping data might provide some insights in the near feature. However, a better comprehensive view could only be reached if consequences of genomic variations and environment on the intermingled epigenetic modifications and spatiotemporal regulation of genetic expression could be defined and meaningfully integrated. This issue of phenotypic heterogeneity is a theoretical and intellectual challenge, but it also represents a serious and frequent medical problem. As long as we remain unable to anticipate individual patients and parents' concerns regarding phenotypic consequences and the severity of phenotypes associated with a given mutation, the practice of medical genetic will remain frustrating and below expectations and needs.

Molecular bases of ID with or without MCD should also integrate emerging compelling evidences demonstrating the contribution of somatic mutations in the diversity and heterogeneity of MCD. Confirmation of the occurrence of de novo mutations after fertilization, and therefore presence of at least two cellular populations differing by the presence or the absence of the genetic defect, came with the identification of somatic mutations in LIS1 and DCX.[74,77,79,138] These findings were further confirmed by Jamuar et al. (2014) using a new high-throughput and deep-targeted sequencing approach.[78] Somatic mutations were also identified in genes encoding proteins of the PI3K−AKT−mTOR pathway in patients with hemimegalencephaly[139,140] and numerous other overgrowth syndromes, including Proteus syndrome and CLOVE syndrome.[141,142] In view of these findings, it is reasonable to hypothesize that somatic mutations in a subset of genes involved in MCD and other types of neurodevelopmental disorders could also cause diseases without structural abnormalities, such as ID, neuropsychiatric diseases, autism spectrum disorders, and epilepsy, in which neuronal connectivity and networking, and synaptic function and plasticity are emerging as essential pathophysiological mechanisms underlying these disorders.

As mentioned in the introduction, the distinction between ID with MCD versus ID with no apparent malformation mainly relies on brain MRI technology. The outstanding contrast resolution of MRI, superimposed on the ability to image in any plane, allows identification of even subtle malformations. Indeed, in the heterogeneous group of epilepsies refractory to treatment, MRI has revealed a higher than expected prevalence of subtle cortical malformations (8−14% of cases). Also, as shown by Guerrini and colleagues in a study focused on patients with PMG, ultra−high-field MRI and 7T imaging can even reveal more anatomic details compared with 3T conventional sequences, with potential implications

for diagnosis, genetic studies, and surgical treatment of associated epilepsy.[143] For other neurodevelopmental disorders, such as ID and epilepsy, in which no obvious cortical malformations are visible by high-resolution MRI, current knowledge suggests that underlying genetic causes lead to neurobiological functional defects involved in the establishment of cortical connectivity and networks. Such abnormalities are generally more difficult to pinpoint than classical malformations. However, because of continuous advances in imaging technologies and their performance, including development of applications to define subtle qualitative and/or quantitative brain anomalies, it stands to reason that one should expect an increased ability to better define subtle malformations and detect subtle brain abnormalities in patients thought to be free of malformations.

The notion of the presence or absence of cortical developmental abnormalities ultimately depends on histological studies that are exceptionally well carried out. The study, highlighted below, on Dravet syndrome cases well illustrates these remarks.

In the same vein, some studies have reported description of patients with malformations of cortical development carrying mutations in genes such as RAI1, SCN1A, and CUL4B, known to be responsible for Smith Magenis (SMS), Dravet, and ID syndromes without MCD, respectively. For instance, Capra et al.[196] reported on two patients harboring deletions of the 17p11.2 region in whom the SMS typical phenotype was associated with bilateral PNH. These observations expand the spectrum of chromosomal rearrangements associated with PNH and indicate that abnormal neuronal migration may contribute to the neurocognitive phenotype of SMS. Barba et al.[197] reported on six patients with SCN1A mutations and malformations of cortical development (MCDs) and described their clinical course, genetic findings, and electrographic, imaging, and neuropathologic features. All patients exhibited electroclinical features consistent with the Dravet syndrome spectrum, cognitive impairment, and autistic features, as well as mutations in SCN1A gene. Brain MRI revealed bilateral PNH in two patients and focal cortical dysplasia (FCD) in three, and disclosed no macroscopic abnormality in one. In the MRI-negative patient, neuropathologic study of the whole brain performed after sudden unexpected death from epilepsy, revealed multifocal micronodular dysplasia in the left temporal lobe. Two patients with FCD underwent epilepsy surgery. Neuropathology revealed FCD type IA and type IIA. This study illustrates that MCDs and SCN1A gene mutations can co-occur. Although epidemiology and frequency of mutations do not support a causative role for SCN1A mutations in MCD, one might suggest that these unexpected phenotypic expression of SCN1A mutations result from a loss or impaired protein function and the effect of susceptibility factors and genetic modifiers.

Another example that illustrates the complexity of the issue of ID and MCD is *CUL4B*-related phenotypes. Variants in Cullin 4B (*CUL4B*) are a known cause of syndromic X-linked ID. In a recent study, we described a series of 25 patients from 11 families with mutations in *CUL4B*.[144] Neuroimaging data available for 15 patients showed the presence of cerebral malformations in 10 patients. The cerebral anomalies were difficult to classify but were composed of MCD such as simplified gyral pattern and bilateral perisylvian PMG, ventriculomegaly, and diminished white matter volume. These heterogeneous *CUL4B*-related phenotypes are mainly related to loss-of-function mutations with no evident genotype phenotype correlation. However, the fact that CUL4B is known to regulate various cellular processes, including neuronal progenitor proliferation, and was shown to interact with *WDR62*,[144] are interesting hints for further understanding of the heterogeneity of cerebral malformations in patients with variants in *CUL4B*.

Malformations of Cortical Development and ID: What Are the Perspectives to Reverse Cellular and Neurodevelopmental Defects?

At first sight, and because of developmental neuroanatomical abnormalities, it is difficult to conceptualize treatment and restoration of defects corresponding to malformations of cortical development disorders; to date, mainly rehabilitation and symptomatic treatments are proposed. However, there have been at least two series of studies based on mouse models suggesting the possibility of reversing cellular and clinical phenotypes.

These two experimentally based model studies, detailed below, reinforce the growing number of cellular and animal model-based studies showing the potential reversibility of defects underlying neurodevelopmental disorders such as ID disorders. As far as genetically related ID is concerned, until the latter half of the twentieth century, it was thought that these disorders were developmentally determined and therefore not accessible to therapeutic approaches. However, this dogma was disproved long ago by pioneering studies regarding phenylketonuria (PKU)-related ID and after breakthroughs associated with newborn screening and metabolic corrections. Phenylketonuria was discovered by the Norwegian physician Ivar Asbjørn Følling in 1934 and was the first disorder to be routinely diagnosed through widespread newborn screening introduced by Robert Guthrie in the early 1960s.[145,146] With the knowledge that PKU could be detected before symptoms were evident and treatment initiated, screening was quickly adopted around the world. Austria started screening

for PKU in 1966, and England in 1968. Prevention and correction of PKU-related deficits were followed by other successes, most still in the field of metabolic and storage disorders.

Moreover, for ID disorders (not related to metabolic disorders), although efficient therapeutic application in humans remains a challenging issue, tremendous progress in the understanding of genetic and cellular mechanisms was achieved and perspectives for therapeutic and intervention options are beginning to emerge for a number of specific conditions. Indeed, advances in understanding disorders such as fragile X, Prader—Willi, Down, and Rett syndromes and PI3K—AKT—mTOR pathway-related disorders are resulting in promising treatment directions (review by Ref. 147).

Surprisingly, this trend regarding potential reversibility of neurodevelopmental defects seems to be possible even for MCDs. In this chapter we propose illustrating these advances using the following two examples. First, Manent et al.[148] showed that neuronal migration defect in a *Dcx*-knockdown rat model mimicking subcortical band heterotopia phenotype could be partially rescued and migration could be induced even after birth.[148] Second, elegant pathophysiological-based studies reported by Wynshaw-Boris and colleagues led to the identification of therapeutic intervention that resulted in phenotypic improvement of heterozygous Lis1 mutant mice (Lis1$^{+/-}$) that exhibit cortical malformation and defects in neuronal migration.[149]

Postnatal rescue of Dcx-related neuronal migration defects. Manent et al.[148] provided the first evidence demonstrating that molecular intervention can induce postnatal migration of Dcx-deficient neurons arrested in the intermediate zone. Indeed, in a rat model of SBH generated by in utero ribonucleic acid (RNA) interference of the *Dcx* gene, they first showed that the model reproduces anatomical features of the malformations present in the human double cortex syndrome.[150] Subsequently, they developed a conditional approach to determine whether delayed intervention after SBH has formed can reduce heterotopia and restore neuronal patterning. Although the effect of *Dcx* small hairpin RNA (shRNA) and neuronal migration phenotype were shown to be partly mediated by off-target effects and endogenous microRNA dysregulation,[151] the study by Manent et al.[148] showed that both laminar displacement of neurons and SBH size are reduced upon delayed expression of Dcx during the early postnatal period. They tested consequences of Dcx re-expression at different developmental stages and found that Dcx re-expression at postnatal day (P)0 induces neuronal migration and marked regression of heterotopia, as well as restoration of neocortical lamination. However, Dcx re-expression at P5 results in partial restoration of neuronal position and heterotopia regression. Moreover, they showed that rats with SBH are more susceptible to seizures induced by the convulsant pentylenetetrazol and that intervention after birth and reduction of SBH restore seizure thresholds to levels similar to those of unaffected controls.[148] Although these studies raise several questions and require further investigations, they suggest that developmentally misplaced neuronal cells maintain the capacity to migrate from deeper to more superficial positions. They also open new perspective for the development of strategies aiming to improve cortical malformations and clinical manifestations.

Rescue of phenotypic defects in Lis1 mutants by inhibiting LIS1 degradation. After the implication of LIS1 gene in lissencephaly, functional studies and animal models showed that LIS1 protein acts within a protein complex (LIS1/ NDEL1/mNUDC) and regulates cytoplasmic dynein function and localization in a kinesin-dependent fashion (see review by Ref. 149). Subsequent investigations carried out by Yamada and colleagues showed that a substantial fraction of LIS1 is degraded at the periphery of the cells after transport to the plus end of microtubules and that calpain inhibitors efficiently prevent LIS1 degradation.[152] The authors assessed the in vivo consequences and showed that the calpain inhibitors (i.e., ALLN-N-acetyl-L-leucyl-L-leucyl-L-norleucinal) protect LIS1 protein from proteolysis and led not only to augmentation of LIS1 level in Lis1$^{+/-}$ mouse embryonic cells but also to rescue of various cellular phenotypes.[153] Interestingly, they also showed that intraperitoneal injection of calpain inhibitor, such as ALLN, to pregnant Lis1$^{+/-}$ mice prevented neuronal cell death and neuronal migration defects, and partially rescued impaired motor behavior and impaired behavioral skills in Lis1$^{+/-}$ offspring. Administration of this treatment to Lis1$^{+/-}$ newborn pups also led to improvement of some of these features.[153,154] To complete their elegant demonstration, the authors used in utero approach and showed that knockdown of calpain by shRNA rescued defective cortical layering in Lis1$^{+/-}$ mice. Altogether, these data suggest that calpain inhibition represents a potential therapeutic approach for LIS1-related developmental abnormalities.

Although these breakthroughs and promising avenues remain far from applicable for patients with MCD, they provide strikingly and unexpected proof of principle for potential reversibility and effective therapeutic strategies for DCX- and LIS1-related neuronal migration disorders.

Acknowledgments

We thank Dr Bahi-buisson for kindly providing us with MRI illustrations of diverse MCD. The research activities of J. Chelly and Y. Saillour are supported by grants from the Fondation pour la Recherche Médicale (Equipe FRM; J.C: DEQ20130326477), the Fondation Maladies Rares, Fondation NRJ — Institut de France, the Agence National de Recherche (ANR Blanc 1103 01, project R11039KK; ANR E-Rare-012-01, project E10107KP; ANR-13-BSV-0009-01), and the EC-FP7 (projects: GENECODYS (grant 241995) and DESIRE (grant agreement 602531); and we are grateful for their support.

References

1. Caviness Jr VS, Takahashi T, Nowakowski RS. Numbers, time and neocortical neuronogenesis: a general developmental and evolutionary model. *Trends Neurosci* September 1995;**18**(9):379—83.
2. Geschwind DH, Rakic P. Cortical evolution: judge the brain by its cover. *Neuron* October 30, 2013;**80**(3):633—47.
3. Rakic P. A small step for the cell, a giant leap for mankind: a hypothesis of neocortical expansion during evolution. *Trends Neurosci* September 1995;**18**(9):383—8.
4. Pavlowsky A, Chelly J, Billuart P. Emerging major synaptic signaling pathways involved in intellectual disability. *Mol Psychiatry* July 2012;**17**(7):682—93.
5. Caviness Jr VS. Neocortical histogenesis in normal and reeler mice: a developmental study based upon [3H]thymidine autoradiography. *Brain Res* July 1982;**256**(3):293—302.
6. Rakic P. Mode of cell migration to the superficial layers of fetal monkey neocortex. *J Comp Neurol* May 1972;**145**(1):61—83.
7. Rakic P. Neurons in rhesus monkey visual cortex: systematic relation between time of origin and eventual disposition. *Science (New York, N.Y.)* February 1, 1974;**183**(4123):425—7.
8. Batista-Brito R, Fishell G. The developmental integration of cortical interneurons into a functional network. *Curr Top Dev Biol* 2009;**87**:81—118.
9. Hansen DV, Lui JH, Parker PR, Kriegstein AR. Neurogenic radial glia in the outer subventricular zone of human neocortex. *Nature* March 25, 2010;**464**(7288):554—61.
10. Kriegstein AR, Noctor SC. Patterns of neuronal migration in the embryonic cortex. *Trends Neurosci* July 2004;**27**(7):392—9.
11. Noctor SC, Martinez-Cerdeno V, Ivic L, Kriegstein AR. Cortical neurons arise in symmetric and asymmetric division zones and migrate through specific phases. *Nat Neurosci* February 2004;**7**(2):136—44.
12. Noctor SC, Flint AC, Weissman TA, Dammerman RS, Kriegstein AR. Neurons derived from radial glial cells establish radial units in neocortex. *Nature* February 8, 2001;**409**(6821):714—20.
13. Francis F, Meyer G, Fallet-Bianco C, et al. Human disorders of cortical development: from past to present. *Eur J Neurosci* February 2006;**23**(4):877—93.
14. Guerrini R, Dobyns WB. Malformations of cortical development: clinical features and genetic causes. *Lancet Neurol* July 2014;**13**(7):710—26.
15. Jaglin XH, Chelly J. Tubulin-related cortical dysgeneses: microtubule dysfunction underlying neuronal migration defects. *Trends Genet* December 2009;**25**(12):555—66.
16. Bystron I, Rakic P, Molnar Z, Blakemore C. The first neurons of the human cerebral cortex. *Nat Neurosci* July 2006;**9**(7):880—6.
17. Hartfuss E, Galli R, Heins N, Gotz M. Characterization of CNS precursor subtypes and radial glia. *Dev Biol* January 1, 2001;**229**(1):15—30.
18. Malatesta P, Hartfuss E, Gotz M. Isolation of radial glial cells by fluorescent-activated cell sorting reveals a neuronal lineage. *Development* December 2000;**127**(24):5253—63.
19. Heins N, Malatesta P, Cecconi F, et al. Glial cells generate neurons: the role of the transcription factor Pax6. *Nat Neurosci* April 2002;**5**(4):308—15.

20. Mo Z, Moore AR, Filipovic R, et al. Human cortical neurons originate from radial glia and neuron-restricted progenitors. *J Neurosci* April 11, 2007;**27**(15):4132–45.

21. Itoh Y, Tyssowski K, Gotoh Y. Transcriptional coupling of neuronal fate commitment and the onset of migration. *Curr Opin Neurobiol* December 2013;**23**(6):957–64.

22. Hippenmeyer S. Molecular pathways controlling the sequential steps of cortical projection neuron migration. *Adv Exp Med Biol* 2014;**800**:1–24.

23. Barnes AP, Polleux F. Establishment of axon-dendrite polarity in developing neurons. *Annu Rev Neurosci* 2009;**32**:347–81.

24. Asada N, Sanada K. LKB1-mediated spatial control of GSK3beta and adenomatous polyposis coli contributes to centrosomal forward movement and neuronal migration in the developing neocortex. *J Neurosci* June 30, 2010;**30**(26):8852–65.

25. Asada N, Sanada K, Fukada Y. LKB1 regulates neuronal migration and neuronal differentiation in the developing neocortex through centrosomal positioning. *J Neurosci* October 24, 2007;**27**(43):11769–75.

26. Sapir T, Sapoznik S, Levy T, et al. Accurate balance of the polarity kinase MARK2/Par-1 is required for proper cortical neuronal migration. *J Neurosci* May 28, 2008;**28**(22):5710–20.

27. Conde C, Caceres A. Microtubule assembly, organization and dynamics in axons and dendrites. *Nat Rev Neurosci* May 2009;**10**(5):319–32.

28. Price TJ, Flores CM, Cervero F, Hargreaves KM. The RNA binding and transport proteins staufen and fragile X mental retardation protein are expressed by rat primary afferent neurons and localize to peripheral and central axons. *Neuroscience* September 15, 2006;**141**(4):2107–16.

29. Barkovich AJ, Kuzniecky RI, Jackson GD, Guerrini R, Dobyns WB. A developmental and genetic classification for malformations of cortical development. *Neurology* December 27, 2005;**65**(12):1873–87.

30. Guerrini R, Dobyns WB, Barkovich AJ. Abnormal development of the human cerebral cortex: genetics, functional consequences and treatment options. *Trends Neurosci* March 2008;**31**(3):154–62.

31. Barkovich AJ, Guerrini R, Kuzniecky RI, Jackson GD, Dobyns WB. A developmental and genetic classification for malformations of cortical development: update 2012. *Brain* May 2012;**135**(Pt 5):1348–69.

32. Kerjan G, Gleeson JG. Genetic mechanisms underlying abnormal neuronal migration in classical lissencephaly. *Trends Genet* December 2007;**23**(12):623–30.

33. Fallet-Bianco C, Laquerriere A, Poirier K, et al. Mutations in tubulin genes are frequent causes of various foetal malformations of cortical development including microlissencephaly. *Acta Neuropathol Commun* 2014;**2**:69.

34. Saillour Y, Broix L, Bruel-Jungerman E, et al. Beta tubulin isoforms are not interchangeable for rescuing impaired radial migration due to Tubb3 knockdown. *Hum Mol Genet* March 15, 2014;**23**(6):1516–26.

35. Bilguvar K, Ozturk AK, Louvi A, et al. Whole-exome sequencing identifies recessive WDR62 mutations in severe brain malformations. *Nature* September 9, 2010;**467**(7312):207–10.

36. Yu TW, Mochida GH, Tischfield DJ, et al. Mutations in WDR62, encoding a centrosome-associated protein, cause microcephaly with simplified gyri and abnormal cortical architecture. *Nat Genet* November 2010;**42**(11):1015–20.

37. Jackson AP, Eastwood H, Bell SM, et al. Identification of microcephalin, a protein implicated in determining the size of the human brain. *Am J Hum Genet* July 2002;**71**(1):136–42.

38. Bond J, Scott S, Hampshire DJ, et al. Protein-truncating mutations in ASPM cause variable reduction in brain size. *Am J Hum Genet* November 2003;**73**(5):1170–7.

39. Bond J, Roberts E, Springell K, et al. A centrosomal mechanism involving CDK5RAP2 and CENPJ controls brain size. *Nat Genet* April 2005;**37**(4):353–5.

40. Kumar A, Girimaji SC, Duvvari MR, Blanton SH. Mutations in STIL, encoding a pericentriolar and centrosomal protein, cause primary microcephaly. *Am J Hum Genet* February 2009;**84**(2):286–90.

41. Guernsey DL, Jiang H, Hussin J, et al. Mutations in centrosomal protein CEP152 in primary microcephaly families linked to MCPH4. *Am J Hum Genet* July 9, 2010;**87**(1):40–51.

42. Sir JH, Barr AR, Nicholas AK, et al. A primary microcephaly protein complex forms a ring around parental centrioles. *Nat Genet* November 2011;**43**(11):1147–53.

43. Hussain MS, Baig SM, Neumann S, et al. A truncating mutation of CEP135 causes primary microcephaly and disturbed centrosomal function. *Am J Hum Genet* May 4, 2012;**90**(5):871–8.

44. Hussain MS, Baig SM, Neumann S, et al. CDK6 associates with the centrosome during mitosis and is mutated in a large Pakistani family with primary microcephaly. *Hum Mol Genet* December 20, 2013;**22**(25):5199–214.

45. Awad S, Al-Dosari MS, Al-Yacoub N, et al. Mutation in PHC1 implicates chromatin remodeling in primary microcephaly pathogenesis. *Hum Mol Genet* June 1, 2013;**22**(11):2200–13.

46. Yang YJ, Baltus AE, Mathew RS, et al. Microcephaly gene links trithorax and REST/NRSF to control neural stem cell proliferation and differentiation. *Cell* November 21, 2012;**151**(5):1097–112.

47. Genin A, Desir J, Lambert N, et al. Kinetochore KMN network gene CASC5 mutated in primary microcephaly. *Hum Mol Genet* December 15, 2012;**21**(24):5306–17.

48. Khan MA, Rupp VM, Orpinell M, et al. A missense mutation in the PISA domain of HsSAS-6 causes autosomal recessive primary microcephaly in a large consanguineous Pakistani family. *Hum Mol Genet* June 20, 2014;**23**(22):5940–9.

49. Mahmood S, Ahmad W, Hassan MJ. Autosomal Recessive Primary Microcephaly (MCPH): clinical manifestations, genetic heterogeneity and mutation continuum. *Orphanet J Rare Dis* 2011;**6**:39.

50. Gruber R, Zhou Z, Sukchev M, Joerss T, Frappart PO, Wang ZQ. MCPH1 regulates the neuroprogenitor division mode by coupling the centrosomal cycle with mitotic entry through the Chk1-Cdc25 pathway. *Nat Cell Biol* November 2011;**13**(11):1325–34.

51. Zhou ZW, Tapias A, Bruhn C, Gruber R, Sukchev M, Wang ZQ. DNA damage response in microcephaly development of MCPH1 mouse model. *DNA Repair (Amst)* August 2013;**12**(8):645–55.

52. Fujimori A, Itoh K, Goto S, et al. Disruption of Aspm causes microcephaly with abnormal neuronal differentiation. *Brain Dev* September 2014;**36**(8):661–9.

53. Lizarraga SB, Margossian SP, Harris MH, et al. Cdk5rap2 regulates centrosome function and chromosome segregation in neuronal progenitors. *Development* June 2010;**137**(11):1907–17.

54. Buchman JJ, Durak O, Tsai LH. ASPM regulates Wnt signaling pathway activity in the developing brain. *Genes Dev* September 15, 2011;**25**(18):1909–14.

55. McIntyre RE, Lakshminarasimhan Chavali P, Ismail O, et al. Disruption of mouse Cenpj, a regulator of centriole biogenesis, phenocopies Seckel syndrome. *PLoS Genet* 2012;**8**(11):e1003022.

56. Evans PD, Anderson JR, Vallender EJ, Choi SS, Lahn BT. Reconstructing the evolutionary history of microcephalin, a gene controlling human brain size. *Hum Mol Genet* June 1, 2004;**13**(11):1139–45.

57. Evans PD, Anderson JR, Vallender EJ, et al. Adaptive evolution of ASPM, a major determinant of cerebral cortical size in humans. *Hum Mol Genet* March 1, 2004;**13**(5):489–94.

58. Feng Y, Chen MH, Moskowitz IP, et al. Filamin A (FLNA) is required for cell-cell contact in vascular development and cardiac morphogenesis. *Proc Natl Acad Sci USA* December 26, 2006;**103**(52):19836–41.

59. Guerrini R, Mei D, Sisodiya S, et al. Germline and mosaic mutations of FLN1 in men with periventricular heterotopia. *Neurology* July 13, 2004;**63**(1):51—6.

60. Sheen VL, Ganesh VS, Topcu M, et al. Mutations in ARFGEF2 implicate vesicle trafficking in neural progenitor proliferation and migration in the human cerebral cortex. *Nat Genet* January 2004;**36**(1):69—76.

61. Cardoso C, Boys A, Parrini E, et al. Periventricular heterotopia, mental retardation, and epilepsy associated with 5q14.3-q15 deletion. *Neurology* March 3, 2009;**72**(9):784—92.

62. Guerrini R, Parrini E. Neuronal migration disorders. *Neurobiol Dis* May 2010;**38**(2):154—66.

63. Shu T, Ayala R, Nguyen MD, Xie Z, Gleeson JG, Tsai LH. Ndel1 operates in a common pathway with LIS1 and cytoplasmic dynein to regulate cortical neuronal positioning. *Neuron* October 14, 2004; **44**(2):263—77.

64. Francis F, Koulakoff A, Boucher D, et al. Doublecortin is a developmentally regulated, microtubule-associated protein expressed in migrating and differentiating neurons. *Neuron* June 1999; **23**(2):247—56.

65. Moores CA, Perderiset M, Francis F, Chelly J, Houdusse A, Milligan RA. Mechanism of microtubule stabilization by doublecortin. *Mol Cell* June 18, 2004;**14**(6):833—9.

66. Kappeler C, Dhenain M, Phan Dinh Tuy F, et al. Magnetic resonance imaging and histological studies of corpus callosal and hippocampal abnormalities linked to doublecortin deficiency. *J Comp Neurol* January 10, 2007;**500**(2):239—54.

67. Kappeler C, Saillour Y, Baudoin JP, et al. Branching and nucleokinesis defects in migrating interneurons derived from doublecortin knockout mice. *Hum Mol Genet* May 1, 2006;**15**(9):1387—400.

68. Corbo JC, Deuel TA, Long JM, et al. Doublecortin is required in mice for lamination of the hippocampus but not the neocortex. *J Neurosci* September 1, 2002;**22**(17):7548—57.

69. Pilz DT, Matsumoto N, Minnerath S, et al. LIS1 and XLIS (DCX) mutations cause most classical lissencephaly, but different patterns of malformation. *Hum Mol Genet* December 1998;**7**(13): 2029—37.

70. Dobyns WB, Truwit CL, Ross ME, et al. Differences in the gyral pattern distinguish chromosome 17-linked and X-linked lissencephaly. *Neurology* July 22, 1999;**53**(2):270—7.

71. des Portes V, Pinard JM, Billuart P, et al. A novel CNS gene required for neuronal migration and involved in X-linked subcortical laminar heterotopia and lissencephaly syndrome. *Cell* January 9, 1998;**92**(1):51—61.

72. Gleeson JG, Allen KM, Fox JW, et al. Doublecortin, a brain-specific gene mutated in human X-linked lissencephaly and double cortex syndrome, encodes a putative signaling protein. *Cell* January 9, 1998;**92**(1):63—72.

73. Bahi-Buisson N, Souville I, Fourniol FJ, et al. New insights into genotype-phenotype correlations for the doublecortin-related lissencephaly spectrum. *Brain* January 2013;**136**(Pt 1):223—44.

74. Gleeson JG. Classical lissencephaly and double cortex (subcortical band heterotopia): LIS1 and doublecortin. *Curr Opin Neurol* April 2000;**13**(2):121—5.

75. Matsumoto N, Leventer RJ, Kuc JA, et al. Mutation analysis of the DCX gene and genotype/phenotype correlation in subcortical band heterotopia. *Eur J Hum Genet* January 2001;**9**(1):5—12.

76. Poolos NP, Das S, Clark GD, et al. Males with epilepsy, complete subcortical band heterotopia, and somatic mosaicism for DCX. *Neurology* May 28, 2002;**58**(10):1559—62.

77. Quelin C, Saillour Y, Souville I, et al. Mosaic DCX deletion causes subcortical band heterotopia in males. *Neurogenetics* November 2012;**13**(4):367—73.

78. Jamuar SS, Lam AT, Kircher M, et al. Somatic mutations in cerebral cortical malformations. *N Engl J Med* August 21, 2014; **371**(8):733—43.

79. Pilz DT, Kuc J, Matsumoto N, et al. Subcortical band heterotopia in rare affected males can be caused by missense mutations in DCX (XLIS) or LIS1. *Hum Mol Genet* September 1999;**8**(9):1757—60.

80. Kielar M, Tuy FP, Bizzotto S, et al. Mutations in Eml1 lead to ectopic progenitors and neuronal heterotopia in mouse and human. *Nat Neurosci* July 2014;**17**(7):923—33.

81. Keays DA, Tian G, Poirier K, et al. Mutations in alpha-tubulin cause abnormal neuronal migration in mice and lissencephaly in humans. *Cell* January 12, 2007;**128**(1):45—57.

82. Bahi-Buisson N, Poirier K, Boddaert N, et al. Refinement of cortical dysgeneses spectrum associated with TUBA1A mutations. *J Med Genet* October 2008;**45**(10):647—53.

83. Breuss M, Heng JI, Poirier K, et al. Mutations in the beta-tubulin gene TUBB5 cause microcephaly with structural brain abnormalities. *Cell Rep* December 27, 2012;**2**(6):1554—62.

84. Jaglin XH, Poirier K, Saillour Y, et al. Mutations in the beta-tubulin gene TUBB2B result in asymmetrical polymicrogyria. *Nat Genet* June 2009;**41**(6):746—52.

85. Poirier K, Saillour Y, Bahi-Buisson N, et al. Mutations in the neuronal tubulin subunit TUBB3 result in malformation of cortical development and neuronal migration defects. *Hum Mol Genet* November 15, 2010;**19**(22):4462—73.

86. Poirier K, Lebrun N, Broix L, et al. Mutations in TUBG1, DYNC1H1, KIF5C and KIF2A cause malformations of cortical development and microcephaly. *Nat Genet* June 2013;**45**(6): 639—47.

87. Raymond AA, Fish DR, Sisodiya SM, Alsanjari N, Stevens JM, Shorvon SD. Abnormalities of gyration, heterotopias, tuberous sclerosis, focal cortical dysplasia, microdysgenesis, dysembryoplastic neuroepithelial tumour and dysgenesis of the archicortex in epilepsy. Clinical, EEG and neuroimaging features in 100 adult patients. *Brain* June 1995;**118**(Pt 3):629—60.

88. Glaser T, Jepeal L, Edwards JG, Young SR, Favor J, Maas RL. PAX6 gene dosage effect in a family with congenital cataracts, aniridia, anophthalmia and central nervous system defects. *Nat Genet* August 1994;**7**(4):463—71.

89. Baala L, Briault S, Etchevers HC, et al. Homozygous silencing of T-box transcription factor EOMES leads to microcephaly with polymicrogyria and corpus callosum agenesis. *Nat Genet* April 2007; **39**(4):454—6.

90. Brooks AS, Bertoli-Avella AM, Burzynski GM, et al. Homozygous nonsense mutations in KIAA1279 are associated with malformations of the central and enteric nervous systems. *Am J Hum Genet* July 2005;**77**(1):120—6.

91. Cantagrel V, Lossi AM, Lisgo S, et al. Truncation of NHEJ1 in a patient with polymicrogyria. *Hum Mutat* April 2007;**28**(4):356—64.

92. Aligianis IA, Johnson CA, Gissen P, et al. Mutations of the catalytic subunit of RAB3GAP cause Warburg Micro syndrome. *Nat Genet* March 2005;**37**(3):221—3.

93. Roll P, Rudolf G, Pereira S, et al. SRPX2 mutations in disorders of language cortex and cognition. *Hum Mol Genet* April 1, 2006;**15**(7): 1195—207.

94. Villard L, Nguyen K, Cardoso C, et al. A locus for bilateral perisylvian polymicrogyria maps to Xq28. *Am J Hum Genet* April 2002; **70**(4):1003—8.

95. Robin NH, Taylor CJ, McDonald-McGinn DM, et al. Polymicrogyria and deletion 22q11.2 syndrome: window to the etiology of a common cortical malformation. *Am J Med Genet A* November 15, 2006;**140**(22):2416—25.

96. Dobyns WB, Mirzaa G, Christian SL, et al. Consistent chromosome abnormalities identify novel polymicrogyria loci in 1p36.3, 2p16.1-p23.1, 4q21.21-q22.1, 6q26-q27, and 21q2. *Am J Med Genet A* July 1, 2008;**146A**(13):1637—54.

97. Bahi-Buisson N, Poirier K, Fourniol F, et al. The wide spectrum of tubulinopathies: what are the key features for the diagnosis? *Brain* June 2014;**137**(Pt 6):1676—700.

98. Piao X, Hill RS, Bodell A, et al. G protein-coupled receptor-dependent development of human frontal cortex. *Science* March 26, 2004;**303**(5666):2033–6.

99. Bahi-Buisson N, Poirier K, Boddaert N, et al. GPR56-related bilateral frontoparietal polymicrogyria: further evidence for an overlap with the cobblestone complex. *Brain* November 2010;**133**(11):3194–209.

100. Li S, Jin Z, Koirala S, et al. GPR56 regulates pial basement membrane integrity and cortical lamination. *J Neurosci* May 28, 2008;**28**(22):5817–26.

101. Cushion TD, Dobyns WB, Mullins JG, et al. Overlapping cortical malformations and mutations in TUBB2B and TUBA1A. *Brain* February 2013;**136**(Pt 2):536–48.

102. Kumar RA, Pilz DT, Babatz TD, et al. TUBA1A mutations cause wide spectrum lissencephaly (smooth brain) and suggest that multiple neuronal migration pathways converge on alpha tubulins. *Hum Mol Genet* July 15, 2010;**19**(14):2817–27.

103. Barkovich AJ, Kjos BO. Schizencephaly: correlation of clinical findings with MR characteristics. *Am J Neuroradiol* January–February 1992;**13**(1):85–94.

104. Barkovich AJ, Norman D. MR imaging of schizencephaly. *Am J Roentgenol* June 1988;**150**(6):1391–6.

105. Brunelli S, Faiella A, Capra V, et al. Germline mutations in the homeobox gene EMX2 in patients with severe schizencephaly. *Nat Genet* January 1996;**12**(1):94–6.

106. Faiella A, Brunelli S, Granata T, et al. A number of schizencephaly patients including 2 brothers are heterozygous for germline mutations in the homeobox gene EMX2. *Eur J Hum Genet* July–August 1997;**5**(4):186–90.

107. Mallamaci A, Muzio L, Chan CH, Parnavelas J, Boncinelli E. Area identity shifts in the early cerebral cortex of Emx2-/- mutant mice. *Nat Neurosci* July 2000;**3**(7):679–86.

108. Merello E, Swanson E, De Marco P, et al. No major role for the EMX2 gene in schizencephaly. *Am J Med Genet A* May 1, 2008;**146A**(9):1142–50.

109. Pellegrini M, Mansouri A, Simeone A, Boncinelli E, Gruss P. Dentate gyrus formation requires Emx2. *Development* December 1996;**122**(12):3893–8.

110. Hehr U, Pineda-Alvarez DE, Uyanik G, et al. Heterozygous mutations in SIX3 and SHH are associated with schizencephaly and further expand the clinical spectrum of holoprosencephaly. *Hum Genet* March 2010;**127**(5):555–61.

111. Schell-Apacik CC, Ertl-Wagner B, Panzel A, et al. Maternally inherited heterozygous sequence change in the sonic hedgehog gene in a male patient with bilateral closed-lip schizencephaly and partial absence of the corpus callosum. *Am J Med Genet A* July 2009;**149A**(7):1592–4.

112. Yoneda Y, Haginoya K, Kato M, et al. Phenotypic spectrum of COL4A1 mutations: porencephaly to schizencephaly. *Ann Neurol* January 2013;**73**(1):48–57.

113. Nakano I, Funahashi M, Takada K, Toda T. Are breaches in the glia limitans the primary cause of the micropolygyria in Fukuyama-type congenital muscular dystrophy (FCMD)? Pathological study of the cerebral cortex of an FCMD fetus. *Acta Neuropathol* 1996;**91**(3):313–21.

114. Dobyns WB, Pagon RA, Armstrong D, et al. Diagnostic criteria for Walker-Warburg syndrome. *Am J Med Genet* February 1989;**32**(2):195–210.

115. Santavuori P, Somer H, Sainio K, et al. Muscle-eye-brain disease (MEB). *Brain Dev* 1989;**11**(3):147–53.

116. Fukuyama Y, Osawa M, Suzuki H. Congenital progressive muscular dystrophy of the Fukuyama type – clinical, genetic and pathological considerations. *Brain Dev* 1981;**3**(1):1–29.

117. Vuillaumier-Barrot S, Bouchet-Seraphin C, Chelbi M, et al. Identification of mutations in TMEM5 and ISPD as a cause of severe cobblestone lissencephaly. *Am J Hum Genet* December 7, 2012;**91**(6):1135–43.

118. Beltran-Valero de Bernabe D, Currier S, Steinbrecher A, et al. Mutations in the O-mannosyltransferase gene POMT1 give rise to the severe neuronal migration disorder Walker-Warburg syndrome. *Am J Hum Genet* November 2002;**71**(5):1033–43.

119. van Reeuwijk J, Janssen M, van den Elzen C, et al. POMT2 mutations cause alpha-dystroglycan hypoglycosylation and Walker-Warburg syndrome. *J Med Genet* December 2005;**42**(12):907–12.

120. Yoshida A, Kobayashi K, Manya H, et al. Muscular dystrophy and neuronal migration disorder caused by mutations in a glycosyltransferase, POMGnT1. *Dev Cell* November 2001;**1**(5):717–24.

121. Longman C, Brockington M, Torelli S, et al. Mutations in the human LARGE gene cause MDC1D, a novel form of congenital muscular dystrophy with severe mental retardation and abnormal glycosylation of alpha-dystroglycan. *Hum Mol Genet* November 1, 2003;**12**(21):2853–61.

122. Kondo-Iida E, Kobayashi K, Watanabe M, et al. Novel mutations and genotype-phenotype relationships in 107 families with Fukuyama-type congenital muscular dystrophy (FCMD). *Hum Mol Genet* November 1999;**8**(12):2303–9.

123. Brockington M, Blake DJ, Prandini P, et al. Mutations in the fukutin-related protein gene (FKRP) cause a form of congenital muscular dystrophy with secondary laminin alpha2 deficiency and abnormal glycosylation of alpha-dystroglycan. *Am J Hum Genet* December 2001;**69**(6):1198–209.

124. Stevens E, Carss KJ, Cirak S, et al. Mutations in B3GALNT2 cause congenital muscular dystrophy and hypoglycosylation of alpha-dystroglycan. *Am J Hum Genet* March 7, 2013;**92**(3):354–65.

125. Buysse K, Riemersma M, Powell G, et al. Missense mutations in beta-1,3-N-acetylglucosaminyltransferase 1 (B3GNT1) cause Walker-Warburg syndrome. *Hum Mol Genet* May 1, 2013;**22**(9):1746–54.

126. Manzini MC, Tambunan DE, Hill RS, et al. Exome sequencing and functional validation in zebrafish identify GTDC2 mutations as a cause of Walker-Warburg syndrome. *Am J Hum Genet* September 7, 2012;**91**(3):541–7.

127. Di Costanzo S, Balasubramanian A, Pond HL, et al. POMK mutations disrupt muscle development leading to a spectrum of neuromuscular presentations. *Hum Mol Genet* November 1, 2014;**23**(21):5781–92.

128. Radmanesh F, Caglayan AO, Silhavy JL, et al. Mutations in LAMB1 cause cobblestone brain malformation without muscular or ocular abnormalities. *Am J Hum Genet* March 7, 2013;**92**(3):468–74.

129. Willer T, Lee H, Lommel M, et al. ISPD loss-of-function mutations disrupt dystroglycan O-mannosylation and cause Walker-Warburg syndrome. *Nat Genet* May 2012;**44**(5):575–80.

130. Roscioli T, Kamsteeg EJ, Buysse K, et al. Mutations in ISPD cause Walker-Warburg syndrome and defective glycosylation of alpha-dystroglycan. *Nat Genet* May 2012;**44**(5):581–5.

131. Liu J, Yang Y, Li X, Zhang P, Qi Y, Hu H. Cellular and molecular characterization of abnormal brain development in protein o-mannose N-acetylglucosaminyltransferase 1 knockout mice. *Methods Enzymol* 2010;**479**:353–66.

132. Satz JS, Barresi R, Durbeej M, et al. Brain and eye malformations resembling Walker-Warburg syndrome are recapitulated in mice by dystroglycan deletion in the epiblast. *J Neurosci* October 15, 2008;**28**(42):10567–75.

133. Hu H, Li J, Gagen CS, et al. Conditional knockout of protein O-mannosyltransferase 2 reveals tissue-specific roles of O-mannosyl glycosylation in brain development. *J Comp Neurol* May 1, 2011;**519**(7):1320–37.

134. Wright KM, Lyon KA, Leung H, Leahy DJ, Ma L, Ginty DD. Dystroglycan organizes axon guidance cue localization and axonal pathfinding. *Neuron* December 6, 2012;**76**(5):931–44.

135. Chiyonobu T, Sasaki J, Nagai Y, et al. Effects of fukutin deficiency in the developing mouse brain. *Neuromuscul Disord* June 2005; **15**(6):416–26.

136. Kitamura K, Yanazawa M, Sugiyama N, et al. Mutation of ARX causes abnormal development of forebrain and testes in mice and X-linked lissencephaly with abnormal genitalia in humans. *Nat Genet* November 2002;**32**(3):359–69.

137. Shoubridge C, Fullston T, Gecz J. ARX spectrum disorders: making inroads into the molecular pathology. *Hum Mutat* August 2010;**31**(8):889–900.

138. Sicca F, Kelemen A, Genton P, et al. Mosaic mutations of the LIS1 gene cause subcortical band heterotopia. *Neurology* October 28, 2003;**61**(8):1042–6.

139. Poduri A, Evrony GD, Cai X, et al. Somatic activation of AKT3 causes hemispheric developmental brain malformations. *Neuron* April 12, 2012;**74**(1):41–8.

140. Lee JH, Huynh M, Silhavy JL, et al. De novo somatic mutations in components of the PI3K-AKT3-mTOR pathway cause hemimegalencephaly. *Nat Genet* August 2012;**44**(8):941–5.

141. Kurek KC, Luks VL, Ayturk UM, et al. Somatic mosaic activating mutations in PIK3CA cause CLOVES syndrome. *Am J Hum Genet* June 8, 2012;**90**(6):1108–15.

142. Lindhurst MJ, Parker VE, Payne F, et al. Mosaic overgrowth with fibroadipose hyperplasia is caused by somatic activating mutations in PIK3CA. *Nat Genet* August 2012;**44**(8):928–33.

143. De Ciantis A, Barkovich AJ, Cosottini M, et al. Ultra-high-field MR imaging in polymicrogyria and epilepsy. *Am J Neuroradiol* September 25, 2014;**36**(2):309–16.

144. Vulto-van Silfhout AT, Nakagawa T, Bahi-Buisson N, et al. Variants in CUL4B are associated with cerebral malformations. *Hum Mutat* January 2015;**36**(1):106–17.

145. Mitchell JJ, Trakadis YJ, Scriver CR. Phenylalanine hydroxylase deficiency. *Genet Med* August 2011;**13**(8):697–707.

146. Folling I. The discovery of phenylketonuria. *Acta Paediatr Suppl* December 1994;**407**:4–10.

147. Picker JD, Walsh CA. New innovations: therapeutic opportunities for intellectual disabilities. *Ann Neurol* September 2013;**74**(3): 382–90.

148. Manent JB, Wang Y, Chang Y, Paramasivam M, LoTurco JJ. Dcx reexpression reduces subcortical band heterotopia and seizure threshold in an animal model of neuronal migration disorder. *Nat Med* January 2009;**15**(1):84–90.

149. Wynshaw-Boris A, Pramparo T, Youn YH, Hirotsune S. Lissencephaly: mechanistic insights from animal models and potential therapeutic strategies. *Semin Cell Dev Biol* October 2010;**21**(8): 823–30.

150. Ramos RL, Bai J, LoTurco JJ. Heterotopia formation in rat but not mouse neocortex after RNA interference knockdown of DCX. *Cereb Cortex* September 2006;**16**(9):1323–31.

151. Baek ST, Kerjan G, Bielas SL, et al. Off-target effect of doublecortin family shRNA on neuronal migration associated with endogenous microRNA dysregulation. *Neuron* June 18, 2014;**82**(6): 1255–62.

152. Yamada M, Toba S, Yoshida Y, et al. LIS1 and NDEL1 coordinate the plus-end-directed transport of cytoplasmic dynein. *EMBO J* October 8, 2008;**27**(19):2471–83.

153. Yamada M, Yoshida Y, Mori D, et al. Inhibition of calpain increases LIS1 expression and partially rescues in vivo phenotypes in a mouse model of lissencephaly. *Nat Med* October 2009; **15**(10):1202–7.

154. Toba S, Tamura Y, Kumamoto K, et al. Post-natal treatment by a blood-brain-barrier permeable calpain inhibitor, SNJ1945 rescued defective function in lissencephaly. *Sci Rep* 2013;**3**:1224.

155. Liang Y, Gao H, Lin SY, et al. BRIT1/MCPH1 is essential for mitotic and meiotic recombination DNA repair and maintaining genomic stability in mice. *PLoS Genet* January 2010;**6**(1):e1000826.

156. Pulvers JN, Bryk J, Fish JL, et al. Mutations in mouse Aspm (abnormal spindle-like microcephaly associated) cause not only microcephaly but also major defects in the germline. *Proc Natl Acad Sci USA* September 21, 2010;**107**(38):16595–600.

157. Fish JL, Kosodo Y, Enard W, Paabo S, Huttner WB. Aspm specifically maintains symmetric proliferative divisions of neuroepithelial cells. *Proc Natl Acad Sci USA* July 5, 2006;**103**(27):10438–43.

158. Buchman JJ, Tseng HC, Zhou Y, Frank CL, Xie Z, Tsai LH. Cdk5rap2 interacts with pericentrin to maintain the neural progenitor pool in the developing neocortex. *Neuron* May 13, 2010; **66**(3):386–402.

159. Bogoyevitch MA, Yeap YY, Qu Z, et al. WD40-repeat protein 62 is a JNK-phosphorylated spindle pole protein required for spindle maintenance and timely mitotic progression. *J Cell Sci* November 1, 2012;**125**(Pt 21):5096–109.

160. Reiner O, Carrozzo R, Shen Y, et al. Isolation of a Miller-Dieker lissencephaly gene containing G protein beta-subunit-like repeats. *Nature* August 19, 1993;**364**(6439):717–21.

161. Hirotsune S, Fleck MW, Gambello MJ, et al. Graded reduction of Pafah1b1 (Lis1) activity results in neuronal migration defects and early embryonic lethality. *Nat Genet* August 1998;**19**(4):333–9.

162. Gopal PP, Simonet JC, Shapiro W, Golden JA. Leading process branch instability in Lis1+/- nonradially migrating interneurons. *Cereb Cortex* June 2010;**20**(6):1497–505.

163. Tsai JW, Chen Y, Kriegstein AR, Vallee RB. LIS1 RNA interference blocks neural stem cell division, morphogenesis, and motility at multiple stages. *J Cell Biol* September 12, 2005;**170**(6):935–45.

164. Koizumi H, Higginbotham H, Poon T, Tanaka T, Brinkman BC, Gleeson JG. Doublecortin maintains bipolar shape and nuclear translocation during migration in the adult forebrain. *Nat Neurosci* June 2006;**9**(6):779–86.

165. Bai J, Ramos RL, Ackman JB, Thomas AM, Lee RV, LoTurco JJ. RNAi reveals doublecortin is required for radial migration in rat neocortex. *Nat Neurosci* December 2003;**6**(12):1277–83.

166. Homma N, Takei Y, Tanaka Y, et al. Kinesin superfamily protein 2A (KIF2A) functions in suppression of collateral branch extension. *Cell* July 25, 2003;**114**(2):229–39.

167. Maor-Nof M, Homma N, Raanan C, Nof A, Hirokawa N, Yaron A. Axonal pruning is actively regulated by the microtubule-destabilizing protein kinesin superfamily protein 2A. *Cell Rep* April 25, 2013;**3**(4):971–7.

168. Yuba-Kubo A, Kubo A, Hata M, Tsukita S. Gene knockout analysis of two gamma-tubulin isoforms in mice. *Dev Biol* June 15, 2005;**282**(2):361–73.

169. Colasante G, Simonet JC, Calogero R, et al. ARX regulates cortical intermediate progenitor cell expansion and upper layer neuron formation through repression of Cdkn1c. *Cereb Cortex* August 22, 2013;**25**(2):322–35.

170. Friocourt G, Kanatani S, Tabata H, et al. Cell-autonomous roles of ARX in cell proliferation and neuronal migration during corticogenesis. *J Neurosci* May 28, 2008;**28**(22):5794–805.

171. Hong SE, Shugart YY, Huang DT, et al. Autosomal recessive lissencephaly with cerebellar hypoplasia is associated with human RELN mutations. *Nat Genet* September 2000;**26**(1):93–6.

172. Gulsuner S, Tekinay AB, Doerschner K, et al. Homozygosity mapping and targeted genomic sequencing reveal the gene responsible for cerebellar hypoplasia and quadrupedal locomotion in a consanguineous kindred. *Genome Res* December 2011;**21**(12): 1995–2003.

173. Trommsdorff M, Gotthardt M, Hiesberger T, et al. Reeler/Disabled-like disruption of neuronal migration in knockout mice lacking the VLDL receptor and ApoE receptor 2. *Cell* June 11, 1999;**97**(6):689–701.

174. Sheen VL, Dixon PH, Fox JW, et al. Mutations in the X-linked filamin 1 gene cause periventricular nodular heterotopia in males as well as in females. *Hum Mol Genet* August 15, 2001;**10**(17):1775–83.

175. Nagano T, Morikubo S, Sato M. Filamin A and FILIP (Filamin A-interacting protein) regulate cell polarity and motility in neocortical subventricular and intermediate zones during radial migration. *J Neurosci* October 27, 2004;**24**(43):9648–57.

176. Lian G, Lu J, Hu J, et al. Filamin a regulates neural progenitor proliferation and cortical size through Wee1-dependent Cdk1 phosphorylation. *J Neurosci* May 30, 2012;**32**(22):7672–84.

177. Carabalona A, Beguin S, Pallesi-Pocachard E, et al. A glial origin for periventricular nodular heterotopia caused by impaired expression of Filamin-A. *Hum Mol Genet* March 1, 2012;**21**(5):1004–17.

178. Zhang J, Neal J, Lian G, Shi B, Ferland RJ, Sheen V. Brefeldin A-inhibited guanine exchange factor 2 regulates filamin A phosphorylation and neuronal migration. *J Neurosci* September 5, 2012;**32**(36):12619–29.

179. Willer T, Prados B, Falcon-Perez JM, et al. Targeted disruption of the Walker-Warburg syndrome gene Pomt1 in mouse results in embryonic lethality. *Proc Natl Acad Sci USA* September 28, 2004;**101**(39):14126–31.

180. Li J, Yu M, Feng G, Hu H, Li X. Breaches of the pial basement membrane are associated with defective dentate gyrus development in mouse models of congenital muscular dystrophies. *Neurosci Lett* November 7, 2011;**505**(1):19–24.

181. Shaheen R, Faqeih E, Ansari S, Alkuraya FS. A truncating mutation in B3GNT1 causes severe Walker-Warburg syndrome. *Neurogenetics* July 23, 2013;**14**(3–4):243–5.

182. Miner JH, Li C, Mudd JL, Go G, Sutherland AE. Compositional and structural requirements for laminin and basement membranes during mouse embryo implantation and gastrulation. *Development* May 2004;**131**(10):2247–56.

183. Chan YM, Keramaris-Vrantsis E, Lidov HG, et al. Fukutin-related protein is essential for mouse muscle, brain and eye development and mutation recapitulates the wide clinical spectrums of dystroglycanopathies. *Hum Mol Genet* October 15, 2010;**19**(20):3995–4006.

184. Koirala S, Jin Z, Piao X, Corfas G. GPR56-regulated granule cell adhesion is essential for rostral cerebellar development. *J Neurosci* June 10, 2009;**29**(23):7439–49.

185. Harada A, Takei Y, Kanai Y, Tanaka Y, Nonaka S, Hirokawa N. Golgi vesiculation and lysosome dispersion in cells lacking cytoplasmic dynein. *J Cell Biol* April 6, 1998;**141**(1):51–9.

186. Hafezparast M, Klocke R, Ruhrberg C, et al. Mutations in dynein link motor neuron degeneration to defects in retrograde transport. *Science* May 2, 2003;**300**(5620):808–12.

187. Valence S, Poirier K, Lebrun N, et al. Homozygous truncating mutation of the KBP gene, encoding a KIF1B-binding protein, in a familial case of fetal polymicrogyria. *Neurogenetics* November 2013;**14**(3–4):215–24.

188. Stottmann RW, Donlin M, Hafner A, Bernard A, Sinclair DA, Beier DR. A mutation in Tubb2b, a human polymicrogyria gene, leads to lethality and abnormal cortical development in the mouse. *Hum Mol Genet* June 19, 2013;**22**(20):4053–63.

189. Tischfield MA, Baris HN, Wu C, et al. Human TUBB3 mutations perturb microtubule dynamics, kinesin interactions, and axon guidance. *Cell* January 8, 2010;**140**(1):74–87.

190. Sisodiya SM, Free SL, Williamson KA, et al. PAX6 haploinsufficiency causes cerebral malformation and olfactory dysfunction in humans. *Nat Genet* July 2001;**28**(3):214–6.

191. Stoykova A, Hatano O, Gruss P, Gotz M. Increase in reelin-positive cells in the marginal zone of Pax6 mutant mouse cortex. *Cereb Cortex* June 2003;**13**(6):560–71.

192. Kroll TT, O'Leary DD. Ventralized dorsal telencephalic progenitors in Pax6 mutant mice generate GABA interneurons of a lateral ganglionic eminence fate. *Proc Natl Acad Sci USA* May 17, 2005;**102**(20):7374–9.

193. Arnold SJ, Huang GJ, Cheung AF, et al. The T-box transcription factor Eomes/Tbr2 regulates neurogenesis in the cortical subventricular zone. *Genes Dev* September 15, 2008;**22**(18):2479–84.

194. Komada M, Saitsu H, Kinboshi M, Miura T, Shiota K, Ishibashi M. Hedgehog signaling is involved in development of the neocortex. *Development* August 2008;**135**(16):2717–27.

195. Rizzoti K, Brunelli S, Carmignac D, Thomas PQ, Robinson IC, Lovell-Badge R. SOX3 is required during the formation of the hypothalamo-pituitary axis. *Nat Genet* March 2004;**36**(3):247–55.

196. Capra V, Biancheri R, Morana G, et al. Periventricular nodular heterotopia in Smith-Magenis syndrome. *Am J Med Genet A* December 2014;**164A**(12):3142–7.

197. Barba C, Parrini E, Coras R, et al. Co-occurring malformations of cortical development and SCN1A gene mutations. *Epilepsia* July 2014;**55**(7):1009–19.

5

Immune Dysfunction in Autism Spectrum Disorder

Natalia V. Malkova, Elaine Y. Hsiao

Division of Biology and Biological Engineering, California Institute of Technology, Pasadena, CA, USA

INTRODUCTION

Autism spectrum disorder (ASD) is a pervasive neurodevelopmental disorder diagnosed based on core impairments in social interaction and communication, and the presence of repetitive or stereotyped behaviors. In addition to the spectrum of particular types and severities of these cardinal diagnostic criteria, there is also a spectrum in the diversity of medical comorbidities associated with ASD. Immune dysregulation is of particular interest in light of increasing evidence that immunological abnormalities are seen across several body sites, including the brain, blood, peripheral lymphoid organs, and gastrointestinal (GI) tract, in ASD individuals. Overt immune dysfunction is comorbid in an estimated 15–60% of ASD children.[128] Immune alterations in ASD are further seen at various levels of biological examination, including gene expression analysis, cytokine profiling, and cellular functional assays. Not just a widespread symptom of ASD, immune dysregulation is also implicated in the etiopathogenesis of the disorder. Maternal infection, autoantibody production, and autoimmune diseases are associated with increased risk for ASD in the offspring. In addition, various genetic and environmental risk factors for ASD are known to alter immune function, and as such, may converge on immune dysregulation as a common pathological element (Figure 1).

Here we review neural, peripheral, and enteric immune abnormalities seen in ASD. We further discuss immune-related genetic and environmental risk factors for ASD, and preclinical investigations into the role of immune-related gene—environment interactions in increasing risk for ASD-related behavioral and neuropathological abnormalities. Finally, we review evidence supporting immunomodulatory treatments for ASD and

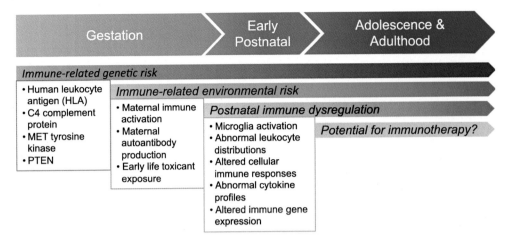

FIGURE 1   Immune contributions to ASD.

consider future directions for understanding the role of immune factors in neurodevelopment and the etiology of ASD.

IMMUNE ABNORMALITIES IN ASD

The Neuroimmune System

A number of studies demonstrate striking immune abnormalities in brains from individuals with ASD.[100,173] Neuroglia are particularly affected, and are composed of microglia, the resident monocyte-derived leukocytes in the brain, as well as astrocytes, star-shaped glial cells that have an important role in the secretion or absorption of neurotransmitters, blood—brain barrier (BBB) maintenance, neuronal migration, and brain repair. Both microglia and astrocytes are activated in the brains of ASD patients.[100,117,118,160,165,173] Microgliosis and astrogliosis are detected in many brain areas, but the cerebellum exhibits the most prominent neuroglial responses that occur predominantly in the Purkinje cell layer. Consistent with these findings, positron emission tomography imaging studies reveal increased binding of a microglial ligand in various brain regions, suggesting ongoing microglial activation in brains of living ASD individuals.[160] Interestingly, microglial and astroglial activation is observed in the absence of overt lymphocyte infiltration or immunoglobulin deposition in the central nervous system (CNS).

Morphological detection of neuroglial activation is further associated with signs of elevated functional activity, in which various regions of the ASD postnatal brain exhibit increased levels of cytokines, such as monocyte chemoattractant protein (MCP)-1, insulin-like growth factor-binding protein 1 (IGFBP-1), interleukin (IL)-6, IL-8, transforming growth factor (TGF)-β1, tumor necrosis factor (TNF)-α, granulocyte-macrophage colony stimulating factor, and interferon (IFN)-gamma.[104,173] Analysis of cerebrospinal fluid (CSF) from living patients with ASD also reveals a proinflammatory-like profile characterized by marked increases in MCP-1, IL-6, IL-8, IFN-gamma, macrophage inflammatory protein (MIP)-1, IFN-gamma inducing protein-10 (IP-10), and TNF-α, as well alterations in levels of growth factors, such as macrophage migration inhibitory factor (MIF), vascular endothelial growth factor, leukemia inhibitory factor, osteoprotegerin, hepatocyte growth factor (HGF), fibroblast growth factor (FGF)-4, FGF-9, IGFBP3, and IGFBP4.[40,173,195] These cytokine signatures in the CSF are consistent with the observation of activated microglia and astroglia in the ASD postmortem brain, suggesting ongoing CNS inflammation in ASD.

Transcriptomic analyses further reveal significant overexpression of immune response pathways in the frontal and temporal cortices of ASD brains.[65,174] Immune response genes are among the most significantly dysregulated in a whole-genome analysis study of the ASD prefrontal cortex.[42] Changes in the expression of gene modules related to inflammation and immune activation are reported to correlate with the severity of particular ASD-related behaviors,[66] pointing to a potential contribution of neuroimmune dysregulation to the development of core ASD symptoms.

The Peripheral Immune System

Outside the CNS, a variety of systemic immune abnormalities have been detected in ASD individuals, including changes in the abundance of immune cell subtypes,[190] aberrant cytokine and chemokine production,[5,7,72,151,159,195] and alterations in cellular immune function at rest and in response to immunological challenge[54,60] (Table 1). Notably, many of these systemic immune changes correlate with the severity of

TABLE 1   Abnormal Peripheral Immune Functions in ASD Patients

Component of Immune System	Abnormalities	References
T cells	Low number of T cells	177,181,190
T helper cells (CD4+)	Low number of CD4+ T cells	53,77,141,177,181,190
	Low Fas expression on CD4+ T cells	58
Cytotoxic T cells (CD8+)	Low number of CD8+ T cells	77,141
	No changes in number of CD8+ T cells	177,181
Regulatory T cells (CD4+CD25+)	Decreased number of regulatory T cells (Tregs)	119
	No changes in number of Tregs	182
Natural killer (NK) cells (CD3−CD56+)	Low NK activity resulting from low intracellular levels of glutathione, IL-2, and IL-15	175
	No changes in number of NK cells	177,181
	Increased expression of NK cell associated genes in blood	59,60,71
	Increased number but decreased activity of NK cells; increased NK production of perforin, granzyme B, and IFN-alfa	59,60
B cells	Low number of B cells	190
	No changes in number of B cells	177,181
	Increased number of D8/17-positive B cells positively correlated with severity of repetitive behaviors	83
	Increased number of activated CD19/CD23 B cells	182
Monocytes/ macrophages	Increased number of monocytes and high level of neopterin and NO that indicates activation of cell-mediated immune response	113,162,163,170
	Increased production of TNF-α, IL-4, IL-5, and IL-13 by unstimulated and stimulated monocytes	92,114,115
	Decreased production of IL-23 by stimulated monocytes	126
Mast cells	Increased release of mitochondrial DNA by activated mast cells	196
Immune-related genes	Increased frequency of complement protein C4B null allele	124,176,180
	Prevalence of HLA-DRB1*04	103,169
	Polymorphism of MIF associated with stereotypic behavior	72
	Increased frequency of MET receptor tyrosine C allele	35,36,197
	Single-nucleotide polymorphism in PRKCB1 gene that results in decreased gene expression and protein production	106,133
	Mutations in protein phosphatase and tensin homolog (PTEN)	198,108
	Increased RNA gene expression of 11 genes involved in mediated cytotoxicity pathway including perforin and granzyme B	59,60,71
Cytokines	Increased plasma IFN-gamma, MIF, TNF-α, IL-1β, IL-1RA, IL-4, IL-5, IL-6, IL-8, IL-12, IL-13, IL-17, MCP-1, RANTES, eotaxin, and GRO-α levels	5−7,59,60,72,159,170,195
	Decreased plasma level for TGF-β1	125
Ig	Diminished level of IgA but not IgG and IgE	182,199
	Reduced levels of plasma immunoglobulin (Ig)G and IgM correlated with behavioral severity	82
	Increased level of IgG4 positively correlated with stereotypical behavior and lethargy	59,60

Continued

I. AUTISM SPECTRUM DISORDERS AND INTELLECTUAL DISABILITY: GENETIC AND NON-GENETIC CAUSES

TABLE 1   Abnormal Peripheral Immune Functions in ASD Patients—cont'd

Component of Immune System	Abnormalities	References
	Increased IgG level	47,171
	Increased IgE level	76
	Increased levels of autoantibodies to NAFP, GFAP, MBP, and BDNF	43,152,153
	Serum autoantibodies to basal ganglia and frontal lobe cingulate gyrus and cerebellum	136,149,186,184

NK, natural killers; IL, interleukin; CD, cluster of differentiation; IFN, interferon; Treg, regulatory T cell; NO, nitric oxide; TNF, tumor necrosis factor; Ig, immunoglobulin; HLA, human leukocyte antigen; MIF, macrophage migration inhibitory factor; MCP-1, monocyte chemoattractant protein-1; RANTES, regulated on activation normal T cell expressed and secreted; TGF, transforming growth factor; NAFP, neuron-axon filament protein; GFAP, glial fibrillary acidic protein; MBP, myelin basic protein; BDNF, brain-derived neurotrophic factor.

impairments in core behavioral phenotypes of ASD,[5,6,72,82,83] which raises the important question of whether immune abnormalities contribute to the development or persistence of ASD or whether they are an epiphenomenon or side effect of primary neural dysfunction.

Cellular Immunity

Altered abundances of various subtypes of T cells, including CD4+ T helper cells, which assist in the maturation, activation, and proliferation of other leukocytes, and CD8+ cytotoxic T cells, which have a pivotal role in destroying virally infected and tumor cells, have been identified in ASD individuals. Statistically significant decreases in blood levels of CD4+ and CD8+ T cells,[141,181,190] as well as abnormal distributions of CD4+ and CD8+ T cells,[53,77,178] have been reported in ASD. In addition, ASD patients display decreased levels of IFN-gamma and IL-2 synthesizing CD4+ and CD8+ T cells but increased IL-4–containing T cells, further supporting ASD-associated alterations in particular T cell subsets. Interestingly, decreased levels of CD4+ cells that express IL-2 receptor are reported to correlate with the severity of ASD symptoms.[53] Reduced Fas expression by CD4+ T cells and higher plasma levels of soluble Fas have been described in ASD patients,[58] which mirrors similar findings in autoimmune disease.[67,123,166] Fas is a cell-surface protein involved in the initiation of apoptosis in immune cells. Autism spectrum disorder patients also display a significantly lower number of CD4+CD25 + Tregs, which have a key role in immunosuppression and immune tolerance. These cells are deficient in 73.3% of children with ASD, a phenotype that is similarly seen in individuals with allergy (40%) or with a family history of autoimmunity (53.3%).[119]

Altered levels of NK cells, leukocytes that contribute to host antimicrobial and antitumor defense, are also reported in ASD. In a study of 1027 autistic children, 45% exhibited low blood CD3−CD56+ NK cell activity, with low intracellular level of glutathione, IL-2, and IL-15.[175] Increased numbers of blood NK cells but decreased cytolytic activity are also seen in another study of ASD patients.[60] Interestingly, unstimulated NK cells from ASD children contain high levels of the cytolytic proteins perforin and granzyme B as well as IFN-gamma, indicating baseline NK cell abnormalities in ASD individuals.

Studies examining levels of B cells, which contribute humoral immunity by making antibodies and providing immunological memory, have yielded inconsistent results in ASD patients, from decreased[190] or unchanged[181] to elevated[83] B cell levels. Increased numbers of activated CD23/19 B cells and reduced levels of IgA have also been reported in ASD.[182] One study in particular reported increased abundance of D8/17-positive B cells in ASD individuals, which positively correlates with the severity of repetitive behavior.[83] D8/17 is a B cell antigen with unknown function, although it is increased in B cells of patients with autoimmune diseases (rheumatic fever and Sydenham chorea) and subgroups of patients with obsessive-compulsive disorder and Tourette disorder who exhibit highly repetitive behavior.[161]

Altered abundance and function of macrophages, which derive from monocytes, phagocytize pathogens, and present antigens to T lymphocytes to stimulate cell-mediated immunity, is also reported in ASD. Increased absolute monocyte counts and significantly higher levels of neopterin and nitric oxide (NO) are seen in blood samples from ASD individuals.[113,162,163,170] High neopterin concentration is an indicator of monocyte/macrophage activation[17] and is similarly observed in neurodegenerative diseases.[101] Elevated NO is associated with inflammatory diseases, including multiple sclerosis, rheumatoid arthritis, and acquired immunodeficiency syndrome.[68,69] Autism spectrum disorder monocytes also produce higher levels of TNF-α,[92] IL-4, IL-5, and IL-13[115] but decreased levels of IL-23.[126]

Blood Cytokines

Consistent with alterations in peripheral leukocyte profiles and functional responses, numerous studies report that ASD patients exhibit abnormal levels of plasma cytokines, including increases in IFN-gamma, MIF, MIP-1β, TNF-α, IL-1β, IL-1RA, IL-4, IL-5, IL-6, IL-8, IL-12, IL-13, IL-17, MCP-1, RANTES, eotaxin, and GRO-α.[5,7,60,72,159,170,195] Interestingly, plasma levels of TGF-β1, known to inhibit functions of T cells, B cells, and macrophages, are decreased in ASD patients,[125] providing one potential mechanism that contributes to the increased activation and production of proinflammatory cytokines by peripheral immune cells in ASD. There is also a strong positive correlation between increased levels of IL-1β, IL-6, IL-8, IL-12, RANTES, MIP-1α, MCP-1, MIF, and eotaxin and the severity of ASD behavioral traits, including lethargy, stereotypy, hyperactivity, impaired communication, and abnormal socialization.[5,7,72] These findings suggest that ongoing inflammatory responses may be linked to disturbances in ASD-related behavior, and raise the question of whether cytokines and their receptors might be tractable targets for ASD therapies.

Immunoglobulins

Altered levels of immunoglobulins (Igs), antibodies produced by B cells to identify and neutralize foreign antigens, are commonly reported in ASD,[59,82] but the data are diverse and often contradictory. Both increased[47,171] and decreased blood IgG levels[82] have been reported for ASD individuals compared with typically developing controls. Immunoglobulin M has also been reported to be both increased[171] and decreased,[82] whereas IgA has been reported to be either decreased[179,182] or unchanged.[171] Furthermore, one study finds that levels of IgG and IgM are negatively correlated with the severity of particular ASD behaviors,[82] whereas another study reports positive correlations between levels of IgG4 and the severity of behavioral abnormalities in ASD.[47,59] Aside from differences in experimental design, the inconsistency between experiments may be contributed by heterogeneity of the sample ASD cohort, in which symptom severity, genetic background, medical comorbidities, medicinal treatments, and dietary effects may be confounding factors.

Despite differential findings on gross levels of Ig subtypes in ASD, there is growing evidence for a link between ASD and increases in particular serum autoantibodies (IgG isotype) in both ASD individuals and their mothers.[9,136,150,152,184−186,194] Unique 37/73-kDa autoantibodies are observed specifically in sera from ASD mothers and are reported to react against fetal brain antigens. The autoantibodies identified in ASD children also exhibit reactivity to CNS structures, including the basal ganglia, frontal lobe cingulate gyrus, and cerebellum. In the cerebellum, immunoreactivity is localized to Golgi cells, GABAergic inhibitory neurons that have an integral role in cerebellar function.[88,136] Additional studies report that ASD children exhibit elevated levels of autoantibodies reactive to neuron-axon filament protein, glial fibrillary acidic protein, myelin basic protein, and brain-derived neurotrophic factor.[43,152,153] Subjects with plasma brain-reactive autoantibodies demonstrate greater emotional and behavioral difficulties[136] compared with controls. Preclinical studies demonstrate that autoantibody injection in rodents or monkeys can sufficiently cause abnormalities in brain and behavior, as discussed subsequently. Altogether, these data support the notion that brain-reactive autoimmunity may contribute to the etiopathogenesis or manifestations of disease symptoms in subsets of ASD individuals. These findings further contribute to a growing number of behavioral and psychiatric disorders rooted in autoantibody reactivity to brain antigens, including anti-N-methyl-D-aspartate encephalitis and pediatric autoimmune neuropsychiatric disorders associated with streptococcal infections.

The Enteric Immune System

Autism spectrum disorder individuals with comorbid GI abnormalities represent one clinical subtype that may be particularly relevant to the presence of immune abnormalities in ASD. Gastrointestinal disturbances such as constipation/diarrhea, gastroesophageal reflux, and abdominal pain are commonly observed in individuals with ASD, although the precise prevalences of particular GI symptoms in ASD are unclear.[30,45,85] Consistent with this, several abnormalities in the enteric immune system are seen in subsets of individuals with ASD, including leukocyte infiltration into the intestinal epithelium, altered abundances of immune cell subtypes, and nodular hyperplasia. Abnormal intestinal permeability and alterations in the composition of the GI microbiota are also reported, both of which can influence or be influenced by the immune system. An increasing number of studies are extending investigations of the gut−brain axis to explore the prospect that GI abnormalities may contribute to the severity of core ASD symptoms, and likewise, that correcting particular GI disruptions can improve features of ASD.

Neuroimmune Interactions

Overall, a preponderance of evidence supports widespread dysfunction of innate and adaptive immunity in ASD individuals. The vast majority of phenotypes are consistent with a proinflammatory-like state of the neuroimmune, peripheral, and enteric immune systems in ASD, in which particular leukocyte subtypes exhibit increased activation and/or elevated responses to stimulation. Interestingly, similar immune abnormalities have been reported for Rett syndrome and fragile X syndrome, neurodevelopmental disorders that involve features of ASD and well-defined genetic causes.[8,37,172] Many of these symptoms are also reported in neurodegenerative and inflammatory diseases, which suggests common inflammatory pathways relevant to diverse neurological, neurodevelopmental, and neurodegenerative diseases. Whether immune abnormalities and other ASD-related medical comorbidities are enriched particularly in ASD individuals with specific genetic signatures is a key question for future research. In addition, whether particular immune abnormalities contribute to the development or persistence of core ASD behaviors is unclear. However, a great body of literature supports the importance of neuroimmune and gut–brain interactions in modulating brain development and behavior.

It is now well established that the CNS is a highly immunologically active organ.[99] In addition to resident microglia and macrophages, there is increasing evidence that several other innate and adaptive immune cell subtypes are found in the healthy brain. Furthermore, resident leukocytes, astrocytes, and neurons themselves are known to produce and secrete various chemokines and cytokines.[63,98] Neurons express receptors for IL-1, TNF-α, IL-6, and IL-10, among several other cytokines, and cytokine-mediated signal transduction modulates neuronal excitability,[44] hormone release, and behavioral responses.[16,57] Canonical immune molecules and cell subtypes in the brain are being increasingly appreciated for their roles in normal neurodevelopment. Major histocompatibility complex (MHC) I and complement proteins fundamentally regulate synaptic transmission, plasticity, and network modeling. Resident microglia, in addition to regulating immune surveillance and activation, have a key role in synaptic pruning and connectivity during development. Moreover, cytokines produced by microglia influence neuronal proliferation and differentiation, neural repair, and BBB integrity. Overall, there are dynamic interactions between neurons and canonical immune cells, during normal neurodevelopment and inflammation-related conditions.

Peripheral Immune System–Brain Interactions

Products of immune activation in the periphery have extensive effects on brain activity and behavior.[135] Whereas some studies demonstrate that particular cytokines may cross the BBB and enter the CNS directly through the circumventricular organs, several effects of peripheral immune activation on the brain are conferred through long-range interactions. Peripheral cytokines modulate vagal nerve activity, and cytokine-mediated activation of afferent vagal neurons is known to cause sickness behavior in response to infection. In addition, peripheral cytokines and chemokines influence each process that comprises the hypothalamic–pituitary–adrenal (HPA) axis: (1) paraventricular nucleus of the hypothalamus releases corticotrophin-releasing hormone (CRH) and vasopressin; (2) the pituitary secretes adrenocorticotropic hormone (ACTH); and (3) the adrenal cortex produces glucocorticosteroids in response to stimulation by ACTH.[16] Glucocorticoids in turn suppress CRH and ACTH production in a negative feedback loop. Enhanced release of glucocorticosteroids also decreases release of proinflammatory cytokines from macrophages in the periphery, providing effective control over overactive inflammatory immune response.[193] Compared with controls, ASD patients are reported to exhibit altered HPA responses, with elevated levels of salivary cortisol[91] and higher plasma levels of ACTH.[164] Altogether, cytokines and hormones have an important role in regulating homeostasis between the CNS, the neuroendocrine system, and the immune system.

Disruptions in various pathways linking the nervous system, the neuroendocrine system, and the immune system have been implicated in mental disorders, including depression and neurodevelopmental disorders.[98] One of the proposed neuroimmune-based mechanistic hypotheses for the etiology of ASD emphasizes a role of proinflammatory cytokines aroused from maternal inflammation, infection, and possibly autoimmunity during pregnancy.[29,114] Increases in cytokines, or the "cytokine storm," could stimulate microglia and astrocytes, affecting neuronal growth and plasticity in the fetal brain. Such activation of neuroglia could also lead to a positive feedback loop, facilitating the development of a chronic inflammatory environment in the fetus and predisposing it to long-term psychiatric and systemic pathologies.[29] Whereas several studies demonstrate immune abnormalities in the periphery and brains of ASD individuals, more research is needed to investigate how these immune changes may alter neurodevelopment and brain function.

IMMUNE-RELATED SUSCEPTIBILITY FACTORS FOR ASD

Immune-Related Environmental Risk Factors

Although the precise etiologies of ASDs are largely unknown, genetic susceptibility factors are often considered primary contributors to the pathophysiological mechanisms underlying ASD.[70,131,132] Early twin studies reported 73–95% concordance for ASD in monozygotic twins compared with 0–10% in dizygotic twins.[14,157] However, a study of a large twin population (202 pairs) revealed an important contribution of environmental risk to ASD, in which genetic background contributed an estimated 38% whereas shared environmental factors explained approximately 55% of the liability to ASD.[78] This study provides evidence that the rate of concordance in dizygotic twins may have been underestimated in previous studies and reports 21–27% concordance for patients with strict autism and 31–36% for ASD. Moreover, another study that analyzed a population-based cohort of 2,049,973 Swedish children born in 1982 through 2006 estimated 50% heritability of ASD and autistic disorder.[139] Moreover, still unknown is the extent to which epigenetic alterations may contribute to the heritability of ASD. Altogether, these data indicate that environmental risk factors need to be considered alongside genetic susceptibility in the etiopathogenesis of ASD.

Maternal Immune Activation

Consistent with a role for environmental influences on the development of ASD, several environmental risk factors have been identified to increase ASD risk.[95,137,158] Maternal immune activation (MIA) during gestation is regarded as a principal nongenetic risk factor of ASD.[84,95] Early evidence that MIA increases the risk for ASD in the offspring was reported after the 1964 rubella pandemic, in which 8–13% of children born to infected mothers developed autism, which represented an over 200-fold increase in ASD prevalence at the time.[38] These results initiated more extensive epidemiological studies with other potential infectious agents leading to a seminal study, in which over 10,000 ASD cases out of all children born in Denmark from 1980 to 2005 were examined and a significant link between maternal infection during first trimester of pregnancy and increased risk of ASD was reported.[11] Another large epidemiological study that included 24,414 ASD cases from all residents of Stockholm County, Sweden reported similar findings.[102] Moreover, various types of infections including influenza, cytomegalovirus, measles, mumps, varicella, and rubella each have been associated with an increased risk for ASDs.[105] Consistent with this, elevated levels of several inflammatory markers in maternal serum and amniotic fluid are associated with increased ASD risk in the offspring, as are maternal fever and antibiotic treatment.[1,10,28,129,191] Altogether, these findings have led to the understanding that a generalized activation of the maternal immune system, rather than a site- or pathogen-specific infection, is responsible for increasing susceptibility for ASD in the offspring.

Based on the strong epidemiological and clinical studies linking MIA to ASD, several animal models of MIA have been developed to study the molecular bases of ASD-related endophenotypes. Several variations of MIA have been studied in rodents and monkeys, including direct infection with influenza virus and immune activation with the double-stranded RNA, poly(I:C), as a viral mimic,[87,109,148,155,187] or the cell wall antigen, lipopolysaccharide, as a bacterial mimic.[13,81,94] Remarkably, inducing MIA in pregnant mice, rats, or rhesus macaques yields offspring with core behavioral abnormalities that are relevant to ASD. Rodent offspring of MIA mothers exhibit deficits in auditory and olfactory communication, decreased social interaction, and highly repetitive behavior, in addition to elevated anxiety and deficient sensorimotor gating[87,109,148,155] (Table 2). Moreover, poly(I:C)-induced MIA in rhesus monkeys yields offspring with decreased communication and social activity as well as abnormal repetitive behavior.[15]

In addition to displaying behavioral features of ASD, rodent MIA offspring exhibit several neuropathologies relevant to ASD. Adult offspring born to immune-activated mice exhibit a spatially localized deficit in PCs in lobule VII of the cerebellum that aligns distinctly with a hallmark neuropathology of ASD, in which up to 70% of ASD individuals display hypoplasia of cerebellar lobules VI and VII and localized PC loss.[202,203] Maternal immune activation offspring also exhibit delayed migration of granule cells in lobules VI and VII,[201] which could contribute to the deficits in communication and social interaction observed in the MIA model, because the cerebellum is known to contribute to learning, language, sociability, and emotionality.[204,205] Consistent with this, cerebellar abnormalities in ASD are associated with alterations in novel object exploration and stereotyped behavior.[206,207] Moreover, functional magnetic resonance imaging reveals abnormal cerebellar activation during motor and cognitive tasks in ASD subjects,[208,209] and behavioral abnormalities in ASD, such as abnormal eye blink conditioning and visual saccades are particularly relevant for the known functions of lobules VI and VII.[210,211]

The MIA model exhibits face validity for ASD-related behavioral and neuropathological abnormalities, and also for ASD-associated immunological alterations.[6,7,100,173,190] Consistent with the finding that ASD individuals display alterations in T cell subsets and decreased levels of Tregs,[119] MIA offspring display altered immune profiles and function, characterized by a systemic deficit in Treg abundance. Maternal immune activation offspring also exhibit persistently hyperresponsive CD4+ T cells, which produce increased levels of IL-6 and IL-17 in response to stimulation,[86,110] which suggests a long-lasting, proinflammatory phenotype analogous to immune alterations reported in ASD

TABLE 2   Characterization of Environmental Rodent Models Relevant to ASD

Phenotype	MIA Model	Maternal AB	VPA
Behavior			
Social	Decreased social interaction[81,87,94,109,155]	Decreased sociability[25,149]	Decreased social interaction[143]
Communicative	Decreased ultrasonic vocalizations in young and adult mice[87,109,13]		Decreased ultrasonic vocalizations in response to female[183]
	Low olfactory communication[109]		
Repetitive	Highly repetitive behavior[87,109]		Highly repetitive behavior[144]
	Perseverative behavior[200]		
Other	Low exploratory activity[155,200]	Hyperactivity, impaired motor and sensory development, increased anxiety[49,149]	Low exploratory activity[143]
	Deficit in PPI[109,155]		High anxiety, memory deficits, lower sensitivity to pain and high sensitivity to painless stimuli and deficit in PPI[93,112,143]
	Impaired associative learning[13]		
	Increased anxiety[81]		
Brain pathology	Purkinje cell loss and delayed migration of granule cells in the VII lobule of cerebellum[201]	Microglial activation and increased fetal brain BDNF levels at E18[149]	Deficit in cerebellar Purkinje cells (PCs)[89]
			Activation of microglia and increased level of proinflammatory cytokines in brain[50,107]
			Increased apoptosis and cell loss in cortex[80,93,189]
Immune dysfunction	Deficit in Tregs, elevated levels of Gr-1—positive cells, elevated CD4+ T cell responsiveness, which produce increased IL-6 and IL-17 levels[86]		
Gut dysfunction	Increased gut permeability, abnormal intestinal cytokine profiles and altered microbial composition[87]		Changes in microbial composition, intestinal inflammation, loss of epithelial cells, and reduced level of serotonin in intestines[50,51]

patients.[5,7] Moreover, MIA during fetal development alters distributions of other leukocyte subtypes in the offspring, shifting hematopoietic stem cell differentiation toward the myeloid lineage and resulting in increased levels of monocytic and neutrophilic Gr-1+ cells. Granulocytes are major effectors of acute inflammation and contribute to chronic inflammatory conditions and adaptive immune responses.[96] High levels of monocytes and increased activity of these cells are also reported for ASD children.[92,113,115,162,163] Whether immune abnormalities actually contribute to the manifestation of core ASD symptoms is still unclear. Several studies demonstrate that the severity of particular immune alterations in ASD correlate with the severity of specific behavioral abnormalities, which suggests that there may be an interaction between immunological and behavioral traits.

In addition to behavioral, neurological, and immunological abnormalities, MIA offspring exhibit GI impairments similar to those observed in subsets of ASD.[30,45] In particular, MIA offspring display increased intestinal permeability, abnormal intestinal cytokine profiles, and altered composition of the gut microbiota.[87] It is becoming increasingly appreciated that the gut microbiota communicates with the nervous system through neural, endocrine, and immune pathways, conferring important effects on brain function and behavior.[48,116] As with particular immune alterations, some GI problems correlate with severity of core behavioral symptoms of ASD,[2] which suggests a possible interaction between GI symptoms and manifestation of ASD. Interestingly, probiotic therapy with the human commensal bacterium *Bacteroides fragilis* successfully corrects gut permeability, particularly changes in the gut microbiota, and ameliorates defects in communicative, stereotypic, anxiety-like, and sensorimotor behaviors in MIA offspring, suggesting that the gut microbiota can regulate behaviors relevant to neurodevelopmental disorders. Overall, modeling the MIA environmental risk factor in animals effectively yields offspring displaying cardinal behavioral, neuropathological, immunological, and GI symptoms of ASD. As such, the MIA model serves as a valuable tool for investigating mechanisms underlying how acute maternal immune challenge leads to persistent system-wide dysfunctions relevant to ASD and further enables exploration into potential therapies for ASD symptoms.

Autoantibody Production

Contributing to the substantial evidence that maternal immune status affects ASD risk, several autoantibodies reactive against CNS proteins have been identified in sera from ASD children.[150,184–186] In addition, studies have shown that mothers of children with ASD often have antibodies reactive to antigens on lymphocytes and in the CNS of their affected children.[27,177] One of the early case–control studies (61 mothers of ASD children and 102 control mothers) reported a highly specific pattern of autoantibody reactivity to fetal human brain proteins in the serum of mothers who had a child with ASD.[23] Immunoglobulin G reactivity to 37- and 73-kDa proteins in human fetal brain tissue is found in 8–12% of mothers with ASD children, whereas this phenomenon is not observed in mothers of typically developing children. Moreover, the presence of this immunoreactive IgG in the maternal serum highly correlated with abnormal brain enlargement in ASD children.[121] In addition, a population-based case–control study nested within a cohort of infants born between July 2000 and September 2001 demonstrated immunoreactivity to 39-kDa or a complex of 39- and 73-kDa proteins from human fetal brain tissue in 7% of mothers of ASD children.[46] Notably, autoantibodies from mothers of ASD children bind to fetal and adult mouse and rat brain, as well as fetal rhesus macaque brain.[24,149,194] The particular brain antigens that are targeted by ASD-associated maternal autoantibodies include lactate dehydrogenase A and B (LDH), cypin, stress-induced phosphoprotein 1 (STIP1), collapsin response mediator proteins 1 and 2 (CRMP1 and CRMP2), and Y-box-binding protein.[26] The proteins are known to have an important role in neurodevelopment, but interestingly are not specifically expressed in the brain.[26] Notably, ASD children from mothers with specific reactivity to LDH, STIP1, and CRMP1 and/or cypin (7% versus 0% in controls) demonstrate elevated stereotypical behaviors compared with ASD children from mothers lacking these antibodies. It is still unclear what initiates ASD-related production of autoantibodies, and furthermore, how these autoantibodies are generated, because the identified antigens from fetal brain are cytoplasmic. Although significantly higher levels of autoantibodies are detected in individuals with ASD compared with controls, the pathogenic significance of these particular antibodies is not yet understood.

Importantly, several studies demonstrate that injecting autoantibodies from mothers of ASD children into rodents or primates sufficiently causes behavioral and neuropathological abnormalities relevant to ASD, revealing a potential role for autoantibody production in the etiology of ASD (Table 2). In mice, prenatal exposure to antibodies from women with ASD children results in offspring with altered behavior, including hyperactivity, significantly impaired motor and sensory development, increased anxiety, and decreased sociability.[25,49,149] Moreover, maternal autoantibody injection leads to the activation of microglia in the fetal brain[25] and cerebellar abnormalities,[49] well-replicated characteristics of ASD. Similar results have been reported in rhesus monkey animal models, in which exposure to ASD-associated autoantibodies causes abnormal social behavior, reduced peer contact, increased nonsocial activity, hyperactivity, and whole-body stereotypies.[15,111] Moreover, male monkeys displaying ASD-related behavioral symptoms also exhibit enlarged brain volume, consistent with human neuroimaging data demonstrating increased brain size in boys with ASD.[122] Together, these studies demonstrate that in a significant number of ASD cases, maternal antibodies developed against certain fetal brain proteins may disturb embryonic brain development, possibly resulting in behavioral features of ASD. The exact mechanisms by which this may occur are still known, but would likely involve maternal synthesis of autoantibodies that cross the placenta and immature fetal BBB and bind to targets in the developing fetal brain. The implications of these findings are promising in their suggestion that the presence of ASD-related maternal autoantibodies can be used as reliable diagnostic markers and therapeutic targets for ASD.

Valproic Acid and Other Toxicants

Clinical studies over the past 40 years reveal that maternal use of the antiseizure drug valproic acid (VPA) is associated with birth defects, cognitive deficits, and increased risk of ASD in offspring.[127,137] In rodents, similar to MIA model, male offspring born to mothers injected during gestation with VPA display several ASD-related behaviors including increased stereotypic behaviors and decreased social interaction and communication[50,51,93,112,138,143,144,183] (Table 2). In addition, VPA offspring exhibit higher anxiety, memory deficits, lower sensitivity to pain, and higher sensitivity to painless stimuli and diminished acoustic prepulse inhibition.[93,112,143] Valproic acid mice also present with ASD-related neuropathologies, including deficient numbers of cerebellar PCs,[89] activation of microglia, and increased expression of proinflammatory cytokines in the brain.[50,107] Moreover, VPA exposure results in increased apoptosis and cell loss in both prefrontal and somatosensory cortices.[80,93,189] Interestingly, similar to MIA offspring, VPA mice also have disrupted gut microbiota[50,51] and changes in the microbial composition are negatively correlated with social behavior. These alterations in the microbiota are associated with intestinal inflammation, loss of epithelial cells, and reduced levels of serotonin in the intestines of VPA offspring. Thus, maternal exposure to VPA sufficiently leads to behavioral and neuropathological impairments in offspring that are relevant to ASD-related endophenotypes, rendering the VPA model with strong face and construct validity for ASD.

Environmental exposures to other toxicants, including organophosphates[61] and the teratogen thimerosal,[90] have been also linked epidemiologically to ASD,[212] but additional research is needed to corroborate these associations and to evaluate the effect of such toxicants in preclinical models.

Overall, an etiological role for environmental factors in ASD has been demonstrated in rodent models for MIA induced by viral and bacterial agents, maternal antibodies reactive to fetal tissues, and prenatal exposure to VPA. All three of these risk factors and models involve maternal and early-life immunological perturbations as potential causes of ASD-related behavioral, neuropathological, and comorbid medical symptoms. Maternal immune activation in rodents and monkeys effectively models cardinal social, communicative, and stereotypic features of ASD in addition to several brain pathologies, including localized PC deficits, and ASD-related immune and GI dysfunction. Exposure to maternal reactive autoantibodies or VPA in preclinical models also results in ASD-related features, but additional behavioral and biochemical abnormalities remain to be assessed (Table 2). Altogether, these environmental models provide evidence that immune-related environmental factors have an important role in the etiology of ASD.

Immune-Related Genetic Risk Factors

In addition to immune-related environmental risk factors, several immune-related genetic susceptibility factors have been identified to increase ASD risk (Table 1). In particular, human leukocyte antigen (HLA) genes are often associated with ASD.[103,169] This group of genes resides within a large genomic region known as the MHC on chromosome 6, which encodes cell-surface antigen-presenting proteins. Various HLA haplotypes, including *HLA-DR4*, occur more often in children with ASD compared with the general population.[103,169] Another gene located in MHC locus, which encodes the complement protein C4, is also associated with ASD. Autism spectrum disorder patients display an increased frequency of the C4B null allele that results in significant decrease in plasma C4B concentrations,[124,168,176,180] which could lead to deficient activation of complement pathway and humoral defense. In addition, polymorphisms in the *MIF* gene, and resultant increases plasma MIF levels, have been found in ASD and are positively correlated with behavioral indicators of ASD.[72] Moreover, 11 genes involved in NK-mediated cytotoxicity are altered in ASD children,[60,71] which suggests that there may be genetic bases for ASD-related immune abnormalities.[56]

Another ASD linkage region spans chromosome 7q21-q36, which includes the *MET* locus on chromosome 7q31.8–13 and several immune-related genes. The *MET* gene encodes a receptor tyrosine kinase that mediates HGF signaling in brain circuit formation, immune function, and GI repair.[130] The *MET* promoter common variant rs1858830 allele C is strongly associated with ASD and results in systemic transcriptional dysregulation and activation of the MET signaling pathway.[35,36,82] Additional studies reveal particular single nucleotide polymorphisms (SNPs) in the promoter of *MET* gene that are predominant in ASD patients.[213] The *Reelin* gene is also localized on chromosome 7q, with several genetic variants and SNPs associated with ASD,[64,65,145,214] many of which result in decreased protein production.[62] Reelin has a major role in synaptic plasticity, which may explain its involvement in such diverse neurological disorders as ASD, schizophrenia, bipolar disorder, and major depression.[62,73] In the periphery, reelin regulates the proliferation of T cells, B cells, and monocytes, with important implications for intestinal function and liver repair.[154,167]

A significant genetic association with ASD is also reported for *protein kinase C β1* (*PRKCB1*) gene that is located on human chromosome 16p11.2 and is involved in signal transduction, regulation of gene expression, and control of cell division in the CNS, immune system, digestive tract, and kidney.[106,133] The particular SNPs observed in ASD alter *PRKCB1* splicing, resulting in decreased PRKCB1 protein production and disrupted *PRKCB1*-regulated gene expression patterns, as observed in postmortem neocortical tissue.[106,133] In addition, mutations in *PRKCB1* in ASD patients lead to excessive renal oligopeptiduria.[106]

Tumor suppressor phosphatase and tensin homolog (PTEN) germline mutations are found in a small subset of ASD children with macrocephaly.[34,108,192] The PTEN homolog is an important regulator of the host immune response against melanoma cells that is responsible for repressing the expression of immunosuppressive cytokines by blocking the phosphatidylinositide 3-kinase pathway.[55] In ASD patients, mutations in *PTEN* result in dysfunction of neuronal cells and are hypothesized to contribute to abnormalities in social behavior.[34,108,192]

Collectively, that several genetic and environmental risk factors for ASD affect immune function raises the question of whether there are converging immune-related pathways that are disrupted in ASD. Studying the basic mechanisms underlying how these risk factors may lead to ASD-related phenotypes will help uncover functional overlaps among these various risk factors, and potential molecular targets for treatment development. Because immune dysregulation is a common co-morbidity of ASD, peripheral functional signatures may serve as useful molecular diagnostics for the sub-classification of ASD into well-defined subtypes. Moreover, genomic analysis of peripheral blood cells can reveal insight into relevant transcriptomic and functional alterations in the nervous system.

IMMUNE-RELATED TREATMENTS FOR ASD

Although there is a substantial body of literature demonstrating that peripheral and central immune abnormalities can alter brain development and behavior, whether the particular immune alterations seen in ASD actually contribute to core symptoms is unclear. Interestingly, a variety of immunomodulatory therapies have been evaluated for efficacy in treatment of ASD. Corticosteroids have shown some promise in improving ASD behavioral features, presumably through their physiological effects on stress and the immune response.[147,156] Treatment with a synthetic corticosteroid prednisolone advanced social interaction and speech in two separate studies. Moreover, two open-label studies including 11 and 44 children with ASD demonstrated that corticosteroid treatment improved speech, attention, and emotional abilities.[41,120] Moreover, treatment with ACTH that stimulates the release of corticosteroids from the adrenal cells enhanced social interaction and improved stereotypic behavior in ASD individuals.[31–33]

Lenalidomide, an immunomodulatory agent and analog of thalidomide, is commonly used in hematology and cancer therapy. It is known to inhibit production of the proinflammatory cytokines IL-1, IL-6, IL-12, and TNF-α while increasing release of the anti-inflammatory cytokine IL-10.[97] To date, there has been one open-label study of lenalidomide treatment in seven children with ASD, who also demonstrated elevated level of TNF-α in the CSF.[39] Treatment of ASD children with lenalidomide decreased serum and CSF levels of TNF-α and improved expressive and receptive language. Pioglitazone, another immunomodulator commonly used to treat diabetes mellitus and various autoimmune disorders, and spironolactone, a potassium sparing diuretic and aldosterone antagonist, resulted in significant improvement in

irritability, social withdrawal, stereotypy, and hyperactivity in ASD patients.[19,22]

Notably, combined therapy of risperidone, one of two current Food and Drug Administration–approved treatments for ASD, with immunomodulators such as the cyclooxygenase-2 inhibitors celecoxib and pentoxifylline, yielded a beneficial effect on ASD symptoms. Compared with control (risperidone plus placebo), an adjunctive treatment of risperidone and celecoxib or pentoxifylline resulted in significant improvement in irritability, social withdrawal, and stereotypic behavior,[3,4] as well as hyperactivity, and improvement in inappropriate speech for risperidone and pentoxifylline.[3] These findings reveal that risperidone and immunosuppressive treatments may target separate, albeit important pathways regulating ASD-associated behavioral symptoms.

Intravenous immune globulin (IVIG) treatment, used to treat autoimmune disorders and antibody deficiency,[75] yielded mixed results in ASD individuals. In a group of 10 ASD children with comorbid IgG deficiency,[76] IVIG treatment for 6 months resulted in clinical improvements, including increased eye contact, calmer behavior, decreased echolalia, and increased expressive speech. Similar results were reported in another retrospective study involving 26 ASD children, in whom IVIG treatment for 6 months resulted in improvements in irritability, social withdrawal, stereotypy, hyperactivity, and speech.[20] However, other attempts to use IVIG therapy reported no significant benefit.[52,134] Oral therapy with panglobulin, an encapsulated human immunoglobulin known for its immunomodulatory effects on mucosal immunity, also resulted in mixed results for treatment of ASD.[79,142] In a study of 12 ASD patients, 8-week treatment resulted in decreased GI abnormalities and improved social interaction and speech in 50% of patients.[142] However, a subsequent randomized double-blind, placebo-controlled trial with 125 ASD children[79] reported no significant effects of oral human immunoglobulin therapy in reducing ASD or GI symptoms.

In light of the comorbidity of ASD with GI abnormalities, in addition to an increasing appreciation that the gut microbiota fundamentally impacts brain development and behavior, microbe-based treatments for ASD have been of interest. Early studies revealed that in some ASD cases, antibiotic treatment resulted in behavioral improvement.[18,140] In particular, vancomycin treatment was associated with decreased levels of *Clostridia* spp. and related metabolic signatures, which have been implicated in ASD.[146] Similar findings were reported for metronidazole and ketoconazole therapy. Consistent with this association between microbial status and ASD behavior, a preclinical study revealed beneficial effects of treatment with the immunomodulatory bacterium *B. fragilis* on ASD-related behavior in the MIA mouse model.[87] Based on the notion that microbiota changes may contribute to the severity of ASD symptoms, clinical trials of fecal transplants, which successfully treat *Clostridium difficile* infection,[12,21] are currently being investigated for ASD.

Altogether, these studies of immunomodulatory and anti-inflammatory drugs for the treatment of ASD are promising, but there are some limitations. First, most such clinical trials were underpowered, carried out in small cohorts of ASD individuals. Second, many studies relied on retrospective reports from parents or guardians, and as such, may be confounded by reporting bias. In addition, longitudinal or long-term effects of immune treatment were often not evaluated. Third, immunological profiles were often not documented before or after treatment. Additional research is needed to examine whether immune-based treatments for ASD may be effective for the treatment of ASD.

CONCLUSION

Immune abnormalities are increasingly implicated in ASD. Several immune-related environmental insults, including MIA and maternal autoantibody production, are associated with increased ASD risk. Preclinical models of these factors sufficiently induce neuropathological and behavioral features, in addition to associated medical comorbidities, which suggests that early-life immune alterations may be involved in the etiopathogenesis of ASD. In addition, genome-wide association studies have identified several immune-related common gene variants, SNPs, and CNVs that are linked to elevated risk for ASD.[74,188] Translation of these immune-related genetic risk factors to animal models will be interesting to investigate whether ASD-associated immune abnormalities may be genetically encoded, and furthermore, whether they contribute to the development or manifestation of ASD-related endophenotypes.

Whether any of the immune-related environmental and/or genetic risk factors for ASD converge on similar pathogenic mechanisms is unclear. Additional studies comparing and contrasting the effects of various ASD-associated risk factors could reveal commonly modulated pathways and potential targets for intervention. Furthermore, the question of whether environmental risk for ASD can lead to epigenetic modifications that contribute to the high heritability of the disorder is intriguing but poorly understood. Indeed, epigenetic modifications and early-life programming of later-life disease is implicated in various other chronic diseases including asthma, allergy, and metabolic disorders, which raises the interesting question of analogous perturbations influence ASD etiology.

In addition to the impact of immune alterations in the form of environmental and genetic influence during early life, widespread immune dysfunction is observed in children and adults with ASD. Several phenotypic and functional abnormalities spanning various types of innate and adaptive immune cells are associated with ASD, leading to the hypothesis that immune dysregulation may be a useful parameter for defining subsets of ASD that exhibit phenotypic similarities. Although several immune abnormalities have been identified in ASD patients, the findings are often inconsistent because of methodological limitations and inherent heterogeneity in the disorder. Well-controlled studies on well-delineated subclasses of individuals with ASD are needed to bring clarity to the precise cellular immune signatures seen in subsets of individuals with ASD and to further guide preclinical studies on effects of ASD-related immune abnormalities in behavioral and neurodevelopment. Further investigation into the roles of immune factors and effects of immune alterations in brain and behavioral development will advance understanding of the molecular underpinnings of ASD, as well as the numerous other neurological and neurodegenerative diseases involving immune dysregulation.

References

1. Abdallah MW, Hougaard DM, Norgaard-Pedersen B, Grove J, Bonefeld-Jorgensen EC, Mortensen EL. Infections during pregnancy and after birth, and the risk of autism spectrum disorders: a register-based study utilizing a Danish historic birth cohort. *Turk Psikiyatri Derg* 2012;**23**:229–35.
2. Adams JB, Johansen LJ, Powell LD, Quig D, Rubin RA. Gastrointestinal flora and gastrointestinal status in children with autism—comparisons to typical children and correlation with autism severity. *BMC Gastroenterol* 2011;**11**:22.
3. Akhondzadeh S, Fallah J, Mohammadi MR, Imani R, Mohammadi M, Salehi B, et al. Double-blind, placebo-controlled trial of pentoxifylline added to risperidone: effects on aberrant behavior in children with autism. *Prog Neuropsychopharmacol Biol Psychiatry* 2010;**34**:32–6.
4. Asadabadi M, Mohammadi MR, Ghanizadeh A, Ashrafi M, Hassanzadeh E, Forghani S, et al. Celecoxib as adjunctive treatment to risperidone in children with autistic disorder: a randomized, double-blind, placebo-controlled trial. *Psychopharmacology (Berlin)* 2013;**225**:51–9.
5. Ashwood P, Krakowiak P, Hertz-Picciotto I, Hansen R, Pessah I, Van de Water J. Elevated plasma cytokines in autism spectrum disorders provide evidence of immune dysfunction and are associated with impaired behavioral outcome. *Brain Behav Immun* 2011a;**25**:40–5.
6. Ashwood P, Krakowiak P, Hertz-Picciotto I, Hansen R, Pessah IN, Van de Water J. Altered T cell responses in children with autism. *Brain Behav Immun* 2011b;**25**:840–9.
7. Ashwood P, Krakowiak P, Hertz-Picciotto I, Hansen R, Pessah IN, Van de Water J. Associations of impaired behaviors with elevated plasma chemokines in autism spectrum disorders. *J Neuroimmunol* 2011c;**232**:196–9.
8. Ashwood P, Nguyen DV, Hessl D, Hagerman RJ, Tassone F. Plasma cytokine profiles in fragile X subjects: is there a role for cytokines in the pathogenesis? *Brain Behav Immun* 2010;**24**:898–902.

9. Ashwood P, Van de Water J. A review of autism and the immune response. *Clin Dev Immunol* 2004;**11**:165—74.

10. Atladottir HO, Henriksen TB, Schendel DE, Parner ET. Autism after infection, febrile episodes, and antibiotic use during pregnancy: an exploratory study. *Pediatrics* 2012;**130**:e1447—1454.

11. Atladottir HO, Thorsen P, Ostergaard L, Schendel DE, Lemcke S, Abdallah M, et al. Maternal infection requiring hospitalization during pregnancy and autism spectrum disorders. *J Autism Dev Disord* 2010;**40**:1423—30.

12. Austin M, Mellow M, Tierney WM. Fecal microbiota transplantation in the treatment of clostridium difficile infections. *Am J Med* 2014;**127**:479—83.

13. Baharnoori M, Bhardwaj SK, Srivastava LK. Neonatal behavioral changes in rats with gestational exposure to lipopolysaccharide: a prenatal infection model for developmental neuropsychiatric disorders. *Schizophr Bull* 2012;**38**:444—56.

14. Bailey A, Le Couteur A, Gottesman I, Bolton P, Simonoff E, Yuzda E, et al. Autism as a strongly genetic disorder: evidence from a British twin study. *Psychol Med* 1995;**25**:63—77.

15. Bauman MD, Iosif AM, Smith SE, Bregere C, Amaral DG, Patterson PH. Activation of the maternal immune system during pregnancy alters behavioral development of rhesus monkey offspring. *Biol Psychiatry* 2014;**75**:332—41.

16. Bellavance MA, Rivest S. The HPA—immune axis and the immunomodulatory actions of glucocorticoids in the brain. *Front Immunol* 2014;**5**:136.

17. Berdowska A, Zwirska-Korczala K. Neopterin measurement in clinical diagnosis. *J Clin Pharm Ther* 2001;**26**:319—29.

18. Bolte ER. Autism and clostridium tetani. *Med Hypotheses* 1998;**51**:133—44.

19. Boris M, Kaiser CC, Goldblatt A, Elice MW, Edelson SM, Adams JB, et al. Effect of pioglitazone treatment on behavioral symptoms in autistic children. *J Neuroinflamm* 2007;**4**.

20. Boris M, Goldblatt A, Edelson SM. Improvement in children with autism treated with intravenous gamma globulin. *J Nutr Environ Med* 2006;**15**:1—8.

21. Borody TJ, Paramsothy S, Agrawal G. Fecal microbiota transplantation: indications, methods, evidence, and future directions. *Curr Gastroenterol Rep* 2013;**15**:337.

22. Bradstreet JJ, Smith S, Granpeesheh D, El-Dahr JM, Rossignol D. Spironolactone might be a desirable immunologic and hormonal intervention in autism spectrum disorders. *Med Hypotheses* 2007;**68**:979—87.

23. Braunschweig D, Ashwood P, Krakowiak P, Hertz-Picciotto I, Hansen R, Croen LA, et al. Autism: maternally derived antibodies specific for fetal brain proteins. *Neurotoxicology* 2008;**29**:226—31.

24. Braunschweig D, Duncanson P, Boyce R, Hansen R, Ashwood P, Pessah IN, et al. Behavioral correlates of maternal antibody status among children with autism. *J Autism Dev Disord* 2012a;**42**:1435—45.

25. Braunschweig D, Golub MS, Koenig CM, Qi L, Pessah IN, Van de Water J, et al. Maternal autism-associated IgG antibodies delay development and produce anxiety in a mouse gestational transfer model. *J Neuroimmunol* 2012b;**252**:56—65.

26. Braunschweig D, Krakowiak P, Duncanson P, Boyce R, Hansen RL, Ashwood P, et al. Autism-specific maternal autoantibodies recognize critical proteins in developing brain. *Transl Psychiatry* 2013;**3**:e277.

27. Braunschweig D, Van de Water J. Maternal autoantibodies in autism. *Arch Neurol* 2012;**69**:693—9.

28. Brown AS. Epidemiologic studies of exposure to prenatal infection and risk of schizophrenia and autism. *Dev Neurobiol* 2012;**72**:1272—6.

29. Buehler MR. A proposed mechanism for autism: an aberrant neuroimmune response manifested as a psychiatric disorder. *Med Hypotheses* 2011;**76**:863—70.

30. Buie T, Campbell DB, Fuchs 3rd GJ, Furuta GT, Levy J, Van de water J, et al. Evaluation, diagnosis, and treatment of gastrointestinal disorders in individuals with ASDs: a consensus report. *Pediatrics* 2010;**125**(Suppl. 1):S1—18.

31. Buitelaar JK, van Engeland H, de Kogel K, de Vries H, van Hooff J, van Ree J. The adrenocorticotrophic hormone (4—9) analog ORG 2766 benefits autistic children: report on a second controlled clinical trial. *J Am Acad Child Adolesc Psychiatry* 1992a;**31**:1149—56.

32. Buitelaar JK, van Engeland H, de Kogel KH, de Vries H, van Hooff JA, van Ree JM. The use of adrenocorticotrophic hormone (4—9) analog ORG 2766 in autistic children: effects on the organization of behavior. *Biol Psychiatry* 1992b;**31**:1119—29.

33. Buitelaar JK, van Engeland H, van Ree JM, de Wied D. Behavioral effects of Org 2766, a synthetic analog of the adrenocorticotrophic hormone (4—9), in 14 outpatient autistic children. *J Autism Dev Disord* 1990;**20**:467—78.

34. Buxbaum JD, Cai G, Chaste P, Nygren G, Goldsmith J, Reichert J, et al. Mutation screening of the PTEN gene in patients with autism spectrum disorders and macrocephaly. *Am J Med Genet B Neuropsychiatr Genet* 2007;**144b**:484—91.

35. Campbell DB, D'Oronzio R, Garbett K, Ebert PJ, Mirnics K, Levitt P, et al. Disruption of cerebral cortex MET signaling in autism spectrum disorder. *Ann Neurol* 2007;**62**:243—50.

36. Campbell DB, Sutcliffe JS, Ebert PJ, Militerni R, Bravaccio C, Trillo S, et al. A genetic variant that disrupts MET transcription is associated with autism. *Proc Natl Acad Sci USA* 2006;**103**:16834—9.

37. Careaga M, Noyon T, Basuta K, Van de Water J, Tassone F, Hagerman RJ, et al. Group I metabotropic glutamate receptor mediated dynamic immune dysfunction in children with fragile X syndrome. *J Neuroinflammation* 2014;**11**:110.

38. Chess S. Autism in children with congenital rubella. *J Autism Child Schizophr* 1971;**1**:33—47.

39. Chez M, Low R, Parise C, Donnel T. Safety and observations in a pilot study of lenalidomide for treatment in autism. *Autism Res Treat* 2012:291601.

40. Chez MG, Dowling T, Patel PB, Khanna P, Kominsky M. Elevation of tumor necrosis factor-alpha in cerebrospinal fluid of autistic children. *Pediatr Neurol* 2007;**36**:361—5.

41. Chez MG, Loeffel M, Buchanan CP, Field-Chez M. Pulse high dose steroids as combination therapy with valproic acid in epileptic aphasia patients with pervasive developmental delay or autism. *Ann Neurol* 1998;**44**:539.

42. Chow ML, Pramparo T, Winn ME, Barnes CC, Li HR, Weiss L, et al. Age-dependent brain gene expression and copy number anomalies in autism suggest distinct pathological processes at young versus mature ages. *PLoS Genet* 2012;**8**:e1002592.

43. Connolly AM, Chez M, Streif EM, Keeling RM, Golumbek PT, Kwon JM, et al. Brain-derived neurotrophic factor and autoantibodies to neural antigens in sera of children with autistic spectrum disorders, Landau-Kleffner syndrome, and epilepsy. *Biol Psychiatry* 2006;**59**:354—63.

44. Conti B, Tabarean I, Sanchez-Alavez M, Davis C, Brownell S, Behrens M, et al. Cytokine receptors in the brain. *Neuroimmune Biol* 2008;**6**(19):21—38.

45. Coury DL, Ashwood P, Fasano A, Fuchs G, Geraghty M, Kaul A, et al. Gastrointestinal conditions in children with autism spectrum disorder: developing a research agenda. *Pediatrics* 2012;**130**(Suppl. 2):S160—8.

46. Croen LA, Braunschweig D, Haapanen L, Yoshida CK, Fireman B, Grether JK, et al. Maternal mid-pregnancy autoantibodies to fetal brain protein: the early markers for autism study. *Biol Psychiatry* 2008;**64**:583—8.

47. Croonenberghs J, Wauters A, Devreese K, Verkerk R, Scharpe S, Bosmans E, et al. Increased serum albumin, gamma globulin, immunoglobulin IgG, and IgG2 and IgG4 in autism. *Psychol Med* 2002;**32**:1457—63.

48. Cryan JF, Dinan TG. Mind-altering microorganisms: the impact of the gut microbiota on brain and behaviour. *Nat Rev Neurosci* 2012; **13**:701–12.

49. Dalton P, Deacon R, Blamire A, Pike M, McKinlay I, Stein J, et al. Maternal neuronal antibodies associated with autism and a language disorder. *Ann Neurol* 2003;**53**:533–7.

50. de Theije CG, Koelink PJ, Korte-Bouws GA, Lopes da Silva S, Korte SM, Olivier B, et al. Intestinal inflammation in a murine model of autism spectrum disorders. *Brain Behav Immun* 2014a; **37**:240–7.

51. de Theije CG, Wopereis H, Ramadan M, van Eijndthoven T, Lambert J, Knol J, et al. Altered gut microbiota and activity in a murine model of autism spectrum disorders. *Brain Behav Immun* 2014b;**37**:197–206.

52. DelGiudice-Asch G, Simon L, Schmeidler J, Cunningham-Rundles C, Hollander E. Brief report: a pilot open clinical trial of intravenous immunoglobulin in childhood autism. *J Autism Dev Disord* 1999;**29**:157–60.

53. Denney DR, Frei BW, Gaffney GR. Lymphocyte subsets and interleukin-2 receptors in autistic children. *J Autism Dev Disord* 1996;**26**:87–97.

54. Depino AM. Peripheral and central inflammation in autism spectrum disorders. *Mol Cell Neurosci* 2013;**53**:69–76.

55. Dong Y, Richards JA, Gupta R, Aung PP, Emley A, Kluger Y, et al. PTEN functions as a melanoma tumor suppressor by promoting host immune response. *Oncogene* 2014;**33**:4632–42.

56. Du X, Tang Y, Xu H, Lit L, Walker W, Ashwood P, et al. Genomic profiles for human peripheral blood T cells, B cells, natural killer cells, monocytes, and polymorphonuclear cells: comparisons to ischemic stroke, migraine, and Tourette syndrome. *Genomics* 2006;**87**:693–703.

57. Dunn AJ. Effects of cytokines and infections on brain neurochemistry. *Clin Neurosci Res* 2006;**6**:52–68.

58. Engstrom HA, Ohlson S, Stubbs EG, Maciulis A, Caldwell V, Odell JD, et al. Decreased expression of CD95 (FAS/APO-1) on CD4+ T-lymphocytes from participants with autism. *J Dev Phys Disabil* 2003;**15**:155–63.

59. Enstrom A, Krakowiak P, Onore C, Pessah IN, Hertz-Picciotto I, Hansen RL, et al. Increased IgG4 levels in children with autism disorder. *Brain Behav Immun* 2009a;**23**:389–95.

60. Enstrom AM, Lit L, Onore CE, Gregg JP, Hansen RL, Pessah IN, et al. Altered gene expression and function of peripheral blood natural killer cells in children with autism. *Brain Behav Immun* 2009b;**23**:124–33.

61. Eskenazi B, Marks AR, Bradman A, Harley K, Barr DB, Johnson C, et al. Organophosphate pesticide exposure and neurodevelopment in young Mexican-American children. *Environ Health Perspect* 2007;**115**:792–8.

62. Fatemi SH, Snow AV, Stary JM, Araghi-Niknam M, Reutiman TJ, Lee S, et al. Reelin signaling is impaired in autism. *Biol Psychiatry* 2005;**57**:777–87.

63. Filiano AJ, Gadani SP, Kipnis J. Interactions of innate and adaptive immunity in brain development and function. *Brain Res* 2014.

64. Fu X, Mei Z, Sun L. Association between the g.296596G > A genetic variant of *RELN* gene and susceptibility to autism in a Chinese Han population. *Genet Mol Biol* 2013;**36**:486–9.

65. Garbett K, Ebert PJ, Mitchell A, Lintas C, Manzi B, Mirnics K, et al. Immune transcriptome alterations in the temporal cortex of subjects with autism. *Neurobiol Dis* 2008;**30**:303–11.

66. Ginsberg MR, Rubin RA, Falcone T, Ting AH, Natowicz MR. Brain transcriptional and epigenetic associations with autism. *PLoS One* 2012;**7**:e44736.

67. Giordano C, De Maria R, Stassi G, Todaro M, Richiusa P, Giordano M, et al. Defective expression of the apoptosis-inducing CD95 (Fas/APO-1) molecule on T and B cells in IDDM. *Diabetologia* 1995;**38**:1449–54.

68. Giovannoni G. Cerebrospinal fluid and serum nitric oxide metabolites in patients with multiple sclerosis. *Mult Scler (Houndmills, Basingstoke, England)* 1998;**4**:27–30.

69. Giovannoni G, Silver NC, O'Riordan J, Miller RF, Heales SJ, Land JM, et al. Increased urinary nitric oxide metabolites in patients with multiple sclerosis correlates with early and relapsing disease. *Mult Scler (Houndmills, Basingstoke, England)* 1999;**5**:335–41.

70. Goldani AA, Downs SR, Widjaja F, Lawton B, Hendren RL. Biomarkers in autism. *Front Psychiatry* 2014;**5**:100.

71. Gregg JP, Lit L, Baron CA, Hertz-Picciotto I, Walker W, Davis RA, et al. Gene expression changes in children with autism. *Genomics* 2008;**91**:22–9.

72. Grigorenko EL, Han SS, Yrigollen CM, Leng L, Mizue Y, Anderson GM, et al. Macrophage migration inhibitory factor and autism spectrum disorders. *Pediatrics* 2008;**122**:e438–445.

73. Guidotti A, Auta J, Davis JM, Di-Giorgi-Gerevini V, Dwivedi Y, Grayson DR, et al. Decrease in reelin and glutamic acid decarboxylase67 (GAD67) expression in schizophrenia and bipolar disorder: a postmortem brain study. *Arch Gen Psychiatry* 2000;**57**:1061–9.

74. Gupta AR, State MW. Recent advances in the genetics of autism. *Biol Psychiatry* 2007;**61**:429–37.

75. Gupta S. Immunological treatments for autism. *J Autism Dev Disord* 2000;**30**:475–9.

76. Gupta S, Aggarwal S, Heads C. Dysregulated immune system in children with autism: beneficial effects of intravenous immune globulin on autistic characteristics. *J Autism Dev Disord* 1996;**26**:439–52.

77. Gupta S, Aggarwal S, Rashanravan B, Lee T. Th1- and Th2-like cytokines in CD4+ and CD8+ T cells in autism. *J Neuroimmunol* 1998;**85**:106–9.

78. Hallmayer J, Cleveland S, Torres A, Phillips J, Cohen B, Torigoe T, et al. Genetic heritability and shared environmental factors among twin pairs with autism. *Arch Gen Psychiatry* 2011;**68**:1095–102.

79. Handen BL, Melmed RD, Hansen RL, Aman MG, Burnham DL, Bruss JB, et al. A double-blind, placebo-controlled trial of oral human immunoglobulin for gastrointestinal dysfunction in children with autistic disorder. *J Autism Dev Disord* 2009;**39**:796–805.

80. Hara Y, Maeda Y, Kataoka S, Ago Y, Takuma K, Matsuda T. Effect of prenatal valproic acid exposure on cortical morphology in female mice. *J Pharmacol Sci* 2012;**118**:543–6.

81. Hava G, Vered L, Yael M, Mordechai H, Mahoud H. Alterations in behavior in adult offspring mice following maternal inflammation during pregnancy. *Dev Psychobiol* 2006;**48**:162–8.

82. Heuer L, Ashwood P, Schauer J, Goines P, Krakowiak P, Hertz-Picciotto I, et al. Reduced levels of immunoglobulin in children with autism correlates with behavioral symptoms. *Autism Res Off J Int Soc Autism Res* 2008;**1**:275–83.

83. Hollander E, DelGiudice-Asch G, Simon L, Schmeidler J, Cartwright C, DeCaria CM, et al. B lymphocyte antigen D8/17 and repetitive behaviors in autism. *Am J Psychiatry* 1999;**156**:317–20.

84. Hsiao EY. Immune dysregulation in autism spectrum disorder. *Int Rev Neurobiol* 2013;**113**:269–302.

85. Hsiao EY. Gastrointestinal issues in autism spectrum disorder. *Harv Rev Psychiatry* 2014;**22**:104–11.

86. Hsiao EY, McBride SW, Chow J, Mazmanian SK, Patterson PH. Modeling an autism risk factor in mice leads to permanent immune dysregulation. *Proc Natl Acad Sci USA* 2012;**109**:12776–81.

87. Hsiao EY, McBride SW, Hsien S, Sharon G, Hyde ER, McCue T, et al. Microbiota modulate behavioral and physiological abnormalities associated with neurodevelopmental disorders. *Cell* 2013;**155**:1451–63.

88. Hull C, Regehr WG. Identification of an inhibitory circuit that regulates cerebellar golgi cell activity. *Neuron* 2012;**73**:149–58.

89. Ingram JL, Peckham SM, Tisdale B, Rodier PM. Prenatal exposure of rats to valproic acid reproduces the cerebellar anomalies associated with autism. *Neurotoxicol Teratol* 2000;**22**:319–24.

90. Institute of Medicine Immunization Safety Review Committee. In: Stratton K, Gable A, McCormick MC, editors. *Immunization safety review: thimerosal-containing vaccines and neurodevelopmental disorders*. Washington (DC): National Academies Press (US); 2001. Copyright 2001 by the National Academy of Sciences. All rights reserved.

91. Jansen LM, Gispen-de Wied CC, van der Gaag RJ, van Engeland H. Differentiation between autism and multiple complex developmental disorder in response to psychosocial stress. *Neuropsychopharmacology* 2003;**28**:582–90.

92. Jyonouchi H, Sun S, Le H. Proinflammatory and regulatory cytokine production associated with innate and adaptive immune responses in children with autism spectrum disorders and developmental regression. *J Neuroimmunol* 2001;**120**:170–9.

93. Kataoka S, Takuma K, Hara Y, Maeda Y, Ago Y, Matsuda T. Autism-like behaviours with transient histone hyperacetylation in mice treated prenatally with valproic acid. *Int J Neuropsychopharmacol* 2013;**16**:91–103.

94. Kirsten TB, Taricano M, Florio JC, Palermo-Neto J, Bernardi MM. Prenatal lipopolysaccharide reduces motor activity after an immune challenge in adult male offspring. *Behav Brain Res* 2010; **211**:77–82.

95. Knuesel I, Chicha L, Britschgi M, Schobel SA, Bodmer M, Hellings JA, et al. Maternal immune activation and abnormal brain development across CNS disorders. *Nat Rev Neurol* 2014; **10**:643–60.

96. Kolaczkowska E, Kubes P. Neutrophil recruitment and function in health and inflammation. *Nat Rev Immunol* 2013;**13**:159–75.

97. Kotla V, Goel S, Nischal S, Heuck C, Vivek K, Das B, et al. Mechanism of action of lenalidomide in hematological malignancies. *J Hematol Oncol* 2009;**2**:36.

98. Kraneveld AD, de Theije CG, van Heesch F, Borre Y, de Kivit S, Olivier B, et al. The neuro-immune axis: prospect for novel treatments for mental disorders. *Basic Clin Pharmacol Toxicol* 2014;**114**:128–36.

99. Lampron A, Elali A, Rivest S. Innate immunity in the CNS: redefining the relationship between the CNS and its environment. *Neuron* 2013;**78**:214–32.

100. Laurence JA, Fatemi SH. Glial fibrillary acidic protein is elevated in superior frontal, parietal and cerebellar cortices of autistic subjects. *Cerebellum (London, England)* 2005;**4**:206–10.

101. Leblhuber F, Walli J, Demel U, Tilz GP, Widner B, Fuchs D. Increased serum neopterin concentrations in patients with Alzheimer's disease. *Clin Chem Lab Med* 1999;**37**:429–31.

102. Lee BK, Magnusson C, Gardner RM, Blomstrom S, Newschaffer CJ, Burstyn I, et al. Maternal hospitalization with infection during pregnancy and risk of autism spectrum disorders. *Brain Behav Immun* 2014.

103. Lee LC, Zachary AA, Leffell MS, Newschaffer CJ, Matteson KJ, Tyler JD, et al. HLA-DR4 in families with autism. *Pediatr Neurol* 2006;**35**:303–7.

104. Li X, Chauhan A, Sheikh AM, Patil S, Chauhan V, Li XM, et al. Elevated immune response in the brain of autistic patients. *J Neuroimmunol* 2009;**207**:111–6.

105. Libbey JE, Sweeten TL, McMahon WM, Fujinami RS. Autistic disorder and viral infections. *J Neurovirol* 2005;**11**:1–10.

106. Lintas C, Sacco R, Garbett K, Mirnics K, Militerni R, Bravaccio C, et al. Involvement of the PRKCB1 gene in autistic disorder: significant genetic association and reduced neocortical gene expression. *Mol Psychiatry* 2009;**14**:705–18.

107. Lucchina L, Depino AM. Altered peripheral and central inflammatory responses in a mouse model of autism. *Autism Res* 2014; **7**:273–89.

108. Lv JW, Cheng TL, Qiu ZL, Zhou WH. Role of the PTEN signaling pathway in autism spectrum disorder. *Neurosci Bull* 2013;**29**: 773–8.

109. Malkova NV, Yu CZ, Hsiao EY, Moore MJ, Patterson PH. Maternal immune activation yields offspring displaying mouse versions of the three core symptoms of autism. *Brain Behav Immun* 2012;**26**: 607–16.

110. Mandal M, Marzouk AC, Donnelly R, Ponzio NM. Maternal immune stimulation during pregnancy affects adaptive immunity in offspring to promote development of TH17 cells. *Brain Behav Immun* 2011;**25**:863–71.

111. Martin LA, Ashwood P, Braunschweig D, Cabanlit M, Van de Water J, Amaral DG. Stereotypies and hyperactivity in rhesus monkeys exposed to IgG from mothers of children with autism. *Brain Behav Immun* 2008;**22**:806–16.

112. Mehta MV, Gandal MJ, Siegel SJ. mGluR5-antagonist mediated reversal of elevated stereotyped, repetitive behaviors in the VPA model of autism. *PloS One* 2011;**6**:e26077.

113. Messahel S, Pheasant AE, Pall H, Ahmed-Choudhury J, Sungum-Paliwal RS, Vostanis P. Urinary levels of neopterin and biopterin in autism. *Neurosci Lett* 1998;**241**:17–20.

114. Molloy CA, Morrow AL, Meinzen-Derr J, Dawson G, Bernier R, Dunn M, et al. Familial autoimmune thyroid disease as a risk factor for regression in children with autism spectrum disorder: a CPEA study. *J Autism Dev Disord* 2006a;**36**:317–24.

115. Molloy CA, Morrow AL, Meinzen-Derr J, Schleifer K, Dienger K, Manning-Courtney P, et al. Elevated cytokine levels in children with autism spectrum disorder. *J Neuroimmunol* 2006b;**172**: 198–205.

116. Moloney RD, Desbonnet L, Clarke G, Dinan TG, Cryan JF. The microbiome: stress, health and disease. *Mamm Genome* 2014;**25**: 49–74.

117. Morgan JT, Chana G, Abramson I, Semendeferi K, Courchesne E, Everall IP. Abnormal microglial-neuronal spatial organization in the dorsolateral prefrontal cortex in autism. *Brain Res* 2012;**1456**: 72–81.

118. Morgan JT, Chana G, Pardo CA, Achim C, Semendeferi K, Buckwalter J, et al. Microglial activation and increased microglial density observed in the dorsolateral prefrontal cortex in autism. *Biol Psychiatry* 2010;**68**:368–76.

119. Mostafa GA, Al Shehab A, Fouad NR. Frequency of CD4+CD25high regulatory T cells in the peripheral blood of Egyptian children with autism. *J Child Neurol* 2010;**25**:328–35.

120. Mott SH, Weinstein SL, Conry JA, Kenworthy LE, Lockwood S, Wagner A, et al. Pervasive developmental disorder/autism versus Landau–Kleffner syndrome: steroid-responsive encephalopathy characterized by language and social interactive impairment. *Ann Neurol* 1996;**42**:332.

121. Nordahl CW, Braunschweig D, Iosif AM, Lee A, Rogers S, Ashwood P, et al. Maternal autoantibodies are associated with abnormal brain enlargement in a subgroup of children with autism spectrum disorder. *Brain Behav Immun* 2013;**30**:61–5.

122. Nordahl CW, Lange N, Li DD, Barnett LA, Lee A, Buonocore MH, et al. Brain enlargement is associated with regression in preschool-age boys with autism spectrum disorders. *Proc Natl Acad Sci USA* 2011;**108**:20195–200.

123. Nozawa K, Kayagaki N, Tokano Y, Yagita H, Okumura K, Hasimoto H. Soluble Fas (APO-1, CD95) and soluble Fas ligand in rheumatic diseases. *Arthritis Rheum* 1997;**40**:1126–9.

124. Odell D, Maciulis A, Cutler A, Warren L, McMahon WM, Coon H, et al. Confirmation of the association of the C4B null allele in autism. *Hum Immunol* 2005;**66**:140–5.

125. Okada K, Hashimoto K, Iwata Y, Nakamura K, Tsujii M, Tsuchiya KJ, et al. Decreased serum levels of transforming growth factor-beta1 in patients with autism. *Prog Neuro-Psychopharmacol Biol Psychiatry* 2007;**31**:187–90.

126. Onore C, Enstrom A, Krakowiak P, Hertz-Picciotto I, Hansen R, Van de Water J, et al. Decreased cellular IL-23 but not IL-17 production in children with autism spectrum disorders. *J Neuroimmunol* 2009;**216**:126–9.

127. Ornoy A. Valproic acid in pregnancy: how much are we endangering the embryo and fetus? *Reprod Toxicol (Elmsford, NY)* 2009;**28**:1–10.

128. Pardo CA, Vargas DL, Zimmerman AW. Immunity, neuroglia and neuroinflammation in autism. *Int Rev Psychiatry (Abingdon, England)* 2005;**17**:485–95.

129. Parker-Athill EC, Tan J. Maternal immune activation and autism spectrum disorder: interleukin-6 signaling as a key mechanistic pathway. *Neuro-Signals* 2010;**18**:113–28.

130. Peng Y, Huentelman M, Smith C, Qiu S. MET receptor tyrosine kinase as an autism genetic risk factor. *Int Rev Neurobiol* 2013;**113**:135–65.

131. Persico AM, Bourgeron T. Searching for ways out of the autism maze: genetic, epigenetic and environmental clues. *Trends Neurosci* 2006;**29**:349–58.

132. Persico AM, Napolioni V. Autism genetics. *Behav Brain Res* 2013;**251**:95–112.

133. Philippi A, Roschmann E, Tores F, Lindenbaum P, Benajou A, Germain-Leclerc L, et al. Haplotypes in the gene encoding protein kinase c-beta (PRKCB1) on chromosome 16 are associated with autism. *Mol Psychiatry* 2005;**10**:950–60.

134. Plioplys AV. Intravenous immunoglobulin treatment of children with autism. *J Child Neurol* 1998;**13**:79–82.

135. Procaccini C, Pucino V, De Rosa V, Marone G, Matarese G. Neuroendocrine networks controlling immune system in health and disease. *Front Immunol* 2014;**5**:143.

136. Rossi CC, Van de Water J, Rogers SJ, Amaral DG. Detection of plasma autoantibodies to brain tissue in young children with and without autism spectrum disorders. *Brain Behav Immun* 2011;**25**:1123–35.

137. Roullet FI, Lai JK, Foster JA. In utero exposure to valproic acid and autism—a current review of clinical and animal studies. *Neurotoxicol Teratol* 2013;**36**:47–56.

138. Roullet FI, Wollaston L, Decatanzaro D, Foster JA. Behavioral and molecular changes in the mouse in response to prenatal exposure to the anti-epileptic drug valproic acid. *Neuroscience* 2010;**170**:514–22.

139. Sandin S, Lichtenstein P, Kuja-Halkola R, Larsson H, Hultman CM, Reichenberg A. The familial risk of autism. *Jama* 2014;**311**:1770–7.

140. Sandler RH, Finegold SM, Bolte ER, Buchanan CP, Maxwell AP, Vaisanen ML, et al. Short-term benefit from oral vancomycin treatment of regressive-onset autism. *J Child Neurol* 2000;**15**:429–35.

141. Saresella M, Marventano I, Guerini FR, Mancuso R, Ceresa L, Zanzottera M, et al. An autistic endophenotype results in complex immune dysfunction in healthy siblings of autistic children. *Biol Psychiatry* 2009;**66**:978–84.

142. Schneider CK, Melmed RD, Barstow LE, Enriquez FJ, Ranger-Moore J, Ostrem JA. Oral human immunoglobulin for children with autism and gastrointestinal dysfunction: a prospective, open-label study. *J Autism Dev Disord* 2006a;**36**:1053–64.

143. Schneider T, Przewlocki R. Behavioral alterations in rats prenatally exposed to valproic acid: animal model of autism. *Neuropsychopharmacology* 2005;**30**:80–9.

144. Schneider T, Turczak J, Przewlocki R. Environmental enrichment reverses behavioral alterations in rats prenatally exposed to valproic acid: issues for a therapeutic approach in autism. *Neuropsychopharmacology* 2006b;**31**:36–46.

145. Serajee FJ, Zhong H, Mahbubul Huq AH. Association of Reelin gene polymorphisms with autism. *Genomics* 2006;**87**:75–83.

146. Shaw W. Increased urinary excretion of a 3-(3-hydroxyphenyl)-3-hydroxypropionic acid (HPHPA), an abnormal phenylalanine metabolite of *Clostridia* spp. in the gastrointestinal tract, in urine samples from patients with autism and schizophrenia. *Nutr Neurosci* 2010;**13**:135–43.

147. Shenoy S, Arnold S, Chatila T. Response to steroid therapy in autism secondary to autoimmune lymphoproliferative syndrome. *J Pediatr* 2000;**136**:682–7.

148. Shi L, Fatemi SH, Sidwell RW, Patterson PH. Maternal influenza infection causes marked behavioral and pharmacological changes in the offspring. *J Neurosci* 2003;**23**:297–302.

149. Singer HS, Morris C, Gause C, Pollard M, Zimmerman AW, Pletnikov M. Prenatal exposure to antibodies from mothers of children with autism produces neurobehavioral alterations: a pregnant dam mouse model. *J Neuroimmunol* 2009;**211**:39–48.

150. Singer HS, Morris CM, Williams PN, Yoon DY, Hong JJ, Zimmerman AW. Antibrain antibodies in children with autism and their unaffected siblings. *J Neuroimmunol* 2006;**178**:149–55.

151. Singh VK. Plasma increase of interleukin-12 and interferon-gamma. Pathological significance in autism. *J Neuroimmunol* 1996;**66**:143–5.

152. Singh VK, Warren R, Averett R, Ghaziuddin M. Circulating autoantibodies to neuronal and glial filament proteins in autism. *Pediatr Neurol* 1997;**17**:88–90.

153. Singh VK, Warren RP, Odell JD, Warren WL, Cole P. Antibodies to myelin basic protein in children with autistic behavior. *Brain Behav Immun* 1993;**7**:97–103.

154. Smalheiser NR, Costa E, Guidotti A, Impagnatiello F, Auta J, Lacor P, et al. Expression of reelin in adult mammalian blood, liver, pituitary pars intermedia, and adrenal chromaffin cells. *Proc Natl Acad Sci USA* 2000;**97**:1281–6.

155. Smith SE, Li J, Garbett K, Mirnics K, Patterson PH. Maternal immune activation alters fetal brain development through interleukin-6. *J Neurosci Off J Soc Neurosci* 2007;**27**:10695–702.

156. Stefanatos GA, Grover W, Geller E. Case study: corticosteroid treatment of language regression in pervasive developmental disorder. *J Am Acad Child Adolesc Psychiatry* 1995;**34**:1107–11.

157. Steffenburg S, Gillberg C, Hellgren L, Andersson L, Gillberg IC, Jakobsson G, et al. A twin study of autism in Denmark, Finland, Iceland, Norway and Sweden. *J Child Psychol Psychiatry Allied Discip* 1989;**30**:405–16.

158. Stigler KA, Sweeten TL, Posey DJ, McDougle CJ. Autism and immune factors: a comprehensive review. *Res Autism Spectr Disord* 2009;**3**:840–60.

159. Suzuki K, Matsuzaki H, Iwata K, Kameno Y, Shimmura C, Kawai S, et al. Plasma cytokine profiles in subjects with high-functioning autism spectrum disorders. *PloS One* 2011;**6**:e20470.

160. Suzuki K, Sugihara G, Ouchi Y, Nakamura K, Futatsubashi M, Takebayashi K, et al. Microglial activation in young adults with autism spectrum disorder. *JAMA Psychiatry* 2013;**70**:49–58.

161. Swedo SE, Leonard HL, Mittleman BB, Allen AJ, Rapoport JL, Dow SP, et al. Identification of children with pediatric autoimmune neuropsychiatric disorders associated with streptococcal infections by a marker associated with rheumatic fever. *Am J Psychiatry* 1997;**154**:110–2.

162. Sweeten TL, Posey DJ, McDougle CJ. High blood monocyte counts and neopterin levels in children with autistic disorder. *Am J Psychiatry* 2003;**160**:1691–3.

163. Sweeten TL, Posey DJ, Shankar S, McDougle CJ. High nitric oxide production in autistic disorder: a possible role for interferon-gamma. *Biol Psychiatry* 2004;**55**:434–7.

164. Tani P, Lindberg N, Matto V, Appelberg B, Nieminen-von Wendt T, von Wendt L, et al. Higher plasma ACTH levels in adults with asperger syndrome. *J Psychosom Res* 2005;**58**:533–6.

165. Tetreault NA, Hakeem AY, Jiang S, Williams BA, Allman E, Wold BJ, et al. Microglia in the cerebral cortex in autism. *J Autism Dev Disord* 2012;**42**:2569–84.

166. Tokano Y, Miyake S, Kayagaki N, Nozawa K, Morimoto S, Azuma M, et al. Soluble Fas molecule in the serum of patients with systemic lupus erythematosus. *J Clin Immunol* 1996;**16**:261–5.

167. Torrente F, Murch S. P0870 expression of the reelin signalling pathway on intestinal epithelium and peripheral blood lymphocytes. *J Pediatr Gastroenterol Nutr* 2004;**39**:S388.

168. Torres AR, Maciulis A, Odell D. The association of MHC genes with autism. *Front Biosci J Virtual Libr* 2001;**6**:D936–43.

169. Torres AR, Westover JB, Rosenspire AJ. HLA immune function genes in autism. *Autism Res Treat* 2012;**2012**:959073.

170. Tostes MH, Teixeira HC, Gattaz WF, Brandao MA, Raposo NR. Altered neurotrophin, neuropeptide, cytokines and nitric oxide levels in autism. *Pharmacopsychiatry* 2012;**45**:241–3.

171. Trajkovski V, Ajdinski L, Spiroski M. Plasma concentration of immunoglobulin classes and subclasses in children with autism in the Republic of Macedonia: retrospective study. *Croat Med J* 2004;**45**:746–9.

172. Valacchi G, Ashwood P. ASD: biochemical mechanisms behind behavioral disorders. *Mediat Inflamm* 2014;**2014**:758473.

173. Vargas DL, Nascimbene C, Krishnan C, Zimmerman AW, Pardo CA. Neuroglial activation and neuroinflammation in the brain of patients with autism. *Ann Neurol* 2005;**57**:67–81.

174. Voineagu I, Wang X, Johnston P, Lowe JK, Tian Y, Horvath S, et al. Transcriptomic analysis of autistic brain reveals convergent molecular pathology. *Nature* 2011;**474**:380–4.

175. Vojdani A, Mumper E, Granpeesheh D, Mielke L, Traver D, Bock K, et al. Low natural killer cell cytotoxic activity in autism: the role of glutathione, IL-2 and IL-15. *J Neuroimmunol* 2008;**205**: 148–54.

176. Warren RP, Burger RA, Odell D, Torres AR, Warren WL. Decreased plasma concentrations of the C4B complement protein in autism. *Arch Pediatr Adolesc Med* 1994;**148**:180–3.

177. Warren RP, Cole P, Odell JD, Pingree CB, Warren WL, White E, et al. Detection of maternal antibodies in infantile autism. *J Am Acad Child Adolesc Psychiatry* 1990a;**29**:873–7.

178. Warren RP, Margaretten NC, Pace NC, Foster A. Immune abnormalities in patients with autism. *J Autism Dev Disord* 1986;**16**: 189–97.

179. Warren RP, Odell JD, Warren WL, Burger RA, Maciulis A, Daniels WW, et al. Brief report: immunoglobulin A deficiency in a subset of autistic subjects. *J Autism Dev Disord* 1997;**27**:187–92.

180. Warren RP, Singh VK, Averett RE, Odell JD, Maciulis A, Burger RA, et al. Immunogenetic studies in autism and related disorders. *Mol Chem Neuropathol* 1996;**28**:77–81.

181. Warren RP, Yonk LJ, Burger RA, Cole P, Odell JD, Warren WL, et al. Deficiency of suppressor-inducer (CD4+CD45RA+) T cells in autism. *Immunol Invest* 1990b;**19**:245–51.

182. Wasilewska J, Kaczmarski M, Stasiak-Barmuta A, Tobolczyk J, Kowalewska E. Low serum IgA and increased expression of CD23 on B lymphocytes in peripheral blood in children with regressive autism aged 3–6 years old. *Arch Med Sci* 2012;**8**:324–31.

183. Wellmann KA, Varlinskaya EI, Mooney SM. d-Cycloserine ameliorates social alterations that result from prenatal exposure to valproic acid. *Brain Res Bull* 2014;**108c**:1–9.

184. Wills S, Cabanlit M, Bennett J, Ashwood P, Amaral D, Van de Water J. Autoantibodies in autism spectrum disorders (ASD). *Ann NY Acad Sci* 2007;**1107**:79–91.

185. Wills S, Cabanlit M, Bennett J, Ashwood P, Amaral DG, Van de Water J. Detection of autoantibodies to neural cells of the cerebellum in the plasma of subjects with autism spectrum disorders. *Brain Behav Immun* 2009;**23**:64–74.

186. Wills S, Rossi CC, Bennett J, Martinez Cerdeno V, Ashwood P, Amaral DG, et al. Further characterization of autoantibodies to GABAergic neurons in the central nervous system produced by a subset of children with autism. *Mol Autism* 2011;**2**:5.

187. Xuan IC, Hampson DR. Gender-dependent effects of maternal immune activation on the behavior of mouse offspring. *PloS One* 2014;**9**:e104433.

188. Yang MS, Gill M. A review of gene linkage, association and expression studies in autism and an assessment of convergent evidence. *Int J Dev Neurosci* 2007;**25**:69–85.

189. Yochum CL, Bhattacharya P, Patti L, Mirochnitchenko O, Wagner GC. Animal model of autism using GSTM1 knockout mice and early post-natal sodium valproate treatment. *Behav Brain Res* 2010;**210**:202–10.

190. Yonk LJ, Warren RP, Burger RA, Cole P, Odell JD, Warren WL, et al. CD4+ helper T cell depression in autism. *Immunol Lett* 1990;**25**:341–5.

191. Zerbo O, Iosif AM, Walker C, Ozonoff S, Hansen RL, Hertz-Picciotto I. Is maternal influenza or fever during pregnancy associated with autism or developmental delays? Results from the CHARGE (CHildhood Autism Risks from Genetics and Environment) study. *J Autism Dev Disord* 2013;**43**:25–33.

192. Zhou J, Parada LF. PTEN signaling in autism spectrum disorders. *Curr Opin Neurobiol* 2012;**22**:873–9.

193. Ziemssen T, Kern S. Psychoneuroimmunology—cross-talk between the immune and nervous systems. *J Neurol* 2007;**254**(Suppl. 2): II8–11.

194. Zimmerman AW, Connors SL, Matteson KJ, Lee LC, Singer HS, Castaneda JA, et al. Maternal antibrain antibodies in autism. *Brain Behav Immun* 2007;**21**:351–7.

195. Zimmerman AW, Jyonouchi H, Comi AM, Connors SL, Milstien S, Varsou A, et al. Cerebrospinal fluid and serum markers of inflammation in autism. *Pediatr Neurol* 2005;**33**:195–201.

196. Theoharides TC, Angelidou A, Alysandratos K-D, Zhang B, Asadi S, Francis K, et al. Mast cell activation and autism. *Biochim Biophys Acta* 2012;**1822**:34–41.

197. Baek JH, Birchmeier C, Zenke M, Hieronymus T. The HGF receptor/Met tyrosine kinase is a key regulator of dendritic cell migration in skin immunity. *J Immunol* 2012;**189**:1699–707.

198. Herman GE, Butter E, Enrile B, Pastore M, Prior TW, Sommer A. Increasing knowledge of PTEN germline mutations: two additional patients with autism and macrocephaly. *Am J Med Genet A* 2007;**143A**:589–93.

199. Warren RP, Foster A, Margaretten NC. Reduced natural killer cell activity in autism. *J Am Acad Child Adolesc Psychiatry* 1987;**26**: 333–5.

200. Meyer U, Nyffeler M, Engler A, Urwyler A, Schedlowski M, Knuesel I, et al. The time of prenatal immune challenge determines the specificity of inflammation-mediated brain and behavioral pathology. *J Neurosci* 2006;**26**:4752–62.

201. Shi L, Smith SE, Malkova N, Tse D, Su Y, Patterson PH. Activation of the maternal immune system alters cerebellar development in the offspring. *Brain Behav Immun* 2009;**23**:116–23.

202. Palmen SJ, van Engeland H, Hof PR, Schmitz C. Neuropathological findings in autism. *Brain* 2004;**127**:2572–83.

203. Amaral DG, Schumann CM, Nordahl CW. Neuroanatomy of autism. *Trends Neurosci* 2008;**31**:137–45.

204. Ito HT, Smith SE, Hsiao E, Patterson PH. Maternal immune activation alters nonspatial information processing in the hippocampus of the adult offspring. *Brain Behav Immun* 2010;**24**:930–41.

205. Thach WT. What is the role of the cerebellum in motor learning and cognition? *Trends Cogn Sci* 1998;**2**:331–7.

206. Pierce K, Courchesne E. Evidence for a cerebellar role in reduced exploration and stereotyped behavior in autism. *Biol Psychiatry* 2001;**49**:655–64.

207. Akshoomoff N, Lord C, Lincoln AJ, Courchesne RY, Carper RA, Townsend J, Courchesne E. Outcome classification of preschool children with autism spectrum disorders using MRI brain measures. *J Am Acad Child Adolesc Psychiatry* 2004;**43**:349–57.

208. Allen G, Courchesne E. Differential effects of developmental cerebellar abnormality on cognitive and motor functions in the cerebellum: an fMRI study of autism. *Am J Psychiatry* 2003;**160**:262–73.

209. Kates WR, Burnette CP, Eliez S, Strunge LA, Kaplan D, Landa R, et al. Neuroanatomic variation in monozygotic twin pairs discordant for the narrow phenotype for autism. *Am J Psychiatry* 2004; **161**:539–46.

210. Nowinski CV, Minshew NJ, Luna B, Takarae Y, Sweeney JA. Oculomotor studies of cerebellar function in autism. *Psychiatry Res* 2005;**137**:11–9.

211. Takarae Y, Minshew NJ, Luna B, Krisky CM, Sweeney JA. Pursuit eye movement deficits in autism. *Brain* 2004;**127**:2584–94.

212. Kalkbrenner AE, Schmidt RJ, Penlesky AC. Environmental chemical exposures and autism spectrum disorders: a review of the epidemiological evidence. *Curr Probl Pediatr Adolesc Health Care* 2014;**44**:277–318.

213. Thanseem I, Nakamura K, Miyachi T, Toyota T, Yamada S, Tsujii M, et al. Further evidence for the role of MET in autism susceptibility. *Neurosci Res* 2010;**68**:137–41.

214. Skaar DA, Shao Y, Haines JL, Stenger JE, Jaworski J, Martin ER, et al. Analysis of the RELN gene as a genetic risk factor for autism. *Mol Psychiatry* 2005;**10**:563–71.

PART II

FUNCTION OF MUTATED GENES IN INTELLECTUAL DISABILITY (ID) AND AUTISM

6

Synapse Proteomes and Disease: The MASC Paradigm

Àlex Bayés[1,2], Seth G.N. Grant[3]

[1]Molecular Physiology of the Synapse Laboratory, Biomedical Research Institute Sant Pau (IIB Sant Pau), Barcelona, Spain; [2]Universitat Autònoma de Barcelona, Cerdanyola del Vallès, Spain; [3]Genes to Cognition Programme, Centre for Clinical Brain Science, University of Edinburgh, Edinburgh, UK

The synapse has long been known to be of central importance to all behaviors, from the simplest reflexes to complex cognitive functions. It also controls our mood, fears, and other feelings. Physiologists uncovered the basis of neurotransmission and revealed that release of neurotransmitters from the presynaptic terminal activates receptors on the postsynaptic terminal, thereby permitting electrical activity in one neuron to be transmitted to the next. The molecular biology and biochemistry of these processes led to the discovery of the molecular machinery causing neurotransmitter vesicle release in the presynaptic terminal and the varieties of ion channels and receptors responsible for electrical events activated on the postsynaptic terminal.

These proteins are only the tip of the synapse proteome iceberg. In the past 10—15 years, proteomic studies of the synaptic proteome have uncovered its molecular constituents, identifying a much larger molecular complexity than originally anticipated.[1,2] Although new proteins are still being added to the synaptic proteome, it is reasonable to state that most genes expressed at the synapse have already been identified. The current estimate of the total number of proteins in mammalian synapses is about 2000.[1,2]

This complexity represents a new and exciting scenario and provides an important basis for our understanding of the molecular mechanisms underpinning cognition and other behaviors. One of the most important contributions of proteomic studies, so far, has been to identify the gene products of mutations that cause many brain diseases and disorders of behavior. These disorders are now known as synaptopathies,[3] or pathologies of the synapse. Many different brain disorders converge on synapse proteins, including forms of intellectual disability (ID), which although genetically characterized many years earlier, had no known mechanisms until it was discovered that they encoded synapse proteins.[4,5] More recent large-scale genetic studies of complex behavioral conditions, such as autism spectrum disorders (ASDs) and schizophrenia, have associated many synaptic genes to these disorders, unraveling the synapse as a key structure in their pathophysiology.

Proteomic studies of the synapse have been facilitated by the fact that biochemical methods used to isolate these neuronal structures and their protein complexes had been previously developed.[6,7] Most synapse proteomic research has focused on postsynaptic supramolecular complexes such as the postsynaptic density,[8–14] although the presynaptic proteome has also been well studied.[15–18] In this chapter we will focus on a family of postsynaptic protein complexes, which we named membrane-associated guanylate kinases (MAGUK)-associated signaling complexes (MASC); these complexes are key components of the postsynaptic density.[7]

MASC AS A PARADIGM FOR POSTSYNAPTIC SUPRAMOLECULAR ORGANIZATION

It is well accepted that proteins work within molecular ensembles, named protein complexes, rather than on their own.[19,20] Proteins in the same complex normally participate in the same biological process or molecular pathway.[19,20] Several protein complexes have been identified at glutamatergic synapses,[4,7,8,21–23] most of them at the postsynaptic terminal. The first synaptic complexes to be studied at the proteomic level were those associated with the N-methyl-D-aspartate (NMDA) glutamate receptor and postsynaptic MAGUK proteins.[7] Because the NMDA receptor and MAGUKs co-assemble, these two complexes showed a highly similar composition.

Membrane-associated guanylate kinases are postsynaptic scaffolding molecules found in all vertebrates.[24] Scaffolding, or adaptor, proteins are actively involved in bringing together the different components of protein complexes.[19,20,25] In many instances these proteins lack any enzymatic or signaling activity, just mediating protein–protein interactions that assemble the complexes. Scaffolding molecules are multidomain proteins containing different types of protein–protein interaction domains.[25] Membrane-associated guanylate kinases are characterized by three main types of protein–protein interaction domains: PDZ, SH3, and guanylate kinase.[26]

This last domain has been used to name the family, yet these proteins have no kinase activity because they have lost the ability to bind adenosine triphosophate.[26] The family of mammalian MAGUKs has five members, currently named DLG1 to DLG5. A role for the first four members in synaptic function has been known for some time[26]; hence, they are more widely known by their original names: SAP97 (DLG1), PSD93/CHAPSIN-110 (DLG2), SAP102 (DLG3), and PSD95 (DLG4). The fifth member (DLG5) was shown to be involved in synaptic biology.[27]

The first proteomic profiling[7] of the MAGUK protein complexes identified many proteins important for molecular signaling; for this reason, this complex was named MAGUK-associated signaling complex (MASC). Although the number of MASC proteins has grown as proteomics methods improved, the seminal study performed in 2000[7] had already identified its key components and molecular functions. MAGUK-associated signaling complexes were found to contain ionotropic glutamate receptors, both α-amino-3-hydroxy-5-methyl-4-isoxazolepropionic acid (AMPA) and NMDA types, metabotropic glutamate receptors, protein kinases from the PKA, PKC, FYN, MAPK, or CAMKII families as well as protein phosphatases, adaptor proteins including the four MAGUKs listed above, small G-proteins and their modulators, and cytoskeletal and cell adhesion molecules.

The advancement of mass spectrometry–based proteomics and the improvement in biochemical methods to isolate MASCs allowed to identify an increasing number of MASC components with higher confidence. A total of four proteomic analyses of MASC have been performed to date[4,7,8,28], the most recent being published in 2014. The original complexes contained a total of 79 proteins[7] and subsequent studies have increased this number to 473 (Supplementary Table 1 and Figure 1).

The large numbers of proteins associated with MASC reflect the existence of different MASC complexes residing in independent synapses. Indeed, the mean size of MASC complexes measured using gel filtration or native electrophoresis is about 2 MDa,[29] which indicates that different combinations of proteins form distinct MASCs. Taking into consideration that proteomics methods require the use of large numbers of cells and synapses, we hypothesize that the actual number of MASC components has to be understood as the maximum molecular complexity that MASC can accommodate across the brain. In other words, individual synapses will have smaller sets of MASC complexes, with fewer components, and that these complexes will likely be dynamic. These will also change during brain development, across brain regions, or as a function of synaptic activity.

TABLE 1   Number of Genes Expressed in MASC Related to Human Disease

		Molecular Basis Known	Molecular Basis Unknown	All
All disease types	Gene 2 disease[a]	254	99	353
	Disease number	250	54	304
	Gene number	146	67	188[b]
NSDs	Gene 2 disease[a]	155	89	244
	Disease number	153	44	197
	Gene number	104	68	145[b]
Non-NSDs	Gene 2 disease[a]	99	10	109
	Disease number	97	10	107
	Gene number	60	10	67[b]

[a]Contains all relations found between diseases and genes expressed at MASC. As some genes are linked to more than one disease and several diseases are related to more than one MASC gene; numbers in this row are higher than values in Disease number or Gene number.
[b]The number of genes in this column is lower than the addition of values in the two previous columns because occasionally the same gene is related to both groups of disease. All diseases—gene relationships are in Supplementary Table 2.

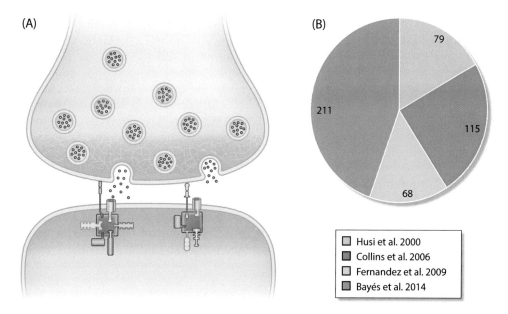

FIGURE 1   **Postsynaptic MASCs and its successive proteomic profiles.** (A) Schematic of synapse showing postsynaptic multiprotein complex associated with MAGUKs (MASC). (B) Pie chart showing the numbers of MASC proteins added with each new profiling experiment. A total of 473 proteins have been identified.

Unfortunately, the spatial resolution at which we can currently study the synaptic proteome does not yet allow us to test these hypotheses. For this reason, in this chapter when referring to MASC we will consider all 473 proteins.

Classifying the protein classes found among MASC proteins is a useful way to make this proteomic complexity more manageable and comprehensible. Indeed, bioinformatics analysis[30] of protein classes among MASC members unravels the key molecular characteristics (Figure 2). Although all protein classes identified in 2000 are found among the most relevant ones, the increase in MASC components has incorporated additional molecular functions to these

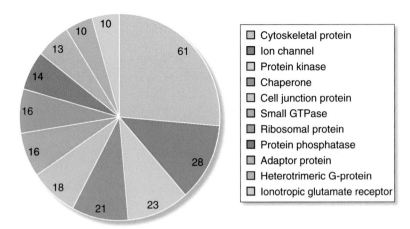

FIGURE 2   **Key protein classes among MASC components.** Pie chart representing the main protein classes among MASC components and their relative abundance. The digit in each section corresponds with the number of MASC proteins for that class. Analysis performed with PANTHER classification system.[30]

complexes. The current list of key MASC protein classes includes: (1) membrane proteins as cell junction proteins, heterotrimeric G-proteins, and ion channels, especially ionotropic glutamate receptors; (2) signaling molecules, especially those belonging to the system of kinases and phosphatase and small G-proteins; (3) proteins involved in protein synthesis and turnover (ribosomal proteins and chaperons); (4) cytoskeletal proteins related to both actin and tubulin; and (5) adaptor proteins that mediate protein–protein interactions, particularly between membrane proteins and signaling molecules.

This updated analysis essentially involves the MASC complex in three new molecular functions: (1) signaling through heterotrimeric G-proteins, likely transducing information from the G-protein–coupled receptors found at MASC, chiefly class I metabotropic glutamate receptors and brain-specific angiogenesis inhibitor 2; (2) acting upon voltage-gated potassium and calcium ion channels; and (3) participating in local protein synthesis and turnover through ribosomal components involved in translational control (RPS3, RPS14, or RPS27) and protein chaperones.

When comparing functions performed by MASC proteins with those undertaken by proteins from the whole postsynaptic proteome, where MASC is integrated, it becomes clear that MASC participates in most key postsynaptic functions,[28] which indicates that MASC is a core component of the postsynaptic machinery. This central role of MASC in synaptic biology and ultimately in cognition and behavior, is corroborated by the large numbers of genes expressed in this complex that are linked to nervous system disorders (NSDs).

A HIGH NUMBER OF GENES ENCODING MASC PROTEINS HAVE BEEN LINKED TO NSDs

In this chapter we evaluate the relevance of the MASC complex in nervous system disorders using available proteomic and genetic data. We have placed particular interest on ASD and ID. For simplicity, we refer to all genes whose corresponding protein product has been identified in MASC as the set of MASC genes. To study MASC relevance in NSDs we have investigated which MASC genes have been involved in brain disorders by genetic studies. By doing so, we have focused our work on conditions with a well-accepted genetic origin. Within these disorders we have considered separately those with a known causal gene from those that, despite having a well-established genetic basis, have not been unambiguously matched to a causal gene. We refer to the first group of conditions as *molecular basis known*, and to the second as *molecular basis unknown*. We have taken this nomenclature from the databases of inherited diseases, Online Mendelian Inheritance in Man[31] (OMIM). Table 1 summarizes the numbers of diseases and MASC genes identified in this study. All brain disorders with a known molecular basis have been collected from OMIM. The curation of the relevant literature has allowed us to incorporate into this study complex genetic disorders such as ASD and schizophrenia.

As many as 353 gene–disease relationships have been found among MASC genes; of these, 244 involve the nervous system. Because some genes are related to more than one condition and the same disorder is related to different genes, the total number of MASC genes and NSDs identified is smaller. In total, 145

TABLE 2   MASC Genes Related to Four or More NSDs

Gene Symbol	Gene Name	Number of Diseases	Disease/Disorder Name
GRIN2B	Glutamate receptor, ionotropic, NMDA 2B	8	Attention-deficit hyperactivity disorder; ASD; bipolar disorder; epileptic encephalopathy, early infantile, 27; Huntington; mental retardation, autosomal dominant 6; obsessive-compulsive disorder; schizophrenia
FLNA	Filamin A, alpha	8	FG syndrome 2; frontometaphyseal dysplasia; heterotopia, periventricular; heterotopia, periventricular, ED variant; intestinal pseudo-obstruction, neuronal; Melnick-Needles syndrome; otopalatodigital syndrome, type I; otopalatodigital syndrome, type II
SLC2A1	Solute carrier family 2 (facilitated glucose transporter), member 1	7	Dystonia 9; epilepsy, idiopathic generalized, susceptibility to, 12; GLUT1 deficiency syndrome 1; GLUT1 deficiency syndrome 2; microcephaly; migraine; paroxysmal exercise-induced dyskinesia
L1CAM	L1 cell adhesion molecule	6	Corpus callosum, partial agenesis of; CRASH syndrome; hydrocephalus due to aqueductal stenosis; hydrocephalus with congenital idiopathic intestinal pseudo-obstruction; hydrocephalus with Hirschsprung disease; MASA syndrome
GNAS	Guanine nucleotide binding protein (G protein)	5	Adrenocorticotropic hormone-independent macronodular adrenal hyperplasia; pseudohypoparathyroidism Ia; pseudohypoparathyroidism Ib; pseudohypoparathyroidism Ic; pseudopseudohypoparathyroidism
GDAP1	Ganglioside induced differentiation associated protein 1	4	Charcot-Marie-Tooth disease, axonal, type 2K; Charcot-Marie-Tooth disease, axonal, with vocal cord paresis; Charcot-Marie-Tooth disease, recessive intermediate, A; Charcot-Marie-Tooth disease, type 4A
GRIN1	Glutamate receptor, ionotropic, NMDA 1	4	Bipolar disorder; mental retardation, autosomal dominant 8; multiple sclerosis; schizophrenia
GRIN2A	Glutamate receptor, ionotropic, NMDA 2A	4	Alcoholism; encephalopathies; epilepsy, focal, with speech disorder and with or without mental retardation; Huntington; speech disorder
NF1	Neurofibromin 1	4	Neurofibromatosis—Noonan syndrome; neurofibromatosis, familial spinal; neurofibromatosis, type 1; Watson syndrome
NRXN1	Neurexin 1	4	ASD; mental disability; Pitt—Hopkins-like syndrome 2; schizophrenia
SNCA	Synuclein, alpha (non A4 component of amyloid precursor)	4	Dementia, Lewy body; multiple system atrophy; Parkinson disease 1; Parkinson disease 4
NMDA receptor (GRIN1, GRIN2A, GRIN2B, GRIN2D)[a]		14	Bipolar disorder; mental retardation, autosomal dominant 8; multiple sclerosis; schizophrenia; alcoholism; encephalopathies; epilepsy, focal, with speech disorder and with or without mental retardation; Huntington, age of onset; speech disorder; attention-deficit hyperactivity disorder; ASD; epileptic encephalopathy, early infantile, 27; mental retardation, autosomal dominant 6; obsessive-compulsive disorder
AMPA receptor (GRIA1, GRIA2, GRIA3)[a]		5	Mental retardation; migraine with aura; schizophrenia; mental retardation, X-linked 94; migraine

[a]Genes coding for subunits of ionotropic glutamate receptors are considered together. The names of the genes related to diseases are between parentheses.

MASC genes have been related to 197 nervous system conditions (listed in Supplementary Table 2), meaning that 30% of the MASC proteome has been involved in NSDs, a number that is likely to grow with future genetic studies. Of all MASC genes involved in NSDs 104 (22%) cause inherited disorders. The same analysis for the entire postsynaptic density proteome revealed that 10% of its proteome causes NSDs,[28] which indicates that the figure obtained for MASC is particularly high.

MASC GENES RELATED TO A LARGE NUMBER OF NSDs

As mentioned, some of the 145 MASC genes related to NSDs are involved in more than one condition; 54 MASC genes are related to two or more of these conditions (Table 2 lists all genes involved in four or more NSDs). The highest number of NSDs associated with a single MASC gene is eight. Both the 2B subunit of the NMDA glutamate receptor (GRIN2B) and filamin A (FLNA), a protein involved in actin cytoskeleton dynamics, have been related to eight NSDs. The nature of the diseases related to these genes is different. Whereas GRIN2B is related more to mental and behavioral disorders, including ASD and ID, FLNA is involved in neurological diseases usually involving gross anatomical malformations. This difference could be related to the distinctive expression patterns and functional characteristics of these two genes. GRIN2B expression and function are highly restricted to the synapse, whereas FLNA has a much wider expression, participating in various cellular functions related to actin dynamics, including neuronal migration. This difference suggests that disorders caused by genes with a function restricted to glutamatergic synapses are most relevant to disorders involving cognitive impairment. Our research on this particular matter indicates that proteins found at postsynaptic complexes are more often related to mental and behavioral disorders, especially to ID, than to other groups of disorders.[5,28] Membrane-associated guanylate kinase—associated signaling complexes would be a paradigmatic example of this observation, because they are further enriched in proteins causing ID than the bulk of the postsynaptic proteome.[5,28] Yet, more data will have to be gathered to fully demonstrate the hypothesis that proteins with an expression pattern restricted to the synapse are especially relevant to mental and behavioral disorders.

The number of NSDs involved with genes coding for subunits of the NMDA glutamate receptor is particularly striking (Table 2). As many as 14 conditions such as ASD, ID, schizophrenia, and bipolar disorder have been related to this key receptor for synaptic plasticity and cognition. These NSDs are mainly mental and behavioral disorders, although mutations causing epileptic and neurodegenerative diseases have also been reported. Most associations between the NMDA receptor and cognitive disorders have been discovered in the past few years[32] with the use of new-generation DNA sequencing technologies to study complex genetic disorders. We anticipate that with the future realization of larger genetic screenings of these disorders, many new mutations will be related to NMDA glutamate receptor.

SYNAPSE PROTEOMICS AND HUMAN GENOME SEQUENCING HAVE DRIVEN THE INCREASE IN MASC DISEASES

During the past 15 years there has been a dramatic increase in the number of new MASC genes related to NSDs. Whereas in 2000 around 10 MASC genes had been involved in NSD, by 2014 this number had risen to 145. Similarly, the number of NSDs related to MASC genes had grown from 4 to 197. This analysis indicates that there has been an important and steady rise in the number of MASC genes related to diseases (Figure 3). Notably, this increase has mainly occurred on NSD, whereas the number of non-NSD related to MASC genes has hardly grown (Figure 3). We wanted to determine whether the increase in MASC genes relevant to disease was proportional to the increase in the size of MASC proteome (Figure 1) or whether it was higher. To answer this question, we calculated the fraction of MASC genes involved in disease relative to MASC size (Figure 3(B)). This analysis also retrieved a steady increase in the number of MASC genes related to NSDs. We found that from 2000 to 2014, the fraction of MASC genes related to NSD had grown by a factor of 6, from 5% to 30% of its proteome. This increase is even more noticeable if we consider, for instance, that in the same period the OMIM database of mendelian diseases only doubled its number of diseases with known molecular basis (according to OMIM statistics). Overall, this analysis indicates that MASC genes have been implicated in NSDs at a high pace over the past 15 years, which speaks to MASC relevance in brain function and pathology.

LARGE-SCALE GENETIC STUDIES HAVE INVOLVED MASC IN NSDs WITH COMPLEX GENETIC BACKGROUND

In this chapter we have considered diseases with a well-known causal gene as well as genetically complex disorders, which we label *molecular basis unknown*.

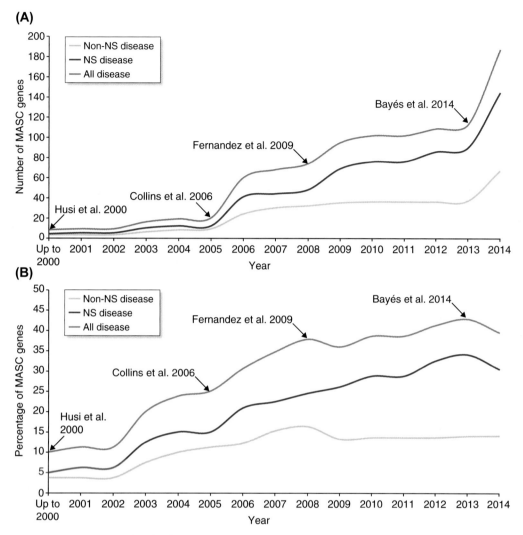

FIGURE 3 **Increase in MASC genes related to human diseases.** (A) Number of new MASC genes implicated in disease is shown per year. Nervous system (NS) and non-NS diseases are plotted independently. The sum of both disease groups is also shown (purple line). The publication of each of the four MASC proteomics studies is also indicated. (B) Percentage of MASC genes involved in disease relative to MASC size. Nervous system and non-NS diseases are plotted independently. The sum of both disease groups is also shown (purple line). The publication of each of the four MASC proteomics studies is also indicated.

Disorders causing ID belong mostly to the first group[33–36] whereas ASD belongs to the second group.[37–39] Many important brain disorders, especially mental and behavioral, have a clear genetic component,[40,41] although the exact genes involved are not always identified.[40] Some of these genetically complex disorders include ASD, schizophrenia, bipolar disorder, and obsessive compulsive disorders. The genetic study of these disorders has become feasible with the development of next-generation DNA sequencing, which make it affordable to sequence DNA from large cohorts of individuals.[42]

The fact that MASC and postsynaptic density supramolecular complexes are significantly enriched in genes causing ID has been previously established.[5,28]

Yet, until recently it has not been possible to address whether they are similarly related to ASDs, which are closest to IDs than to any other NSD.[43,44] In the past few years a number of important genetic studies have screened large cohorts of individuals with ASD, identifying genes giving high risk to these disorders. We investigated whether MASC genes are also associated with ASD and other psychiatric and neurodevelopmental conditions of complex genetic background.

The percentage of MASC genes implicated with disorders of an unknown molecular basis has been growing since 2000. In the past 5 years, around 40% of all new MASC genes implicated in NSDs have belonged to this group (Figure 4). These studies have

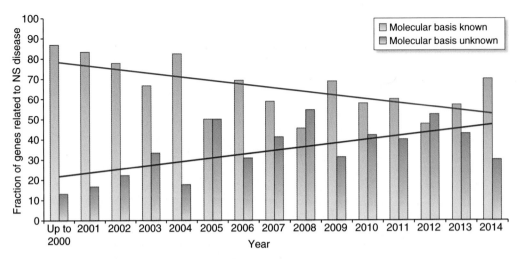

FIGURE 4   **Genetics basis of NSDs related to MASC genes.** Bar charts and trend lines for the proportion of new MASC genes related to NSDs with a well-known genetic cause (molecular basis known, in blue) and for diseases with an unknown molecular basis (in red). Trend lines show opposed tendencies for these two groups, with an increase in the fraction of MASC genes related to disorders without an unknown causal gene.

involved MASC in conditions such as depression, speech disorder, alcoholism and schizophrenia, but above all, these studies have involved MASC in ASDs. Between 2010 and 2014 as many as eight MASC genes have been associated with ASD, while the total number of MASC genes related to ASD is eleven (Table 3 and Supplementary Table 2). Most of these molecules have well-established synaptic functions with expression highly restricted to the synapse. Six of these genes are primarily expressed at the post-synaptic side: SHANK1, SHANK2, HOMER1, SYNGAP1, GRIN2B, and DLGAP2; genes with a predominantly presynaptic expression are NEUREXIN1, NEUREXIN2, and SNAP25.

TYPES OF DISEASE INVOLVING MASCs

We have shown that a large proportion of MASC proteins are involved in NSDs. We have also stated that MASC genes are often related to IDs and ASDs. Here, we more systematically investigated the types of NSDs with which MASC genes have been associated. We organized all NSDs found in this study according to the International Classification of Diseases (version 10) (ICD-10), which is published by the United Nations World Health Organization. This classification system is divided in 22 chapters, each of which is further organized into blocks.

This categorization reveals that MASC genes are relevant to only four of the 22 ICD-10 chapters (Figure 5(A)): endocrine, nutritional and metabolic diseases (Chapter IV); mental and behavioral disorders

(Chapter V); diseases of the nervous system (Chapter VI); and congenital malformations, deformations, and chromosomal abnormalities (Chapter XVII). Furthermore, NSDs in Chapters V and VI account for over 75% of all diseases. The chapter on Diseases of the Nervous System includes both neurological and neurodegenerative diseases (Figure 5(B)). Among neurological diseases, those that predominate are related to epilepsies and movement disorders such as ataxias or dystonias. In the group of neurodegenerative diseases, there are genes conferring higher risk to Alzheimer's disease and multiple sclerosis and others causing rare forms of Parkinson's disease and amyotrophic lateral sclerosis. Mental and behavioral disorders are the second most abundant ICD-10 chapter (Figure 5(C)). Within this chapter we found three main groups of mental disorders: (1) ASDs (included in the block of disorders of psychological development), IDs (referred to in Figure 5(C)) as Mental Retardation as this is the nomenclature still used by ICD-10), and schizophrenia. All MASC genes related to disorders of psychological development and mental retardation are listed in Table 3.

We wanted to analyze which of these disease classes has accumulated more MASC genes over the years. This study revealed that the number of genes causing NSDs did not grow similarly in all disease types. Instead, certain ICD-10 chapters have grown more than others (Figure 6). This is the case of the " Diseases of the Nervous System" and "Mental and Behavioral Disorders" chapters (Figure 6(A)), which kept increasing with time while the others remained more or less constant. If we now ask, within these two chapters, which blocks (or types) of disorders

TABLE 3   Membrane-Associated Guanylate Kinase—Associated Signaling Complex (MASC) Genes Related to ASDs or ID

HGNC Gene Name	Disorder/OMIM Phenotype	Date of First Nervous System Implication	References	Molecular Basis Known (OMIM)[a]
Disorders of Psychological Development				
SHANK2	Autism susceptibility 17	01/06/10	54	y
GRIN2A	Speech disorder	01/09/13	55	n
HOMER1	ASD	01/04/12	56	n
GRIN2B	ASD	01/11/11	57	n
SNAP25	ASD	01/09/11	58	n
SYNGAP1	ASD	01/05/11	59,60	n
DLGAP2	Autism susceptibility 1	01/07/10	61	n
PRKCB	ASD	01/07/09	62	n
SHANK1	ASD	01/05/12	63	(y)
NRXN2	ASD	01/10/11	64	(y)
SLC25A12	ASD	01/04/04	65	(y)
MAP2	Rett syndrome	01/12/03	66	(y)
NBEA	ASD	01/05/03	67	(y)
NRXN1	ASD	01/03/07	68,69	(y)
ID (Mental Retardation)				
PURA	Mental retardation, autosomal dominant 31	01/11/14	70	y
CTNNB1	Mental retardation, autosomal dominant 19	01/11/12	71	y
CACNG2	Mental retardation, autosomal dominant 10	01/03/11	72	y
GRIN1	Mental retardation, autosomal dominant 8	01/03/11	72	y
GRIN2B	Mental retardation, autosomal dominant 6	01/11/10	73	y
IQSEC2	Mental retardation, X-linked 1	01/06/10	74	y
SYNGAP1	Mental retardation, autosomal dominant 5	01/02/09	75	y
GRIA3	Mental retardation, X-linked 94	01/11/07	76	y
GRIK2	Mental retardation, autosomal recessive, 6	01/10/07	77	y
DLG3	Mental retardation, X-linked 90	01/08/04	78,79	y
RPS6KA3	Mental retardation, X-linked 19	01/12/96	80	y
GPD2	Mental disability	01/05/13	81	n
TNR	Mental disability	01/07/12	82	n
CLTC	Mental retardation	01/03/97	83	n
MAPK10	Mental retardation	01/01/13	84	(y)
CAMK2G	Mental retardation	01/11/12	71	(y)
GRIA1	Mental retardation	01/11/12	85	(y)
PSMA7	Mental retardation	01/11/12	71	(y)
NRXN1	Mental disability	01/06/10	86—89	(y)

[a]*A "y" is used when OMIM database establishes a causal relationship between gene and disease; "(y)" is used when OMIM describes a potential relation between gene and disease; this information is contained in the Molecular Genetics section of OMIM information about the gene; "n" is used to indicate that no relationship between gene and disease has been reported in OMIM.*

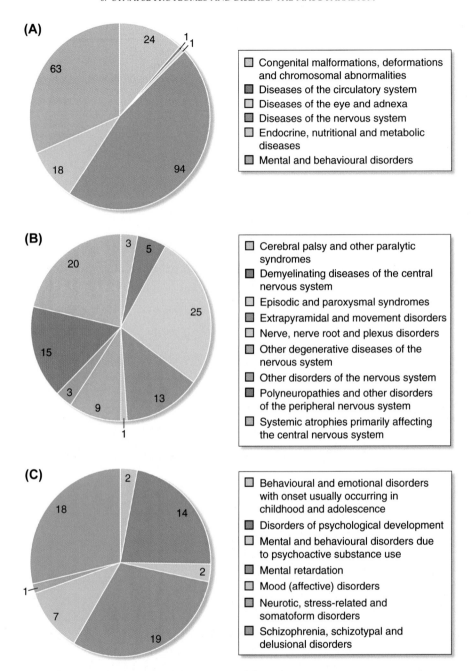

FIGURE 5 **Classification of NSDs related to MASC genes according to the International Classification of Diseases (ICD-10).** (A) Classification of NSDs related to MASC genes in ICD-10 chapters. Number of NSD per chapter is indicated. (B) Types of "Diseases of the Nervous System" related to MASC genes. (C) Types of "Mental and Behavioral Disorders" related to MASC genes.

experienced larger growth, we again find differences. Both chapters contain 11 blocks, but only four in each case continued to accumulate MASC genes related to their disorders (Figure 6(B) and (C)). These include both ID (in the block defined by ICD-10 as mental retardation) and ASD (included in the block of disorders of psychological development) but also schizophrenia (Figure 6(C)), which accumulates almost as many MASC genes as ID, or epileptic conditions (included in episodic and paroxysmal syndromes, Figure 6(B)), which has accumulated many MASC genes in the past few years. As we have shown throughout this chapter, the current data indicates that MASC genes are predominantly involved with mental and behavioral disorders, especially with ID, ASD, and schizophrenia.

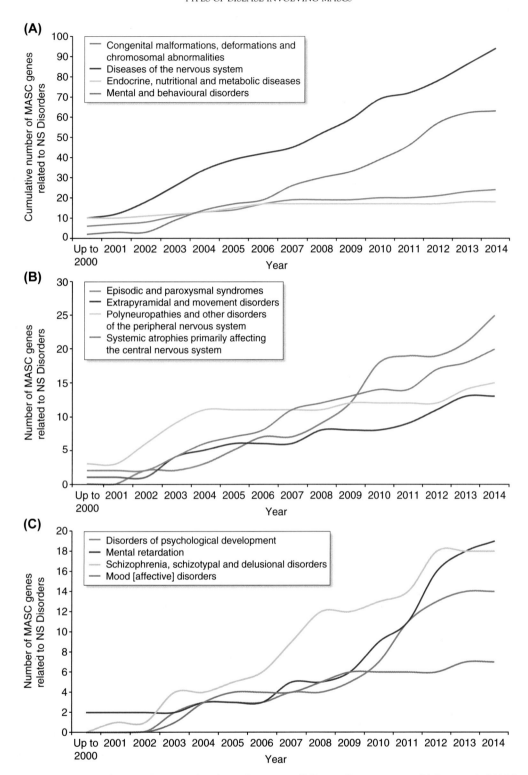

FIGURE 6 **Comparative increase in MASC genes related to NSD among different disease groups.** (A) Increase in MASC genes related to NSD among ICD-10 chapters. (B) Increase in MASC genes related to NSD among ICD-10 blocks from the chapter on Diseases of the Nervous System. (C) Increase in MASC genes related to NSD among ICD-10 blocks from the chapter on Mental and Behavioral Disorders.

SUMMARY AND CONCLUSIONS

Through the study of MASCs a number of general findings regarding the molecular complexity of synapses and the synaptic basis of disease become apparent. First, synapse proteomic studies have importantly contributed to establishing a synaptic role for many NSDs. Second, multiprotein complexes comprising MASCs are disrupted by many different gene mutations that result in multiple diseases. Third, cognitive behavioral disorders are prominent among these disorders, especially ID, autism and schizophrenia. An extensive body of literature in mice has also demonstrated that mutations in MASC proteins result in cognitive impairment.[45–51] Interestingly, studies of intelligence quotient (IQ) variation in the population show that genetic variation in MASC significantly contributes to variation in IQ.[52] Membrane-associated guanylate kinase–associated signaling complexes are clearly of central importance to human brain function.

There is an important need to study MASCs isolated directly from the brain of humans; our studies have demonstrated the feasibility of this in neurosurgical and postmortem tissue.[28] In addition, it is important to enhance our understanding of the subtypes of MASCs and the mechanisms for assembly of the combinations of proteins into discrete molecular machines. It is also important to study how these different MASCs are distributed into different synapses.

Human genetics is uncovering mutations in MASC and other synapse proteins at an unprecedented rate. The variation in alleles, single nucleotide polymorphisms, and copy number variations raise new questions about the roles of gene dosage and subtle changes in protein function in disease. These are likely to be important in the context of MASCs, as multimeric protein complexes carry proteins encoded by both autosomal alleles. Hence, protein stoichiometry will have an influence in the disease relevance of a given mutation, and its understanding will necessarily require the combined used of genetics and biochemistry.

Finally, the remarkable proteome complexity of the mammalian synapse and MASCs arose from eukaryotic components that were amplified by genome duplications in the vertebrate lineage.[24,53] This genomic evolution, which generated the proteome complexity, is the foundation for both our behavioral repertoire and its susceptibility to mutations and disease.

Acknowledgments

We thank Michelle McNab and Mike Croning for the literature search and curation. Àlex Bayés was funded by Proyectos de investigación no orientada, (Ref. BFU2012-34398), Career Integration grant CIG, (Ref. 304111) and Subprograma Ramón y Cajal, (Ref. RYC-2011-08391). Seth GN Grant was supported by the Medical Research Council, the Wellcome Trust, and European Union programs (Project GENCODYS no. 241995, Project EUROSPIN no. 242498, and Project SYNSYS no. 242167).

References

1. Bayés A, Grant SGN. Neuroproteomics: understanding the molecular organization and complexity of the brain. *Nat Rev Neurosci* 2009;**10**(9):635–46. http://dx.doi.org/10.1038/nrn2701.
2. O'Rourke NA, Weiler NC, Micheva KD, Smith SJ. Deep molecular diversity of mammalian synapses: why it matters and how to measure it. *Nat Rev Neurosci* 2012;**13**. http://dx.doi.org/10.1038/nrn3170.
3. Grant SG. Synaptopathies: diseases of the synaptome. *Curr Opin Neurobiol* 2012;**22**:522–9. http://dx.doi.org/10.1016/j.conb.2012.02.002.
4. Fernandez E, Collins MO, Uren RT, Kopanitsa MV, Komiyama NH, Croning MD, et al. Targeted tandem affinity purification of PSD-95 recovers core postsynaptic complexes and schizophrenia susceptibility proteins. *Mol Syst Biol* 2009;**5**:269. http://dx.doi.org/10.1038/msb.2009.27.
5. Bayés A, Van De Lagemaat LN, Collins MO, Croning MDR, Whittle IR, Choudhary JS, et al. Characterization of the proteome, diseases and evolution of the human postsynaptic density. *Nat Neurosci* 2011;**14**(1):19–21. http://dx.doi.org/10.1038/nn.2719.
6. Carlin RK, Grab DJ, Cohen RS, Siekevitz P. Isolation and characterization of postsynaptic densities from various brain regions: enrichment of different types of postsynaptic densities. *J Cell Biol* 1980;**86**(3):831–45.
7. Husi H, Ward MA, Choudhary JS, Blackstock WP, Grant SG. Proteomic analysis of NMDA receptor-adhesion protein signaling complexes. *Nat Neurosci* 2000;**3**(7):661–9.
8. Collins MO, Husi H, Yu L, Brandon JM, Anderson CNG, Blackstock WP, et al. Molecular characterization and comparison of the components and multiprotein complexes in the postsynaptic proteome. *J Neurochem* 2006;**97**(Suppl. 1):16–23. http://dx.doi.org/10.1111/j.1471-4159.2005.03507.x.
9. Dosemeci A, Makusky AJ, Jankowska-Stephens E, Yang X, Slotta DJ, Markey SP. Composition of the synaptic PSD-95 complex. *Mol Cell Proteomics* 2007;**6**(10):1749–60.
10. Trinidad JC, Thalhammer A, Specht CG, Lynn AJ, Baker PR, Schoepfer R, et al. Quantitative analysis of synaptic phosphorylation and protein expression. *Mol Cell Proteomics* 2008;**7**(4):684–96. http://dx.doi.org/10.1074/mcp.M700170-MCP200.
11. Bayés A, Collins MO, Croning MDR, Van De Lagemaat LN, Choudhary JS, Grant SGN. Comparative study of human and mouse postsynaptic proteomes finds high compositional conservation and abundance differences for key synaptic proteins. *PLoS One* 2012;**7**(10):e46683. http://dx.doi.org/10.1371/journal.pone.0046683.
12. Peng J, Kim MJ, Cheng D, Duong DM, Gygi SP, Sheng M. Semiquantitative proteomic analysis of rat forebrain postsynaptic density fractions by mass spectrometry. *J Biol Chem* 2004;**279**(20):21003–11.
13. Cheng D, Hoogenraad CC, Rush J, Ramm E, Schlager MA, Duong DM, et al. Relative and absolute quantification of postsynaptic density proteome isolated from rat forebrain and cerebellum. *Mol Cell Proteomics* 2006;**5**(6):1158–70.
14. Li KW, Hornshaw MP, van der Schors RC, Watson R, Tate S, Casetta B, et al. Proteomics analysis of rat brain postsynaptic density. Implications of the diverse protein functional groups for the integration of synaptic physiology. *J Biol Chem* 2004;**279**(2):987–1002.

15. Burre J, Beckhaus T, Schagger H, Corvey C, Hofmann S, Karas M, et al. Analysis of the synaptic vesicle proteome using three gel-based protein separation techniques. *Proteomics* 2006;**6**(23): 6250–62.

16. Takamori S, Holt M, Stenius K, Lemke EA, Gronborg M, Riedel D, et al. Molecular anatomy of a trafficking organelle. *Cell* 2006;**127**(4): 831–46.

17. Phillips GR, Huang JK, Wang Y, Tanaka H, Shapiro L, Zhang W, et al. The presynaptic particle web: ultrastructure, composition, dissolution, and reconstitution. *Neuron* 2001;**32**(1):63–77.

18. Volknandt W, Karas M. Proteomic analysis of the presynaptic active zone. *Exp Brain Res* 2012;**217**(3–4):449–61. http://dx.doi.org/10.1007/s00221-012-3031-x.

19. Sahni N, Yi S, Taipale M, Fuxman Bass JI, Coulombe-Huntington J, Yang F, et al. Widespread macromolecular interaction perturbations in human genetic disorders. *Cell* 2015;**161**(3):647–60. http://dx.doi.org/10.1016/j.cell.2015.04.013.

20. Rolland T, Tasan M, Charloteaux B, Pevzner SJ, Zhong Q, Sahni N, et al. A proteome-scale map of the human interactome network. *Cell* 2014;**159**(5):1212–26. http://dx.doi.org/10.1016/j.cell.2014. 10.050.

21. Klemmer P, Smit AB, Li KW. Proteomics analysis of immuno-precipitated synaptic protein complexes. *J Proteomics* 2009;**72**(1): 82–90. Epub November 5, 2008.

22. Farr CD, Gafken PR, Norbeck AD, Doneanu CE, Stapels MD, Barofsky DF, et al. Proteomic analysis of native metabotropic glutamate receptor 5 protein complexes reveals novel molecular constituents. *J Neurochem* 2004;**91**(2):438–50.

23. Li X, Xie C, Jin Q, Liu M, He Q, Cao R, et al. Proteomic screen for multiprotein complexes in synaptic plasma membrane from rat hippocampus by blue native gel electrophoresis and tandem mass spectrometry. *J Proteome Res* 2009;**8**(7):3475–86. http://dx.doi.org/10.1021/pr900101d.

24. Emes RD, Grant SGN. Evolution of synapse complexity and diversity. *Annu Rev Neurosci* 2012;**35**(1):111–31. http://dx.doi.org/10.1146/annurev-neuro-062111-150433.

25. Good MC, Zalatan JG, Lim WA. Scaffold proteins: hubs for controlling the flow of cellular information. *Science* 2011;**332**(6030):680–6. http://dx.doi.org/10.1126/science.1198701.

26. Oliva C, Escobedo P, Astorga C, Molina C, Sierralta J. Role of the MAGUK protein family in synapse formation and function. *Dev Neurobiol* 2012;**72**(1):57–72. http://dx.doi.org/10.1002/dneu.20949.

27. Wang S-HJ, Celic I, Choi S-Y, Riccomagno M, Wang Q, Sun LO, et al. Dlg5 regulates dendritic spine formation and synaptogenesis by controlling subcellular N-cadherin localization. *J Neurosci* 2014; **34**(38):12745–61. http://dx.doi.org/10.1523/JNEUROSCI.1280-14.2014.

28. Bayés A, Collins MO, Galtrey CM, Simonnet C, Roy M, Croning MD, et al. Human post-mortem synapse proteome integrity screening for proteomic studies of postsynaptic complexes. *Mol Brain* 2014;**7**(1):88. http://dx.doi.org/10.1186/s13041-014-0088-4.

29. Husi H, Grant SG. Isolation of 2000-kDa complexes of N-methyl-D-aspartate receptor and postsynaptic density 95 from mouse brain. *J Neurochem* 2001;**77**(1):281–91.

30. Mi H, Muruganujan A, Thomas PD. PANTHER in 2013: modeling the evolution of gene function, and other gene attributes, in the context of phylogenetic trees. *Nucleic Acids Res* 2013;**41**(Database issue):D377–86. http://dx.doi.org/10.1093/nar/gks1118.

31. McKusick VA. Mendelian inheritance in man and its online version, OMIM. *Am J Hum Genet* 2007;**80**(4):588–604. http://dx.doi.org/10.1086/514346.

32. Soto D, Altafaj X, Sindreu C, Bayés A. Glutamate receptor mutations in psychiatric and neurodevelopmental disorders. *Commun Integr Biol* 2014;**7**(1):e27887. http://dx.doi.org/10.4161/cib.27887.

33. Musante L, Ropers HH. Genetics of recessive cognitive disorders. *Trends Genet* 2013;**30**(1):32–9. http://dx.doi.org/10.1016/j.tig. 2013.09.008.

34. Bassani S, Zapata J, Gerosa L, Moretto E, Murru L, Passafaro M. The neurobiology of X-linked intellectual disability. *Neuroscientist* 2013;**19**:541–52. http://dx.doi.org/10.1177/1073858413493972.

35. Ellison JW, Rosenfeld JA, Shaffer LG. Genetic basis of intellectual disability. *Annu Rev Med* 2013;**64**(1):441–50. http://dx.doi.org/10.1146/annurev-med-042711-140053.

36. Ropers HH. Genetics of early onset cognitive impairment. *Annu Rev Genomics Hum Genet* 2010;**11**:161–87. http://dx.doi.org/10.1146/annurev-genom-082509-141640.

37. Ronemus M, Iossifov I, Levy D, Wigler M. The role of de novo mutations in the genetics of autism spectrum disorders. *Nat Rev* 2014; **15**(2):133–41. http://dx.doi.org/10.1038/nrg3585.

38. Krumm N, O'Roak BJ, Shendure J, Eichler EE. A de novo convergence of autism genetics and molecular neuroscience. *Trends Neurosci* 2014;**37**(2):95–105. http://dx.doi.org/10.1016/j.tins.2013.11.005.

39. Talkowski ME, Minikel EV, Gusella JF. Autism spectrum disorder genetics: diverse genes with diverse clinical outcomes. *Harv Rev Psychiatry* 2014;**22**(2):65–75. http://dx.doi.org/10.1097/HRP. 0000000000000002.

40. Sullivan PF, Daly MJ, O'Donovan M. Genetic architectures of psychiatric disorders: the emerging picture and its implications. *Nat Rev* 2012;**13**(8):537–51. http://dx.doi.org/10.1038/nrg3240.

41. Gejman PV, Sanders AR, Kendler KS. Genetics of schizophrenia: new findings and challenges. *Annu Rev Genomics Hum Genet* 2011; **12**:121–44. http://dx.doi.org/10.1146/annurev-genom-082410-101459.

42. Koboldt DC, Steinberg KM, Larson DE, Wilson RK, Mardis ER. The next-generation sequencing revolution and its impact on genomics. *Cell* 2013;**155**(1):27–38. http://dx.doi.org/10.1016/j.cell.2013.09.006.

43. Srivastava AK, Schwartz CE. Intellectual disability and autism spectrum disorders: causal genes and molecular mechanisms. *Neurosci Biobehav Rev* 2014;**46**. http://dx.doi.org/10.1016/j.neubiorev.2014.02.015.

44. Matson JL, Shoemaker M. Intellectual disability and its relationship to autism spectrum disorders. *Res Dev Disabil* 2009;**30**(6): 1107–14. http://dx.doi.org/10.1016/j.ridd.2009.06.003.

45. Migaud M, Charlesworth P, Dempster M, Webster LC, Watabe AM, Makhinson M, et al. Enhanced long-term potentiation and impaired learning in mice with mutant postsynaptic density-95 protein. *Nature* 1998;**396**(6710):433–9.

46. Komiyama NH, Watabe AM, Carlisle HJ, Porter K, Charlesworth P, Monti J, et al. SynGAP regulates ERK/MAPK signaling, synaptic plasticity, and learning in the complex with postsynaptic density 95 and NMDA receptor. *J Neurosci* 2002; **22**(22):9721–32.

47. Cuthbert PC, Stanford LE, Coba MP, Ainge JA, Fink AE, Opazo P, et al. Synapse-associated protein 102/dlgh3 couples the NMDA receptor to specific plasticity pathways and learning strategies. *J Neurosci* 2007;**27**(10):2673–82. http://dx.doi.org/10.1523/JNEUROSCI.4457-06.2007.

48. Schmeisser MJ, Ey E, Wegener S, Bockmann J, Stempel AV, Kuebler A, et al. Autistic-like behaviours and hyperactivity in mice lacking ProSAP1/Shank2. *Nature* 2012;**486**(7402):256–60. http://dx.doi.org/10.1038/nature11015.

49. Ronesi JA, Collins KA, Hays SA, Tsai N-P, Guo W, Birnbaum SG, et al. Disrupted Homer scaffolds mediate abnormal mGluR5 function in a mouse model of fragile X syndrome. *Nat Neurosci* 2012; **15**(3):431–40. http://dx.doi.org/10.1038/nn.3033.

50. Wöhr M, Roullet FI, Hung AY, Sheng M, Crawley JN. Communication impairments in mice lacking Shank1: reduced levels of ultrasonic vocalizations and scent marking behavior. *PLoS One* 2011; **6**(6):e20631. http://dx.doi.org/10.1371/journal.pone.0020631.

51. Peça J, Feliciano C, Ting JT, Wang W, Wells MF, Venkatraman TN, et al. Shank3 mutant mice display autistic-like behaviours and striatal dysfunction. *Nature* 2011;**472**(7344):437—42. http://dx.doi.org/10.1038/nature09965.

52. Hill WD, Davies G, van de Lagemaat LN, Christoforou A, Marioni RE, Fernandes CPD, et al. Human cognitive ability is influenced by genetic variation in components of postsynaptic signalling complexes assembled by NMDA receptors and MAGUK proteins. *Transl Psychiatry* 2014;**4**:e341. http://dx.doi.org/10.1038/tp.2013.114.

53. Emes RD, Pocklington AJ, Anderson CNG, Bayés A, Collins MO, Vickers CA, et al. Evolutionary expansion and anatomical specialization of synapse proteome complexity. *Nat Neurosci* 2008;**11**(7): 799—806. http://dx.doi.org/10.1038/nn.2135.

54. Berkel S, Marshall CR, Weiss B, Howe J, Roeth R, Moog U, et al. Mutations in the SHANK2 synaptic scaffolding gene in autism spectrum disorder and mental retardation. *Nat Genet* 2010;**42**(6): 489—91. http://dx.doi.org/10.1038/ng.589.

55. Lesca G, Rudolf G, Bruneau N, Lozovaya N, Labalme A, Boutry-Kryza N, et al. GRIN2A mutations in acquired epileptic aphasia and related childhood focal epilepsies and encephalopathies with speech and language dysfunction. *Nat Genet* 2013;**45**(9):1061—6. http://dx.doi.org/10.1038/ng.2726.

56. Kelleher RJ, Geigenmüller U, Hovhannisyan H, Trautman E, Pinard R, Rathmell B, et al. High-throughput sequencing of mGluR signaling pathway genes reveals enrichment of rare variants in autism. *PLoS One* 2012;**7**(4):e35003. http://dx.doi.org/10.1371/journal.pone.0035003.

57. Tarabeux J, Kebir O, Gauthier J, Hamdan FF, Xiong L, Piton A, et al., S2D Team. Rare mutations in N-methyl-D-aspartate glutamate receptors in autism spectrum disorders and schizophrenia. *Transl Psychiatry* 2011;**1**:e55. http://dx.doi.org/10.1038/tp.2011.52.

58. Guerini FR, Bolognesi E, Chiappedi M, Manca S, Ghezzo A, Agliardi C, et al. SNAP-25 single nucleotide polymorphisms are associated with hyperactivity in autism spectrum disorders. *Pharmacol Res* 2011;**64**(3):283—8. http://dx.doi.org/10.1016/j.phrs.2011.03.015.

59. Berryer MH, Hamdan FF, Klitten LL, Møller RS, Carmant L, Schwartzentruber J, et al. Mutations in SYNGAP1 cause intellectual disability, autism and a specific form of epilepsy by inducing haploinsufficiency. *Hum Mutat* 2012;**34**(2):385—99. http://dx.doi.org/10.1002/humu.22248. n/a—n/a.

60. Hamdan FF, Daoud H, Piton A, Gauthier J, Dobrzeniecka S, Krebs MO, et al. De Novo SYNGAP1 mutations in nonsyndromic intellectual disability and autism. *Biol Psychiatry* 2011;**69**:898—901. http://dx.doi.org/10.1016/j.biopsych.2010.11.015.

61. Pinto D, Pagnamenta AT, Klei L, Anney R, Merico D, Regan R, et al. Functional impact of global rare copy number variation in autism spectrum disorders. *Nature* 2010;**466**(7304):368—72. http://dx.doi.org/10.1038/nature09146.

62. Lintas C, Sacco R, Garbett K, Mirnics K, Militerni R, Bravaccio C, et al. Involvement of the PRKCB1 gene in autistic disorder: significant genetic association and reduced neocortical gene expression. *Mol Psychiatry* 2009;**14**(7):705—18. http://dx.doi.org/10.1038/mp.2008.21.

63. Sato D, Lionel AC, Leblond CS, Prasad A, Pinto D, Walker S, et al. SHANK1 deletions in males with autism spectrum disorder. *Am J Hum Genet* 2012;**90**(5). http://dx.doi.org/10.1016/j.ajhg.2012.03.017.

64. Gauthier J, Siddiqui TJ, Huashan P, Yokomaku D, Hamdan FF, Champagne N, et al. Truncating mutations in NRXN2 and NRXN1 in autism spectrum disorders and schizophrenia. *Hum Genet* 2011; **130**(4):563—73. http://dx.doi.org/10.1007/s00439-011-0975-z.

65. Ramoz N, Reichert JG, Smith CJ, Silverman JM, Bespalova IN, Davis KL, et al. Linkage and association of the mitochondrial aspartate/glutamate carrier SLC25A12 gene with autism. *Am J Psychiatry* 2004;**161**(4):662—9.

66. Pescucci C, Meloni I, Bruttini M, Ariani F, Longo I, Mari F, et al. Chromosome 2 deletion encompassing the MAP2 gene in a patient with autism and Rett-like features. *Clin Genet* 2003;**64**(6):497—501.

67. Castermans D, Wilquet V, Parthoens E, Huysmans C, Steyaert J, Swinnen L, et al. The neurobeachin gene is disrupted by a translocation in a patient with idiopathic autism. *J Med Genet* 2003;**40**(5):352—6.

68. Autism Genome Project Consortium, Szatmari P, Paterson AD, Zwaigenbaum L, Roberts W, Brian J, Liu X-Q, et al. Mapping autism risk loci using genetic linkage and chromosomal rearrangements. *Nat Genet* 2007;**39**(3):319—28. http://dx.doi.org/10.1038/ng1985.

69. Kim HG, Kishikawa S, Higgins AW, Seong IS, Donovan DJ, Shen Y, et al. Disruption of neurexin 1 associated with autism spectrum disorder. *Am J Hum Genet* 2008;**82**(1):199—207. http://dx.doi.org/10.1016/j.ajhg.2007.09.011.

70. Lalani SR, Zhang J, Schaaf CP, Brown CW, Magoulas P, Tsai AC-H, et al. Mutations in PURA cause profound neonatal hypotonia, seizures, and encephalopathy in 5q31.3 microdeletion syndrome. *Am J Hum Genet* 2014;**95**(5):579—83. http://dx.doi.org/10.1016/j.ajhg.2014.09.014.

71. de Ligt J, Willemsen MH, van Bon BWM, Kleefstra T, Yntema HG, Kroes T, et al. Diagnostic exome sequencing in persons with severe intellectual disability. *N Engl J Med* 2012;**367**(20):1921—9. http://dx.doi.org/10.1056/NEJMoa1206524.

72. Hamdan FF, Gauthier J, Araki Y, Lin DT, Yoshizawa Y, Higashi K, et al. Excess of de novo deleterious mutations in genes associated with glutamatergic systems in nonsyndromic intellectual disability. *Am J Hum Genet* 2011;**88**(3):306—16. http://dx.doi.org/10.1016/j.ajhg.2011.02.001.

73. Endele S, Rosenberger G, Geider K, Popp B, Tamer C, Stefanova I, et al. Mutations in GRIN2A and GRIN2B encoding regulatory subunits of NMDA receptors cause variable neurodevelopmental phenotypes. *Nat Genet* 2010;**42**(11):1021—6. http://dx.doi.org/10.1038/ng.677.

74. Shoubridge C, Tarpey PS, Abidi F, Ramsden SL, Rujirabanjerd S, Murphy JA, et al. Mutations in the guanine nucleotide exchange factor gene IQSEC2 cause nonsyndromic intellectual disability. *Nat Genet* 2010;**42**(6):486—8. http://dx.doi.org/10.1038/ng.588.

75. Hamdan FF, Gauthier J, Spiegelman D, Noreau A, Yang Y, Pellerin S, et al. Mutations in SYNGAP1 in autosomal nonsyndromic mental retardation. *N Engl J Med* 2009;**360**(6):599—605.

76. Wu Y, Arai AC, Rumbaugh G, Srivastava AK, Turner G, Hayashi T, et al. Mutations in ionotropic AMPA receptor 3 alter channel properties and are associated with moderate cognitive impairment in humans. *Proc Natl Acad Sci* 2007;**104**(46):18163—8. http://dx.doi.org/10.1073/pnas.0708699104.

77. Motazacker MM, Rost BR, Hucho T, Garshasbi M, Kahrizi K, Ullmann R, et al. A defect in the ionotropic glutamate receptor 6 gene (GRIK2) is associated with autosomal recessive mental retardation. *Am J Hum Genet* 2007;**81**(4):792—8. http://dx.doi.org/10.1086/521275.

78. Clinton SM, Meador-Woodruff JH. Abnormalities of the NMDA receptor and associated intracellular molecules in the thalamus in schizophrenia and bipolar disorder. *Neuropsychopharmacology* 2004;**29**(7):1353—62. http://dx.doi.org/10.1038/sj.npp.1300451.

79. Tarpey P, Parnau J, Blow M, Woffendin H, Bignell G, Cox C, et al. Mutations in the DLG3 gene cause nonsyndromic X-linked mental retardation. *Am J Hum Genet* 2004;**75**(2):318—24. http://dx.doi.org/10.1086/422703.

80. Merienne K, Jacquot S, Pannetier S, Zeniou M, Bankier A, Gecz J, et al. A missense mutation in RPS6KA3 (RSK2) responsible for non-specific mental retardation. *Nat Genet* 1999;**22**(1):13—4. http://dx.doi.org/10.1038/8719.

81. Barge-Schaapveld DQCM, Ofman R, Knegt AC, Alders M, Höhne W, Kemp S, et al. Intellectual disability and hemizygous GPD2 mutation. *Am J Med Genet A* 2013;**161A**(5):1044—50. http://dx.doi.org/10.1002/ajmg.a.35873.

II. FUNCTION OF MUTATED GENES IN INTELLECTUAL DISABILITY (ID) AND AUTISM

82. Dufresne D, Hamdan FF, Rosenfeld JA, Torchia B, Rosenblatt B, Michaud JL, et al. Homozygous deletion of Tenascin-R in a patient with intellectual disability. *J Med Genet* 2012;**49**(7):451−4. http://dx.doi.org/10.1136/jmedgenet-2012-100831.

83. Holmes SE, Riazi MA, Gong W, McDermid HE, Sellinger BT, Hua A, et al. Disruption of the clathrin heavy chain-like gene (CLTCL) associated with features of DGS/VCFS: a balanced (21;22)(p12;q11) translocation. *Hum Mol Genet* 1997;**6**(3):357−67.

84. Kunde S-A, Rademacher N, Tzschach A, Wiedersberg E, Ullmann R, Kalscheuer VM, et al. Characterisation of de novo MAPK10/JNK3 truncation mutations associated with cognitive disorders in two unrelated patients. *Hum Genet* 2013;**132**(4):461−71. http://dx.doi.org/10.1007/s00439-012-1260-5.

85. Kang WS, Park JK, Kim SK, Park HJ, Lee SM, Song JY, et al. Genetic variants of GRIA1 are associated with susceptibility to schizophrenia in Korean population. *Mol Biol Rep* 2012;**39**(12):10697−703. http://dx.doi.org/10.1007/s11033-012-1960-x.

86. Ching MSL, Shen Y, Tan W-H, Jeste SS, Morrow EM, Chen X, et al. Children's Hospital Boston Genotype Phenotype Study Group. Deletions of NRXN1 (neurexin-1) predispose to a wide spectrum of developmental disorders. *Am J Med Genet B Neuropsychiatr Genet* 2010;**153B**(4):937−47. http://dx.doi.org/10.1002/ajmg.b.31063.

87. Béna F, Bruno DL, Eriksson M, van Ravenswaaij-Arts C, Stark Z, Dijkhuizen T, et al. Molecular and clinical characterization of 25 individuals with exonic deletions of NRXN1 and comprehensive review of the literature. *Am J Med Genet B Neuropsychiatr Genet* 2013;**162B**(4):388−403. http://dx.doi.org/10.1002/ajmg.b.32148.

88. Gregor A, Albrecht B, Bader I, Bijlsma EK, Ekici AB, Engels H, et al. Expanding the clinical spectrum associated with defects in CNTNAP2 and NRXN1. *BMC Med Genet* 2011;**12**:106. http://dx.doi.org/10.1186/1471-2350-12-106.

89. Schaaf CP, Boone PM, Sampath S, Williams C, Bader PI, Mueller JM, et al. Phenotypic spectrum and genotype-phenotype correlations of NRXN1 exon deletions. *Eur J Hum Genet* 2012;**20**(12):1240−7. http://dx.doi.org/10.1038/ejhg.2012.95.

7

The Function of MeCP2 and Its Causality in Rett Syndrome

Janine M. Lamonica, Zhaolan Zhou

Department of Genetics, Perelman School of Medicine, University of Pennsylvania, Philadelphia, PA, USA

RETT SYNDROME

Rett syndrome (RTT) is a neurodevelopmental disorder first described by the Austrian pediatrician Andreas Rett in 1965.[1] Affecting about 1 in 10,000 females, RTT is the leading cause of intellectual disability in young girls. Patients develop normally for the first 6—18 months of age, followed by a period of regression characterized by loss of learned language skills and purposeful hand movements. During this period, development of autistic-like traits and a marked deceleration of head growth, eventually leading to microcephaly, are common. After the regression stage, development reaches a plateau, at which time additional symptoms often emerge, including hand stereotypies, seizures, respiratory abnormalities, and profound cognitive impairment. In later life, patients undergo a steep decline in motor performance and often lose the ability to walk[2] (see also Chapter 19).

Mutations in the X-linked gene encoding methyl-CpG binding protein 2 (MeCP2) account for approximately 95% of classical RTT cases.[3] In a small subset of patients, mutations have been identified in the related genes cyclin-dependent kinase—like 5 (*CDKL5*) and forkhead box G1 (*FOXG1*), which are associated with the early-onset seizure and congenital variants of RTT, respectively. Most *MECP2* mutations are de novo, arising spontaneously in the paternal germ line. Heterozygous female offspring are somatic mosaics owing to random X chromosome inactivation (XCI) and have a roughly 1:1 mixture of wild-type and mutant *MECP2*-expressing cells. Skewed expression toward the wild-type or mutant allele can happen when XCI is nonrandom, leading to milder or more severe phenotypes, respectively. Hemizygous males present with neonatal encephalopathy and rarely survive beyond 2 years of age.[4]

Several hundred pathogenic mutations that span the entire *MECP2* gene have been identified and include missense, frameshift, nonsense, and splice-site mutations.[5—8] Several of these mutations occur at higher

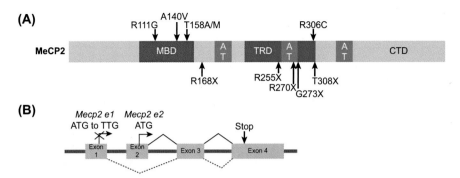

FIGURE 1   Rett syndrome (RTT)-associated patient mutations modeled in mice. (A) The structural domains of methyl-CpG binding protein 2 (MeCP2) and the locations of RTT-causing missense and nonsense mutations. MBD, Methyl-CpG binding domain; AT, AT-hook domain; TRD, transcription repression domain; CTD, C-terminal domain. (B) Translation of the *Mecp2-e1* isoform is eliminated by a missense mutation in the ATG start site, whereas *Mecp2-e2* translation remains intact.

frequency (T158M, R168X, R255X, R270X, R294X, R306C, and R133C) (RettBASE, http://mecp2.chw.edu.au). Typically, early truncating mutations as well as missense mutations in the methyl-CpG binding domain (MBD) of MeCP2 lead to complete loss-of-function and are associated with more severe phenotypes, whereas C-terminal truncations likely lead to partial loss-of-function and cause milder symptoms (Figure 1(A)). Disease phenotype is therefore affected by the particular pathogenic mutation, as well as by nonrandom XCI in mosaic females.

MeCP2 AS A MULTIFACETED PROTEIN

Cloned and purified in 1992, MeCP2 is the founding member of the MBD family of proteins that have binding affinity for methylated deoxyribonucleic acid (DNA).[9] Although expressed ubiquitously, MeCP2 levels are highest in postmitotic neurons of the central nervous system (CNS).[10] Methyl-CpG binding protein 2 contains an 84-amino-acid domain, the MBD, which is necessary and sufficient for binding to methylated DNA in vitro.[11] Methyl-CpG binding protein 2 also binds to chromatin in a methylation-dependent manner in vivo.[12,13] Methyl-CpG binding protein 2 was proposed to act as a transcriptional repressor owing to the well-established correlation between DNA methylation and gene repression.[14] Indeed, MeCP2 represses transcription from methylated templates in vitro and in heterologous cells.[15] Repressive activity was subsequently mapped to a second domain, the transcriptional repression domain (TRD), which associates with repressors such as mSin3A,[15] c-Ski,[16] and NCoR/SMRT,[16–18] and their associated histone deacetylase activity. These findings support a model in which MeCP2 exerts its repressive functions by recruiting corepressor complexes to methylated DNA to generate a hypoacetylated, locally repressive chromatin environment.

Although traditionally studied in the context of gene repression, the role of MeCP2 as a bona fide transcriptional repressor has been the subject of controversy. If MeCP2 acts as a transcriptional repressor, one prediction is that the absence of MeCP2 would result in the upregulation of downstream targets. This prediction, however, is not supported by microarray studies from whole brain tissue, which revealed only subtle changes in gene expression in the absence of MeCP2.[19] Such modest changes may be a consequence of the cellular heterogeneity of the mammalian brain, which might obscure cell type–specific differences in gene expression. To partially circumvent this problem, gene expression was profiled specifically in the hypothalamus,[20] cerebellum,[21] and striatum.[22] These studies found that the absence of MeCP2 led to changes in the expression of hundreds of genes, although most changes were subtle. Surprisingly, most differentially expressed genes were downregulated by MeCP2 ablation, which suggests a previously unappreciated role for MeCP2 in gene activation. In support of this finding, MeCP2 has been reported to interact with the transcriptional activator CREB and to recruit it to activated gene targets.[20] More recently, human neurons derived from embryonic stem cells containing a loss-of-function *MECP2* allele were found to have reduced genome-wide levels of ribonucleic acid (RNA). Coupled with global transcriptional downregulation, *MECP2* mutant neurons displayed impaired protein synthesis, mitochondrial function, and AKT/mTOR signaling.[23] Given these data, a role for MeCP2 in global gene activation has been proposed (also see Chapter 7).

In addition, the genes regulated by MeCP2 appear to depend on cell type or brain region. For example, upon MeCP2 deletion in the striatum, a region of the brain composed almost exclusively of inhibitory medium spiny neurons, a number of differentially expressed genes were identified; however, most of these genes were not differentially expressed upon MeCP2 deletion in the hypothalamus or cerebellum.[22] Thus, it appears that MeCP2 regulates different sets of genes in different cell types or brain regions.[22] Together, these studies highlight the complexity of MeCP2-dependent gene regulation, with MeCP2 both activating and repressing genes depending on cellular context. Although technically challenging, expression profiling of pure subpopulations of neuronal cells in the absence of MeCP2 would help to address the contribution of MeCP2 to gene regulation throughout the brain.

Methyl-CpG binding protein 2 binds preferentially to methylated DNA in vitro[9,24] and is reported to track with methylated DNA in vivo.[25] Nevertheless, MeCP2 has only a threefold greater affinity for methylated versus nonmethylated DNA in vitro[26,27] and associates with both methylated and nonmethylated promoters in neuronal cell lines.[28] In brain nuclei, a large fraction of MeCP2 localizes to nuclease-accessible regions, which are likely regions of transcriptional activity.[29] These data further support a role for MeCP2 in both repressing and activating gene transcription. More recently, evidence has emerged that MeCP2 associates with 5-hydroxymethylcytosine (5hmC), a DNA modification that is highly enriched in the gene bodies of active genes.[30] In vitro studies suggest that MeCP2's affinity for 5hmC is similar to that of methylated DNA (5mC).[30] Methyl-CpG binding protein 2 might therefore regulate transcription bidirectionally through dynamic association with 5mC and 5hmC. Moreover, in the absence of MeCP2, 5hmC-enriched DNA exists in a more compact, repressive conformation.[30] Thus, it has been proposed that when bound to 5hmC along gene bodies, MeCP2 facilitates transcription by regulating chromatin accessibility.

Additional studies suggest a role for MeCP2 in the maintenance of chromatin structure. Methyl-CpG binding protein 2 binds broadly throughout the genome in a histone-like manner, and in neuronal nuclei, the abundance of MeCP2 is comparable to that of nucleosomes.[25] Moreover, MeCP2 and linker histone H1 both induce marked condensation of nucleosomal arrays, with MeCP2 competing with histone H1 for nucleosome binding sites.[15,27] These observations suggest that MeCP2 might serve as an alternative linker histone. Rather than repressing transcription in a gene-specific manner, MeCP2 might instead regulate chromatin structure globally. To test this idea, Skene et al.[25] examined the levels of histone H3 acetylation (H3Ac) in Mecp2-null brains and found increased levels, both globally and at specific loci, relative to wild-type controls. This increase in H3Ac levels was accompanied by an increase in spurious transcription of repetitive elements throughout the genome. Methyl-CpG binding protein 2 thus may have a structural role in chromatin organization, which in part may serve to dampen transcriptional noise emanating from repetitive elements.[25] These data suggest that MeCP2 might have a more global role in the modulation of gene expression by mediating changes in chromatin configuration.

Methyl-CpG binding protein 2 has been implicated in additional cellular roles by virtue of its interacting partners. One MeCP2 cofactor is α-thalassemia/mental retardation, X-linked (ATRX), a SWI2/SNF2 DNA helicase/ATPase that is mutated in X-linked mental retardation with α-thalassemia syndrome.[31] Methyl-CpG binding protein 2 recruits the helicase domain of ATRX to heterochromatin-rich foci in a DNA methylation-dependent manner.[31] Several disease-associated mutations in MeCP2 disrupt its interaction with ATRX, which can be used as a marker of disease severity.[31–33] It has been proposed that MeCP2 and ATRX function together to regulate nucleosome positioning at specific CTCF binding sites, thus facilitating local chromatin looping configurations.[34] Another MeCP2 cofactor is Y box-binding protein 1 (YB-1), a conserved protein involved in the regulation of RNA splicing. In vivo, abnormal alternative splicing events have been reported in MeCP2 mutant animals.[35] In addition, MeCP2 directly interacts with DGCR8, an essential component of the microRNA (miRNA)-processing machinery.[36] In the absence of MeCP2, the levels of mature miRNAs are increased, which suggests that MeCP2 inhibits the expression of miRNAs posttranscriptionally.[36] Collectively, these studies demonstrate that MeCP2 is a multifunctional protein that mediates many downstream events depending on the cellular context.

MeCP2 POSTTRANSLATIONAL MODIFICATIONS

Methyl-CpG binding protein 2 undergoes numerous posttranslational modifications (PTMs) that regulate its functional versatility. One MeCP2 phosphorylation event that has been studied extensively is activity-dependent phosphorylation at serine 421 located in the C-terminal domain (CTD).[37,38] This residue becomes phosphorylated selectively in the brain in response to sensory stimuli. In cultured neurons, phosphorylation at S421 correlates with Bdnf expression and is required for proper dendritic and synaptic development, which suggests that this modification is necessary to establish proper connectivity in the nervous system.[37] Interestingly, this phosphorylation event also regulates certain aspects of cognitive function because its loss in mice results in abnormal behavioral responses to novel experiences.[38] Chromatin immunoprecipitation (ChIP) followed by massively parallel sequencing (ChIP-seq) experiments do not support a role for activity-dependent S421 phosphorylation in regulating the binding of MeCP2 to DNA; rather, it has been proposed that this modification contributes to MeCP2-mediated structural changes in chromatin architecture.[38]

A more recent study set out to identify additional sites of activity-dependent phosphorylation on MeCP2 using phosphotryptic mapping.[39] Using this method, residues S86, S274, T308, and S421 were found to be newly phosphorylated in response to membrane depolarization; of these, S86 and T308 had not been previously identified by mass spectrometry. Owing to its close proximity to the RTT-associated R306C mutation, the authors focused on phosphorylation at T308, located at the C-terminal edge of the TRD. Activity-dependent phosphorylation of T308 was found to abrogate the MeCP2-NCoR/SMRT interaction, whereas the absence of phosphorylation at T308 led to constitutive MeCP2 binding to NCoR/SMRT. To examine the in vivo consequence of constitutive MeCP2-NCoR binding, T308A knock-in mice were generated. They displayed several neurological impairments including reduced brain weight, motor problems, hind-limb clasping, and increased seizures and lower seizure threshold. Moreover, these animals displayed reduced activity-dependent activation of several genes, including *Bdnf* and *Npas4*. Altered transcription of these genes could explain the increased numbers of seizures, which could lead to loss of excitatory/inhibitory cellular balance, and consequent hyperexcitability of neuronal networks.[39] Phosphorylation at T308 upon sensory stimulation may thus function to dampen the repressive activity of MeCP2 by regulating the association of MeCP2 with NCoR/SMRT. Interestingly, R306C mutations also disrupt phosphorylation at T308, which lends support to the idea that loss of activity-dependent phosphorylation at T308 could contribute in part to the RTT symptoms seen in individuals with T306C mutations.[18,39]

Serines 80 and 229 of MeCP2 are also modified by phosphorylation.[40] It has been reported that these modifications regulate the interaction of MeCP2 with distinct combinations of binding partners, which may be a mechanism by which MeCP2 alters its activities.[40] For example, phosphorylation at S80 enhances the interaction of MeCP2 with DGCR8[36] and the splicing factor YB-1.[40] Moreover, phosphorylation at serine 30[40] has been reported to regulate MeCP2's in vivo localization.[41] A fraction of MeCP2 not phosphorylated at S30 is localized to the nucleoplasm where it associates with YB-1 and various components of the nuclear matrix.[41] This unmodified form of MeCP2 may thus function predominantly in the nucleoplasm, whereas the phosphorylated form might function when bound to DNA. Aside from

phosphorylation, MeCP2 is also modified by acetylation[42] and small ubiquitin-like modifiers.[43] Methyl-CpG binding protein 2 is also ubiquitylated at multiple sites, the in vivo functional consequences of which are unclear.[40] These studies demonstrate that MeCP2 can be dynamically regulated via PTMs at multiple sites.

MOUSE MODELS OF RTT

Mecp2 mouse models hold great promise for understanding the molecular events underlying RTT pathogenesis, as well as shedding light on and rigorously testing new translational directions. Overall, these mouse models display construct validity, the degree to which a model reproduces the pathophysiology of the disorder, as well as face validity, the degree to which the model recapitulates the symptoms of the disorder. The first established RTT mouse models consisted of *Mecp2*-null alleles, generated by deletion of exons 3 and/or 4 of *Mecp2*, producing a functionally inactive protein.[44,45] Because *Mecp2* is an X-linked gene, hemizygous male mice are fully penetrant for the *Mecp2* mutation, whereas heterozygous females are variably penetrant owing to XCI. As in the human condition, symptoms in *Mecp2* mutant males progress more rapidly and are more severe than those of *Mecp2*-null females. After normal early postnatal development, *Mecp2*-null male begin to display many of the neurological features reminiscent of RTT: abnormal gait, hypoactivity, irregular breathing, hind-limb clasping, learning and memory impairments, increased anxiety, and ultimately death by about 10 weeks of age.[44] *Mecp2*-null males have reduced overall brain size (microcephaly), and depending on the genetic background, either increased or decreased body weight.[45] Female heterozygotes are fertile and develop a similar set of symptoms, including tremor, hind-limb clasping, abnormal gait, and hypoactivity by 4–12 months of age.[44]

MeCP2 CONDITIONAL KNOCKOUT STUDIES

A number of conditional knockout studies have been undertaken to examine the requirement for MeCP2 in various cell types. Because the symptoms of RTT are primarily neurological and MeCP2 is highly abundant in neurons, *Mecp2* was deleted specifically in neurons using *Nestin*-cre.[45] Neuron-specific ablation of *Mecp2* resulted in a spectrum of phenotypes similar to those of the constitutive *Mecp2* knockout, indicating that loss of MeCP2 in neurons primarily underlies RTT pathology. However, RTT is not exclusively caused by the loss of MeCP2 from neurons, because several labs have implicated mutant glia as a contributing factor in RTT pathogenesis. Preferential re-expression of MeCP2 in the astrocytes of *Mecp2*-deficient mice leads to significant improvements in locomotion, respiratory function, and longevity.[46] Moreover, restoration of MeCP2 function in astrocytes positively influences the morphology of nearby neurons in a noncell autonomous fashion.[46] Whereas MeCP2 ablation from oligodendrocytes, the myelin-producing glial cells of the brain, results in only a mild RTT-like phenotype, restoration of MeCP2 expression in the oligodendrocytes of *Mecp2*-null animals extends the lifespan, significantly rescues motor function and hind-limb clasping in male and female mice, and fully restores body weight in male mice.[47] Impaired phagocytic activity of microglia, the tissue-resident macrophages of the brain, has also been implicated in the pathogenesis of RTT and represents a novel therapeutic avenue for the condition.[48]

Considerable effort has been made to identify the specific brain region or subsets of neurons disrupted in RTT. Although these studies have been instrumental in identifying which cell types mediate certain phenotypes upon loss of MeCP2, for the most part, conditional deletion of *Mecp2* from specific subpopulations of neuronal cells is not sufficient to recapitulate the full spectrum or severity of phenotypes observed in constitutive *Mecp2*-null animals. The absence of MeCP2 from tyrosine hydroxylase-expressing dopaminergic neurons causes motor dysfunction,[49] whereas loss from serotonergic neurons leads to hyperactivity and increased aggression.[49] Moreover, mice lacking MeCP2 from Sim1-expressing neurons in the hypothalamus exhibit increased aggression, hyperphagia, and obesity.[50] Deletion of MeCP2 from the brain stem and spinal cord revealed crucial roles for MeCP2 in the control of heart rate, respiratory response to hypoxia, and longevity.[51] Thus, specific features of RTT are associated with dysfunction of MeCP2 in specific neuronal populations or brain regions.

Notably, conditional knockouts of *Mecp2* have revealed that MeCP2 function is particularly important in inhibitory GABAergic neurons, a type of interneuron that contributes to the essential balance between excitatory and inhibitory inputs. The absence of MeCP2 from GABAergic and glycinergic neurons of the brain using *Viaat1*-cre reproduces most of the behavioral deficits found in *Mecp2*-null mice, as well as those not normally seen in *Mecp2*-null mice, including forelimb clasping and overgrooming, resulting in self-injury.[52] Consistent with these findings, loss of MeCP2 function from forebrain GABAergic, but not glutamatergic interneurons, led to significant deficits in auditory event related potentials (ERPs), hyperexcitability, and behavioral seizures.[53] Because inhibitory neurons make up only about 20% of neurons, these studies suggest a selective impact of MeCP2 on this neuronal subtype.

Additional studies have addressed the temporal requirement for MeCP2 in RTT pathogenesis. Tamoxifen-inducible *cre-ER*—expressing mice were crossed to mice expressing a floxed *Mecp2* allele, permitting tamoxifen-dependent excision of the *loxP* sites and formation of a loss-of-function *Mecp2* allele.[54,55] Inactivation of *Mecp2* at different postnatal time points (from late juvenile to adult) in an otherwise healthy animal resulted in severe RTT-like phenotypes, including motor dysfunction, learning and memory deficits, and premature death. At the anatomical level, conditional deletion of *Mecp2* in adult animals led to morphological abnormalities such as loss of dendritic complexity and spine density.[54] These studies revealed two important aspects of MeCP2 function. First, normal MeCP2 function during early postnatal life is not sufficient to prevent symptoms in adult animals, and second, MeCP2 is required in the adult brain to maintain neurons in a fully functional state.

MODELING PATIENT-ASSOCIATED RTT MUTATIONS IN MICE

Patient-associated MeCP2 mutations span the entire protein and include missense, frameshift, nonsense, and splice-site mutations.[5,6] Several hundred mutations in MeCP2 have been identified, with certain mutations occurring at higher frequency (T158M, R168X, R255X, R270X, R294X, R306C, and R133C) (RettBASE, http://mecp2.chw.edu.au). Most MeCP2 mutations are caused by C > T transitions at hypermutable CpG dinucleotides within the gene.[56] Missense mutations provide clues about functionally important regions of the protein because only one amino acid is altered. Rett syndrome—causing missense mutations localize predominantly to two clusters mapping to the MBD and the C-terminal portion of the TRD (RettBASE, http://mecp2.chw.edu.au), which suggests that these two regions of the protein are critical for MeCP2 function. The development of mouse models recapitulating RTT-associated MeCP2 mutations has expanded our understanding of MeCP2 function and RTT pathogenesis, and provides the opportunity to study the phenotypic differences between distinct mutation types (Figure 1). In the subsequent discussion, we will examine the behavioral and functional consequences of several of these disease-causing mutations when modeled in mice.

Missense Mutations

Mecp2^{T158A}: Missense mutations at residue threonine 158, converting it to either an alanine or a methionine, are the most frequent missense mutations associated with human RTT and are often associated with severe symptom presentation. To elucidate the causal role for this mutation in the etiology of RTT, T158A knock-in mice were generated.[57] $Mecp2^{T158A/y}$ male mice develop normally for the first 4 weeks of life and become progressively symptomatic after 5 weeks of age, with 50% dying by 16 weeks. $Mecp2^{T158A/y}$ display many key clinical features of RTT, including microcephaly, motor dysfunction, and learning and memory deficits. Moreover, auditory ERP recordings in $Mecp2^{T158A/y}$ mice were significantly altered relative to wild-type littermates. Presymptomatic mice did not display altered ERPs, which suggests that neural networks underlying information processing are disrupted in an age-dependent manner by MePC2 dysfunction, corresponding to the onset of behavioral phenotypes. The phenotypes observed in $Mecp2^{T158A/y}$ mice are similar to those observed in $Mecp2$-null animals, although not as severe, which suggests that the T158A mutation is a partial loss-of-function mutation. $Mecp2^{T158A/+}$ female mice also develop RTT-like symptoms, but with a delayed time course.[57] Female mice also display respiratory phenotypes, although with decreased severity relative to other $Mecp2$ mutant mouse models.[58]

Mutation at T158 reduces the affinity for MeCP2 for mCpG in vitro. It is believed that loss of the hydroxyl group in threonine destabilizes the tandem Asx-ST motif in the MBD and reduces the affinity of MeCP2 for mCpG.[59] To examine the biological consequences of the T158A in vivo, ChIP was performed, revealing a reduction in MeCP2 T158A binding to several known target genes, including $Bdnf$, $Xist$, $Snrpn$, and Crh.[57] Moreover, the T158A mutation disrupted the association of MeCP2 with heterochromatin-rich foci, which further highlights the importance of this residue in binding to methylated DNA. In addition to the DNA binding defect, the T158A mutation also destabilizes MeCP2 protein in vivo, as evidenced by a reduction in steady-state MeCP2 T158A protein levels in the brain, and increased MeCP2 turnover in cycloheximide-treated cortical neurons. Together, these results demonstrate that the patient-associated MeCP2 T158A mutation leads to RTT-like phenotypes through reduced binding of MeCP2 to methylated DNA and decreased MeCP2 protein stability.[57] These data further suggest that interventions that increase MeCP2 protein stability and/or binding to methylated DNA may be of therapeutic value.

$Mecp2^{R306C}$: Approximately 5% of RTT cases are caused by mutation in the C-terminal portion of the TRD at residue 306, converting an arginine to a cysteine (R306C).[60] Two independent labs have generated and characterized $Mecp2^{R306C}$ mutant mice.[18,33] $Mecp2^{R306C}$ mice display microcephaly, increased weight, hindlimb clasping, and a median lifespan of about 18 weeks. More detailed behavioral characterization revealed increased anxiety and deficits in locomotion, motor coordination, and learning and memory.[18,33] The phenotypes were milder than those of $Mecp2$-null mice, indicating that MeCP2 R306C is not a complete loss-of-function mutation.[33]

In vitro and in vivo mapping experiments pinpointed an approximate 25-amino-acid region including R306 as the NCoR/SMRT corepressor interaction domain (NID). In $Mecp2^{R306C}$ mice, the interaction between MeCP2 and NCoR/SMRT was lost, resulting in failure of MeCP2 to recruit NCoR/SMRT to heterochromatic foci and loss of MeCP2-mediated transcriptional repression.[18] This is the first example of a RTT-causing mutation disrupting the interaction of MeCP2 with one of its binding partners. It further pinpoints NCoR/SMRT recruitment as one critical function of MeCP2. In addition to interfering with the MeCP2—NCoR/SMRT interaction, MeCP2 R306C also has reduced affinity for DNA in vitro and in vivo, which might be consequence of disruption of the highly conserved basic cluster of amino acids flanking R306.[33] As discussed above, the interaction of NCoR/SMRT with MeCP2 is regulated by a phosphorylation event at T308. Because of the requirement by kinases of a basophilic residue near the site of phosphorylation, R306C mutations also abrogate activity-dependent phosphorylation at T308.[39]

$Mecp2^{R111G}$: A known RTT-causing mutation occurs at residue 111, converting an arginine to a glycine (R111G).[61] R111 is located in the MBD and is critical for binding to methylated DNA.[62,63] Mice with the R111G mutation exhibit severe phenotypes and have a median lifespan of about 11 weeks, comparable to that of $Mecp2$-null mice.[33] Thus, $Mecp2^{R111G}$ is essentially a null allele, which underscores the importance of methyl-CpG binding for MeCP2 function.

$Mecp2^{A140V}$: In females, most mutations in $MECP2$ result in classical or variant RTT phenotypes. Methyl-CpG binding protein 2 mutations are also associated with a less severe phenotype, described as X-linked mental retardation (XLMR), which occurs in both boys and girls and is somewhat clinically distinct from RTT.[64–66] One such XLMR-associated mutation, $MECP2^{A140V}$, is located in the MBD and accounts for about 0.6% of all MeCP2 mutations (RettBASE, http://mecp2.chw.edu.au). $Mecp2^{A140V}$ mice display no obvious phenotypes; however, anatomical studies revealed increased cell-packing density and reduced dendritic branching, consistent with phenotypes reported in RTT patients as well as other $Mecp2$ mutant mouse models.[67] In addition, electrophysiological studies found deficits in neuronal signaling, although these impairments were milder than those reported for $Mecp2$-null mice.[68] Specifically, $Mecp2^{A140V}$ mutant neurons have reduced frequency and amplitude of spontaneous inhibitory postsynaptic potentials (IPSCs), suggesting neuronal hyperexcitability as well as deficits in short-term and long-term potentiation of CA3-CA1 synapses in adult animals.[68] Interestingly, mutation at A140V disrupts the association of MeCP2 with ATRX without interfering with MeCP2's ability to bind mCpG.[31]

Nonsense Mutations

Mecp2^{R168X}: The most common patient-associated truncation mutation occurs at residue R168, which eliminates the TRD and both of MeCP2's nuclear localization signals. Typically, R168X mutations are more clinically severe, with more prominent deficits in motor and purposeful hand movements reported in patients.[8,69,70] *Mecp2^{R168X}* mice exhibit a progressive neurological phenotype characterized by respiratory abnormalities, decreased anxiety, motor dysfunction, and learning deficits.[71,72] Overall, *Mecp2^{R168X}* and *Mecp2*-null males display phenotypes of similar severity.[71] By contrast, *Mecp2^{R168X}* females, except for the presence of spontaneous seizures, display a milder phenotype relative to *Mecp2*-null females, which indicates that MeCP2 R168X might retain partial function.[44,71] Significant respiratory phenotypes in *Mecp2^{R168X}* females have been reported; these breathing abnormalities are more severe than those of female *Mecp2^{T158A}* mice,[58] demonstrating functional differences between distinct MeCP2 mutations.

Mecp2^{R270X} and Mecp2^{G273X}: Although rare, *MECP2* mutations have also been reported in boys. An interesting observation is that boys with MeCP2 R270X mutations present with severe symptoms, neonatal encephalopathy, and death before 4 years of age,[73,74] whereas a boy with the MeCP2 G273X mutation lived longer with a comparatively milder set of neuropsychiatric symptoms.[75] How does the addition of just three amino acids in MeCP2 lead to such a considerable difference in disease severity? To answer these questions, Baker et al. modeled both of these truncating mutations in mice.[32] *Mecp2^{R270X}* mutant mice exhibited severe impairments, age-dependent neurological abnormalities, microcephaly, increased body weight, and reduced longevity (median survival of 85 days). By contrast, *Mecp2^{G273X}* mice were leaner, maintained a higher average brain weight, and lived significantly longer (median survival of 201 days) than *Mecp2^{R270X}* mice. Thus, the phenotypic disparity observed in *MECP2^{R270X}* and *MECP2^{G273X}* patients was successfully recapitulated using mouse models.

Methyl-CpG binding protein 2 R270X and G273X bind equally well to DNA and have similar impairments in repressor activity; therefore, neither can explain the observed phenotypic disparity. To identify new functional domains in the MeCP2 protein, interspecies sequence alignments were performed, leading to the identification of three well-conserved AT-hook domains, one of which terminates after G273. AT-hooks bind to AT-rich sequences and are found in proteins of the high-mobility-group AT-hook family, which function to alter chromatin structure.[76] Although the MBD is primarily responsible for the localization of MeCP2 to DNA, it is hypothesized that the AT-hook domain located in the TRD might allow MeCP2 to manipulate the nearby chromatin architecture so as to stabilize its association with DNA. In support of this, MeCP2 R270X failed to facilitate oligomerization of nucleosomal arrays and had reduced binding to certain DNA sequences by native ChIP. It is proposed that disruption of the AT-hook domain in *MECP2^{R270X}* but not *MECP2^{G273X}* might result in the inability of MeCP2 to alter chromatin structure properly, leading to the more severe deficits in *MECP2^{R270X}* patients.

Mecp2^{R255X}: Methyl-CpG binding protein 2 R255X, the second most common RTT-associated nonsense mutation, lies within the TRD of MeCP2. Similar to RTT patients, knock-in mice carrying this mutation fail to express a truncated protein, indicating that this mutation is likely a null allele.[77] Indeed, *Mecp2^{R255X}* mice have a significantly reduced lifespan, breathing and heart abnormalities, and impairments in motor function, learning, and anxiety. These deficits can be rescued by expression of a wild-type copy of *MECP2* (*MECP2^{Tg}*). *Mecp2^{R255X}* mice also display decreased evoked field excitatory postsynaptic potentials in the CA1 region of the hippocampus; however, the presence of *MECP2^{Tg}* failed to rescue this impairment in long-term potentiation (LTP).[77] Importantly, the finding that MeCP2 R255X does not behave as a dominant negative in these genetic rescue experiments suggests that this mutation is amenable to treatment approaches that use read-through compounds.

Mecp2^{T308X}: The *Mecp2^{T308X}* mouse model expresses a truncated protein containing the MBD and terminating at the C-terminal edge of the NID. Normal for the first 6 weeks of life, *Mecp2^{T308X}* mice develop a progressive neurological disease reminiscent of RTT: tremors, motor impairments, hypoactivity, increased anxiety-related behavior, seizures, kyphosis, and stereotypic forelimb motions.[78] Deficits in learning and memory were observed at later ages.[79,80] In line with clinical data from RTT patients, this truncation mutation leads to milder phenotypes, a delayed onset of symptoms, and a prolonged lifespan compared with *Mecp2*-null mice.[44] The milder symptoms might be a result of retention of the MBD and partial binding to NCoR/SMRT.[18] Electrophysiological studies on glutamatergic neurons differentiated from female heterozygous *Mecp2$^{T308X/+}$* induced pluripotent stem cells (iPSCs) revealed deficits in intrinsic excitability and excitatory synaptic transmission relative to wild-type controls. The overall reduced numbers of action potentials and reduced peak inward currents in $Mecp2^{T308X/+}$ differentiated neurons further suggest impaired Na+ channel function[81] (also see Chapter 18).

Other RTT Mouse Models

Mecp2 **hypo/hypermorphs**: Methyl-CpG binding protein 2 levels need to be precisely controlled, because mice expressing approximately 50% less *Mecp2* mRNA and about 50% less protein display an array of neurological phenotypes including motor impairments, decreased anxiety, abnormal social interaction, respiratory irregularities, and deficits in learning.[82,83] At the opposite end of the spectrum, an overabundance of MeCP2 also has detrimental effects. A modest approximately onefold overexpression of MeCP2 in transgenic mice leads to a neurological phenotype overlapping with RTT.[84] *Mecp2* transgenic mice are normal up until 10–12 months of age, after which they begin to develop phenotypes that include forepaw stereotypy, seizures, aggression, hypoactivity, ataxia, and premature death by 12 months of age. The latter mouse model mimics the human *MECP2* duplication syndrome, with patients typically showing a range of neurological symptoms including altered head growth rates, ataxia, frequent respiratory infections, seizures and intellectual disability.[85,86] *Mecp2* transgenic mice have increased numbers of dendritic spines, enhanced glutamatergic neurotransmission, and increased LTP.[84,87] Thus, *Mecp2* transgenic mice and *Mecp2*-null mice display opposite synaptic phenotypes, which suggests a bidirectional role for MeCP2 in controlling excitatory neurotransmission.

Mecp2 **exon 1 deletion**: *MECP2/Mecp2* is alternatively spliced to generate two isoforms, MeCP2-e1 and MeCP2-e2, with distinct translation start sites at their N-termini. The MeCP2-e1 isoform is encoded by exons 1, 3, and 4, whereas the MeCP2-e2 isoform is encoded by exons 2, 3, and 4. The two isoforms are identical except for their N-termini: the e1 isoform has 21 unique N-terminal amino acids whereas the e2 isoform has 9. Several lines of evidence implicate Mecp2-e1 as the isoform most relevant for RTT. First, MeCP2-e1 is more abundantly expressed in the adult brain.[6] Second, mutations in exon 1, but not exon 2, have been identified in RTT patients.[88–90] Indeed, neurons derived from iPSCs from a patient with a severely truncated *MECP2-e1* have reduced soma size and defects in generating action potentials and excitatory synaptic responses.[91] Third, ablation of MeCP2-e2 fails to produce RTT-like phenotypes in mice, suggesting a nonessential role for this isoform in the brain.[92] To examine the role of MeCP2-e1 in the etiology of RTT, mice were engineered to express

a known RTT-causing mutation that converts the translational start site in exon 1 from ATG to TTG (Figure 1(B)). This missense mutation prevents translation of *Mecp2-e1* whereas *Mecp2-e2* translation remains intact.[41] By 6 weeks of age, MeCP2-e1–deficient male mice develop neurological phenotypes that include gait abnormalities, hind-limb clasping, seizures, reduced anxiety, and impaired sociability, with 50% surviving until about 16 weeks. Female mice also develop mild neurological deficits by 30 weeks of age.[41] These data implicate MeCP2-e1 as a key contributor to RTT pathogenesis and suggest nonredundant functions for these isoforms.

SYNAPTIC DYSFUNCTION IN RTT MOUSE MODELS

It has been proposed that reduced cortical connectivity between glutamatergic excitatory pyramidal neurons in part underlies RTT pathology. In RTT patients, deficits in connectivity are reflected by alterations in neuronal structure, which include reduced dendritic complexity and reduced dendritic spine density in cortical pyramidal neurons.[93,94] In addition, neurons differentiated from iPSCs from RTT patients possess fewer synapses and dendritic spines and exhibit decreased amplitude and frequency of spontaneous postsynaptic currents.[95]

Likewise, the brains of *Mecp2* mutant mice exhibit a similar array of morphological and electrophysiological deficits. *Methyl-CpG binding protein 2*-null animals have a smaller cortical neuron size with increased cell-packing density,[96] reduced dendritic spine density,[97] and reduced complexity of dendritic branching.[96,98] *Mecp2*-null pyramidal neurons within cortical layer II/III and layer V have a reduced spontaneous firing rate, caused in part by decreased glutamatergic quantal amplitude and reduced numbers of excitatory synapses on pyramidal neurons.[99–101] Decreased glutamatergic neurotransmission leads to a shift in excitatory/inhibitory (E/I) synaptic balance and a concomitant increase in inhibitory neurotransmission in layer V pyramidal neurons.[99] Loss of proper E/I balance can lead to hyperexcitability of neuronal networks, a phenomenon that often manifests as seizures, a common RTT symptom. The observed synaptic dysfunctions, moreover, lead to impairments in long-term potentiation (LTP) and long-term depression (LTD), two forms of synaptic plasticity associated with long-term memory formation and circuit refinement during development. In *Mecp2* mutant mice, reduced LTP was found at CA3-to-CA1 synapses in the hippocampus,[102] and in layer II/III of the primary somatosensory cortex,[103] whereas reduced LTD was found in area

CA1.[79,102] Notably, ablation of MeCP2 from GABAergic neurons, which recapitulates most RTT-like symptoms, leads to reduced GABA levels, decreased IPSC amplitude and charge in striatum and cortex, and disrupted E/I balance.[52,53] Together, these studies illustrate the importance of MeCP2 for proper neuronal morphology, and synaptic function and plasticity.

TOWARD A THERAPY FOR RTT

To date, there is no cure for RTT and treatment is limited to management of symptoms. Historically, RTT has been classified as a neurodevelopmental disorder rather than a neurodegenerative disorder, because patients exhibit abnormal, immature neuronal morphology, but not neuronal death.[93] A critical question for translational studies is whether the observed behavioral and structural deficits can be reversed. To test this, mice were generated containing a *lox-stop* cassette inserted into intron 2 of the mouse *Mecp2* gene, creating a null allele. Crossing these mice to mice expressing a *cre-ER* fusion allowed tamoxifen-dependent re-expression of *Mecp2* in adult mice. Reactivation of *Mecp2* in symptomatic *Mecp2*-deficient mice leads to significant phenotypic rescue, including increased lifespan, normalized respiratory measures, and improved sensorimotor skills.[104] Importantly, phenotypic rescue was accompanied by rescue of the underlying neuronal morphology, including neuronal size, dendritic complexity, and spine density.[105] These results demonstrate that RTT is reversible and, at least in mice, can be treated even at late stages of the disease. It further suggests that early developmental absence of MeCP2 does no lasting damage to neurons, challenging the categorization of RTT as a neurodevelopmental disorder. Instead of being required for early development, MeCP2 might instead be essential for the maintenance and stabilization of the mature neuronal state.

This important study raises the possibility that simply expressing a functional copy of MeCP2 might cure RTT. Therefore, identifying strategies to restore normal MeCP2 function in patients has been a central focus. To this end, gene therapy approaches that increase the expression of MeCP2 have been successful in mice,[106] whereas administration of aminoglycosides that read through nonsense mutations has restored MeCP2 levels in vitro.[77,107,108] Targeting microglia is also a promising approach because bone marrow transplantation of wild-type microglia into *Mecp2*-deficient mice significantly improves symptoms.[48] Targeting pathways that are downstream of MeCP2 function, such as treating with insulin-like growth factor[109] and cholesterol-lowering statins,[110] also hold great potential.

CONCLUDING REMARKS

Despite major advances in our understanding of MeCP2 function over the years, the full extent of MeCP2 activity and how its disruption contributes to RTT remain to be further investigated. Current progress supports the notion that MeCP2 is a multifunctional protein that modulates gene expression in a cell type–specific manner, depending on the local distribution of unmethylated, methylated, and hydroxymethylated DNA. The function of MeCP2 is further regulated by PTMs and numerous binding partners. The development of mouse models of RTT has been instrumental in dissecting the role of MeCP2 in brain development and revealing the synaptic mechanisms underlying RTT-like behavioral phenotypes. This has helped to lay the groundwork for the identification of new therapeutic avenues for RTT.

References

1. Rett A. On a unusual brain atrophy syndrome in hyperammonemia in childhood. *Wien Med Wochenschr* September 10, 1966; **116**(37):723–6.
2. Chahrour M, Zoghbi HY. The story of Rett syndrome: from clinic to neurobiology. *Neuron* November 8, 2007;**56**(3):422–37.
3. Amir RE, Van den Veyver IB, Wan M, Tran CQ, Francke U, Zoghbi HY. Rett syndrome is caused by mutations in X-linked MECP2, encoding methyl-CpG-binding protein 2. *Nat Genet* October 1999;**23**(2):185–8.
4. Neul JL, Kaufmann WE, Glaze DG, et al. Rett syndrome: revised diagnostic criteria and nomenclature. *Ann Neurol* December 2010;**68**(6):944–50.
5. Bienvenu T, Chelly J. Molecular genetics of Rett syndrome: when DNA methylation goes unrecognized. *Nat Rev Genet* June 2006; **7**(6):415–26.
6. Kriaucionis S, Bird A. The major form of MeCP2 has a novel N-terminus generated by alternative splicing. *Nucleic Acids Res* 2004;**32**(5):1818–23.
7. Cuddapah VA, Pillai RB, Shekar KV, et al. Methyl-CpG-binding protein 2 (MECP2) mutation type is associated with disease severity in Rett syndrome. *J Med Genet* March 2014;**51**(3):152–8.
8. Neul JL, Fang P, Barrish J, et al. Specific mutations in methyl-CpG-binding protein 2 confer different severity in Rett syndrome. *Neurology* April 15, 2008;**70**(16):1313–21.
9. Lewis JD, Meehan RR, Henzel WJ, et al. Purification, sequence, and cellular localization of a novel chromosomal protein that binds to methylated DNA. *Cell* June 12, 1992;**69**(6):905–14.
10. Shahbazian MD, Antalffy B, Armstrong DL, Zoghbi HY. Insight into Rett syndrome: MeCP2 levels display tissue- and cell-specific differences and correlate with neuronal maturation. *Hum Mol Genet* January 15, 2002;**11**(2):115–24.
11. Nan X, Meehan RR, Bird A. Dissection of the methyl-CpG binding domain from the chromosomal protein MeCP2. *Nucleic Acids Res* October 25, 1993;**21**(21):4886–92.
12. Nguyen CT, Gonzales FA, Jones PA. Altered chromatin structure associated with methylation-induced gene silencing in cancer cells: correlation of accessibility, methylation, MeCP2 binding and acetylation. *Nucleic Acids Res* November 15, 2001;**29**(22): 4598–606.

13. Nan X, Tate P, Li E, Bird A. DNA methylation specifies chromosomal localization of MeCP2. *Mol Cell Biol* January 1996;**16**(1): 414–21.

14. Bird AP. CpG-rich islands and the function of DNA methylation. *Nature* May 15-21, 1986;**321**(6067):209–13.

15. Nan X, Campoy FJ, Bird A. MeCP2 is a transcriptional repressor with abundant binding sites in genomic chromatin. *Cell* February 21, 1997;**88**(4):471–81.

16. Kokura K, Kaul SC, Wadhwa R, et al. The Ski protein family is required for MeCP2-mediated transcriptional repression. *J Biol Chem* September 7, 2001;**276**(36):34115–21.

17. Stancheva I, Collins AL, Van den Veyver IB, Zoghbi H, Meehan RR. A mutant form of MeCP2 protein associated with human Rett syndrome cannot be displaced from methylated DNA by notch in Xenopus embryos. *Mol Cell* August 2003;**12**(2):425–35.

18. Lyst MJ, Ekiert R, Ebert DH, et al. Rett syndrome mutations abolish the interaction of MeCP2 with the NCoR/SMRT corepressor. *Nat Neurosci* July 2013;**16**(7):898–902.

19. Tudor M, Akbarian S, Chen RZ, Jaenisch R. Transcriptional profiling of a mouse model for Rett syndrome reveals subtle transcriptional changes in the brain. *Proc Natl Acad Sci USA* November 26, 2002;**99**(24):15536–41.

20. Chahrour M, Jung SY, Shaw C, et al. MeCP2, a key contributor to neurological disease, activates and represses transcription. *Science* May 30, 2008;**320**(5880):1224–9.

21. Ben-Shachar S, Chahrour M, Thaller C, Shaw CA, Zoghbi HY. Mouse models of MeCP2 disorders share gene expression changes in the cerebellum and hypothalamus. *Hum Mol Genet* July 1, 2009;**18**(13):2431–42.

22. Zhao YT, Goffin D, Johnson BS, Zhou Z. Loss of MeCP2 function is associated with distinct gene expression changes in the striatum. *Neurobiol Dis* November 2013;**59**:257–66.

23. Li Y, Wang H, Muffat J, et al. Global transcriptional and translational repression in human-embryonic-stem-cell-derived Rett syndrome neurons. *Cell Stem Cell* October 3, 2013;**13**(4):446–58.

24. Meehan RR, Lewis JD, Bird AP. Characterization of MeCP2, a vertebrate DNA binding protein with affinity for methylated DNA. *Nucleic Acids Res* October 11, 1992;**20**(19):5085–92.

25. Skene PJ, Illingworth RS, Webb S, et al. Neuronal MeCP2 is expressed at near histone-octamer levels and globally alters the chromatin state. *Mol Cell* February 26, 2010;**37**(4):457–68.

26. Fraga MF, Ballestar E, Montoya G, Taysavang P, Wade PA, Esteller M. The affinity of different MBD proteins for a specific methylated locus depends on their intrinsic binding properties. *Nucleic Acids Res* March 15, 2003;**31**(6):1765–74.

27. Ishibashi T, Thambirajah AA, Ausio J. MeCP2 preferentially binds to methylated linker DNA in the absence of the terminal tail of histone H3 and independently of histone acetylation. *FEBS Lett* April 2, 2008;**582**(7):1157–62.

28. Yasui DH, Peddada S, Bieda MC, et al. Integrated epigenomic analyses of neuronal MeCP2 reveal a role for long-range interaction with active genes. *Proc Natl Acad Sci USA* December 4, 2007;**104**(49):19416–21.

29. Thambirajah AA, Ng MK, Frehlick LJ, et al. MeCP2 binds to nucleosome free (linker DNA) regions and to H3K9/H3K27 methylated nucleosomes in the brain. *Nucleic Acids Res* April 2012;**40**(7):2884–97.

30. Mellen M, Ayata P, Dewell S, Kriaucionis S, Heintz N. MeCP2 binds to 5hmC enriched within active genes and accessible chromatin in the nervous system. *Cell* December 21, 2012;**151**(7):1417–30.

31. Nan X, Hou J, Maclean A, et al. Interaction between chromatin proteins MECP2 and ATRX is disrupted by mutations that cause inherited mental retardation. *Proc Natl Acad Sci USA* February 20, 2007;**104**(8):2709–14.

32. Baker SA, Chen L, Wilkins AD, Yu P, Lichtarge O, Zoghbi HY. An AT-hook domain in MeCP2 determines the clinical course of Rett syndrome and related disorders. *Cell* February 28, 2013;**152**(5): 984–96.

33. Heckman LD, Chahrour MH, Zoghbi HY. Rett-causing mutations reveal two domains critical for MeCP2 function and for toxicity in MECP2 duplication syndrome mice. *Elife* 2014;**3**.

34. Kernohan KD, Vernimmen D, Gloor GB, Berube NG. Analysis of neonatal brain lacking ATRX or MeCP2 reveals changes in nucleosome density, CTCF binding and chromatin looping. *Nucleic Acids Res* 2014;**42**(13):8356–68.

35. Young JI, Hong EP, Castle JC, et al. Regulation of RNA splicing by the methylation-dependent transcriptional repressor methyl-CpG binding protein 2. *Proc Natl Acad Sci USA* December 6, 2005;**102**(49):17551–8.

36. Cheng TL, Wang Z, Liao Q, et al. MeCP2 suppresses nuclear microRNA processing and dendritic growth by regulating the DGCR8/Drosha complex. *Dev Cell* March 10, 2014;**28**(5): 547–60.

37. Zhou Z, Hong EJ, Cohen S, et al. Brain-specific phosphorylation of MeCP2 regulates activity-dependent Bdnf transcription, dendritic growth, and spine maturation. *Neuron* October 19, 2006;**52**(2): 255–69.

38. Cohen S, Gabel HW, Hemberg M, et al. Genome-wide activity-dependent MeCP2 phosphorylation regulates nervous system development and function. *Neuron* October 6, 2011;**72**(1):72–85.

39. Ebert DH, Gabel HW, Robinson ND, et al. Activity-dependent phosphorylation of MeCP2 threonine 308 regulates interaction with NCoR. *Nature* July 18, 2013;**499**(7458):341–5.

40. Gonzales ML, Adams S, Dunaway KW, LaSalle JM. Phosphorylation of distinct sites in MeCP2 modifies cofactor associations and the dynamics of transcriptional regulation. *Mol Cell Biol* July 2012; **32**(14):2894–903.

41. Yasui DH, Gonzales ML, Aflatooni JO, et al. Mice with an isoform-ablating Mecp2 exon 1 mutation recapitulate the neurologic deficits of Rett syndrome. *Hum Mol Genet* May 1, 2014;**23**(9):2447–58.

42. Zocchi L, Sassone-Corsi P. SIRT1-mediated deacetylation of MeCP2 contributes to BDNF expression. *Epigenetics* July 2012; **7**(7):695–700.

43. Cheng J, Huang M, Zhu Y, et al. SUMOylation of MeCP2 is essential for transcriptional repression and hippocampal synapse development. *J Neurochem* March 2014;**128**(6):798–806.

44. Guy J, Hendrich B, Holmes M, Martin JE, Bird A. A mouse Mecp2-null mutation causes neurological symptoms that mimic Rett syndrome. *Nat Genet* March 2001;**27**(3):322–6.

45. Chen RZ, Akbarian S, Tudor M, Jaenisch R. Deficiency of methyl-CpG binding protein-2 in CNS neurons results in a Rett-like phenotype in mice. *Nat Genet* March 2001;**27**(3):327–31.

46. Lioy DT, Garg SK, Monaghan CE, et al. A role for glia in the progression of Rett's syndrome. *Nature* July 28, 2011;**475**(7357): 497–500.

47. Nguyen MV, Felice CA, Du F, et al. Oligodendrocyte lineage cells contribute unique features to Rett syndrome neuropathology. *J Neurosci* November 27, 2013;**33**(48):18764–74.

48. Derecki NC, Cronk JC, Lu Z, et al. Wild-type microglia arrest pathology in a mouse model of Rett syndrome. *Nature* April 5, 2012; **484**(7392):105–9.

49. Samaco RC, Mandel-Brehm C, Chao HT, et al. Loss of MeCP2 in aminergic neurons causes cell-autonomous defects in neurotransmitter synthesis and specific behavioral abnormalities. *Proc Natl Acad Sci USA* December 22, 2009;**106**(51):21966–71.

50. Fyffe SL, Neul JL, Samaco RC, et al. Deletion of Mecp2 in Sim1-expressing neurons reveals a critical role for MeCP2 in feeding behavior, aggression, and the response to stress. *Neuron* September 25, 2008;**59**(6):947–58.

51. Ward CS, Arvide EM, Huang TW, Yoo J, Noebels JL, Neul JL. MeCP2 is critical within HoxB1-derived tissues of mice for normal lifespan. *J Neurosci* July 13, 2011;**31**(28):10359−70.

52. Chao HT, Chen H, Samaco RC, et al. Dysfunction in GABA signalling mediates autism-like stereotypies and Rett syndrome phenotypes. *Nature* November 11, 2010;**468**(7321):263−9.

53. Goffin D, Brodkin ES, Blendy JA, Siegel SJ, Zhou Z. Cellular origins of auditory event-related potential deficits in Rett syndrome. *Nat Neurosci* June 2014;**17**(6):804−6.

54. Nguyen MV, Du F, Felice CA, et al. MeCP2 is critical for maintaining mature neuronal networks and global brain anatomy during late stages of postnatal brain development and in the mature adult brain. *J Neurosci* July 18, 2012;**32**(29): 10021−34.

55. McGraw CM, Samaco RC, Zoghbi HY. Adult neural function requires MeCP2. *Science* July 8, 2011;**333**(6039):186.

56. Wan M, Lee SS, Zhang X, et al. Rett syndrome and beyond: recurrent spontaneous and familial MECP2 mutations at CpG hotspots. *Am J Hum Genet* December 1999;**65**(6):1520−9.

57. Goffin D, Allen M, Zhang L, et al. Rett syndrome mutation MeCP2 T158A disrupts DNA binding, protein stability and ERP responses. *Nat Neurosci* February 2012;**15**(2):274−83.

58. Bissonnette JM, Schaevitz LR, Knopp SJ, Zhou Z. Respiratory phenotypes are distinctly affected in mice with common Rett syndrome mutations MeCP2 T158A and R168X. *Neuroscience* May 16, 2014;**267**:166−76.

59. Ho KL, McNae IW, Schmiedeberg L, Klose RJ, Bird AP, Walkinshaw MD. MeCP2 binding to DNA depends upon hydration at methyl-CpG. *Mol Cell* February 29, 2008;**29**(4):525−31.

60. Fyfe S, Cream A, de Klerk N, Christodoulou J, Leonard H. InterRett and RettBASE: International Rett Syndrome Association databases for Rett syndrome. *J Child Neurol* October 2003;**18**(10): 709−13.

61. Laccone F, Huppke P, Hanefeld F, Meins M. Mutation spectrum in patients with Rett syndrome in the German population: evidence of hot spot regions. *Hum Mutat* March 2001;**17**(3):183−90.

62. Free A, Wakefield RI, Smith BO, Dryden DT, Barlow PN, Bird AP. DNA recognition by the methyl-CpG binding domain of MeCP2. *J Biol Chem* February 2, 2001;**276**(5):3353−60.

63. Kudo S, Nomura Y, Segawa M, et al. Heterogeneity in residual function of MeCP2 carrying missense mutations in the methyl CpG binding domain. *J Med Genet* July 2003;**40**(7):487−93.

64. Couvert P, Bienvenu T, Aquaviva C, et al. MECP2 is highly mutated in X-linked mental retardation. *Hum Mol Genet* April 15, 2001;**10**(9):941−6.

65. Meloni I, Bruttini M, Longo I, et al. A mutation in the rett syndrome gene, MECP2, causes X-linked mental retardation and progressive spasticity in males. *Am J Hum Genet* October 2000;**67**(4): 982−5.

66. Imessaoudene B, Bonnefont JP, Royer G, et al. MECP2 mutation in non-fatal, non-progressive encephalopathy in a male. *J Med Genet* March 2001;**38**(3):171−4.

67. Jentarra GM, Olfers SL, Rice SG, et al. Abnormalities of cell packing density and dendritic complexity in the MeCP2 A140V mouse model of Rett syndrome/X-linked mental retardation. *BMC Neurosci* 2010;**11**:19.

68. Ma LY, Wu C, Jin Y, et al. Electrophysiological phenotypes of MeCP2 A140V mutant mouse model. *CNS Neurosci Ther* May 2014;**20**(5):420−8.

69. Colvin L, Leonard H, de Klerk N, et al. Refining the phenotype of common mutations in Rett syndrome. *J Med Genet* January 2004; **41**(1):25−30.

70. Downs J, Bebbington A, Jacoby P, et al. Level of purposeful hand function as a marker of clinical severity in Rett syndrome. *Dev Med Child Neurol* September 2010;**52**(9):817−23.

71. Schaevitz LR, Gomez NB, Zhen DP, Berger-Sweeney JE. MeCP2 R168X male and female mutant mice exhibit Rett-like behavioral deficits. *Genes Brain Behav* October 2013;**12**(7):732−40.

72. Wegener E, Brendel C, Fischer A, Hulsmann S, Gartner J, Huppke P. Characterization of the MeCP2R168X knockin mouse model for Rett syndrome. *PLoS One* 2014;**9**(12):e115444.

73. Venancio M, Santos M, Pereira SA, Maciel P, Saraiva JM. An explanation for another familial case of Rett syndrome: maternal germline mosaicism. *Eur J Hum Genet* August 2007;**15**(8):902−4.

74. Kankirawatana P, Leonard H, Ellaway C, et al. Early progressive encephalopathy in boys and MECP2 mutations. *Neurology* July 11, 2006;**67**(1):164−6.

75. Ravn K, Nielsen JB, Uldall P, Hansen FJ, Schwartz M. No correlation between phenotype and genotype in boys with a truncating MECP2 mutation. *J Med Genet* January 2003;**40**(1):e5.

76. Grasser KD. Chromatin-associated HMGA and HMGB proteins: versatile co-regulators of DNA-dependent processes. *Plant Mol Biol* October 2003;**53**(3):281−95.

77. Pitcher MR, Herrera JA, Buffington SA, et al. Rett syndrome like phenotypes in the R255X Mecp2 mutant mouse are rescued by MECP2 transgene. *Hum Mol Genet* January 29, 2015;**24**(9):2662−72.

78. Shahbazian M, Young J, Yuva-Paylor L, et al. Mice with truncated MeCP2 recapitulate many Rett syndrome features and display hyperacetylation of histone H3. *Neuron* July 18, 2002;**35**(2):243−54.

79. Moretti P, Levenson JM, Battaglia F, et al. Learning and memory and synaptic plasticity are impaired in a mouse model of Rett syndrome. *J Neurosci* January 4, 2006;**26**(1):319−27.

80. De Filippis B, Ricceri L, Laviola G. Early postnatal behavioral changes in the Mecp2-308 truncation mouse model of Rett syndrome. *Genes Brain Behav* March 1, 2010;**9**(2):213−23.

81. Farra N, Zhang WB, Pasceri P, Eubanks JH, Salter MW, Ellis J. Rett syndrome induced pluripotent stem cell-derived neurons reveal novel neurophysiological alterations. *Mol Psychiatry* December 2012;**17**(12):1261−71.

82. Samaco RC, Fryer JD, Ren J, et al. A partial loss of function allele of methyl-CpG-binding protein 2 predicts a human neurodevelopmental syndrome. *Hum Mol Genet* June 15, 2008;**17**(12):1718−27.

83. Kerr B, Alvarez-Saavedra M, Saez MA, Saona A, Young JI. Defective body-weight regulation, motor control and abnormal social interactions in Mecp2 hypomorphic mice. *Hum Mol Genet* June 15, 2008;**17**(12):1707−17.

84. Collins AL, Levenson JM, Vilaythong AP, et al. Mild overexpression of MeCP2 causes a progressive neurological disorder in mice. *Hum Mol Genet* November 1, 2004;**13**(21):2679−89.

85. Van Esch H, Bauters M, Ignatius J, et al. Duplication of the MECP2 region is a frequent cause of severe mental retardation and progressive neurological symptoms in males. *Am J Hum Genet* September 2005;**77**(3):442−53.

86. Meins M, Lehmann J, Gerresheim F, et al. Submicroscopic duplication in Xq28 causes increased expression of the MECP2 gene in a boy with severe mental retardation and features of Rett syndrome. *J Med Genet* February 2005;**42**(2):e12.

87. Na ES, Nelson ED, Adachi M, et al. A mouse model for MeCP2 duplication syndrome: MeCP2 overexpression impairs learning and memory and synaptic transmission. *J Neurosci* February 29, 2012;**32**(9):3109−17.

88. Amir RE, Fang P, Yu Z, et al. Mutations in exon 1 of MECP2 are a rare cause of Rett syndrome. *J Med Genet* February 2005;**42**(2):e15.

89. Quenard A, Yilmaz S, Fontaine H, et al. Deleterious mutations in exon 1 of MECP2 in Rett syndrome. *Eur J Med Genet* Jul-Aug 2006; **49**(4):313−22.

90. Saunders CJ, Minassian BE, Chow EW, Zhao W, Vincent JB. Novel exon 1 mutations in MECP2 implicate isoform MeCP2_e1 in classical Rett syndrome. *Am J Med Genet A* May 2009;**149A**(5): 1019−23.

91. Djuric U, Cheung AY, Zhang W, et al. MECP2e1 isoform mutation affects the form and function of neurons derived from Rett syndrome patient iPS cells. *Neurobiol Dis* January 30, 2015;**76C**:37−45.

92. Itoh M, Tahimic CG, Ide S, et al. Methyl CpG-binding protein isoform MeCP2_e2 is dispensable for Rett syndrome phenotypes but essential for embryo viability and placenta development. *J Biol Chem* April 20, 2012;**287**(17):13859−67.

93. Armstrong D, Dunn JK, Antalffy B, Trivedi R. Selective dendritic alterations in the cortex of Rett syndrome. *J Neuropathol Exp Neurol* March 1995;**54**(2):195−201.

94. Armstrong DD, Dunn K, Antalffy B. Decreased dendritic branching in frontal, motor and limbic cortex in Rett syndrome compared with trisomy 21. *J Neuropathol Exp Neurol* November 1998;**57**(11):1013−7.

95. Marchetto MC, Carromeu C, Acab A, et al. A model for neural development and treatment of Rett syndrome using human induced pluripotent stem cells. *Cell* November 12, 2010;**143**(4): 527−39.

96. Wang IT, Reyes AR, Zhou Z. Neuronal morphology in MeCP2 mouse models is intrinsically variable and depends on age, cell type, and Mecp2 mutation. *Neurobiol Dis* October 2013;**58**:3−12.

97. Belichenko PV, Wright EE, Belichenko NP, et al. Widespread changes in dendritic and axonal morphology in Mecp2-mutant mouse models of Rett syndrome: evidence for disruption of neuronal networks. *J Comp Neurol* May 20, 2009;**514**(3):240−58.

98. Kishi N, Macklis JD. MECP2 is progressively expressed in postmigratory neurons and is involved in neuronal maturation rather than cell fate decisions. *Mol Cell Neurosci* November 2004;**27**(3): 306−21.

99. Dani VS, Chang Q, Maffei A, Turrigiano GG, Jaenisch R, Nelson SB. Reduced cortical activity due to a shift in the balance between excitation and inhibition in a mouse model of Rett syndrome. *Proc Natl Acad Sci USA* August 30, 2005;**102**(35): 12560−5.

100. Dani VS, Nelson SB. Intact long-term potentiation but reduced connectivity between neocortical layer 5 pyramidal neurons in a mouse model of Rett syndrome. *J Neurosci* September 9, 2009; **29**(36):11263−70.

101. Wood L, Shepherd GM. Synaptic circuit abnormalities of motor-frontal layer 2/3 pyramidal neurons in a mutant mouse model of Rett syndrome. *Neurobiol Dis* May 2010;**38**(2):281−7.

102. Asaka Y, Jugloff DG, Zhang L, Eubanks JH, Fitzsimonds RM. Hippocampal synaptic plasticity is impaired in the Mecp2-null mouse model of Rett syndrome. *Neurobiol Dis* January 2006; **21**(1):217−27.

103. Lonetti G, Angelucci A, Morando L, Boggio EM, Giustetto M, Pizzorusso T. Early environmental enrichment moderates the behavioral and synaptic phenotype of MeCP2 null mice. *Biol Psychiatry* April 1, 2010;**67**(7):657−65.

104. Guy J, Gan J, Selfridge J, Cobb S, Bird A. Reversal of neurological defects in a mouse model of Rett syndrome. *Science* February 23, 2007;**315**(5815):1143−7.

105. Robinson L, Guy J, McKay L, et al. Morphological and functional reversal of phenotypes in a mouse model of Rett syndrome. *Brain* September 2012;**135**(Pt 9):2699−710.

106. Garg SK, Lioy DT, Cheval H, et al. Systemic delivery of MeCP2 rescues behavioral and cellular deficits in female mouse models of Rett syndrome. *J Neurosci* August 21, 2013;**33**(34):13612−20.

107. Popescu AC, Sidorova E, Zhang G, Eubanks JH. Aminoglycoside-mediated partial suppression of MECP2 nonsense mutations responsible for Rett syndrome in vitro. *J Neurosci Res* August 15, 2010;**88**(11):2316−24.

108. Brendel C, Belakhov V, Werner H, et al. Readthrough of nonsense mutations in Rett syndrome: evaluation of novel aminoglycosides and generation of a new mouse model. *J Mol Med Berl* April 2011; **89**(4):389−98.

109. Castro J, Garcia RI, Kwok S, et al. Functional recovery with recombinant human IGF1 treatment in a mouse model of Rett Syndrome. *Proc Natl Acad Sci USA* July 8, 2014;**111**(27):9941−6.

110. Buchovecky CM, Turley SD, Brown HM, et al. A suppressor screen in Mecp2 mutant mice implicates cholesterol metabolism in Rett syndrome. *Nat Genet* September 2013;**45**(9):1013−20.

8

FMRP and the Pathophysiology of Fragile X Syndrome

Stephanie A. Barnes, Sophie R. Thomson, Peter C. Kind,
Emily K. Osterweil

Centre for Integrative Physiology/Patrick Wild Centre, University of Edinburgh, Edinburgh, UK

The increasing diagnosis of autism spectrum disorders (ASD) has created an urgent need to identify novel targeted treatments. For this to occur, a clear mechanistic understanding of the underlying pathophysiology is required. Unfortunately, a direct relationship genetic mutation and disease pathology has been hampered by the sheer number of genes that have been identified as risk factors for developing ASD. One way forward is to study the cellular and physiological consequences of single gene mutations that account for a significant proportion of ASD cases.

Mutation of the *FMR1* gene results in Fragile X syndrome (FXS), a neurodevelopmental disorder with a high incidence of ASD (approximately 18–33%).[1,2]

In this chapter we will briefly review what is known about the *FMR1* gene and its product, Fragile X mental retardation protein (FMRP). We will then discuss the cellular and physiological consequences that arise from FMRP loss, including pathological alterations in cerebral protein synthesis, dendritic spine morphology, excitation of neuronal circuits, and synaptic plasticity. In subsequent sections, we will summarize evidence supporting the mGluR theory of Fragile X, which states that protein synthesis downstream of Gp1 metabotropic glutamate receptors (mGluRs) is central to the pathophysiology of FXS.[3] We will conclude by discussing the clinical relevance of the mGluR theory and the broader implications of this research for the study of ASD.

Neuronal and Synaptic Dysfunction in Autism Spectrum Disorder and Intellectual Disability
http://dx.doi.org/10.1016/B978-0-12-800109-7.00008-X

FRAGILE X SYNDROME AND FMRP

Fragile X Syndrome

Many studies have been devoted to the neurological and psychiatric symptoms of FXS and the development of potential treatment strategies. A comprehensive review of this work can be found in Chapter 20. In brief, FXS is a prevalent neurodevelopmental disorder characterized by multiple cognitive and behavioral deficits.[4,5] The psychiatric symptoms of FXS are highly variable, but affected individuals share a defining feature of intellectual disability (ID). The severity of ID ranges from moderate to severe and IQ is found to decline further with age.[6] Patients with FXS usually present with language delay and can have additional behavioral symptoms that include hyperactivity, social anxiety, impulsivity, attention-deficit hyperactivity disorder, and autistic-like behaviors such as shyness, poor eye contact, and hypersensitivity to sensory stimuli.[7] The predominant physical feature observed in FXS is macroorchidism (observed in >80% of FXS males) with a variable presence of an elongated face, large and prominent ears, macrocephaly, prominent jaw and forehead, high-arched palate, and loose connective tissue leading to hyperextensible joints, flat feet, and soft skin.[8] Additional medical problems include childhood seizures, sleep disorders, strabismus, a susceptibility to ear and sinus infections, and gastrointestinal problems.[8] For female carriers of the full mutation, symptoms tend to be more variable and milder, depending on the proportion of cells that inactivate the X-chromosome carrying the functional copy of the FMR1 allele.[9]

FMR1 Gene Mutation

Fragile X syndrome is relatively unique among neuropsychiatric disorders in that it is caused by mutation of a single gene, FMR1. The term "fragile X" was first used to identify an abnormality on the X chromosome of certain patients with ID.[10] Indications that a specific syndromic disorder was linked to a heritable mutation on the X chromosome was first described by Martin and Bell in 1943, who recognized an increased prevalence in males versus females.[11] However it was not until 1991 that FMR1 was identified at the fragile site at map position Xq27.3 on the long arm of the X chromosome.[12] Southern blot analysis found that a 40-kb DNA fragment on the X chromosome exhibited a significantly increased size variation, indicating that the FXS mutation may result from the presence of an insertion or amplification event. An unusual number of CGG repeats of varying lengths were observed in the FMR1 gene, which coincided with a hypermethylated CpG island. This led to speculation that the CGG repeat

may influence local methylation and the expansion of this repeat may be responsible for the abnormal methylation status of the FMR1 gene.[12,13] Since these initial observations it is now known that the vast majority of FXS patients have a significant CGG expansion mutation of more than 200 units. This expansion mutation lies in the promoter region of the FMR1 gene leading to hypermethylation of a nearby CpG site.[14−16] As a result, little or no corresponding mRNA is produced and consequently the encoded FMRP is absent. The severity of FXS appears to be negatively correlated with the level of FMRP expression.[17]

In unaffected individuals the CGG repeat upstream of FMR1 is polymorphic, ranging from five to 54 repeats.[18] Although the hypermethylation and silencing of FMR1 occurs with >200 repeats, a premutation of 55−200 repeats leads to separate disorders known as Fragile X—associated tremor/ataxia syndrome and Fragile X—associated primary ovarian insufficiency (for review, see Ref. 19). Because of the instability of this region, the number of trinucleotide repeats can increase with successive generations, increasing the penetrance of FXS.[20] It can also lead to the occurrence of size mosaicism within the FXS population in which individuals exhibit different CGG expansion lengths; some carrying the full mutation of >200 CGG units, whereas others have an expansion repeat of 55−200 repeats that results in the premutation.[21,22] This results in FMRP expression in a subset of cells but not others and is fairly common within the FXS population, affecting approximately 20% of individuals.[23] In addition, some FXS patients present with methylation mosaicism, in which the FMR1 gene carrying the full mutation has a variable methylation status. This leads to some cells carrying the methylated full mutation that is transcriptionally silenced whereas others possess an unmethylated fully mutation that is transcriptional active.[24−26]

Although most FXS cases are the result of a mutant trinucleotide expansion of 200 units or above, there are reports of individuals carrying rare point mutations (I304N and R138Q) in the FMR1 gene that result in a severe form of FXS.[27,28] Examination of the I304N mutation revealed that resides within the coding sequence of the gene, and does not affect the CGG repeat length or methylation status. Instead, this mutation is located within the sequence encoding one of the RNA binding motifs on FMRP. The net result is the production of a mutant FMRP that cannot associate with mRNA.[29] The finding that point mutations also cause FXS confirmed that the syndrome arising from the CGG expansion resulted from the misexpression of FMR1, rather than the regulation of nearby genes.

FMRP Structure and Function

Since its identification as the product of the *FMR1* gene, FMRP has been thoroughly investigated in several different model systems. *FMR1* is highly conserved, and FMRP homologues are found in numerous species including rodents, zebrafish, *Xenopus*, *Drosophila*, and aplysia.[24,30−34] Mammalian FMRP is most abundantly expressed in neurons of the CNS and in testes, with protein expression levels peaking at the end of the first 2 postnatal weeks before gradually declining.[21] It is localized throughout the neuron, including soma, dendrites, and synaptic compartments.[21−23] FMRP belongs to a family of heterogeneous ribonucleoproteins, which function in the regulation of mRNAs.[25,26]

The structure of FMRP can be divided into three main regions: an N-terminal region, containing two Tudor domains that function as a nuclear localization signal; a central region, which contains two RNA-binding K homology (KH) domains and a nuclear export signal (NES); and a C-terminal region, which contains an RGG box RNA-binding domain.[35] The KH and RGG regions may confer some specificity of mRNA binding to FMRP, because they recognize specific "kissing complex" and "G-quartet" sequences found in select mRNAs.[36,37] However, the exact mechanism of mRNA specificity for FMRP is not known.

Initial studies of FMRP explored its role in intracellular mRNA transport. FMRP has been shown to shuttle targets to and from the nuclear compartment, potentially facilitating transcription.[38] Imaging experiments in cultured neurons reveal trafficking of FMRP with mRNPs along dendrites and into synapses.[39−41] The transport of these cargo mRNAs can be regulated by synaptic activation of Gp1 mGluRs.[39,42] Interestingly, the localization and expression levels of many FMRP target mRNAs appear to be largely unaffected in the *Fmr1* mouse model (*Fmr1−/y*).[43] It may be that the trafficking of targets is highly selective or specifically relevant to activity regulation.

Additional work defined what is now considered to be a major role of FMRP: the repression of mRNA translation. The first evidence of this came from in vitro studies showing that most FMRP cosediments with actively translating polyribosome fractions.[29,44−46] Subsequent studies confirmed that FMRP negatively regulates the translation of bound mRNAs.[47,48] The exact mechanism by which FMRP negatively regulates protein synthesis is not known; however, several studies have explored this question. Experiments in mouse brain lysate and cultured cells showed that FMRP sequesters target mRNAs into translationally dormant RNA granules, preventing the association with actively translating polyribosomes.[49,50]

It has been suggested that the localization of FMRP to stalled versus active polysomes is regulated by phosphorylation at serine residue 499, which allows for regulation by synaptic activity.[51] Additional studies of isolated synaptic fractions show that FMRP recruits of cytoplasmic FMRP interacting protein 1 to repress translation by inhibiting the translation initiation complex.[52] FMRP has also been implicated in stalling mRNAs on ribosomes during the elongation step of protein synthesis.[53,54] The binding sites of FMRP occur throughout the coding sequence of target mRNAs, which suggests a potential for significant inhibition of elongation.[53] The most recent evidence of this comes from a study of the fruit fly *Drosophila melanogaster*, which reveals that the FMRP homologue dFMRP directly inhibits tRNA binding to the 80S ribosomal subunit.[54] It is likely that further studies of the ribosomal association of FMRP will yield more specific information about its role in the repression of mRNA translation.

The identification of FMRP target mRNAs has been the focus of several studies. Immunoprecipitation studies from brain lysates and isolated synaptic fractions have estimated that FMRP binds to approximately 4% of total brain mRNAs.[26,55,56] A study using high-throughput cross-linking immunoprecipitation in mouse brain lysates verified over 800 unique transcripts bound to FMRP.[53,55,56] The list includes genes involved in synaptic function and intracellular signaling, and there is a substantial overlap with genes that have been linked to idiopathic autism.[53] The ways in which these targets are dysregulated in FXS and how this contributes to the disease pathology is an area of active investigation and has yet to be established.

PATHOLOGICAL CONSEQUENCES OF THE LOSS OF FMRP

Several studies have been performed in human FXS patients to understand the neurological consequences of FMRP loss; however, there are obvious limitations, especially with regard to mechanistic exploration. To understand the function of FMRP and the pathogenesis of FXS fully, a mouse model was created by deleting the *Fmr1* gene from the genome.[57] Although this model (*Fmr1−/y*) involves deletion of the gene rather than hypermethylation and transcriptional silencing, the resulting loss of FMRP throughout much of brain development is reminiscent of the human disorder.[58] The *Fmr1−/y* mouse has been a valuable tool, and much of what we know about the functional consequences of FMRP loss come from studies using this mouse model of FXS.

Cellular Alterations: Excessive Protein Synthesis

As a brain-enriched repressor of mRNA translation, it is expected that the loss of FMRP should result in changes in the rate of protein synthesis. Surprisingly, this was not directly tested in the $Fmr1^{-/y}$ mouse until 2005 when autoradiographic measurements revealed a small (15–20%) but significant increase in cerebral protein synthesis compared with wild-type (WT) mice.[59] This result was observed in several brain regions including the hippocampus, a critical brain structure involved in learning and memory. Subsequent work recapitulated this finding using metabolic labeling of ex vivo hippocampal slices[60,61] and biochemically isolated cortical synaptoneurosome fractions.[62]

Excessive protein synthesis is now believed to be a core pathophysiology of FXS. Seminal work by Huber et al. provided the first link between exaggerated protein synthesis and altered neural performance in the $Fmr1^{-/y}$ mouse through the study of long-term synaptic depression (LTD).[63] The stimulation of mGluR1/5 in hippocampal CA1 leads to a rapid and sustained LTD that requires de novo protein synthesis.[64] The molecular basis for this mGluR-LTD appears to be the internalization of α-amino-3-hydroxy-5-methyl-4-isoxazolepropionic acid (AMPA)-type glutamate receptors (AMPARs), a process that also requires new translation.[65] In the $Fmr1^{-/y}$ mouse, mGluR-LTD is maintained in the absence of new mRNA translation, which suggests that there is already an abundance of the proteins necessary for synaptic depression.[66] This work was part of the inspiration for the mGluR theory of Fragile X, which posits that many of the pathological changes in FXS can be ameliorated by reduction of protein synthesis downstream of mGluR1/5 activation.[3] We will return to this topic later in the chapter.

The induction and regulation of local mRNA translation is critical for sustaining changes in synaptic strength. Like mGluR-LTD, synaptic late-phase long-term potentiation (L-LTP) requires local protein synthesis.[67] The presence of polyribosomes, translation factors, and mRNAs at individual postsynaptic compartments allows for synapses to respond in a semiautonomous fashion.[68–70] This spatial control is important for specifying which incoming connections will be strengthened or weakened. The timing of mRNA translation in response to activity is also critical. The activation pattern of postsynaptic receptors that induces sustained L-LTP or mGluR-LTD must also induce local protein synthesis.[64,67] It has been suggested that the induction of LTP/D coincides with the translation of a tag that marks the synapses for further strengthening or weakening, thus allowing for synapse specificity.[71]

In the $Fmr1^{-/y}$, stimulus-induced mRNA translation is disrupted. In hippocampal slices, stimulation of either mGluR1/5 or tropomyosin regulated kinase B, under conditions identical to those used to induce LTD or LTP, leads to a robust increase in protein synthesis in WT but fails to elicit a response in the $Fmr1^{-/y}$.[61] A similar lack of stimulus-induced translation is observed in cortical synaptoneurosome preparations, in which activation of glutamatergic transmission results in a significant increase in protein synthesis in WT but not the $Fmr1^{-/y}$.[62] It is possible that the excess protein synthesis in the $Fmr1^{-/y}$ saturates the translation machinery, preventing further stimulus-induced responses. This may explain the variety of synaptic plasticity phenotypes observed throughout the $Fmr1^{-/y}$ brain (discussed later in this section).

Given the impressive list of FMRP mRNA targets, there is likely a significant shift in the translatome of the $Fmr1^{-/y}$.[53] The extent to which the translated products of FMRP target mRNAs are altered in FXS is not yet known, but a number of proteins have been investigated. Among the list of proteins that are aberrantly translated in the $Fmr1^{-/y}$, several are involved in AMPAR endocytosis. These include the microtubule binding protein MAP1B,[72] the immediate early gene Arc/Arg3.1,[73] the phosphatase STEP,[74] and the Alzheimer protein APP.[75] All of these FMRP target mRNAs are localized to synapses and translated in response to mGluR1/5 activation. There is also evidence that the synaptic scaffolding protein PSD-95 and the plasticity protein CaMKII-alpha are overly translated at $Fmr1^{-/y}$ synapses.[61,62,76,77] The matrix metalloproteinase MMP-9 has been identified as an FMRP target that is dysregulated in the $Fmr1^{-/y}$ mouse,[78,79] which has led to investigation of the drug minocycline as a potential treatment strategy for FXS.[80]

It is likely that many other mRNAs are abnormally translated in FXS, and it will be interesting to see what relationship this has to the pathological changes observed in neuronal function. Curiously, many of the proteins overly synthesized in the $Fmr1^{-/y}$ do not appear to be overexpressed in the $Fmr1^{-/y}$ brain.[81] It is possible that the pathology of FXS is not the result of an accumulation of target proteins, but rather an increase in dynamic protein turnover. In this case, typical expression analyses may miss important changes that would only be observed in the newly synthesized population of proteins. A careful investigation of the dynamic regulation of target mRNA translation in $Fmr1^{-/y}$ neurons could reveal more specific information about which targets are contributing to functional abnormalities in FXS.

Neuroanatomical Changes: Altered Dendritic Spines

Because of the close association of FMRP with dendrites and the regulation of mRNAs encoding about one-third of all presynaptic and postsynaptic targets, it is not surprising that many studies have targeted synapses in search for altered structure and function in the $Fmr1^{-/y}$.[53] Dendritic spines are motile short protrusions along neuronal dendrites, and in the cortex they are the primary site of excitatory synapses on excitatory neurons. The morphological properties of dendritic spines have been linked to the efficacy of synaptic function.[82–84] Dendritic spines act as chemical and electrical filters determining the degree to which synaptic activation is coupled to dendrites and nearby synapses.[85,86] Hence they represent a fundamental computation unit for neuronal communication and their number and morphology regulate neuronal function and circuit properties. Although few studies have directly examined spine changes in humans with FXS, alterations in dendritic spine density and morphology in the cortex have been reported.[87–89]

One of the earliest anatomical phenotypes observed in the postmortem brains of patients with FXS was the overabundance of dendritic spines with a thin, tortuous morphology reminiscent of immature synapses.[87,88,90] This abnormal spine phenotype is observed in various cortical regions, which were qualitatively analyzed by rapid Golgi staining. Irwin et al. observed an increase in spine density in the visual and temporal cortices of the FXS brain, which was isolated to the most distal dendritic segments of layer 5 pyramidal neurones.[89] Whereas these findings were based on three individuals with FXS and three control cases (with variable preservation of the postmortem tissue), they suggest that dendritic spines may be affected in FXS, in agreement with findings of the role of FMRP in local protein synthesis and synaptic plasticity.

Analyses of spine density and morphology in mouse models of FXS have been numerous and are largely equivocal (for a detailed review of the literature, see Ref. 91). Although some studies recapitulate spine deficits in the adult neocortex of $Fmr1^{-/y}$ mice[60,92–94] as well as in other brain regions,[95] few studies have found increases in spine density during development.[96–101] Differences in studies include differences in cell type and brain region analyzed, technical approaches, and methods of statistical analysis.

A similar issue of reproducibility is observed in terms of spine shape. Consistent with the human, mouse models of FXS have been reported to have a prevalence of long, thin dendritic spines.[86] Unfortunately, these studies not only have the drawback of technical and statistical issues noted previously regarding spine density, they have an added problem in that they seek to measure morphological features of spines that are below the resolution of the microscopes being employed. Furthermore, many of the studies examining spine morphology artificially classify dendritic spines in different morphological categories (mushroom, long-thin, etc.), which are linked to particular functional outcomes (e.g., synaptic efficacy) to assess differences using particular statistical tests (e.g., chi-square analysis). However, studies using electron microscopy[102,103] and super-resolution fluorescent imaging[85,101] indicate that spine shape forms a continuum without clear structural and functional classes. Thus, categorization of dendritic spines created subjective grouping whose comparison may exaggerate differences in $Fmr1^{-/y}$ mice.

The development of super-resolution microscopy has allowed for more detailed examination of synaptic structure.[85,104] Dendritic spines were examined in $Fmr1^{-/y}$ mice at the nanoscale using stimulated emission depletion (STED) microscopy.[101] STED microscopy has a spatial resolution of about 50 nm, compared with 250 and 400 nm with confocal and two-photon microscopy, respectively. This has enabled a more accurate assessment of dendritic spines, such as head width, neck length, and neck width, which are too small to be measured reliably by diffraction-limited microscopy techniques, but which have crucial roles in regulating synaptic function. This study revealed that between postnatal day (P) 14 and P37, dendritic spines heads dramatically decrease in size whereas spine necks lose their definition, becoming thicker and shorter. Between these two ages, therefore, spines become much more coupled to the dendrite and adjacent synapses. At both ages, spine morphology in the $Fmr1^{-/y}$ is similar to WTs, which indicates that development is proceeding relatively normally in the absence of FMRP. However, some subtle changes were visible in $Fmr1^{-/y}$ in both CA1 pyramidal and layer 5 cortical pyramidal neurons. For example, at P37 CA1 pyramidal neurones in $Fmr1^{-/y}$ have a greater number of spines with larger heads and shorter, narrower necks compared with WT controls, which indicates a subtle immaturity in the hippocampus.[101] These changes, although subtle, suggest that the loss of FMRP may result in spines that are more compartmentalized with less chemical coupling with the dendrites and adjacent synapses. However, whether these subtle changes in morphology result in functional changes in dendritic integration remains to be tested. Nonetheless, these findings indicate that whereas dendritic spine shape and density may be altered in mouse models of FXS, these changes are unlikely to be the primary explanation for the changes in synaptic function and plasticity.

A key feature of dendritic spines is their ability to changes their number and morphology over time. Indeed, spine dynamics are regulated over development, with spine turnover decreasing with age.[91] Studies have suggested that spine dynamics are altered after the loss of FMRP.[98,100] These studies found an increase in spine turnover during development in cortical pyramidal neurons in layer 2/3[98] and layer 5[100] of somatosensory cortex in $Fmr1^{-/y}$ mice, with the former normalizing by 3 weeks of age. Although the timing over which spine turnover was measured was different between the two studies (hours versus days, respectively), these studies suggest that the loss of FMRP prevents synaptic stabilization during cortical development. These findings complement the increase in protein turnover in $Fmr1^{-/y}$s mentioned earlier and are in good agreement with the delay in critical period for the induction of synaptic plasticity observed at thalamocortical synapses in $Fmr1^{-/y}$ somatosensory cortex.[99] Taken together, these studies indicate that delays in synaptic development and plasticity may, in part, underlie the developmental delay associated with FXS.

Because of the function of FMRP in regulating protein synthesis of a range of synaptic proteins and the numerous defects in synaptic function and plasticity, it would be surprising if synaptic structural dynamics and function were not altered in the absence of FMRP. That said, determining the precise relationship between dendritic spine structure and function in an $Fmr1^{-/y}$ animal is not trivial and the precise pathophysiology will likely depend on the age and cell type being examined. Furthermore, although useful, examining static images of dendritic spines will reveal only part of a complex and emerging story that will need to be viewed in the context of spine dynamics if we are to understand how FMRP-dependent changes eventually lead to alterations in neuronal circuits and behavior.

Changes in Neuronal Function: Alterations in Circuit Excitability

Many symptoms of FXS indicate an alteration in the excitability of neuronal circuits including seizures, sensory hypersensitivities, and anxiety.[105] These symptoms of FXS are mirrored by altered circuit activity in $Fmr1^{-/y}$ mice (for a detailed review, see Ref. 106). For example, intracellular recordings of hippocampal CA3 pyramidal neurons in $Fmr1^{-/y}$ hippocampal slices have revealed epileptiform bursting in response to spontaneous synaptic activity.[107,108] These ictal-like responses progress to prolonged synchronized discharges and are comparable to those observed during epileptic seizures. A similar increase in network excitability has also been seen in the cortex.[109,110] These changes in circuit function can arise from a multiple of different sources, from altered intrinsic properties of neurons to altered cellular or circuit homeostasis, including changes to the inhibition-to-excitation ratio. Pinpointing the source of altered excitability in FXS is challenging, especially given the number of mRNA targets of FMRP as well

as findings showing that FMRP directly binds to ion channels to regulate their function.[111–114]

Among the more than 800 identified FMRP targets are mRNAs encoding seven voltage-dependent Ca^{2+} channels, eight voltage-gated K^+ channels, and two voltage-gated Na^+ channels and a myriad of ion transporters and co-transporters.[53] It is not surprising, therefore, that numerous studies have identified alterations in the neuronal excitability in $Fmr1^{-/y}$ mice. However, the relationship between altered translation of these FMRP targets and the pathology of fragile X is not clear. In one study, Lee et al. demonstrated an increase in the translation of the FMRP target mRNA encoding Kv4.2, a K^+ channel implicated in dendritic excitability.[115] This study shows an increased expression of Kv4.2 in dendrites of $Fmr1^{-/y}$ hippocampus, and pharmacological blockade of this channel restores normal levels of LTP. In contrast, Gross et al. showed a decrease in Kv4.2,[116] and a decrease in A-type K+ currents in the dendrites of $Fmr1^{-/y}$ hippocampal neurons was reported.[117] Interestingly, passive properties of cortical layer 4[109] cortical layer 5,[118] and hippocampal CA1[119] neurons are altered in the $Fmr1^{-/y}$; for the latter two studies, however, these resulted from changes in the expression of the HCN1 channel, the mRNA for which has not been identified as a direct target of FMRP. It may be that changes in the expression of HCN1 and other ion channels are due to compensatory changes rather than direct alteration of mRNA translation owing to the loss of FMRP.

There is ample evidence that the loss of FMRP causes significant changes in membrane properties. These include alterations in the expression of voltage-gated calcium channels[120] and in potassium channel function.[111,119,121,122] Together these changes dramatically alter the excitability of individual cells as well as the circuits they form. Surprisingly, a direct role for FMRP in regulating neuronal excitability has been demonstrated that is independent of its canonical function in regulating protein synthesis. FMRP has been shown to directly bind and regulate the channel activity of potassium[111–113] and calcium channels.[114] Indeed, these studies highlight the multiple roles of FMRP in regulating excitability in multiple compartments of neurons demonstrating its role in dendritic integration,[55,111] action potential kinetics,[113,120] and presynaptic vesicle release.[113,114] Future studies are needed to understand the impact of these alterations on specific brain circuits and to assess their overall contribution to the pathology of FXS.

Changes in Synaptic Function: Aberrant Plasticity

For learning to occur, new information must modify existing synaptic connections in a manner that builds on previous experience. It has been proposed that de novo protein synthesis is a cellular mechanism that stabilizes synaptic changes, so neurons can remember previous activity.[123,124] This hypothesis stems from decades of work showing that protein synthesis inhibitors block learning in several different species, and disrupt LTP and LTD in acute brain slices.[64,124−126]

In FXS, where the most prominent phenotype observed is ID, there has been tremendous interest in understanding the relationship between excessive protein synthesis and alterations in protein synthesis—dependent plasticity.

As mentioned previously, induction of mGluR-LTD in the $Fmr1^{-/y}$ leads to an exaggerated level of synaptic depression at CA1 synapses.[63] This occurs in the absence of significant alterations in AMPA receptor—mediated synaptic transmission, which indicates that under basal conditions synapses are functionally intact. A similar exaggeration of mGluR-LTD is seen in parallel fiber to Purkinje cell synapses in the $Fmr1^{-/y}$ cerebellum.[127] Measurements of receptor trafficking in $Fmr1^{-/y}$ neuronal cultures and acute hippocampal slices show that mGluR1/5 stimulation with the agonist (S)-3,5-dihydroxyphenylglycine (DHPG) leads to excessive AMPA receptor internalization from the postsynaptic terminal.[65,73] Both mGluR-LTD and the accompanying internalization of AMPARs require de novo protein synthesis in WT synapses,[64,65] but these processes are unaffected by protein synthesis inhibitors in the $Fmr1^{-/y}$.[66] The prevailing hypothesis is that the proteins required for LTD and AMPAR internalization are excessively translated in the $Fmr1^{-/y}$, and thus do not require de novo synthesis in response to mGluR1/5 activation. Support for this idea can be found in results showing that interruption of de novo Arc/Arg3.1 synthesis using RNA interference (RNAi) restores normal levels of mGluR-LTD and AMPAR internalization in the $Fmr1^{-/y}$ hippocampus.[73]

Whereas multiple studies show that mGluR-LTD is exaggerated in the $Fmr1^{-/y}$, studies of LTP suggest that is either unchanged or reduced in magnitude. Initially, examination of protein synthesis—dependent L-LTP induced by high-frequency stimulation revealed no differences in magnitude between $Fmr1^{-/y}$ and WT mice.[128−132] However, other studies report a reduction of LTP in hippocampal CA1[133−135] or dentate gyrus.[136,137] These discrepancies may be the result of differences in stimulation protocols, which can induce mechanistically distinct forms of LTP.[138] For example, although both tetanic stimulation[128,139] and conventional theta burst[129] produce normal LTP in $Fmr1^{-/y}$ mice, changing the threshold level of theta burst afferent stimulation (from 10 theta bursts to 5) reveals an impairment in LTP.[134] This suggests that the threshold for inducing L-LTP is increased in $Fmr1^{-/y}$ mutants relative to WT mice.

Studies of brain regions have also found evidence of deficient LTP in the $Fmr1^{-/y}$. The critical period for being able to induce LTP at thalamocortical synapses in the primary somatosensory cortex is delayed in $Fmr1^{-/y}$ mice and is mirrored by a delay in the decrease in the NMDA-type glutamate receptor (NMDAR)-to-AMPAR ratio.[99] Despite these changes in the development of synaptic function, the timing of spinogenesis is only mildly affected. These findings raise the possibility that mismatches in developmental events such as synaptic structure and neuronal connectivity may be critical factors in the developmental phenotypes associated with FXS.

An increased LTP threshold is also reported for spike timing—dependent (STD) plasticity, a form of Hebbian plasticity induced by tight temporal correlations between the spikes of the presynaptic and postsynaptic neurones. It is reported that STD-LTP is deficient in $Fmr1^{-/y}$ neurones in somatosensory cortex, prefrontal cortex, and nucleus accumbens.[96,140,141] This form of LTP can be induced if presynaptic stimulation is paired with a stronger postsynaptic stimulation in the medial prefrontal cortex, which suggests that the machinery required for expression of STD-LTP is present in the $Fmr1^{-/y}$ mouse but requires stronger neuronal activity for it to be engaged.[96]

Other forms of LTP that are altered in the $Fmr1^{-/y}$ include homeostatic synaptic scaling,[142] which is deficient, and mGluR1/5 priming of LTP, which no longer requires de novo protein synthesis.[131] Although the overall implications of these changes in plasticity are not yet known, it is clear that deficiencies in synaptic strengthening exist throughout the $Fmr1^{-/y}$ brain.

THE METABOTROPIC GLUTAMATE RECEPTOR THEORY OF FRAGILE X

The broad range of pathological phenotypes seen in the $Fmr1^{-/y}$ animal model shows that FMRP loss results in significant deficits throughout the brain. This complexity is consistent with the multiple behavioral, epileptogenic, and cognitive symptoms associated with FXS. Current therapies for FXS are behavior-modifying and anticonvulsant drugs that target individual symptoms without treating the underlying cause. In contrast, therapeutic strategies that have been suggested based on the mGluR theory of Fragile X are designed to target the core pathophysiology of FXS.

Proposed in 2004 by Bear, Huber, and Warren, the mGluR theory of Fragile X states that antagonism of mGluR1/5 could correct the myriad behavioral and cognitive symptoms of FXS.[3] This hypothesis stemmed from findings that mGluR1/5 activation stimulates mRNA translation at synapses[143] and that mGluR-LTD is exaggerated in the $Fmr1^{-/y}$ hippocampus.[3] The prediction is that a reduction of mGluR1/5 or the associated mRNA translation can correct the pathological changes associated with the loss of FMRP. This has now been validated in numerous studies in multiple species (see Ref. 4 for an extensive review).

In vitro studies in hippocampal slices reveal that the excessive protein synthesis observed in the $Fmr1^{-/y}$ mouse is normalized with genetic reduction of mGluR5, or with acute application of the mGluR5-negative allosteric modulators (NAMs) 2-methyl-6-(phenyl ethynyl)pyridine (MPEP), or 2-chloro-4-((2,5-dimethyl-1-(4-(trifluoromethoxy)phenyl)-1H-imidazol-4-yl)ethynyl)pyridine (CTEP).[60,61,144] Experiments in isolated synaptoneurosome fractions also reveal that MPEP normalizes protein synthesis and corrects abnormal accumulation of mRNA granules in the $Fmr1^{-/y}$ cortex.[50,62] The antagonism of mGluR5 also corrects the LTD phenotype in the $Fmr1^{-/y}$ mouse. Application of MPEP corrects the accelerated AMPAR internalization linked to exaggerated mGluR-LTD in hippocampal cultures where FMRP has been reduced by RNAi.[145] Consistent with these results, genetic reduction of mGluR5 or application of CTEP corrects exaggerated mGluR-LTD in the $Fmr1^{-/y}$ hippocampus.[60,144]

With respect to reducing hyperexcitability, mGluR5 antagonism is particularly effective. In hippocampal CA3, extended stimulation of mGluR1/5 leads to prolonged discharges reminiscent of epileptic seizures.[146] This activity is enhanced in the $Fmr1^{-/y}$ but application of MPEP restores normal levels of activity.[147] Similarly, prolonged periods of persistent activity (UP states) are excessive in $Fmr1^{-/y}$ somatosensory cortex, which are alleviated with genetic reduction of mGluR5 or MPEP application.[148] Studies of audiogenic seizures (AGS) in the $Fmr1^{-/y}$ have also shown a significant reduction in epileptic activity by mGluR5 antagonism. The increased incidence of AGS in $Fmr1^{-/y}$ mice is thought to reflect epilepsy associated with FXS.[105] One of the first studies testing the mGluR theory showed that injection of MPEP reduced both the incidence and severity of AGS in $Fmr1^{-/y}$.[149] Subsequent studies using genetic reduction of mGluR5 or administration of CTEP have similarly shown an impressive suppression of the AGS phenotype in the $Fmr1^{-/y}$ mouse.[60,144]

Many other pathological changes in the $Fmr1^{-/y}$ mouse are either corrected or eliminated with mGluR5 antagonism, including altered dendritic spine morphology, abnormal ocular dominance plasticity in visual cortex, increased locomotor activity, and impaired learning (extensively reviewed in [4,150]). These findings have come from multiple laboratories around the world and have been validated in several animal models including fruit fly, zebrafish, and rat.[151–153] This extraordinary conservation suggests that abnormal function downstream

of mGluR5 is critical to the pathology of FXS. Several treatment strategies that target the mGluR5 pathway have been developed for testing in FXS patients, including direct mGluR5 antagonists, GABA-B receptor antagonists, and inhibitors of downstream signaling molecules (discussed further in Chapter 20).[4,154]

Gp1 mGluR Signaling and Translation Control

Successful validation of the mGluR theory has sparked interest in downstream signaling linking mGluR1/5 to mRNA translation. The canonical signaling pathway associated with mGluR1/5 involves activation of the small G protein Gq, which recruits phospholipase C-beta to release the downstream messengers inositol-1,4,5-trisphosphate and diacylglycerol (see Ref. 155 for review). However, mRNA translation downstream of mGluR1/5 is believed to be independent of this core pathway. Instead, two major translation control signaling pathways have been implicated: the Ras-extracellular signal regulated kinase 1/2 (ERK) pathway and the phosphoinositide 3 kinase (PI3K)-Akt—mammalian target of rapamycin (mTOR) pathway. The signaling mechanisms involved in translation control through these pathways are complex and are summarized in greater detail elsewhere (see Refs 150, 156). In brief, both ERK and mTOR stimulate translation by signaling to regulatory components of the initiation complex, primarily eukaryotic translation initiation factor 4E (eIF4E) and its inhibitor 4E binding protein (4EBP).[157,158] The initiation of protein synthesis involves the association of multiple factors with the 5′-untranslated region of mRNAs, including eIF4E and eIF4G, which together with eIF4A form the eIF4F complex. This complex facilitates the interaction of mRNA with the small ribosomal subunit. Evidence suggests that eIF4F complex formation requires phosphorylation of eIF4E downstream of subsequent activation of ERK and MAPK interacting kinase. In addition, the phosphorylation of 4EBP by mTOR removes it from eIF4E to allow for association with the initiation complex (see Ref. 159). Thus, both pathways activate initiation by promoting eIF4F formation (Figure 1). In addition, ERK and mTOR also stimulate protein synthesis by activating the ribosomal S6 kinase pathway.[159,160] Although it is clear that mGluR1/5 can recruit both ERK and mTOR, the way in which these pathways regulate protein synthesis at the synapse and how this is altered in FXS remain an area of active investigation.

ERK Signaling in FXS

Early studies in cell culture revealed that activation of mGluR1/5 with DHPG resulted in robust activation of

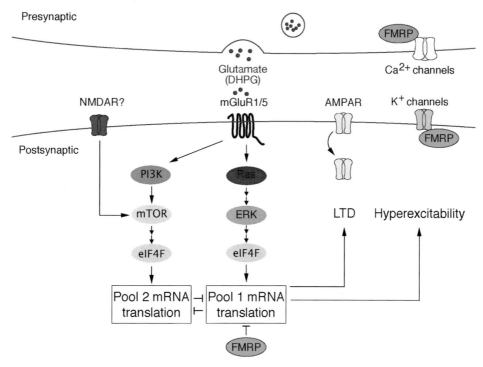

FIGURE 1 **mGluR1/5 signaling and the mGluR theory.** The activation of mGluR1/5 by glutamate or the agonist DHPG stimulates protein synthesis by activating the eIF4F translation initiation complex or the S6K pathway (not shown). When FMRP is lost in FXS, the increased translation of FMRP target mRNAs encoding LTD proteins (i.e., AMPAR endocytic proteins) leads to exaggerated LTD, and the altered synthesis of other proteins (i.e., potassium channels) leads to hyperexcitability. The loss of direct interaction between ion channels and FMRP also contributes to hyperexcitability. Both LTD and hyperexcitability phenotypes, among many others, are corrected by inhibiting mGluR5 or the Ras−MEK−ERK pathway upstream of protein synthesis. Activation of the PI3K−mTOR pathway downstream of mGluR1/5 or other receptors (i.e., NMDARs) may lead to the translation of a different pool of mRNAs, which could inhibit the LTD pool downstream of ERK.

the ERK pathway. Since then, these results have been replicated in a wide variety of systems including cell lines,[161] cultured neurons,[162] striatum,[163] spinal cord,[164] hippocampal slice,[165,166] and retinal pigment epithelial cells.[167] In hippocampal CA1, stimulation of protein synthesis−dependent mGluR-LTD is blocked by the application of the selective MEK-ERK inhibitor U0126.[61,168,169] The induction of epileptiform activity through mGluR1/5 stimulation in hippocampal CA3 is also eliminated with ERK inhibitors U0126 or PD98059.[107] These results show that ERK is required for the protein synthesis−dependent processes downstream of mGluR1/5 at hippocampal synapses.

Although studies of basal ERK signaling in the $Fmr1^{-/y}$ have produced conflicting results, with reports varying from increased activation[170] to no difference[61,133,169] or decreased activation,[171] it is clear that ERK inhibitors normalize the exaggerated protein synthesis downstream of mGluR1/5.[61,108,169] One explanation for this apparent discrepancy is that mRNA translation in the $Fmr1^{-/y}$ brain is hypersensitive to ERK stimulation, with normal levels of signaling producing an exaggerated response at the ribosome.[61] There is ample evidence that inhibition of the ERK pathway is particularly effective in correcting Fragile X pathology. In vitro

application of MEK-ERK inhibitors eliminates epileptiform activity in $Fmr1^{-/y}$ hippocampal CA3,[147] and interperitoneal injection of the brain-penetrant MEK-ERK inhibitor SL-327 greatly diminishes or completely eliminates the AGS phenotype in the $Fmr1^{-/y}$ mouse.[61,172] Correction of several pathological changes in the $Fmr1^{-/y}$ mouse can also be seen by genetic reduction of ERK pathway signaling molecules. In $Fmr1^{-/y}$ bred with a mutation on the ERK-activated eIF4E phosphorylation site, several phenotypes are corrected, including exaggerated protein synthesis, abnormal dendritic spine morphology, exaggerated mGluR-LTD, and deficiencies in social learning.[173] Similar correction of several phenotypes is seen in $Fmr1^{-/y}$ mice bred with mutations in other ERK pathway members, including Mnk1, Mnk2, and S6K1.[173,174] These studies strongly support the idea that ERK inhibition is corrective for FXS.

As a major signaling pathway involved in cell growth, it is difficult to imagine how inhibition of ERK could be used as a treatment strategy for FXS. However, this idea was explored by testing the efficacy of lovastatin, a drug widely prescribed to treat high cholesterol in children and adults, and that also reduces signaling through the Ras-ERK pathway.[175,176] Lovastatin was shown to be remarkably effective in reversing deleterious phenotypes in the mouse model of neurofibromatosis type 1 (NF1), a disorder of hyperactive Ras; it has also been investigated in clinical trials for NF1.[177,178] The idea that lovastatin could be used to correct FXS symptoms was examined by testing pathological phenotypes in the $Fmr1^{-/y}$ mouse model. Results of these experiments show that short-term application of lovastatin corrects excessive hippocampal protein synthesis and mGluR-LTD, eliminates epileptiform activity in hippocampal CA3, and corrects hyperexcitability in $Fmr1^{-/y}$ visual cortical slices.[108] In addition, administration of lovastatin to $Fmr1^{-/y}$ mice in vivo significantly reduces the incidence and severity of AGS, and corrects deficits in visuospatial learning.[61,108,172,179,180] Based on these findings, an open-label clinical trial using lovastatin was performed in a small group of FXS patients, with encouraging results (see Chapter 20 for further details).[181] Further clinical trials will no doubt reveal the extent to which downregulation of ERK by lovastatin or other statins can correct symptoms in FXS.

Dysregulated mTOR Signaling in FXS

Also activated downstream of mGluR1/5, the PI3K-mTOR pathway has a major role in synaptic mRNA translation.[182,183] This pathway is directly linked to mGluR1/5 through association with the PI3K enhancing protein (PIKE) and the scaffolding protein, Homer.[169,182,183] In the $Fmr1^{-/y}$ hippocampus, the mGluR5-Homer complex is destabilized, which results in altered activation of the PI3K—mTOR pathway.[183,184] Enhancing the mGluR—Homer complex by genetically reducing the dominant negative Homer1a isoform restores a number of phenotypes in the $Fmr1^{-/y}$.[169]

Interestingly, both PIKE and the p110-beta subunit of PI3K are mRNA targets of FMRP, and both proteins are overtranslated in the $Fmr1^{-/y}$ brain.[53,185,186] Consistent with these results, upregulation of the PI3K—mTOR pathway has been observed in $Fmr1^{-/y}$ hippocampus and cortex.[185,187] Genetic reduction of PIKE or p110-beta restores normal levels of PI3K—mTOR signaling in the $Fmr1^{-/y}$ and ameliorates several phenotypes, including abnormal dendritic spine morphology, mGluR-LTD, and deficient cognition.[186,188] These results suggest that downregulation of the PI3K—mTOR pathway would be protective for FXS.

Curiously, whereas studies of $Fmr1^{-/y}$ cortical synaptoneurosomes and cultured neurons reveal a correction of protein synthesis with PI3K inhibitors, studies in $Fmr1^{-/y}$ hippocampal slices show that neither application of the PI3K inhibitor wortmannin nor the mTOR inhibitor rapamycin is effective in normalizing exaggerated protein synthesis.[61,169] Pharmacological inhibition mTOR is also ineffective for correcting AGS in the $Fmr1^{-/y}$.[61] These seemingly disparate findings may be due to a difference in preparation or a difference between short-term pharmacological inhibition of PI3K—mTOR and chronic downregulation through genetic deletion of PIKE and/or p110-beta. However, studies using mouse models of tuberous sclerosis complex (TSC), a genetic disorder caused by the loss of the mTOR suppressor complex TSC1/2, suggest that increased mTOR activation could in fact be beneficial for FXS. Experiments performed in the hippocampus of the $Tsc2^{+/-}$ mouse model and in other mouse models of TSC reveal that both LTD and protein synthesis downstream of mGluR1/5 are deficient.[189–191]

It may be that the pool of mRNAs translated downstream of mTOR are inhibitory for the translation of LTD-supporting proteins downstream of mGluR5-ERK (Figure 1). Consistent with this idea, application of either the mTOR inhibitor rapamycin or the mGluR5-positive allosteric modulator CDPPB will correct (raise) deficient LTD and protein synthesis in the $Tsc2^{+/-}$ hippocampus.[189] Moreover, a genetic cross of the $Tsc2^{+/-}$ mouse to the $Fmr1^{-/y}$ mouse corrects deficits in hippocampal LTD and in behavioral measures of learning in both mutants.[189] The suggestion from these studies is that increased mTOR activation is corrective for pathological changes in the $Fmr1^{-/y}$ brain.

Further studies are needed to understand fully how both the reduction of PI3K and the increase in mTOR can lead to similar corrections in $Fmr1^{-/y}$ phenotypes. It may be that the impact of mTOR activation is specific to different postsynaptic receptors (i.e., NMDARs versus mGluRs), and that manipulation of signaling downstream of these receptors should be compared. However, it is clear that inhibition of downstream translational regulators such as S6K, targeted by both the ERK and mTOR pathways, can correct many phenotypes in the $Fmr1^{-/y}$.[174] Reduction of other regulators of mRNA translation such as cytoplasmic polyadenylation element-binding protein will also ameliorate pathological changes in the $Fmr1^{-/y}$ mouse.[192] Thus, future studies to determine new ways to target exaggerated mRNA translation in FXS will be of particular importance.

Clinical Applications of the mGluR Theory

The mGluR theory has been extremely influential to the scientific pursuit of FMRP and FXS, and it has also had a dramatic impact on patients and their families in that there is renewed hope that treatments may be effective even in adults. Preclinical evidence for the mGluR theory has spurred the initiation of several clinical trials that target mGluR5 directly or upstream or downstream regulators of mGluR5 signaling (reviewed in detail in Chapter 20 and discussed in Ref. 154). Unfortunately, translating these studies into successful clinical treatments has been less successful. Two large-scale trials by Hoffmann-La Roche AG and Novartis International AG examining the effectiveness of NAMs of mGluR5 have failed (i.e., did not reach their primary end point; clinicaltrials.gov). There are many possible for this, and a discussion of the limitations of clinical trials for FXS can be found in chapter 20. Two major disadvantages to these studies were the length of time that mGluR5 NAMs could be administered and the age of the participants in the trial. They were also hampered by the lack of specific outcome measures and biomarkers for FXS. It is common for pharmaceutical interventions for psychiatric disorders to help some individuals (responders) and not others (nonresponders) or for people to become tolerant to drugs over time. Finally as noted, FMRP has multiple roles, including those that are independent of a role in protein synthesis; it may emerge that in targeting mGluR5 combined with other targeted interventions, either pharmaceutical will improve outcomes. Similarly, effectiveness may be improved if pharmaceutical intervention and behavioral interventions were paired, the equivalent of teaching a blind person to read after restoring sight.

The combination of advances in human genetics and increased understanding of brain plasticity is generating exciting insights into the pathophysiology of FXS and related neurodevelopmental disorders. Unfortunately, translating fundamental scientific discoveries to the clinic is fraught with pitfalls from translating between species to devising clinical trials with the sensitivity to find clinical efficacy. The treatment of ASDs/IDs such as FXS with tailored interventions is still in its infancy and requires much more research. Nevertheless, there can be little debate that the mGluR theory has stimulated a wealth of research concerning the pathophysiology of FXS, and has highlighted the importance and challenges of translating these findings to the clinic.

BEYOND FMRP: ALTERED PROTEIN SYNTHESIS IN ASD

Research in the FXS field has blossomed, and critical insights into synaptic function are being revisited based on the resulting discoveries. These findings have been essential for the development of novel therapeutics for FXS, and they have also changed our understanding of the role of protein synthesis in synapses and circuits.

Moreover, studies of FXS have suggested that synaptic protein synthesis is a shared pathophysiology of multiple genetic causes of ASD. Of the genes linked to ASD, many are regulators of mRNA translation.[193] Studies of the $Fmr1^{-/y}$ and $Tsc2^{+/-}$ models of FXS and TSC, two of the leading identified single-gene causes of ASD, reveal that both have core deficits in synaptic protein synthesis downstream of mGluR1/5.[189] The suggestion is that dysregulated synaptic protein synthesis is a common disruption in ASD. Supporting this hypothesis, many gain-of-function mutations in the Ras—ERK and PI3K—mTOR pathways are linked to ASD and ID.[193,194] This includes mutations in the SYNGAP1 gene, a negative regulator of the Ras—ERK pathway. Work in the $Syngap1^{+/-}$ mouse model shows that it is highly similar to the $Fmr1^{-/y}$, exhibiting exaggerated mGluR-LTD that is protein synthesis independent and corrected with ERK inhibitors or lovastatin.[195] In addition, mutation of several different translation factors results in phenotypes reminiscent of FXS other ASD mouse models.[196,197] The idea that synaptic mRNA translation is a common point of convergence for multiple genetic causes of ASD may thus lead to future treatments that extend beyond FXS and become relevant to the wider idiopathic autism community.

References

1. Belmonte MK, Bourgeron T. Fragile X syndrome and autism at the intersection of genetic and neural networks. *Nat Neurosci* 2006; **9**(10):1221—5.
2. Zafeiriou DI, Ververi A, Vargiami E. Childhood autism and associated comorbidities. *Brain Dev* 2007;**29**(5):257—72.
3. Bear MF, Huber KM, Warren ST. The mGluR theory of fragile X mental retardation. *Trends Neurosci* 2004;**27**(7):370—7.
4. Krueger DD, Bear MF. Toward fulfilling the promise of molecular medicine in fragile X syndrome. *Annu Rev Med* 2010;**62**:411—29.
5. Lozano R, Rosero CA, Hagerman RJ. Fragile X spectrum disorders. *Intractable Rare Dis Res* 2014;**3**(4):134—46.
6. Kaufmann WE, et al. Genotype, molecular phenotype, and cognitive phenotype: correlations in fragile X syndrome. *Am J Med Genet* 1999;**83**(4):286—95.
7. Hagerman RJ, et al. Advances in the treatment of fragile X syndrome. *Pediatrics* 2009;**123**(1):378—90.
8. Kidd SA, et al. Fragile X syndrome: a review of associated medical problems. *Pediatrics* 2014;**134**(5):995—1005.
9. Mazzocco MM. Advances in research on the fragile X syndrome. *Ment Retard Dev Disabil Res Rev* 2000;**6**(2):96—106.
10. Penagarikano O, Mulle JG, Warren ST. The pathophysiology of fragile X syndrome. *Annu Rev Genomics Hum Genet* 2007;**8**:109—29.
11. Martin JP, Bell J. A pedigree of mental defect showing sex-linkage. *J Neurol Psychiatry* 1943;**6**(3—4):154—7.
12. Verkerk AJ, et al. Identification of a gene (FMR-1) containing a CGG repeat coincident with a breakpoint cluster region exhibiting length variation in fragile X syndrome. *Cell* 1991;**65**(5):905—14.
13. Kremer EJ, et al. Mapping of DNA instability at the fragile X to a trinucleotide repeat sequence p(CCG)n. *Science* 1991;**252**(5013): 1711—4.

14. Oberle I, et al. New polymorphism and a new chromosome breakpoint establish the physical and genetic mapping of DXS369 in the DXS98-FRAXA interval. *Am J Med Genet* 1991;**38**(2–3):336–42.

15. Sutcliffe JS, et al. DNA methylation represses FMR-1 transcription in fragile X syndrome. *Hum Mol Genet* 1992;**1**(6):397–400.

16. Coffee B, et al. Acetylated histones are associated with FMR1 in normal but not fragile X-syndrome cells. *Nat Genet* 1999;**22**(1):98–101.

17. Tassone F, et al. FMRP expression as a potential prognostic indicator in fragile X syndrome. *Am J Med Genet* 1999;**84**(3):250–61.

18. Fu YH, et al. Variation of the CGG repeat at the fragile X site results in genetic instability: resolution of the Sherman paradox. *Cell* 1991;**67**(6):1047–58.

19. Willemsen R, Levenga J, Oostra BA. CGG repeat in the FMR1 gene: size matters. *Clin Genet* 2011;**80**(3):214–25.

20. Sherman SL, et al. Further segregation analysis of the fragile X syndrome with special reference to transmitting males. *Hum Genet* 1985;**69**(4):289–99.

21. Till SM, et al. Altered maturation of the primary somatosensory cortex in a mouse model of fragile X syndrome. *Hum Mol Genet* 2012;**21**(10):2143–56.

22. Devys D, et al. The FMR-1 protein is cytoplasmic, most abundant in neurons and appears normal in carriers of a fragile X premutation. *Nat Genet* 1993;**4**(4):335–40.

23. Feng Y, et al. Fragile X mental retardation protein: nucleocytoplasmic shuttling and association with somatodendritic ribosomes. *J Neurosci* 1997;**17**(5):1539–47.

24. Wan L, et al. Characterization of dFMR1, a *Drosophila melanogaster* homolog of the fragile X mental retardation protein. *Mol Cell Biol* 2000;**20**(22):8536–47.

25. Siomi H, et al. The protein product of the fragile X gene, FMR1, has characteristics of an RNA-binding protein. *Cell* 1993;**74**(2):291–8.

26. Ashley Jr CT, et al. FMR1 protein: conserved RNP family domains and selective RNA binding. *Science* 1993;**262**(5133):563–6.

27. De Boulle K, et al. A point mutation in the FMR-1 gene associated with fragile X mental retardation. *Nat Genet* 1993;**3**(1):31–5.

28. Collins SC, et al. Identification of novel FMR1 variants by massively parallel sequencing in developmentally delayed males. *Am J Med Genet A* 2010;**152A**(10):2512–20.

29. Feng Y, et al. FMRP associates with polyribosomes as an mRNP, and the I304N mutation of severe fragile X syndrome abolishes this association. *Mol Cell* 1997;**1**(1):109–18.

30. Blonden L, et al. Two members of the Fxr gene family, Fmr1 and Fxr1, are differentially expressed in *Xenopus tropicalis*. *Int J Dev Biol* 2005;**49**(4):437–41.

31. Till SM, et al. A presynaptic role for FMRP during protein synthesis-dependent long-term plasticity in Aplysia. *Learn Mem* 2011;**18**(1):39–48.

32. Tucker B, Richards R, Lardelli M. Expression of three zebrafish orthologs of human FMR1-related genes and their phylogenetic relationships. *Dev Genes Evol* 2004;**214**(11):567–74.

33. Faust CJ, et al. Genetic mapping on the mouse X chromosome of human cDNA clones for the fragile X and Hunter syndromes. *Genomics* 1992;**12**(4):814–7.

34. Laval SH, et al. Mapping of FMR1, the gene implicated in fragile X-linked mental retardation, on the mouse X chromosome. *Genomics* 1992;**12**(4):818–21.

35. Bagni C, Oostra BA. Fragile X syndrome: from protein function to therapy. *Am J Med Genet A* 2013;**161A**(11):2809–21.

36. Darnell JC, et al. Kissing complex RNAs mediate interaction between the fragile-X mental retardation protein KH2 domain and brain polyribosomes. *Genes Dev* 2005;**19**(8):903–18.

37. Darnell JC, Warren ST, Darnell RB. The fragile X mental retardation protein, FMRP, recognizes G-quartets. *Ment Retard Dev Disabil Res Rev* 2004;**10**(1):49–52.

38. Eberhart DE, et al. The fragile X mental retardation protein is a ribonucleoprotein containing both nuclear localization and nuclear export signals. *Hum Mol Genet* 1996;**5**(8):1083–91.

39. Antar LN, et al. Metabotropic glutamate receptor activation regulates fragile X mental retardation protein and FMR1 mRNA localization differentially in dendrites and at synapses. *J Neurosci* 2004;**24**(11):2648–55.

40. De Diego Otero Y, et al. Transport of fragile X mental retardation protein via granules in neurites of PC12 cells. *Mol Cell Biol* 2002;**22**(23):8332–41.

41. Dictenberg JB, et al. A direct role for FMRP in activity-dependent dendritic mRNA transport links filopodial-spine morphogenesis to fragile X syndrome. *Dev Cell* 2008;**14**(6):926–39.

42. Wang H, et al. Dynamic association of the fragile X mental retardation protein as a messenger ribonucleoprotein between microtubules and polyribosomes. *Mol Biol Cell* 2008;**19**(1):105–14.

43. Steward O, et al. No evidence for disruption of normal patterns of mRNA localization in dendrites or dendritic transport of recently synthesized mRNA in FMR1 knockout mice, a model for human fragile-X mental retardation syndrome. *Neuroreport* 1998;**9**(3):477–81.

44. Khandjian EW, et al. Biochemical evidence for the association of fragile X mental retardation protein with brain polyribosomal ribonucleoparticles. *Proc Natl Acad Sci USA* 2004;**101**(36):13357–62.

45. Tamanini F, et al. FMRP is associated to the ribosomes via RNA. *Hum Mol Genet* 1996;**5**(6):809–13.

46. Khandjian EW, et al. The fragile X mental retardation protein is associated with ribosomes. *Nat Genet* 1996;**12**(1):91–3.

47. Laggerbauer B, et al. Evidence that fragile X mental retardation protein is a negative regulator of translation. *Hum Mol Genet* 2001;**10**(4):329–38.

48. Li Z, et al. The fragile X mental retardation protein inhibits translation via interacting with mRNA. *Nucleic Acids Res* 2001;**29**(11):2276–83.

49. Mazroui R, et al. Trapping of messenger RNA by fragile X mental retardation protein into cytoplasmic granules induces translation repression. *Hum Mol Genet* 2002;**11**(24):3007–17.

50. Aschrafi A, et al. The fragile X mental retardation protein and group I metabotropic glutamate receptors regulate levels of mRNA granules in brain. *Proc Natl Acad Sci USA* 2005;**102**(6):2180–5.

51. Ceman S, et al. Development and characterization of antibodies that immunoprecipitate the FMR1 protein. *Methods Mol Biol* 2003;**217**:345–54.

52. Napoli I, et al. The fragile X syndrome protein represses activity-dependent translation through CYFIP1, a new 4E-BP. *Cell* 2008;**134**(6):1042–54.

53. Darnell JC, et al. FMRP stalls ribosomal translocation on mRNAs linked to synaptic function and autism. *Cell* 2011;**146**(2):247–61.

54. Chen E, et al. Fragile X mental retardation protein regulates translation by binding directly to the ribosome. *Mol Cell* 2014;**54**(3):407–17.

55. Brown V, et al. Microarray identification of FMRP-associated brain mRNAs and altered mRNA translational profiles in fragile X syndrome. *Cell* 2001;**107**(4):477–87.

56. Darnell JC, et al. Fragile X mental retardation protein targets G quartet mRNAs important for neuronal function. *Cell* 2001;**107**(4):489–99.

57. Fmr1 knockout mice: a model to study fragile X mental retardation. The Dutch-Belgian fragile X consortium. *Cell* 1994;**78**(1):23–33.

58. Willemsen R, Oostra BA. FMRP detection assay for the diagnosis of the fragile X syndrome. *Am J Med Genet* 2000;**97**(3):183–8.

59. Qin M, et al. Postadolescent changes in regional cerebral protein synthesis: an in vivo study in the FMR1 null mouse. *J Neurosci* 2005;**25**(20):5087–95.

60. Dolen G, et al. Correction of fragile X syndrome in mice. *Neuron* 2007;**56**(6):955–62.

61. Osterweil EK, et al. Hypersensitivity to mGluR5 and ERK1/2 leads to excessive protein synthesis in the hippocampus of a mouse model of fragile X syndrome. *J Neurosci* 2010;**30**(46):15616–27.

62. Muddashetty RS, et al. Dysregulated metabotropic glutamate receptor-dependent translation of AMPA receptor and postsynaptic density-95 mRNAs at synapses in a mouse model of fragile X syndrome. *J Neurosci* 2007;**27**(20):5338–48.

63. Huber KM, et al. Altered synaptic plasticity in a mouse model of fragile X mental retardation. *Proc Natl Acad Sci USA* 2002;**99**(11):7746–50.

64. Huber KM, Kayser MS, Bear MF. Role for rapid dendritic protein synthesis in hippocampal mGluR-dependent long-term depression. *Science* 2000;**288**(5469):1254–7.

65. Snyder EM, et al. Internalization of ionotropic glutamate receptors in response to mGluR activation. *Nat Neurosci* 2001;**4**(11):1079–85.

66. Nosyreva ED, Huber KM. Metabotropic receptor-dependent long-term depression persists in the absence of protein synthesis in the mouse model of fragile X syndrome. *J Neurophysiol* 2006;**95**(5):3291–5.

67. Kang H, Schuman EM. A requirement for local protein synthesis in neurotrophin-induced hippocampal synaptic plasticity. *Science* 1996;**273**(5280):1402–6.

68. Steward O, Levy WB. Preferential localization of polyribosomes under the base of dendritic spines in granule cells of the dentate gyrus. *J Neurosci* 1982;**2**(3):284–91.

69. Bourne JN, Harris KM. Coordination of size and number of excitatory and inhibitory synapses results in a balanced structural plasticity along mature hippocampal CA1 dendrites during LTP. *Hippocampus* 2011;**21**(4):354–73.

70. Govindarajan A, et al. The dendritic branch is the preferred integrative unit for protein synthesis-dependent LTP. *Neuron* 2011;**69**(1):132–46.

71. Frey U, Morris RG. Synaptic tagging and long-term potentiation. *Nature* 1997;**385**(6616):533–6.

72. Lu R, et al. The fragile X protein controls microtubule-associated protein 1B translation and microtubule stability in brain neuron development. *Proc Natl Acad Sci USA* 2004;**101**(42):15201–6.

73. Waung MW, et al. Rapid translation of Arc/Arg3.1 selectively mediates mGluR-dependent LTD through persistent increases in AMPAR endocytosis rate. *Neuron* 2008;**59**(1):84–97.

74. Goebel-Goody SM, et al. Genetic manipulation of STEP reverses behavioral abnormalities in a fragile X syndrome mouse model. *Genes Brain Behav* 2012;**11**(5):586–600.

75. Westmark CJ, Malter JS. FMRP mediates mGluR5-dependent translation of amyloid precursor protein. *PLoS Biol* 2007;**5**(3):e52.

76. Zalfa F, et al. The fragile X syndrome protein FMRP associates with BC1 RNA and regulates the translation of specific mRNAs at synapses. *Cell* 2003;**112**(3):317–27.

77. Ifrim MF, Williams KR, Bassell GJ. Single-molecule imaging of PSD-95 mRNA translation in dendrites and its dysregulation in a mouse model of fragile X syndrome. *J Neurosci* 2015;**35**(18):7116–30.

78. Bilousova TV, et al. Minocycline promotes dendritic spine maturation and improves behavioural performance in the fragile X mouse model. *J Med Genet* 2009;**46**(2):94–102.

79. Sidhu H, et al. Genetic removal of matrix metalloproteinase 9 rescues the symptoms of fragile X syndrome in a mouse model. *J Neurosci* 2014;**34**(30):9867–79.

80. Paribello C, et al. Open-label add-on treatment trial of minocycline in fragile X syndrome. *BMC Neurol* 2010;**10**:91.

81. Krueger DD, et al. Cognitive dysfunction and prefrontal synaptic abnormalities in a mouse model of fragile X syndrome. *Proc Natl Acad Sci USA* 2010;**108**(6):2587–92.

82. Matsuzaki M, et al. Dendritic spine geometry is critical for AMPA receptor expression in hippocampal CA1 pyramidal neurons. *Nat Neurosci* 2001;**4**(11):1086–92.

83. Nusser Z, et al. Cell type and pathway dependence of synaptic AMPA receptor number and variability in the hippocampus. *Neuron* 1998;**21**(3):545–59.

84. Kasai H, et al. Structural dynamics of dendritic spines in memory and cognition. *Trends Neurosci* 2010;**33**(3):121–9.

85. Tonnesen J, et al. Spine neck plasticity regulates compartmentalization of synapses. *Nat Neurosci* 2014;**17**(5):678–85.

86. Harnett MT, et al. Synaptic amplification by dendritic spines enhances input cooperativity. *Nature* 2012;**491**(7425):599–602.

87. Hinton VJ, et al. Analysis of neocortex in three males with the fragile X syndrome. *Am J Med Genet* 1991;**41**(3):289–94.

88. Rudelli RD, et al. Adult fragile X syndrome. Clinico-neuropathologic findings. *Acta Neuropathol* 1985;**67**(3–4):289–95.

89. Irwin SA, et al. Abnormal dendritic spine characteristics in the temporal and visual cortices of patients with fragile-X syndrome: a quantitative examination. *Am J Med Genet* 2001;**98**(2):161–7.

90. Irwin SA, Galvez R, Greenough WT. Dendritic spine structural anomalies in fragile-X mental retardation syndrome. *Cereb Cortex* 2000;**10**(10):1038–44.

91. He CX, Portera-Cailliau C. The trouble with spines in fragile X syndrome: density, maturity and plasticity. *Neuroscience* 2013;**251**:120–8.

92. Comery TA, et al. Abnormal dendritic spines in fragile X knockout mice: maturation and pruning deficits. *Proc Natl Acad Sci USA* 1997;**94**(10):5401–4.

93. Galvez R, Greenough WT. Sequence of abnormal dendritic spine development in primary somatosensory cortex of a mouse model of the fragile X mental retardation syndrome. *Am J Med Genet A* 2005;**135**(2):155–60.

94. McKinney BC, et al. Dendritic spine abnormalities in the occipital cortex of C57BL/6 Fmr1 knockout mice. *Am J Med Genet B Neuropsychiatr Genet* 2005;**136B**(1):98–102.

95. Grossman AW, et al. Hippocampal pyramidal cells in adult Fmr1 knockout mice exhibit an immature-appearing profile of dendritic spines. *Brain Res* 2006;**1084**(1):158–64.

96. Meredith RM, et al. Increased threshold for spike-timing-dependent plasticity is caused by unreliable calcium signaling in mice lacking fragile X gene FMR1. *Neuron* 2007;**54**(4):627–38.

97. Ruan YW, et al. Diversity and fluctuation of spine morphology in CA1 pyramidal neurons after transient global ischemia. *J Neurosci Res* 2009;**87**(1):61–8.

98. Cruz-Martin A, Crespo M, Portera-Cailliau C. Delayed stabilization of dendritic spines in fragile X mice. *J Neurosci* 2010;**30**(23):7793–803.

99. Harlow EG, et al. Critical period plasticity is disrupted in the barrel cortex of FMR1 knockout mice. *Neuron* 2010;**65**(3):385–98.

100. Pan F, et al. Dendritic spine instability and insensitivity to modulation by sensory experience in a mouse model of fragile X syndrome. *Proc Natl Acad Sci USA* 2010;**107**(41):17768–73.

101. Wijetunge LS, et al. Stimulated emission depletion (STED) microscopy reveals nanoscale defects in the developmental trajectory of dendritic spine morphogenesis in a mouse model of fragile X syndrome. *J Neurosci* 2014;**34**(18):6405–12.

102. Benavides-Piccione R, et al. Cortical area and species differences in dendritic spine morphology. *J Neurocytol* 2002;**31**(3–5):337–46.

103. Arellano JI, et al. Non-synaptic dendritic spines in neocortex. *Neuroscience* 2007;**145**(2):464–9.

104. Hell SW, Wichmann J. Breaking the diffraction resolution limit by stimulated emission: stimulated-emission-depletion fluorescence microscopy. *Opt Lett* 1994;**19**(11):780–2.

105. Berry-Kravis E. Epilepsy in fragile X syndrome. *Dev Med Child Neurol* 2002;**44**(11):724–8.

106. Contractor A, Klyachko VA, Portera-Cailliau C. Altered neuronal and circuit excitability in fragile X syndrome. *Neuron* 2015;**87**(4): 699–715.

107. Zhao W, et al. Extracellular signal-regulated kinase 1/2 is required for the induction of group I metabotropic glutamate receptor-mediated epileptiform discharges. *J Neurosci* 2004;**24**(1): 76–84.

108. Osterweil EK, et al. Lovastatin corrects excess protein synthesis and prevents epileptogenesis in a mouse model of fragile X syndrome. *Neuron* 2013;**77**(2):243–50.

109. Gibson JR, et al. Imbalance of neocortical excitation and inhibition and altered UP states reflect network hyperexcitability in the mouse model of fragile X syndrome. *J Neurophysiol* 2008;**100**(5): 2615–26.

110. Knoth IS, Lippe S. Event-related potential alterations in fragile X syndrome. *Front Hum Neurosci* 2012;**6**:264.

111. Brown MR, et al. Fragile X mental retardation protein controls gating of the sodium-activated potassium channel Slack. *Nat Neurosci* 2010;**13**(7):819–21.

112. Myrick LK, et al. Independent role for presynaptic FMRP revealed by an FMR1 missense mutation associated with intellectual disability and seizures. *Proc Natl Acad Sci USA* 2015;**112**(4): 949–56.

113. Deng PY, et al. FMRP regulates neurotransmitter release and synaptic information transmission by modulating action potential duration via BK channels. *Neuron* 2013;**77**(4):696–711.

114. Ferron L, et al. Fragile X mental retardation protein controls synaptic vesicle exocytosis by modulating N-type calcium channel density. *Nat Commun* 2014;**5**:3628.

115. Lee HY, et al. Bidirectional regulation of dendritic voltage-gated potassium channels by the fragile X mental retardation protein. *Neuron* 2011;**72**(4):630–42.

116. Gross C, et al. Fragile X mental retardation protein regulates protein expression and mRNA translation of the potassium channel Kv4.2. *J Neurosci* 2011;**31**(15):5693–8.

117. Routh BN, Johnston D, Brager DH. Loss of functional A-type potassium channels in the dendrites of CA1 pyramidal neurons from a mouse model of fragile X syndrome. *J Neurosci* 2013; **33**(50):19442–50.

118. Zhang Y, et al. Dendritic channelopathies contribute to neocortical and sensory hyperexcitability in Fmr1(-/y) mice. *Nat Neurosci* 2014;**17**(12):1701–9.

119. Brager DH, Akhavan AR, Johnston D. Impaired dendritic expression and plasticity of h-channels in the Fmr1(−/y) mouse model of fragile X syndrome. *Cell Rep* 2012;**1**(3):225–33.

120. Chen L, Toth M. Fragile X mice develop sensory hyperreactivity to auditory stimuli. *Neuroscience* 2001;**103**(4):1043–50.

121. Strumbos JG, et al. Fragile X mental retardation protein is required for rapid experience-dependent regulation of the potassium channel Kv3.1b. *J Neurosci* 2010;**30**(31):10263–71.

122. Zhang Y, et al. Regulation of neuronal excitability by interaction of fragile X mental retardation protein with slack potassium channels. *J Neurosci* 2012;**32**(44):15318–27.

123. Holt CE, Schuman EM. The central dogma decentralized: new perspectives on RNA function and local translation in neurons. *Neuron* 2013;**80**(3):648–57.

124. Davis HP, Squire LR. Protein synthesis and memory: a review. *Psychol Bull* 1984;**96**(3):518–59.

125. Krug M, Lossner B, Ott T. Anisomycin blocks the late phase of long-term potentiation in the dentate gyrus of freely moving rats. *Brain Res Bull* 1984;**13**(1):39–42.

126. Frey U, et al. Anisomycin, an inhibitor of protein synthesis, blocks late phases of LTP phenomena in the hippocampal CA1 region in vitro. *Brain Res* 1988;**452**(1–2):57–65.

127. Koekkoek SK, et al. Deletion of FMR1 in Purkinje cells enhances parallel fiber LTD, enlarges spines, and attenuates cerebellar eyelid conditioning in Fragile X syndrome. *Neuron* 2005;**47**(3): 339–52.

128. Godfraind JM, et al. Long-term potentiation in the hippocampus of fragile X knockout mice. *Am J Med Genet* 1996;**64**(2):246–51.

129. Larson J, et al. Age-dependent and selective impairment of long-term potentiation in the anterior piriform cortex of mice lacking the fragile X mental retardation protein. *J Neurosci* 2005; **25**(41):9460–9.

130. Li J, et al. Reduced cortical synaptic plasticity and GluR1 expression associated with fragile X mental retardation protein deficiency. *Mol Cell Neurosci* 2002;**19**(2):138–51.

131. Auerbach BD, Bear MF. Loss of the fragile X mental retardation protein decouples metabotropic glutamate receptor dependent priming of long-term potentiation from protein synthesis. *J Neurophysiol* 2010;**104**(2):1047–51.

132. Zhang J, et al. Altered hippocampal synaptic plasticity in the FMR1 gene family knockout mouse models. *J Neurophysiol* 2009; **101**(5):2572–80.

133. Hu H, et al. Ras signaling mechanisms underlying impaired GluR1-dependent plasticity associated with fragile X syndrome. *J Neurosci* 2008;**28**(31):7847–62.

134. Lauterborn JC, et al. Brain-derived neurotrophic factor rescues synaptic plasticity in a mouse model of fragile X syndrome. *J Neurosci* 2007;**27**(40):10685–94.

135. Shang Y, et al. Fragile X mental retardation protein is required for chemically-induced long-term potentiation of the hippocampus in adult mice. *J Neurochem* 2009;**111**(3):635–46.

136. Eadie BD, et al. NMDA receptor hypofunction in the dentate gyrus and impaired context discrimination in adult Fmr1 knockout mice. *Hippocampus* 2012;**22**(2):241–54.

137. Bostrom CA, et al. Rescue of NMDAR-dependent synaptic plasticity in Fmr1 knock-out mice. *Cereb Cortex* 2013;**25**(1).

138. Abraham WC, Williams JM. Properties and mechanisms of LTP maintenance. *Neuroscientist* 2003;**9**(6):463–74.

139. Li XL, et al. Impairment of long-term potentiation and spatial memory in leptin receptor-deficient rodents. *Neuroscience* 2002; **113**(3):607–15.

140. Desai NS, et al. Early postnatal plasticity in neocortex of Fmr1 knockout mice. *J Neurophysiol* 2006;**96**(4):1734–45.

141. Neuhofer D, et al. Functional and structural deficits at accumbens synapses in a mouse model of Fragile X. *Front Cell Neurosci* 2015; **9**:100.

142. Soden ME, Chen L. Fragile X protein FMRP is required for homeostatic plasticity and regulation of synaptic strength by retinoic acid. *J Neurosci* 2010;**30**(50):16910–21.

143. Weiler IJ, Greenough WT. Metabotropic glutamate receptors trigger postsynaptic protein synthesis. *Proc Natl Acad Sci USA* 1993;**90**(15):7168–71.

144. Michalon A, et al. Chronic pharmacological mGlu5 inhibition corrects fragile X in adult mice. *Neuron* 2012;**74**(1):49–56.

145. Nakamoto M, et al. Fragile X mental retardation protein deficiency leads to excessive mGluR5-dependent internalization of AMPA receptors. *Proc Natl Acad Sci USA* 2007;**104**(39): 15537–42.

146. Bianchi R, Wong RK. Excitatory synaptic potentials dependent on metabotropic glutamate receptor activation in guinea-pig hippocampal pyramidal cells. *J Physiol* 1995;**487**(Pt 3):663–76.

147. Chuang SC, et al. Prolonged epileptiform discharges induced by altered group I metabotropic glutamate receptor-mediated synaptic responses in hippocampal slices of a fragile X mouse model. *J Neurosci* 2005;**25**(35):8048–55.

148. Hays SA, Huber KM, Gibson JR. Altered neocortical rhythmic activity states in Fmr1 KO mice are due to enhanced mGluR5 signaling and involve changes in excitatory circuitry. *J Neurosci* 2011;**31**(40):14223–34.

149. Yan QJ, et al. Suppression of two major Fragile X syndrome mouse model phenotypes by the mGluR5 antagonist MPEP. *Neuropharmacology* 2005;**49**(7):1053–66.

150. Bhakar AL, Dolen G, Bear MF. The pathophysiology of fragile X (and what it teaches us about synapses). *Annu Rev Neurosci* 2012;**35**:417–43.

151. McBride SM, et al. Pharmacological rescue of synaptic plasticity, courtship behavior, and mushroom body defects in a Drosophila model of fragile X syndrome. *Neuron* 2005;**45**(5):753–64.

152. Tucker B, Richards RI, Lardelli M. Contribution of mGluR and Fmr1 functional pathways to neurite morphogenesis, craniofacial development and fragile X syndrome. *Hum Mol Genet* 2006;**15**(23): 3446–58.

153. Till SM, et al. Conserved hippocampal cellular pathophysiology but distinct behavioural deficits in a new rat model of FXS. *Hum Mol Genet* 2015;**24**(21):5977–84.

154. Wijetunge LS, et al. Fragile X syndrome: from targets to treatments. *Neuropharmacology* 2013;**68**:83–96.

155. Luscher C, Huber KM. Group 1 mGluR-dependent synaptic long-term depression: mechanisms and implications for circuitry and disease. *Neuron* 2010;**65**(4):445–59.

156. Gao B, Roux PP. Translational control by oncogenic signaling pathways. *Biochim Biophys Acta* 2015;**1849**(7):753–65.

157. Gingras AC, et al. Hierarchical phosphorylation of the translation inhibitor 4E-BP1. *Genes Dev* 2001;**15**(21):2852–64.

158. Waskiewicz AJ, et al. Phosphorylation of the cap-binding protein eukaryotic translation initiation factor 4E by protein kinase Mnk1 in vivo. *Mol Cell Biol* 1999;**19**(3):1871–80.

159. Proud CG. Mnks, eIF4E phosphorylation and cancer. *Biochim Biophys Acta* 2015;**1849**(7):766–73.

160. Buffington SA, Huang W, Costa-Mattioli M. Translational control in synaptic plasticity and cognitive dysfunction. *Annu Rev Neurosci* 2014;**37**:17–38.

161. Ferraguti F, et al. Activation of the extracellular signal-regulated kinase 2 by metabotropic glutamate receptors. *Eur J Neurosci* 1999;**11**(6):2073–82.

162. Mao L, et al. The scaffold protein Homer1b/c links metabotropic glutamate receptor 5 to extracellular signal-regulated protein kinase cascades in neurons. *J Neurosci* 2005;**25**(10):2741–52.

163. Choe ES, Wang JQ. Group I metabotropic glutamate receptors control phosphorylation of CREB, Elk-1 and ERK via a CaMKII-dependent pathway in rat striatum. *Neurosci Lett* 2001;**313**(3): 129–32.

164. Adwanikar H, Karim F, Gereau RWT. Inflammation persistently enhances nocifensive behaviors mediated by spinal group I mGluRs through sustained ERK activation. *Pain* 2004;**111**(1–2): 125–35.

165. Berkeley JL, Levey AI. Cell-specific extracellular signal-regulated kinase activation by multiple G protein-coupled receptor families in hippocampus. *Mol Pharmacol* 2003;**63**(1):128–35.

166. Gallagher SM, et al. Extracellular signal-regulated protein kinase activation is required for metabotropic glutamate receptor-dependent long-term depression in hippocampal area CA1. *J Neurosci* 2004;**24**(20):4859–64.

167. Garcia S, Lopez E, Lopez-Colome AM. Glutamate accelerates RPE cell proliferation through ERK1/2 activation via distinct receptor-specific mechanisms. *J Cell Biochem* 2008;**104**(2): 377–90.

168. Banko JL, et al. Regulation of eukaryotic initiation factor 4E by converging signaling pathways during metabotropic glutamate receptor-dependent long-term depression. *J Neurosci* 2006;**26**(8): 2167–73.

169. Ronesi JA, et al. Disrupted Homer scaffolds mediate abnormal mGluR5 function in a mouse model of fragile X syndrome. *Nat Neurosci* 2012;**15**(3):431–40, S1.

170. Hou L, et al. Dynamic translational and proteasomal regulation of fragile X mental retardation protein controls mGluR-dependent long-term depression. *Neuron* 2006;**51**(4):441–54.

171. Matic K, et al. Quantitative phosphoproteomics of murine Fmr1-KO cell lines provides new insights into FMRP-dependent signal transduction mechanisms. *J Proteome Res* 2014;**13**(10): 4388–97.

172. Wang X, et al. Activation of the extracellular signal-regulated kinase pathway contributes to the behavioral deficit of fragile X-syndrome. *J Neurochem* 2012;**121**(4):672–9.

173. Gkogkas CG, et al. Pharmacogenetic inhibition of eIF4E-dependent Mmp9 mRNA translation reverses fragile X syndrome-like phenotypes. *Cell Rep* 2014;**9**(5):1742–55.

174. Bhattacharya A, et al. Genetic removal of p70 S6 kinase 1 corrects molecular, synaptic, and behavioral phenotypes in fragile X syndrome mice. *Neuron* 2012;**76**(2):325–37.

175. Mendola CE, Backer JM. Lovastatin blocks N-ras oncogene-induced neuronal differentiation. *Cell Growth Differ* 1990;**1**(10): 499–502.

176. Lambert M, et al. Treatment of familial hypercholesterolemia in children and adolescents: effect of lovastatin. Canadian lovastatin in children study group. *Pediatrics* 1996;**97**(5): 619–28.

177. Li W, et al. The HMG-CoA reductase inhibitor lovastatin reverses the learning and attention deficits in a mouse model of neurofibromatosis type 1. *Curr Biol* 2005;**15**(21):1961–7.

178. Alabama-Birmingham U, NCI. A randomized placebo-controlled study of lovastatin in children with neurofibromatosis type 1 (STARS). ClinicalTrials.gov [Internet]; 2009 [cited 2010] (identifier: NCT00853580).

179. Sidorov MS, et al. Extinction of an instrumental response: a cognitive behavioral assay in Fmr1 knockout mice. *Genes Brain Behav* 2014;**13**(5).

180. Lipton J, Sahin M. Fragile X syndrome therapeutics: translation, meet translational medicine. *Neuron* 2013;**77**(2):212–3.

181. Caku A, et al. Effect of lovastatin on behavior in children and adults with fragile X syndrome: an open-label study. *Am J Med Genet A* 2014;**164A**(11):2834–42.

182. Hou L, Klann E. Activation of the phosphoinositide 3-kinase-Akt-mammalian target of rapamycin signaling pathway is required for metabotropic glutamate receptor-dependent long-term depression. *J Neurosci* 2004;**24**(28):6352–61.

183. Ronesi JA, Huber KM. Homer interactions are necessary for metabotropic glutamate receptor-induced long-term depression and translational activation. *J Neurosci* 2008;**28**(2):543–7.

184. Giuffrida R, et al. A reduced number of metabotropic glutamate subtype 5 receptors are associated with constitutive homer proteins in a mouse model of fragile X syndrome. *J Neurosci* 2005; **25**(39):8908–16.

185. Gross C, et al. Excess phosphoinositide 3-kinase subunit synthesis and activity as a novel therapeutic target in fragile X syndrome. *J Neurosci* 2010;**30**(32):10624–38.

186. Gross C, et al. Increased expression of the PI3K enhancer PIKE mediates deficits in synaptic plasticity and behavior in fragile X syndrome. *Cell Rep* 2015;**11**(5):727–36.

187. Sharma A, et al. Dysregulation of mTOR signaling in fragile X syndrome. *J Neurosci* 2010;**30**(2):694–702.

188. Gross C, et al. Selective role of the catalytic PI3K subunit p110beta in impaired higher order cognition in fragile X syndrome. *Cell Rep* 2015;**11**(5):681–8.

189. Auerbach BD, Osterweil EK, Bear MF. Mutations causing syndromic autism define an axis of synaptic pathophysiology. *Nature* 2011;**480**(7375):63–8.

190. Bateup HS, et al. Loss of Tsc1 in vivo impairs hippocampal mGluR-LTD and increases excitatory synaptic function. *J Neurosci* 2011;**31**(24):8862−9.

191. Potter WB, et al. Reduced juvenile long-term depression in tuberous sclerosis complex is mitigated in adults by compensatory recruitment of mGluR5 and Erk signaling. *PLoS Biol* 2013;**11**(8): e1001627.

192. Udagawa T, et al. Genetic and acute CPEB1 depletion ameliorate fragile X pathophysiology. *Nat Med* 2013;**19**(11):1473−7.

193. Kelleher 3rd RJ, Bear MF. The autistic neuron: troubled translation? *Cell* 2008;**135**(3):401−6.

194. Krab LC, Goorden SM, Elgersma Y. Oncogenes on my mind: ERK and MTOR signaling in cognitive diseases. *Trends Genet* 2008; **24**(10):498−510.

195. Barnes SA, et al. Convergence of hippocampal pathophysiology in Syngap$^{+/-}$ and Fmr1$^{-/y}$ mice. *J Neurosci* 2015;**35**(45):15073−81.

196. Gkogkas CG, et al. Autism-related deficits via dysregulated eIF4E-dependent translational control. *Nature* 2013;**493**(7432): 371−7.

197. Santini E, et al. Exaggerated translation causes synaptic and behavioural aberrations associated with autism. *Nature* 2013; **493**(7432):411−5.

9

X-Linked ASDs and ID Gene Mutations

Edoardo Moretto, Maria Passafaro, Silvia Bassani

CNR Neuroscience Institute, Milan, Italy; Department of Medical Biotechnology and Translational Medicine, University of Milan, Milan, Italy

INTRODUCTION

The term "intellectual disability" (ID) defines a group of disorders that cause impairment in intellectual performance. Autism spectrum disorders (ASDs), composed of autism, Asperger syndrome, childhood disintegrative disorder, and pervasive developmental disorder, cause deficits in communication and social skills in addition to repetitive and stereotyped behaviors.

In this chapter, we focus our attention on IDs and ASDs that are caused by mutations within the X chromosome, which harbors the highest number of cognition-related genes identified to date. The presence of a single X chromosome in males renders them more susceptible to the pathological phenotypes associated with mutations in these genes. This has largely contributed to the significant attention directed to the X chromosome.[1] In addition, it has been proposed that the peculiar evolution to which sexual chromosomes are subjected favored the concentration of brain-specific genes on the X chromosome.[2]

To date, more than 150 X-linked ID (X-LID) syndromes have been characterized, with 102 causative genes identified.[3] A smaller number of X-linked genes have been implicated in ASDs, such as NLGN3 and NLGN4.[4] Notably, a significant overlap exists between ID and autism in patients, likely mirroring the convergence of molecular pathways by which X-linked gene products regulate brain function. The mutations associated with the most common forms of X-LID and autism hit methyl CpG binding protein 2 gene causing Rett syndrome (see Chapter 7) and fragile X mental retardation 1 (FMR1) gene causing fragile X syndrome (see Chapter 8).

In this chapter, we focus our attention on select X-linked genes that exert their roles specifically at the synapse, omitting genes discussed in detail elsewhere in this book, such as the cell adhesion molecules neuroligins and neurexins, cadherins, IL1RAPL1 (Chapters 11 and 14), and genes involved in transcription regulation (for a complete list, see Refs 5,6).

The pathology of X-LID is complex and difficult to assess. Severity is classified via quantification of the intelligence quotient (IQ): ID is mild when the IQ is between 55 and 70, moderate between 35 and 55, severe between 20 and 35, and extremely severe when lower than 20 (according to the Diagnostic and Statistical Manual*of Mental Disorders—IV*). The disorder is generally classified as either syndromic, in which ID is only one of the symptoms, or nonsyndromic, in which ID is the only phenotype associated with the mutation. Syndromic forms are prevalent; approximately one-half of X-LID patients manifest additional symptoms such as ASD and/or seizures with great heterogeneity in age and time of onset, type of seizures, and response to therapy (for a review, see Ref. 3).

Many genes associated with X-LID are involved in different aspects of synapse formation and function. Synapses are highly specialized structures formed by two distinct compartments known as the presynapse, formed on axons, and the postsynapse, formed on dendrites. The presynapse is characterized by a pool of synaptic vesicles filled with neurotransmitter molecules. These vesicles fuse with specialized regions of the plasma membrane called active zones to release their content into the synaptic cleft upon arrival of an electrical stimulus from the axon. Precise coupling between the stimulus and the release of neurotransmitter at the proper concentration is crucial for signal transmission to the postsynaptic neuron. The postsynapse is characterized by the presence of receptors that are able to bind neurotransmitters released at the presynapse and induce a cascade of events that culminate in propagation of electrical stimuli at the postsynaptic neuron. Receptors are clustered at the postsynaptic membrane facing the active zone, in a region called the postsynaptic density (PSD) in excitatory synapses. They are upstream of intracellular proteins that transduce the signal; a crucial role in these processes is played by the actin cytoskeleton, which physically anchors the proteins and is used as a route for intrasynaptic trafficking.

Synapses are typically classified as excitatory and inhibitory, using glutamate and γ-aminobutyric acid (GABA), respectively, as the main neurotransmitter. The genes described within are implicated in neuronal morphology via cytoskeleton remodeling (genes belonging to the Rho GTPase pathway: OPHN1, ARHGEF6, and PAK3), in function, encoding receptor subunits (GRIA3) or acting to localize receptors and secondary messengers (ARHGEF9, TM4SF2, and the membrane-associated guanylate kinases [MAGUKs] CASK and DLG3), and in presynaptic vesicle release (synaptophysin [SYP], CASK, and genes belonging to the Rab GTPase pathway: RAB39B, GDI1) (Figure 1).

Impaired synapse function disrupts the fine balance that exists between excitatory and inhibitory circuits, which has been demonstrated as fundamental for the central nervous system to integrate external and internal stimuli correctly. Most of the genes described within are implicated in forms of synaptic plasticity such as long-term potentiation (LTP) and long-term depression (LTD), in which a precise activity pattern induces long-term modifications in both the structure and protein composition of pre- and postsynaptic sites, serving to increase or decrease the intensity of the transduced signal.

The proteins described in this chapter exhibit a marked heterogeneity of functions, which underscores the complexity of the pathogenesis of these disorders that nevertheless manifest with similar phenotypes commonly associated with morphological defects of synapses. In particular, modification of the quantity or the morphology (length or width) of excitatory postsynaptic compartments known as dendritic spines is a classical hallmark of ID.[7]

To date, no curative treatments exist for this class of diseases; therapy is mainly based on educational and training approaches that are, at best, only able to moderate the symptoms. Greater efforts are needed to fully understand the defects caused by mutations in X-LIDs and ASDs and the exact pathogenesis of these disorders to develop new experimental treatments.

SMALL GUANINE NUCLEOTIDE BINDING PROTEIN PATHWAY

The Ras superfamily is composed of small guanine nucleotide binding proteins (GTPases) that function as molecular switches cycling between a GDP-bound and a GTP-bound state. With few exceptions, the former is inactive, whereas the GTP-bound state is active and allows for the binding and activation of downstream effectors throughout the signaling cascade.

To start a new cycle, GTPases need to release the bound GDP and bind a new GTP molecule that will undergo hydrolysis. However, both GDP dissociation and GTP hydrolysis are slow processes under basal conditions. As such, GTPases require catalysts to perform efficiently.

Guanine nucleotide exchange factors (GEFs) act as these catalysts and promote GDP dissociation. This is readily followed by spontaneous GTP binding, ensured by its high cytoplasmic concentration. GTPase—activating proteins (GAPs) subsequently enhance GTP hydrolysis. In addition to GDP/GTP alternation, the switch of small GTPases can be regulated by subcellular compartmentalization. Indeed, many small GTPases have a farnesyl or geranylgeranyl group in their C-termini for membrane binding. In these cases, guanine dissociation inhibitors (GDIs) mask the lipids and sequester the small GTPases in the cytosol where they form an inactive pool. An effective switch relies on the orchestrated functioning of small GTPases, GEFs, GAPs, and GDIs. Feedback loops and feed-forward mechanisms, which rely in part on the physical interaction between molecules

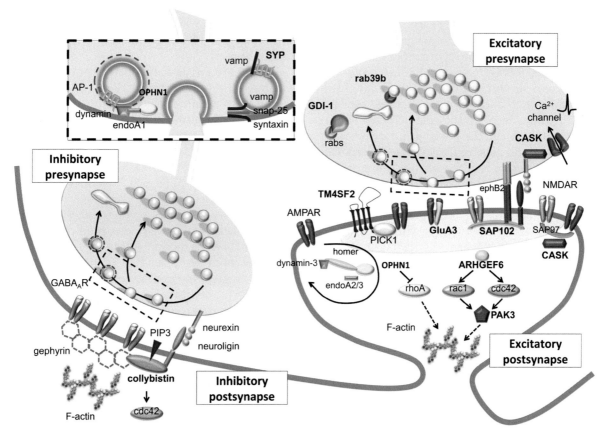

FIGURE 1 X-Linked ID and ASD gene functions at synapse. Pre- and postsynaptic terminals of an excitatory (right) and inhibitory (left) synapse, including magnification of a presynaptic active zone, are shown. OPHN1 encodes oligophrenin 1, a GAP that enhances GTP hydrolysis of Rho proteins. Oligophrenin 1, through RhoA inhibition, regulates actin dynamics and hence dendritic spine structure and AMPAR stability at postsynapses. Furthermore, oligophrenin 1 is involved in AMPAR trafficking with important implications for basal synaptic transmission and plasticity. The binding of oligophrenin 1 with endophilin A2/3 (endoA2/3) is required for AMPAR endocytosis, and the complex composed of oligophrenin 1, Homer 1 and dynamin-3 affords physical coupling between the PSD and the endocytic zone where AMPAR recycling takes place. At the presynapse, oligophrenin 1 interacts with endophilin A1 (endoA1) and regulates neurotransmitter release. ARHGEF6 encodes Cloned-out of library-2 (Cool-2), a Rho GEF active on Rac1 and Cdc42 that promote neurite extension and actin polymerization exerting RhoA opposite function. Cool-2 binds and activates the Rac and Cdc42 downstream kinase Pak3 that is involved in the formation and stabilization of new spines. ARHGEF9 encodes collybistin, a Rho GEF active on Rac1 and Cdc42, crucial for inhibitory synapse structure and function. Collybistin binds PI(3)P in membranes and the scaffolding protein gephyrin, which in turn binds to the cytoskeleton and to GABA$_A$R subunits. Neuroligin-2 binding stabilizes the open configuration of collybistin that is able to bind the membrane and to promote gephyrin postsynaptic clustering. Rab GTPase pathway proteins involved in X-linked cognitive disorders include Rab39b, which is involved in synaptic vesicle trafficking and αGDI, which is involved in the biogenesis and the recycling of synaptic vesicles. In particular, it has been hypothesized that αGDI is crucial to maintain the soluble pool of Rab4 and Rab5, which regulate the transport to and from early endosomes, and to maintain the reserve pool of vesicles. GRIA3 encodes the GluA3 subunit of AMPARs; GluA3 assembles with GluA2, generating a pool of constitutively cycling AMPARs that mediate basal glutamatergic transmission. TM4SF2 encodes tspan7, which belongs to the tetraspanin family of transmembrane proteins. tspan7 regulates AMPAR subcellular distribution through binding with PICK1, a protein known to regulate the trafficking of AMPARs in the synapse. Cask and SAP102 belong to the MAGUK family. Cask is present both in pre- and postsynaptic compartments. In the presynapse, Cask is thought to have a role in active zone formation through its binding to neurexin and N- and P/Q-type calcium channels; in the postsynapse, it binds SAP97 and modulates the trafficking of NMDAR from the ER to the plasma membrane. Synapse-associated protein 102 (SAP102) is an MAGUK highly expressed during neuronal development. SAP102 associates with NMDARs early in the secretory pathway and regulates its trafficking in and out of the synapse. SAP102 was found to interact with many proteins that regulate synapse formation and function, including neuroligins and EphB2. Synaptophysin is a synaptic vesicle marker. It is involved in the biogenesis and in the various phases of exo-endocytic cycling of synaptic vesicles. It has been proposed that the dissociation between synaptophysin and VAMP2 in the priming step regulates the availability of the latter to be inserted in the fusion machinery together with the SNAREs (syntaxin, SNAP-25, and VAMP). Synaptophysin seems to be involved in the fusion/exocytosis step via participation in the formation of the fusion pore, and is crucial for the retrieval of vesicle membranes and protein machinery through its binding with various proteins involved in vesicle endocytosis (e.g., AP-1 and dynamin).

positioned at different levels of the same pathway, complete the complex regulation.[8]

Ras superfamily members can be grouped based on their sequence homology into five subfamilies, exerting similar functions. Ras GTPases regulate cell growth, differentiation, and survival; Rho GTPases are involved in actin dynamics; Rab and Arf act in various aspects of intracellular trafficking; and the small GTPase Ran acts in the transport between the nucleus and cytoplasm.[8]

Several mutations causing ID have been identified in genes encoding members of the small GTPase pathway.

OPHN1 encodes a GAP active on Rho GTPases RhoA, Rac, and Cdc42; ARHGEF6 and ARHGEF9 encode GEFs active on Cdc42 and Rac; Pak3 is a downstream effector of Rac1 and Cdc42, which interacts with the ARHGEF6 protein collybistin. αGDI acts on Rab GTPases, and Rab39b is a small GTPase of the Rab subfamily.

Rho GTPase Pathway: OPHN1, ARHGEF6, PAK3, and ARHGEF9

Rho GTPases are composed of 22 members in mammals that can be subdivided into seven subfamilies (Rho, Rac, Cdc42, Rnd, RhoD, RhoBTD, and RhoH). They are regulated by over 80 GEFs, approximately 70 GAPs, and three GDIs.[8] The most studied Rho GTPases are RhoA, Rac1, and Cdc42.

Rho GTPases are characterized by the presence of a Dbl homology (DH) domain involved in GEF interaction and a pleckstrin homology (PH) domain that mediates membrane binding.[9]

Rho GTPases integrate and translate extracellular stimuli into cytoskeletal remodeling. N-Methyl-D-aspartate receptor (NMDAR) is one of the receptors that signals through Rho GTPases to downstream effectors such as N-WASP, Arp2/3 complex, myosins, cofilin, and actin capping proteins.[7]

These proteins are involved in all aspects of neuronal morphology beginning with neuronal development by means of promoting growth cone dynamics, neuronal polarization, neurite elongation, and synaptogenesis, and during dendritic spine plasticity in mature neurons.[10,11]

Rac1 and Cdc42 promote neurite extension and actin polymerization. Rac1 in particular promotes formation of lamellipodia and Cdc42 filopodia.[12] RhoA exerts an opposite function, via Rho-associated protein kinase (ROCK) effectors and the stimulation of actomyosin-dependent contraction.[13]

Given these juxtaposed roles, dendritic outgrowth requires Rac1 activation and RhoA inhibition, both of which can be achieved through NMDAR-dependent signaling.[10] Similarly, Rac1 promotes spine formation, whereas RhoA activation reduces spine density and causes their retraction.

Identification of the first Rho-linked ID gene OPHN1 dates back to more than 15 years ago. OPHN1 maps onto the long arm of chromosome X (Xq12) and encodes oligophrenin1.[14]

Oligophrenin1 is a Rho GAP that enhances GTP hydrolysis of the Rho proteins RhoA, Rac, and Cdc42. In addition to a central Rho-GAP domain, oligophrenin1 harbors an N-terminal BAR (Bin, amphiphysin, and RSV) domain, which binds curved membranes, followed by a PH domain that binds phosphoinositides. The C-terminus of OPHN1 is characterized by the presence of three proline-rich domains containing SRC homology 3 (SH3)-binding domains.[15,16]

Mutations in OPHN1, either inherited or de novo, can be distinguished as those predicted to be loss-of-function[14] versus those that lead to gene duplication.[17,18] Notably, both types lead to pathological phenotypes, which suggests the dosage sensitivity of OPHN1.

OPHN1 was initially classified among genes that cause a nonsyndromic form of ID[14]; however, the syndromic nature of OPHN1-related ID soon became evident. Patients carrying OPHN1 mutations display moderate to severe ID associated with a defined pattern of clinical and neurological symptoms, a hallmark of which is cerebellar hypoplasia. Lateral ventricle enlargement, early hypotonia, and motor and speech delays are also common features. Occasionally, seizures and strabismus have been reported.[19,20]

Mutations that specifically affect the OPHN1 BAR domain have been reported in two unrelated families. A two—base pair deletion affects OPHN1 messenger ribonucleic acid (RNA) splicing and causes the expression of a protein containing an extra 16—amino acid sequence within the BAR domain.[21] A second mutation causes the loss of 37 amino acids within the BAR domain owing to the in-frame deletion of exon 7. In both cases, the resulting phenotype is similar to that of patients carrying loss-of-function mutations, with the addition of a not previously observed hippocampal alteration in the second family mutation.[22]

The OPHN1 BAR domain is able to mask and inhibit its GAP domain.[23] Among possible explanations, mutations in the BAR domain could indirectly interfere with OPHN1 Rho GAP activity by affecting this autoregulatory element.

Several studies in rodent central nervous system (CNS) primary neurons and mouse models mimicking patient mutations have contributed to the elucidation of OPHN1 function in neurons and synapses and provided an explanation for the pathological consequences of OPHN1 mutations in patients.

OPHN1 is ubiquitously expressed in the brain at both fetal and adult stages. Particularly high expression levels have been observed in the mouse cortex, hippocampus, amygdala, cerebellum, and olfactory bulb.[24]

OPHN1 expression is not limited to neurons because it is also detectable in glia, suggesting a broad role of OPHN1 in brain cells.[15] However, the function of OPHN1 in glia remains unexplored; more information is available regarding the function of OPHN1 in neurons.

In neurons, oligophrenin1 colocalizes with actin[15]; as a Rho GAP, it is involved in the regulation of the cytoskeleton and dendritic spine structure. OPHN1 RNA interference—mediated knockdown in the CA1 region of the hippocampus leads to dendritic spine shortening, a phenotype that can be reversed by inhibitors of RhoA kinase, compensating for the loss of physiological inhibition by oligophrenin1.[16,24] Furthermore, an OPHN1 knockout (KO) mouse model revealed reduced branching and fewer mushroom spines in granule neurons of the dentate gyrus, suggesting a defect in neuronal connections.[25]

In mature neurons, oligophrenin1 localizes at the synapse[16] and regulates excitatory glutamatergic synaptic function by playing crucial roles at both pre- and post-synaptic sites.

OPHN1 is required for hippocampal synapse maturation and for transmission across mature synapses, both under basal conditions and in the context of plasticity.[26]

OPHN1 forms a complex with α-amino-3-hydroxy-5-methyl-4-isoxazolepropionic acid (AMPA) receptors (AMPARs)[26] and is involved in the stabilization and trafficking of AMPARs at synapses. The capability of oligophrenin1 to sustain basal and activity-dependent synapse strengthening relies both on Rho GAP activity and interaction with Homer 1.[16,26,27]

Oligophrenin-mediated RhoA/Rho kinase inhibition favors AMPAR stabilization, likely by affecting actin dynamics.[26]

Postsynaptic scaffolding protein Homer 1 interacts with oligophrenin1 and a second GTPase, dynamin-3, affording physical coupling between the PSD and the endocytic zone (EZ),[28] where clathrin-mediated endocytosis and AMPAR recycling takes place.[29]

Disruption of the interaction between oligophrenin 1 and Homer 1 in the rat hippocampus results in a displacement of the EZ and consequent impairment of AMPAR mobile pool recycling and transmission under basal conditions and LTP.[30]

The amount of oligophrenin 1 at hippocampal synapses is tightly regulated in response to synaptic activity,[26] a common feature of genes that are required for synaptic plasticity.

A positive feedback loop exists between NMDAR activation and oligophrenin 1 synaptic recruitment, which is required for synapse strengthening.[26]

However, oligophrenin 1 also mediates synapse weakening. mGlu-dependent LTD triggers oligophrenin 1 translation in dendrites, which is required for AMPAR endocytosis, a function that relies on oligophrenin 1 binding with endophilin A2/3.[27]

Endophilins are known regulators of the early steps of endocytosis and are involved in both receptor trafficking at the postsynapse and in the recycling of neurotransmitter vesicles at presynapses.[31]

At the presynapse, the proline-rich domains of oligophrenin 1 interact with the SH3 domains of endophilin A1. This complex is recruited to the endocytic sites of synaptic vesicles, where it regulates neurotransmitter release.[32,33] In the absence of OPHN1, phosphate kinase A, and a key effector of RhoA, ROCK, are hyperactive, thus compromising presynaptic plasticity in both the hippocampus and the amygdala. Importantly, pharmacological inhibition of kinases downstream of OPHN1 is able to rescue the phenotype in animal models.[24,32,34]

Additional functions of OPHN1 are emerging. Studies suggest that oligophrenin 1 is implicated in inhibitory transmission. OPHN1 KO mice display defects in synaptic vesicle recycling in the hippocampus, with a decrease in ready releasable pools that is rescued by Rho kinase inhibitors.[25]

Furthermore, OPHN1 is involved in cross-talk between the synapse and the nucleus through its interaction with rev-erb alpha, a transcription repressor involved in circadian rhythms.[35] OPHN1 loss-of-function compromises circadian rhythms in mice, reminiscent of the phenotype observed in intellectual and developmental disabilities.[36]

ARHGEF6 encoding cloned-out of library-2 (Cool-2) or pax-interacting exchange factor (alphaPIX) is a 22-exon gene mapping in Xq26. Mutations in ARHGEF6 cause nonsyndromic ID.

The first male patient reported harbored a chromosomal translocation between the X chromosome and chromosome 21, resulting in a breakpoint between exons 10 and 11 and possibly leading to AHRGEF6 gene disruption. In addition to severe ID, the patient exhibited mild dysmorphic features and sensorineural hearing loss. A second ID-causing mutation has been identified in a Dutch family; it causes skipping of exon 2 that encodes the calponin homology (CH) domain of Cool-2.[37]

Cool-2 is composed of a central DH domain and PH domains, typical of the GEF protein family to which it belongs. These domains are surrounded by a specific CH domain (absent in other Cool proteins), an SH3 domain at the N-terminus, and a leucine zipper at the C-terminus, which allows for dimerization.[37] The SH3 domain binds p21-activated kinase (Pak) and Casitas B-lymphoma (cbl) proteins.

Cool-2 is a Rho GEF, acting specifically on Rac and Cdc42, and unable to activate RhoA.

Cool-2 exists either as monomer or dimer. In its dimeric form, Cool-2 specifically binds GDP-Rac; as a monomer, it binds and activates both GDP-Rac and GDP-Cdc42. As a dimer, a PH domain of one Cool-2 molecule and a DH domain of the second act in trans to create a unique and specific binding site for GDP-Rac. Dimer dissociation is promoted by the binding of PAK in complex with G protein beta-gamma subunits, likely inducing a conformational change. This provides the mechanism by which Cool-2 downstream signaling is regulated by extracellular stimuli through transmembrane receptors coupled to G proteins. Downstream effectors of Cdc24 and Rac include the Pak family. In particular, Cool-2 binds and activates Pak3, likely through Rac and Cdc42.[38,39]

Although Cool-2 expression is ubiquitous and detectable in all brain areas,[37] it is highly enriched in the hippocampus relative to the cortex and cerebellum, especially in CA1 and CA3 regions.[40,41] At the subcellular level, overexpressed Cool-2 localizes within the PSD, reinforcing the involvement of Rho GEF in cognitive processes.[42]

Cool-2 function has been investigated both in cultured neuron in vitro and in a KO mouse model in vivo; the latter study focused on the hippocampus as suggested by expression patterns.

Consistent with its Rho GEF activity and as observed for many ID genes, Cool-2 is involved in cytoskeletal dynamics and has a major role in dendritic spine remodeling and the structure of excitatory synapses.

Cool-2 synthetic RNA (siRNA)-mediated knockdown in vitro shifted dendritic spine morphology toward more thin and elongated spines at the expense of large mushroom-type spines.[42] A prevalence of immature spines was also observed in Pak3 loss-of-function models.[43] As Cool-2 binds and activates Pak3, the two proteins act at different levels of the same pathway, with Rac and Cdc42 in between. This hypothesis was reinforced by the finding that a constitutively active mutant of Pak3 rescued dendritic spine defects in hippocampal neurons.[42]

ARHGEF6 KO in vivo caused the emergence of more elongated spines. In contrast to in vitro observations, the size and relative amount of thin and mushroom-type spines was unaffected. However, Golgi staining of CA1 neurons revealed a global increase in both spine density and the complexity of the dendritic tree, with longer and more branched dendrites in the mutant. More spines and dendrites covering larger areas do not translate into more synaptic contacts. On the contrary, KO of ARHGEF6 results in a decrease in the number of synapses in adult mice. It remains unknown whether this suggests inherent functional defects of spines or compensatory mechanisms that seek to alleviate putative overconnectivity.[41]

In ARHGEF6 KO mice, Hebbian plasticity of hippocampal synapses is compromised. Mice displayed impaired early LTP and increased LTD across CA3—CA1 connections.[41] Although KO animals performed well in simple hippocampal-dependent learning and memory tests, more demanding tasks revealed behavioral defects. In particular, ARHGEF6 KO mice performed worse than wild-type (WT) mice on the complex learning task, were less flexible, and tended to overreact in the context of novelty.[41]

A reduction only of Rac1 and Cdc42 activity levels in the KO hippocampus—the site of enriched ARHGEF6—reinforces the hypothesis that the deleterious effects of ARHGEF6 mutations in patients result from reduced activation of Rac and Cdc42.

However, the effect of ARHGEF6 loss-of-function mutation on dendrites and spines is in apparent contrast with the role proposed for Rac and Cdc42, because they are known to promote branching and spine formation. Less activation of these Rho GAPs, as a consequence of the loss of ARHGEF6 function, results in decreased arborization and spine density.

This discrepancy notes how the relationship between ARHGEF6, Rho GAPs, its downstream effectors, and cytoskeletal dynamics is far from being completely understood. Complex regulatory mechanisms are likely involved, which maintain a fine balance of Rho GAP activation.

PAK3 encodes Pak3, which belongs to the Pak family and, together with two additional isoforms Pak1 and Pak2, forms the mammalian group I of Paks.[44]

Paks associate with the Rho family of GTPases (specifically the Rac and Cdc42 pathway) to control cytoskeleton dynamics and with the mitogen-activated protein kinase (MAPK) pathway to regulate transcription.

Paks exert their regulatory role on the cytoskeleton mainly by activating LIM kinase (LIMK), which in turn phosphorylates and inactivates cofilin/ADF (actin depolymerization factor). As a result, cofilin/ADF is unable to bind and depolymerize F-actin.

A number of kinases involved in neuronal plasticity, such as MAPK, phosphoinositide 3-kinase/protein kinase B (PI3K/Akt), and protein kinase A (PKA), have been found to act downstream of Paks.[45,46]

Paks are characterized by an N-terminal regulatory domain and a C-terminal catalytic domain. The regulatory domain includes a Cdc42/Rac-interacting binding domain (CRIB) and is surrounded by proline-rich sequences that bind SH3 domain-containing proteins such as Nck adaptors (upstream of CRIB) and PIX guanine exchange factors (downstream of CRIB). Pak3 preferentially binds Nck2, which cooperates with ephrinB to regulate dendritic spine morphology.[47]

The CRIB domain partially overlaps with an autoinhibitory domain (AID or KI) of Paks; as inferred from studies on Pak1, it relies on the ability to form dimers in which two Pak proteins inhibit each other via interactions between the catalytic and KI domains. Binding of Rho GTPases induces a conformational switch, promotes dimer disassembly, and allows the phosphorylation events (auto- and trans-phosphorylation) that activate Paks and their downstream effectors.[46]

It has been reported that Pak3 preferentially binds Cdc42 and could be therefore a specific effector of this Rho GTPase.[48] However, Pak3 has different isoforms, some of which are independent from Rho GTPases with respect to their activation. The presence of one or both of two alternatively spliced exons encoding additional amino acids of the auto-inhibitory domain generates Pak3 variants that are constitutively active.[49]

The PAK3 gene is located at Xq23 and is mainly expressed in the CNS, both in the developing and adult rodent brain.[44,50,51] PAK3 mutations are associated with mild to severe nonsyndromic ID, often accompanied by microcephaly or below-average head circumference. Additional symptoms such as dysmorphism, behavioral, and neuropsychiatric problems are reported in a number of patients.

PAK3 mutations identified thus far are mainly point mutations that affect either the catalytic or regulatory region of the protein.[51–55] A splicing mutation has been identified that causes a premature stop codon at position 128.[56]

The first mutation to be identified in patients was nonsense mutation R419X,[51,57] which causes a premature stop codon and, similar to the missense mutation A365E,[53] affects the catalytic domain of Pak3.[48] Missense mutation W446S[54] is expected to impact the phosphotransferase activity of Pak3.

In contrast, the missense mutation R67C falls upstream of the CRIB domain and reduces Rho-GTPase binding, thus impairing Pak3 activation.[52,58]

Missense mutation K389N is responsible for a peculiar neurocutaneous phenotype in which ID is associated with brain structural anomalies and skin defects. Experiments in heterologous cells and zebrafish suggest that the catalytically inactive mutant protein affects MAPK signaling, enhancing the phosphorylation of extracellular signal—regulated kinase.[55]

The most well-characterized function of Pak3 is its regulation of dendritic spine morphology, in accordance with the role of its upstream activator, Cdc42.[48]

In rat hippocampal neurons, siRNA-mediated knockdown of Pak3 or expression of the pathogenic variant R419X results in the appearance of long and immature spines at the expense of mushroom spines.[43] Similarly, mutation A365E affects the kinase activity of Pak3, leading to the formation of elongated spines.[48]

In contrast, the R67C mutation, which maps to the regulatory region of Pak3, significantly reduces the number of spines without affecting morphology. The phenotypic variation associated with PAK3 mutations suggests that Pak3 is able to regulate both spine number and spine morphology, the function of which is ascribable to its different domains.[48]

The multiple roles of Pak3 in regulating dendritic spine morphology have been studied in the context of activity-dependent spine remodeling, which is crucial to sustain the network changes that underlie learning processes.[59] Pak3 is recruited to spines in response to neuronal activity.[60] Inhibition of Pak3 during neuronal activity leads to the formation of clusters of unstable spines. These data suggest that Pak3 regulates both the formation and stabilization of new spines.[60]

Surprisingly, PAK3 KO mice do not display altered neuronal morphology or dendritic spine density or shape, save for a slight increase in the number of short spines.[61] A possible explanation is that other Paks are able to compensate for the loss of Pak3 function, because they have distinct but partially overlapping roles.

Indeed, experiments in hippocampal neurons demonstrate that Pak3 and Pak1 dimerize and colocalize in dendritic spines.[62] Furthermore, a constitutively active Pak1 is able to rescue the phenotype of immature spines caused by Pak3 inhibition.[63]

In support of this hypothesis, double KO mice lacking both PAK1 and PAK3 exhibit defects not found in single KO animals. Dendritic spines are smaller and elongated in double KO mice, which display a large number of spines presenting head protrusions and branches.[64]

The simultaneous KO of PAK3 and PAK1 also recapitulates the reduction in brain size often seen in patients with PAK3 mutations.

Brain size was normal in double KO mice at birth; however, postnatal brain enlargement was severely impaired. The observed reduction in brain size of over 30% does not necessarily implicate neuronal loss. On the contrary, the brain retained its fundamental architecture and cell count. However, the neurons were more densely packed owing to a size reduction in cell bodies and a significant loss of dendritic and axonal complexity. These morphological alterations are associated with aberrant cofilin and actin dynamics, which suggests that Paks regulate cytoskeletal events during postmitotic neuronal morphogenesis and brain development.[64]

Consistent with the strict relationship that exists between morphology and function, PAK3 mutations are associated with impaired synaptic functioning and plasticity.

In vitro experiments performed in rat hippocampal neurons demonstrate that PAK mutations affect glutamatergic transmission and LTP, particularly the stabilization phase of LTP.[43]

Consistent with these findings, PAK3 KO mice display deficits in the late phase of LTP, depending on gene transcription and new protein synthesis[65] and a concomitant reduction in the active form of transcription factor cAMP-responsive element-binding protein. These mice do not exhibit impaired hippocampal-dependent associative memory; however, they are unable to retain taste aversion memories, possibly as a result of amygdala defects.[61] In a mouse model in which the catalytic activity of all Paks is inhibited via expression of autoinhibitory Paks in the postnatal forebrain, the consolidation of both spatial and contextual fear memories is prevented.[66]

PAK1/PAK3 double KO mice display a more severe phenotype. Knockout mice demonstrate impaired LTP, LTD, and spatial learning, in addition to higher anxiety levels and hyperactive behavior.[64] A crucial role of PAKs in cognitive disease is supported by the findings of a cross-talk between Paks and the fragile X mental retardation 1 (FMR1) protein pathways, as well as the involvement of Paks in neurodegenerative diseases such as Alzheimer and Parkinson.[67]

FMR1 gene mutations are a common cause of inherited ID and autism. Interfering with the catalytic activity of Paks partially rescues the pathological phenotype of the Fmr1 KO mouse, including aberrant dendritic spine morphology and plasticity as well as behavioral and learning deficits.[68,69] These findings led the way to a more comprehensive picture of genes and pathways involved in ID and autism.

ARHGEF9 is composed of 11 exons and located on Xq11.1−11.2.[70] It encodes a brain-specific Rho GEF called collybistin in the rat and human homolog of posterior end mark-2 (hPEM-2) in humans.[71]

Mutations in ARHGEF9 result in ID, often in addition to a spectrum of neurological disorders such as epilepsy.

A balanced de novo X chromosome paracentric inversion that abolishes ARHGEF9 expression was identified in a female patient with ID, hyperaroused response to noise and social stimuli, and global developmental delay.[72] De novo chromosomal ARHGEF9 deletions are associated with ID, seizures, hyperactivity with attention deficit and limited social interaction, and delayed psychomotor development.[70,73]

ARHGEF9 point mutations have also been identified. A nonsense mutation has been reported in a boy with ID and epilepsy[70] and a missense mutation in exon 2 (G55A) in a boy with hyperexplexia and early infantile epileptic encephalopathy leading to premature death.[74]

A balanced chromosomal translocation, resulting in the expression of a truncated form of ARHGEF9, has been reported in a female patient with ID and associated with disturbed sleep−wake cycle, seizures, anxiety, and aggressive behavior.[75]

ARHGEF9 transcription is induced in postmitotic neurons in the second half of embryonic development. It is highly expressed in the adult mouse brain, particularly in the hippocampus. This pattern excludes a role in neuronal progenitor proliferation and is often seen in proteins involved in synaptogenesis and neuronal differentiation.[76]

Indeed, ARHGEF9 has emerged as a key molecule for the structural and functional properties of inhibitory synapses.

Collybistin is composed by an N-terminal SH3 domain, central DH, and PH domains and a proline-rich sequence in the C-terminus.[71]

Collybistin undergoes alternative splicing, which generates variants with or without the SH3 domain. However, in both the rat and human, the vast majority of collybistin mRNAs contain the SH3 domain. Furthermore, rat isoforms are distinguishable as a result of distinctive C-termini called CB1, CB2, and CB3 (hPEM-2 like) with a total of four variants, because CB2 alternatively exists with or without the SH3 domain.[74,77]

Crucial to an understanding of the role of collybistin was the finding of its direct interaction with gephyrin.[77] The two molecules interact through the polar amino acids of the linker region between SH3 and the DH domain of collybistin[78] and the C-terminal molybdenum cofactor biosynthesis protein Moea domain of gephyrin in its multimeric form.[74]

Gephyrin is a scaffolding protein found at inhibitory synapses. It is arranged in oligomers at inhibitory postsynapses and has a key role in the structural organization of CNS synapses. It binds to the cytoskeleton, to signaling proteins and in particular to $GABA_A$ receptor ($GABA_AR$) subunits.[79] Gephyrin binds the intracellular loop of $GABA_AR$ $\alpha1$, $\alpha2$, and $\alpha3$ subunits (revised in Ref. 79) as well as beta2 and beta3 subunits.[80] Gephyrin and $GABA_ARs$ reciprocally stabilize themselves at synapses.[81,82]

Gephyrin also associates with high affinity with the beta subunit of glycine receptors (GlyRs), serving to mediate inhibitory transmission in the spinal cord.[83]

Consistent with their patterns of molecular interaction, collybistin and gephyrin colocalize at rodent synapses; collybistin, however, is not present at 100% of gephyrin-positive synapses—the extent of colocalization is specific to brain region.[84]

Collybistin is required for gephyrin clustering at the postsynaptic sites of inhibitory synapses.[74,77] Furthermore, collybistin together with cyclin-dependent kinases has been reported to regulate the phosphorylation of gephyrin.[85]

To promote gephyrin clustering, collybistin requires a functional PH domain in addition to a gephyrin-binding site. The PH domain mediates membrane anchoring via its binding with phosphatidylinositol 3-phosphate (PI[3]P).[74,75]

The SH3 domain of collybistin has an important regulatory role and binds neuroligin-2,[86] neuroligin-4,[87] and the alpha2 subunit of $GABA_AR$.[88] Neuroligins are transmembrane proteins crucial for synaptogenesis and are known to interact with presynaptic neurexins.[89]

Only SH3-lacking isoforms are able to promote the translocation of gephyrin close to the plasma membrane in nonneuronal cells,[77] because the predominant SH3-containing isoform must be activated via protein—protein interactions to exert this function.

Collybistin typically adopts a closed conformation owing to an intramolecular interaction between the SH3 and DH-PH domains.[90] SH3-binding proteins function as activators. Upon neuroligin-2 binding, the open configuration of collybistin is stabilized and activated via membrane binding at the PH domain, thus promoting gephyrin postsynaptic clustering.[90]

Perturbation of the activation mechanism results in compromised gephyrin clustering and impaired clustering of its associated ionotropic receptors. This ultimately leads to impairment in inhibitory transmission.[86,87,91,92]

The auto-inhibition mechanism of SH3 and its release by proteins that reside at the synapse provides a means to compartmentalize gephyrin clustering specifically at postsynapses.[90]

In vitro studies demonstrate that both the G55A substitution mutation that affects the SH3 domain and the chromosomal translocation that causes the loss of the PH domain generate dominant negative collybistin mutants that are unable to target gephyrin properly, and thus GABA$_A$R. Notably, these mutations are characterized by an extremely severe phenotype.[74,75]

Less is known regarding the DH domain and GEF activity of collybistin. Specifically, hPEM2 activates Cdc42 in fibroblasts and promotes actin polymerization and filopodia formation.[71] Although it has been reported that GEF activity is dispensable for the synaptic recruitment of gephyrin,[93] in vitro studies highlight a possible contribution of the Rho GTPase Cdc42 in gephyrin clustering.[94] Overexpression of Cdc42 in cultured hippocampal neurons affects the size of postsynaptic gephyrin clusters. A constitutively active Cdc42 mutant induces the formation of several small gephyrin clusters and is able to rescue the gephyrin mislocalization resulting from expression of a PH-defective collybistin.[94]

The small GTPase GTP-TC10, which is highly similar to Cdc42, was shown to act as an additional collybistin activator. In its active form, GTP-TC10 binds the PH domain of collybistin, thus promoting gephyrin clustering and inhibitory neuronal transmission.[95]

The ARHGEF9 KO mouse represents a suitable model to study patient pathology, because it recapitulates the major neurological deficits. ARHGEF9 KO mice display increased anxiety and impaired spatial learning. Interestingly, KO mice do not exhibit symptoms ascribable to altered glycine-mediated neurotransmission. Because hyperexplexia is not a constant in ARHGEF9 patients, this suggests that ARHGEF9 acts largely to regulate GABAergic synapses. Indeed, the subcellular distribution of gephyrin and GABA$_A$Rs

(but not that of GlyRs) is compromised in KO mice. Impaired gephyrin clustering and inhibitory synapse formation in the KO animal is brain region-specific, most evident in the hippocampus, amygdala, and cerebellum. GABA$_A$R-mediated inhibition is impaired, hippocampal LTD is reduced, and LTP is enhanced.[86]

Rab GTPase Pathway: RAB39B and GDI1

With more than 60 members found in humans, Rab proteins constitute the largest subfamily within the Ras superfamily of small-molecular-weight GTPases. Rab proteins are involved in several steps of trafficking of specific subsets of vesicles along the cytoskeletal tracks constituted by microtubules and actin filaments. Rab proteins work in concert with specific effector proteins (sorting adaptors, kinases, phosphates, and motor proteins) to regulate vesicle tethering and docking, budding, fusion, uncoating, and mobility, thus ensuring proper delivery of various cargoes to different cell compartments.[96] Typically, different Rab members exhibit distinctive subcellular distribution and contribute to membrane identity and function by orchestrating the various steps of membrane vesicle trafficking and the recruitment of regulatory proteins.

Whereas some Rabs are ubiquitously expressed, others are enriched in particular tissues. A subset of Rabs is enriched in the nervous system, where they are important for brain development, neurite outgrowth, and axonal transport (reviewed in Ref. 97).

Synapse functioning largely relies on vesicle trafficking to ensure a regulated release of neurotransmitters at the presynaptic terminal and neurotransmitter receptor cycling at the PSD.

It is therefore not surprising that Rab proteins are implicated in neurological disorders. To date, one X-LID associated with Rab (Rab39b) has been identified[98]; a second (Rab40al) is associated with the neurodevelopmental disorder Martin—Probst syndrome, although the validity of this has been questioned.[99]

Rab proteins are characterized by the presence of a C-terminal geranylgeranyl group and are maintained inactive through the formation of cytoplasmic complexes with GDI proteins. In particular, αGDI is involved in ID.

The gene encoding Rab39b (RAB39B) maps onto the X chromosome at Xq28[98]; the number of RAB39B mutations that cause ID is increasing. Nonsense mutations that cause ID are associated with macrocephaly, epileptic seizures, and ASD.[100] Duplications and triplications involving RAB39B at Xq28 have been reported to result in mild ID and behavioral problems.[101,102]

Symptoms of ID and early-onset Parkinsonism were shared by two unrelated families in which the patients harbored either a missense mutation or a chromosomal deletion resulting in the complete loss of RAB39B.[103] Such findings implicate the protein in a wide spectrum of neurological disorders.

Expression of Rab39 is not specific to the CNS, because it is present in a variety of tissues. That said, it is enriched in brain structures such as the hippocampus, where it is expressed exclusively in neurons.[98]

In cultured mouse hippocampal neurons, Rab39b localizes to growth cones and at the Golgi and trans Golgi network compartments, in sorting and recycling endosomes. It is therefore hypothesized that Rab39b may be involved in the recycling of vesicles from the cell surface to the Golgi.[100]

Consistent with the role of Golgi-derived vesicles in neurite extension, knockdown of Rab39b in neurons impairs the quantity and morphology of growth cones, as well as neuronal branching.[100]

A direct involvement of Rab39b in synaptic function is suggested by a decrease in the density of synaptic contacts in its absence, associated with impairment in synaptic vesicle recycling in the same experimental setting.

Interestingly, Rab39b loss-of-function causes a reduction in the expression of α-synuclein in cultured neurons.[103] α-Synuclein is a major constituent of Lewy bodies in Parkinson disease. It is a presynaptic protein that regulates the activity of several cytoskeletal and synaptic proteins that are implicated in neurotransmitter release, including Rab GTPases. As such, a role of α-synuclein in synaptic plasticity has been proposed.[104]

GDI1 encodes for the GDP-dissociation inhibitor α (αGDI) that, together with βGDI, interacts with and regulates over 40 Rab GTPases in mammals.[105] GDIs bind the GDP-bound form of Rab GTPases and extract them from the membrane of target organelles, thus generating a soluble pool of Rab GTPases that constitute a reserve of Rabs to be loaded onto new membranes.

The GDI1 gene is found on Xq28. Mutations, including nonconservative substitutions and nonsense or frameshift mutations, cause nonsyndromic ID.[106,107]

GDI1 is a candidate causative gene for ASD, said to arise from altered GDI1 dosage. Accordingly, Xq28 duplications that include GDI1 have been reported in two patients with autism and either normal or borderline intellect.[108]

The role of GDI1 has been inferred largely from mouse models in which GDI1 has been deleted.[109,110]

GDI1 constitutive KO mice are characterized by altered sociability and defects in short-term memory. In particular, KO mice are less aggressive relative to WT animals and show impaired spatial working memory and emotional learning, as revealed by radial maze and fear conditioning tests, respectively.[109]

Despite ubiquitous expression of GDI1 in neural and sensory tissues,[111] this phenotype implicates the importance of GDI1 expression in the hippocampus, amygdala, and cortex. Further confirmation is found in the recapitulation of constitutive KO mouse phenotypes in the conditional GDI1 KO mouse, in which GDI1 deletion is confined to postmitotic neurons and glia of the anterior forebrain.[110]

Importantly, the learning gap between KO and WT type animals can be ameliorated using spaced training protocols and pretraining sessions.[112] The capability of GDI1 KO mice to process and store information properly, if trained, has important implications for patients and suggests that learning in the absence of GDI1 is feasible. GDI1 KO mice seem to require a longer time to process and store information.[112]

Which information processing steps are slowed in the absence of GDI1?

GDI1 loss mainly affects the presynapse. Electron microscopy analysis revealed that GDI1 KO presynaptic terminals are normal with respect to area and active zone, but display decreased synaptic vesicle content in both the somatosensory cortex and the CA1 region of the hippocampus. Furthermore, vesicle reduction is not uniformly distributed, but rather is concentrated in the distal region of the presynaptic terminal, indicative of a defect in the reserve pool of vesicles as opposed to the readily releasable pool.[112]

From a functional perspective, KO of GDI1 affects the probability of neurotransmitter release, as suggested by defective glutamate release in response to KCl stimulation in purified synaptosomes and from paired-pulse facilitation experiments in CA1 hippocampal neurons from the same KO mice.[112]

The molecular mechanisms that underlie GDI1 loss-of-function phenotypes have been suggested to involve Rab GTPases, known to be regulated by αGDI.

Rab3a is the most abundant Rab GTPase in the brain and is involved in synaptic vesicle fusion,[113] rendering it a top candidate. However, phenotypes observed in Rab3a KO mice do not overlap with those of GDI1 KO mice[114] and no major defects in Rab3a expression or distribution was identified in GDI KO mice.[109]

Indeed, a different subset of Rab GTPases was affected in GDI1 KO mice. In particular, Rab4 and Rab5 expression was reduced and absent from the synaptosomal fraction; both proteins underwent a shift in favor of the membrane-bound fraction at the expense of the soluble pool,[109] as predicted by the lack of αGDI.

Rab4 and Rab5 both localize at synaptic vesicles and in nonneuronal cells regulate the transport to and from early endosomes.[115,116]

Endosomes are crucial for synaptic vesicle cycling during endo- and exocytosis. They are implicated in both synaptic vesicle maturation[117] and vesicle recycling.[118]

Synaptic vesicle endocytosis is tightly coupled to vesicle exocytosis to maintain a pool of vesicles ready for neurotransmitter release. With the exception of the "kiss and run" mechanism, in which the vesicles form a transient fusion pore with the presynaptic membrane, vesicles are retrieved from the plasma membrane after a complete fusion event via clathrin-mediated endocytosis.[119] They are then able to transit through an intermediate endosomal compartment proposed to serve as a sorting station to check vesicle composition.[120] The endosomal sorting seems to be specific for a slow recycling process that involves the adaptor protein AP3 and takes place after sustained activity to refill the reserve pool of vesicles.[120] At the neuromuscular junction of *Drosophila*, Rab5-mediated passage through the endosomal compartment is a critical rate-limiting step, determining the release probability and recycling pool size.[120]

It has been hypothesized that a loss of GDI1 function associated with reduced Rab4 and Rab5 availability may affect biogenesis and the recycling of synaptic vesicles. In particular, recycling through endosomal compartments would be compromised, as would the refill and maintenance of the reserve pool of vesicles. This would explain the presynaptic defects identified in KO mouse models and associated learning deficits.[112]

GRIA3

GRIA3 encodes AMPAR subunit 3 (GluA3). AMPARs are ion channels that open a central pore in response to the binding of glutamate, leading to the flux of various ions (calcium and sodium enter; potassium exits). Subunit composition of the receptor determines permeability; those lacking the GluA2 subunit are the only ones permeable to calcium.[121]

Cations flux causes depolarization of the postsynaptic membrane and transmittance of the presynaptic electric signal.

The subunits organize in dimers that are mainly GluA1/GluA2, GluA2/GluA3, and GluA1/GluA1; these dimers subsequently assemble into tetramers.[122]

These channels are characterized by fast opening upon glutamate binding and by fast desensitization, and mediate the main part of the fast component of excitatory transmission.[121]

Receptor subunit composition changes during development; mechanisms of RNA editing and posttranslational modification finely regulate transmission properties of the channel.[123,124] In adult mammals, most of the GluA3 subunit is assembled in GluA2/3 dimers, in which GluA2 is mostly edited at the RNA level to become Ca^{2+} impermeable.

AMPARs have been extensively studied since their discovery; they have fundamental roles in both basal transmission and LTP and LTD, which strongly implicates them in learning and memory processes.[125]

In a simplified view, GluA2/3 dimers are part of a pool of receptors that, independent from activity state, cycle from intracellular reservoirs to the plasma membrane and vice versa, chiefly participating in basal transmission. GluA1/2 dimers are predominantly trafficked upon stimulation and are thus more strictly implicated in synaptic plasticity.[126]

Despite the vast knowledge that currently exists about these receptors, little is known specifically about the GluA3 subunit. Nevertheless, GluA3 is the only AMPAR subunit in which mutations have been found that are associated with intellectual disabilities.

Many reports describe patients with deletions, chromosomal translocations, duplications, and point mutations in the GRIA3 gene who present with ID and a variety of other symptoms ranging from facial dysmorphisms and hypotonia to behavioral disturbances such as rage outbursts or self-injury tendencies.[127−133] This pathology is typically found in males, as is often the case for X-linked mutations.

GRIA3 KO mice have been extensively studied and useful for the elucidation of several aspects of pathology, although not all patient-relevant phenotypes are reproduced. Knockout animals exhibit an increased tendency toward aggression in conditions of isolation, similar to a number of patients; interestingly, they display increased sociability and nonaggressive behaviors when not isolated.[134] Increased dopamine in the striatum was observed in KO mice, suggesting enhanced dopaminergic signaling in this region that could account for the observed alterations in social behavior. Adamczyk et al. hypothesized that an increase in dopamine may result from the predominance of GluA1/2 AMPARs in the hippocampal region that innervates the striatum, generated in a compensatory manner for the loss of GluA2/3 dimers. In support of these findings, decreased aggression was reported in GluA1KO animals.[135]

On the other hand GluA3 KO animals exhibit normal cortical and hippocampal transmission, LTP, and paired pulse facilitation.[136,137]

Steenland et al. used electroencephalography recordings to demonstrate reduced power in the low-frequency bands and enhanced seizure susceptibility[138] in GluA3 KO animals. These effects were particularly evident during non−rapid eye movement sleep, in accordance with the involvement of GluA3 in the generation of cortical slow waves.

Wu et al. identified a number of point mutations in highly conserved residues of GRIA3 in patients displaying ID.[129] One such mutation (G833R) leads to a 78% reduction in GluA3 subunit levels, whereas the other two (R631S and M706T) result in deficits in channel current (ranging from minimal to complete) without affecting global protein stability. The authors were unable to determine whether this loss of current was due to altered protein conformation or kinetic properties of the receptors or to inefficient receptor trafficking to the membrane. An additional mutation (R450Q) gives rise to receptors that are properly trafficked and elicit standard currents but exhibit accelerated desensitization and slowed recovery from the desensitized state. Such an effect demonstrates the potential for subtle defects in channel properties to induce ID.

Although GluA1 and GluA2 are generally thought to be the fundamental subunits of AMPARs, the implication of GluA3 in ID calls for a closer investigation of this subunit and its specific role in learning and memory processes.

TM4SF2

The TM4SF2 gene encodes tspan7, which belongs to the tetraspanin family of transmembrane proteins. This family is composed of 33 members in humans that share main structural features. All tetraspanins present four transmembrane domains, short intracellular C- and N-terminal tails and two extracellular loops—namely short extracellular loop (SEL) or EC1 and long extracellular loop (LEL) or EC2.[139] Structural conservation throughout the family is very high; the N and C termini have the widest variation between family members.[140] Subfamily classification is based on the number of cysteine residues present in the LELs that are able to form disulphide bridges and thus to organize the structure of this domain.[141]

The main function of this class of proteins is to organize specific domains of the membrane known as tetraspanin-enriched microdomains via the homohetero interactions across LELs.[142] Tetraspanin-enriched microdomains are thought to function as molecular facilitators, enriching the local concentration and increasing the likelihood of interaction of proteins that cooperate to exert their functions.[143] Tetraspanins regulate cell morphology, motility and signaling in the brain, immune system, and tumors. They have critical roles in oocyte fertilization, neuromuscular synapse formation, lymphocyte activation, and retinal degeneration.[139,144]

Despite their involvement in many fundamental biological functions, few pathological mutations have been reported in humans; this is likely owing to functional, compensatory overlapping across family members.[144]

However, mutations in TM4SF2 have been found in patients affected by ID.[145–152]

In one known case, a mutation resulted in the premature truncation of the protein that removes the last transmembrane domain and the C-terminus.[147]

A brain-specific function of tspan7 has been identified.[153] The C-terminal tail of tspan7 was found to interact with PICK1 (protein interacting with C kinase 1),

a protein known to regulate the trafficking of AMPARs in the synapse.[154] tspan7 was able to influence AMPAR trafficking, regulating its association with PICK1 According to the proposed model, tspan7 and AMPARs compete for PICK1 binding sites. AMPAR binding to PICK1 leads to receptor internalization, whereas the inability of AMPARs to bind a tspan7-bound molecule of PICK1 increases the stability of the receptor at the synaptic plasma membrane. It follows, then, that patients lacking a functional tspan7 or a functional PICK1—binding domain would display reduced levels of surface AMPARs owing to increased receptor internalization.

Short hairpin RNA-mediated knockdown of tspan7 in cultured neurons causes a reduction in dendritic spine width and increases the turnover of existing spines; modification of the morphology and stability of these specialized protrusions is a hallmark of ID. In accordance with these observations, knockdown of tspan7 results in decreased excitatory transmission (mEPSCs amplitude and frequency) and influences the morphological changes that occur upon LTP induction.[153]

These findings, once proven applicable to humans, could pave the way for potential therapeutic treatments in XLID patients.

MEMBRANE-ASSOCIATED GUANYLATE KINASES: CASK AND DLG3

Calmodulin-associated serine kinase (Cask) is a protein belonging to the MAGUK family. It was initially identified in *Caenorhabditis elegans* as a factor regulating epidermal growth factor receptor localization[155] and subsequently in vertebrate neurons as a binding partner of neurexin, a fundamental player in synapse formation.[156]

Two main diseases are caused by mutations in the CASK gene: microcephaly with pontine and cerebellar hypoplasia (MICPCH) and a form of X-LID.

As a member of the MAGUK family, Cask has the hallmark structural features of a C-terminal PSD-95/Dlg/ZO-1 (PDZ) domain and SH3 and guanylate kinase (GUK) domains. Interestingly, it presents some peculiarities, with a unique CaMKII-like domain and two L27 domains.[157]

The kinase activity of the GUK domain is highly reduced. Indeed, it was long believed to be completely absent and to function as intramolecular interactor, keeping the SH3-GUK domain in a closed state. However, Cask is able to phosphorylate both itself and neurexin.[158] It is expressed in two isoforms: one of full length called Cask b and one shorted version termed Cask a, which lacks the CaMKII-like domain and the two L27 domains.[159]

Similar to the other members of the MAGUK family, Cask is predominantly involved in the formation of macromolecular complexes via binding domain-mediated interactions with various proteins.

In vertebrate neurons, Cask is present both in pre- and postsynaptic compartments, where it likely exerts distinctive functions.[160,161]

In the presynapse, the CaMKII domain participates with the L27 domains in the binding of the lin10/X11a/Mint1 family[162] and of Caskin.[163]

The ability of Cask to bind neurexin and N- and P/Q-type calcium channels[164] suggests a likely involvement in the formation of the presynaptic active zone. This is thought to happen via a trafficking mechanism, as suggested by the presence of Cask in intracellular membrane compartments.[165]

A similar mechanism is demonstrated for Cask in the postsynapse, where its ability to bind SAP97 modulates the trafficking of NMDAR from the endoplasmic reticulum (ER) to the plasma membrane via the molecular motor protein KIF17.[166]

Indeed, SAP97 is able to bind and sort AMPARs and NMDARs according to their specific spatiotemporal expression patterns. The ability of SAP97 to discriminate between the two receptors appears to depend on Cask binding, which induces an extended conformation in SAP97, promoting the choice of NMDARs over AMPARs.[167]

Knockdown of Cask alters the transport of NMDARs that, while bound to SAP97, remain in large ER structures and fail to be inserted into vesicles transported via KIF17 motor protein.[168]

Cask enters neuronal nuclei, where it can regulate the transcription of both the NMDAR NR2B subunit and reelin via direct interactions with the T-box transcription factor Tbr1 and the nucleosome assembly protein CINAP/DENTT/TSPY-L2.[169–171] These interactions are likely to result in increased expression owing to the chromatin remodeling activity of CINAP. Both NR2B and reelin have critical functions in the regulation of neuronal activity and brain development. A point mutation in the CASK gene in one patient severely affected by ID has been found to disrupt the C-terminal region of the protein, in which binding to Tbr1 and CINAP occurs.[172] This highlights the importance of this binding function in brain circuit development.

Cask undergoes a series of posttranslational modifications that regulate its activities: The SH3 domain can be SUMOylated[173]; CDK5 is able to phosphorylate Cask, promoting its recruitment to the synaptic membrane[174]; and phosphorylation by protein PKA regulates its interaction with Tbr1 in the nucleus.[175]

Despite what is known with respect to Cask functions, the exact link between mutations and patient symptoms remains unclear. One main reason for this is that mouse models of CASK mutations are lethal at early stages of development owing to a cleft palate,[176] which renders long-term in vivo studies impossible in these animals. Electrophysiological recordings of neurons cultured from these animals reveal impaired glutamate release, consistent with the proposed presynaptic role of Cask. Surprisingly, no changes were observed in postsynaptic basal electrical properties or in evoked transmission. This is in contrast to what is expected based on the hypothetical postsynaptic role of the protein.[176]

Different types of mutations in CASK are found in patients who present ID: Loss-of-function mutations are typically associated with MICPCH, whereas hypomorphic mutations are regularly associated with X-LID.[172] Microcephaly with pontine and cerebellar hypoplasia manifests more often in females, likely because of an embryonic-lethal phenotype in males. It is characterized by microcephaly, moderate to severe ID, absent language, hypotonia or hypertonia, seizures, behavioral abnormalities, short stature, optic nerve hypoplasia, retinopathy, strabismus, hearing loss, and some facial appearance peculiarities.[158] Magnetic resonance imaging typically reveals pontine and cerebellar hypoplasia and, in the case of some patients, low cerebrum/corpus callosum ratio and reduced complexity of the gyri in the frontal cerebral cortex. The few males presenting with this pathology have similar albeit more severe phenotypes than females. The X-LID manifestation of CASK mutations in males is characterized, in addition to ID, by seizures, nystagmus, tremor, unsteady gait, and cerebellar hypoplasia. In contrast, the same CASK mutations are either asymptomatic or cause mild ID and/or mild nystagmus in females.[158] This form of CASK-related disease is generally caused by hypomorphic mutations that are more likely to cause nystagmus if they hit the C-terminus of the protein. This is likely caused by disruption of the interaction of Cask with FRMD7, a 4.1 protein, ezrin, radixin, moesin (FERM) domain protein involved in neurite growth and mutated in idiopathic infantile nystagmus.[177]

Additional efforts are needed to develop animal models harboring CASK mutations to more clearly define the relationship between various synaptic Cask functions and patient phenotypes.

Synapse-associated protein 102 (SAP102) is a member of the MAGUK family encoded by Disk-large 3 (DLG3) gene. Similar to other MAGUKs, it has three N-terminal PDZ domains, an SH3 domain, and a GUK domain. SAP102 is a classical member of the MAGUK family because it is involved in the formation of macromolecular complexes that often contain fundamental postsynaptic receptors and present the ability to associate with cytoskeletal proteins.[161]

The protein is expressed mainly in nonproliferating cells such as neurons, cells of the Langerhans islet of the pancreas, myocytes of the heart, and esophageal epithelium.[178]

In neurons, SAP102 has a peculiar expression pattern. It is the first MAGUK to be expressed at high levels during neuronal development in rodents; it reaches a maximum expression at P10 and is then rapidly substituted by other MAGUKs such as PSD95 and PSD93.[179–181]

This expression pattern strongly parallels that of NR2B, which is mainly replaced by NR2A.[179,181–183] Similar to SAP97, SAP102 can associate with NMDARs early in the secretory pathway and precisely in the ER.[184,185] This complex then travels to the PSD, primarily on actin filaments.[182,183]

Once in spines, SAP102 is highly mobile relative to other MAGUKs such as PSD95, which are trapped at the PSD. It is also found at high levels in the cytoplasmic compartment of spines.[161,186]

SAP102 does not have the ability to oligomerize, nor does it have an N-terminal palmitoylation site or an L27 domain. Thus, it cannot be directly targeted to the plasma membrane.[161]

Chen et al. identified a role for SAP102 in regulating NR2B-containing NMDARs. They proposed a model by which the phosphorylation of a specific residue on NMDARs disrupts interaction with PSD-trapped MAGUKs such as PSD95, thus promoting interaction with SAP102. This interaction, thanks to SAP102 high mobility, translocates the receptors to extrasynaptic sites where standard AP-2-mediated internalization can take place.[187] These findings suggest a general role of SAP102 in trafficking of NMDARs inside and outside the synapse.

SAP102 expression was found to be increased in spines in the rat visual cortex upon eye opening, which suggests activity-dependent regulation.[188]

SAP102 is able to partially rescue the loss of PSD95 and was found at increased levels in PSD95 KO mice. The two proteins were also shown to co-regulate AMPAR activity, either through a direct interaction between the SH3 domain of PSD95 and the GUK domain of SAP102[189–191] or indirectly through their binding to different receptor subunits.[192]

Overexpression of the truncated form of PSD95 in PSD95 KO mice enhanced AMPAR-mediated transmission when SAP102 was present at increased levels.[191] Moreover, the double KO of PSD95 and SAP102 is lethal.[193]

The role of SAP102 in synapse formation was further confirmed by the observation that its removal (via shRNA-mediated knockdown) in cultured neurons increased the number of filopodia, to the detriment of mature dendritic spines. This effect is likely caused by regulation of the actin cytoskeleton by a complex formed by SAP102, NMDARs, EphB2, and Kalirin-7 and via PAK signaling.[194]

Aberrant synapse morphology is a common hallmark of ID. As such, it is not surprising that the loss of this protein induces such a phenotype. A variety of patients who exhibit developmental delays in cognitive function have been found to carry mutations in the DLG3 gene.[133,195]

Most mutations identified cause premature truncation of the protein and thus loss of the C-terminal SH3 and GUK domains, likely altering the ability of SAP102 to bind NMDARs and other partners.

SAP102 was found to interact with many proteins that regulate synapse formation and function. Included in this list are neuroligin,[196] neurobeachin,[197] the GluK2 and GluK6 subunits of the kainate receptor,[198] and A_{2A} adenosine receptor.[199]

This evidence strongly suggests fundamental roles of SAP102 in the development and function of the central nervous system and specifically in the circuits involved in learning and memory processes.

SYNAPTOPHYSIN

Synaptophysin encoded by the SYP gene was first characterized in the 1980s.[200–202]

It is a four-transmembrane protein present at high concentrations exclusively in synaptic vesicles. Synaptophysin is predicted to be present in approximately 32 copies per vesicle, accounting for approximately 10% of vesicle protein content.[203] As such, it is commonly used as a marker for these organelles.

Synaptophysin assembles in hexamers strongly reminiscent of the structure of connexons.[204] It is believed to form a central pore with characteristics similar to voltage-gated potassium channels.[205–208]

Since its discovery, various functions related to synaptic vesicles have been ascribed to synaptophysin.

Synaptophysin is involved in biogenesis and in the various phases of exo-endocytic cycling of synaptic vesicles: targeting to the release site, docking to the plasma membrane, priming, fusion/exocytosis, and retrieval of the membrane by endocytosis.[209]

Synaptophysin binds cholesterol on membranes in addition to a number of proteins[117,210] and is thus likely involved in stabilizing protein complexes on synaptic vesicle membranes.[211]

Synaptophysin is detectable in synaptic vesicles upon their formation in the Golgi apparatus.[212] It has been hypothesized that synaptophysin may act directly in forming synaptic vesicles by inducing membrane curvature.[213] Indeed, synaptophysin overexpression in nonneuronal cells is sufficient to induce the formation of small cytoplasmic vesicles.[214]

Another hypothesis is that synaptophysin is involved in sorting proteins necessary for the formation and maturation of vesicles. Indeed, mislocalization of vesicle-associated membrane protein 2 (VAMP2) upon overexpression can be rescued by ectopic expression of synaptophysin, which restores the physiological sorting of VAMP2 to vesicles.[215] Moreover, the interaction of synaptophysin with VAMP2 and other fundamental proteins of synaptic vesicles begins in the ER before vesicle biogenesis.[216]

In the priming step, during which vesicles are prepared to fuse with the membrane, it is believed that dissociation between synaptophysin and VAMP2 regulates the availability of the latter to be inserted in the fusion machinery together with the SNAP (soluble NSF attachment protein) receptor (SNARE) complex.[217]

Evidence exists that suggests synaptophysin is involved in the fusion/exocytosis step via participation in the formation of the fusion pore that joins two membranes before their complete merging.[209] Indeed, as described above, synaptophysin is able to associate in hexamers with a central pore that dissociates in parallel with the fusion of the vesicle and membrane.[217]

Nevertheless, the process in which synaptophysin seems to be most critically involved is the retrieval of vesicle membranes and protein machinery.

Retrieval is strongly linked to the fusion process. Two general mechanisms are hypothesized. The first implies complete fusion of the synaptic vesicle with the plasma membrane and thus a disruption of the entire lipid/protein machinery that is then retrieved though clathrin-coated vesicles.[218–220] The second, termed "kiss and run," proposes that the vesicle fuses as little as necessary to release its neurotransmitter content and immediately reseals, ready to be filled again.[221–223]

The two models are not mutually exclusive; the kiss-and-run model may be a faster way to replenish the pool of releasable vesicles, useful in the context of prolonged stimulation. Clathrin-mediated retrieval, however, could represent a slower recycling mechanism used under basal conditions.[209]

Kwon et al., however, argued against the latter hypothesis, demonstrating that only 1.3% of vesicles are retrieved in the first second after neuronal stimulation, and suggesting a predominance of clathrin-mediated retrieval.[224] Whereas the relative significance of the two retrieval mechanisms is still a matter of debate, synaptophysin involvement in synaptic vesicle recycling is widely accepted and strongly supported by its interaction with various proteins involved in vesicle endocytosis (e.g., AP-1 and dynamin).[225–227] Moreover, cultured neurons from SYP KO mice reveal defective synaptic vesicle endocytosis both during and after neuronal stimulation.[224]

Several patients affected by ID have been found to carry mutations in the SYP gene.[228] Most of these were frameshift mutations, resulting in a premature termination of the protein. Truncation of the C-terminus has been found to cause slower vesicle endocytosis during neuronal stimulation, whereas no effects were observed after the termination of the stimulus. This suggests that distinct synaptophysin domains may be responsible for respective activities.[224]

SYP KO mice display mild behavioral defects associated with impaired learning and memory.[229,230]

Cultured neurons from KO mice exhibit a strong defect in the retrieval of VAMP2,[231] and X-LID mutations introduced into SYP KO mice were unable to rescue the defect in VAMP2 retrieval.[232] Although VAMP2 is important for vesicle fusion, it has been reported that inefficient VAMP2 retrieval does not impair neurotransmitter release or global synaptic vesicle turnover.[224,231,233] This potentially explains the subtle phenotype observed in KO mice and suggests that more severe defects may manifest under high-intensity stimulation conditions.[232]

References

1. Stevenson RE, Schwartz CE. X-linked intellectual disability: unique vulnerability of the male genome. *Dev Disabil Res Rev* 2009;**15**(4):361–8.
2. Nguyen DK, Disteche CM. High expression of the mammalian X chromosome in brain. *Brain Res* December 18, 2006;**1126**(1):46–9.
3. Stevenson RE, Holden KR, Rogers RC, Schwartz CE. Seizures and X-linked intellectual disability. *Eur J Med Genet* May 2012;**55**(5):307–12.
4. Caglayan AO. Genetic causes of syndromic and non-syndromic autism. *Dev Med Child Neurol* February 2010;**52**(2):130–8.
5. Gecz J, Shoubridge C, Corbett M. The genetic landscape of intellectual disability arising from chromosome X. *Trends Genet* July 2009;**25**(7):308–16.
6. Lubs HA, Stevenson RE, Schwartz CE. Fragile X and X-linked intellectual disability: four decades of discovery. *Am J Hum Genet* April 6, 2012;**90**(4):579–90.
7. Ramakers GJ. Rho proteins, mental retardation and the cellular basis of cognition. *Trends Neurosci* April 2002;**25**(4):191–9.
8. Cherfils J, Zeghouf M. Regulation of small GTPases by GEFs, GAPs, and GDIs. *Physiol Rev* January 2013;**93**(1):269–309.
9. Rossman KL, Der CJ, Sondek J. GEF means go: turning on RHO GTPases with guanine nucleotide-exchange factors. *Nat Rev Mol Cell Biol* February 2005;**6**(2):167–80.
10. Newey SE, Velamoor V, Govek EE, Van Aelst L. Rho GTPases, dendritic structure, and mental retardation. *J Neurobiol* July 2005;**64**(1):58–74.
11. Murakoshi H, Wang H, Yasuda R. Local, persistent activation of Rho GTPases during plasticity of single dendritic spines. *Nature* April 7, 2011;**472**(7341):100–4.
12. Nobes CD, Hall A. Rho, rac, and cdc42 GTPases regulate the assembly of multimolecular focal complexes associated with actin stress fibers, lamellipodia, and filopodia. *Cell* April 7, 1995;**81**(1):53–62.
13. Linseman DA, Loucks FA. Diverse roles of Rho family GTPases in neuronal development, survival, and death. *Front Biosci* 2008;**13**:657–76.
14. Billuart P, Bienvenu T, Ronce N, des Portes V, Vinet MC, Zemni R, et al. Oligophrenin-1 encodes a rhoGAP protein involved in X-linked mental retardation. *Nature* April 30, 1998;**392**(6679):923–6.

15. Fauchereau F, Herbrand U, Chafey P, Eberth A, Koulakoff A, Vinet MC, et al. The RhoGAP activity of OPHN1, a new F-actin-binding protein, is negatively controlled by its amino-terminal domain. *Mol Cell Neurosci* August 2003;**23**(4):574–86.

16. Govek EE, Newey SE, Akerman CJ, Cross JR, Van der Veken L, Van Aelst L. The X-linked mental retardation protein oligophrenin-1 is required for dendritic spine morphogenesis. *Nat Neurosci* April 2004;**7**(4):364–72.

17. Bedeschi MF, Novelli A, Bernardini L, Parazzini C, Bianchi V, Torres B, et al. Association of syndromic mental retardation with an Xq12q13.1 duplication encompassing the oligophrenin 1 gene. *Am J Med Genet Part A* July 1, 2008;**146A**(13):1718–24.

18. Kaya N, Colak D, Albakheet A, Al-Owain M, Abu-Dheim N, Al-Younes B, et al. A novel X-linked disorder with developmental delay and autistic features. *Ann Neurol* April 2012;**71**(4):498–508.

19. Tentler D, Gustavsson P, Leisti J, Schueler M, Chelly J, Timonen E, et al. Deletion including the oligophrenin-1 gene associated with enlarged cerebral ventricles, cerebellar hypoplasia, seizures and ataxia. *Eur J Hum Genet* July 1999;**7**(5):541–8.

20. Zanni G, Saillour Y, Nagara M, Billuart P, Castelnau L, Moraine C, et al. Oligophrenin 1 mutations frequently cause X-linked mental retardation with cerebellar hypoplasia. *Neurology* November 8, 2005;**65**(9):1364–9.

21. Pirozzi F, Di Raimo FR, Zanni G, Bertini E, Billuart P, Tartaglione T, et al. Insertion of 16 amino acids in the BAR domain of the oligophrenin 1 protein causes mental retardation and cerebellar hypoplasia in an Italian family. *Hum Mutat* November 2011;**32**(11):E2294–307.

22. Santos-Reboucas CB, Belet S, Guedes de Almeida L, Ribeiro MG, Medina-Acosta E, Bahia PR, et al. A novel in-frame deletion affecting the BAR domain of OPHN1 in a family with intellectual disability and hippocampal alterations. *Eur J Hum Genet* May 2014;**22**(5):644–51.

23. Eberth A, Lundmark R, Gremer L, Dvorsky R, Koessmeier KT, McMahon HT, et al. A BAR domain-mediated autoinhibitory mechanism for RhoGAPs of the GRAF family. *Biochem J* January 1, 2009;**417**(1):371–7.

24. Khelfaoui M, Denis C, van Galen E, de Bock F, Schmitt A, Houbron C, et al. Loss of X-linked mental retardation gene oligophrenin1 in mice impairs spatial memory and leads to ventricular enlargement and dendritic spine immaturity. *J Neurosci* August 29, 2007;**27**(35):9439–50.

25. Powell AD, Gill KK, Saintot PP, Jiruska P, Chelly J, Billuart P, et al. Rapid reversal of impaired inhibitory and excitatory transmission but not spine dysgenesis in a mouse model of mental retardation. *J Physiol* February 15, 2012;**590**(Pt 4):763–76.

26. Nadif Kasri N, Nakano-Kobayashi A, Malinow R, Li B, Van Aelst L. The Rho-linked mental retardation protein oligophrenin-1 controls synapse maturation and plasticity by stabilizing AMPA receptors. *Genes Dev* June 1, 2009;**23**(11):1289–302.

27. Nadif Kasri N, Nakano-Kobayashi A, Van Aelst L. Rapid synthesis of the X-linked mental retardation protein OPHN1 mediates mGluR-dependent LTD through interaction with the endocytic machinery. *Neuron* October 20, 2011;**72**(2):300–15.

28. Lu J, Helton TD, Blanpied TA, Racz B, Newpher TM, Weinberg RJ, et al. Postsynaptic positioning of endocytic zones and AMPA receptor cycling by physical coupling of dynamin-3 to Homer. *Neuron* September 20, 2007;**55**(6):874–89.

29. Petrini EM, Lu J, Cognet L, Lounis B, Ehlers MD, Choquet D. Endocytic trafficking and recycling maintain a pool of mobile surface AMPA receptors required for synaptic potentiation. *Neuron* July 16, 2009;**63**(1):92–105.

30. Nakano-Kobayashi A, Tai Y, Nadif Kasri N, Van Aelst L. The X-linked mental retardation protein OPHN1 interacts with Homer1b/c to control spine endocytic zone positioning and expression of synaptic potentiation. *J Neurosci* June 25, 2014;**34**(26):8665–71.

31. Kjaerulff O, Brodin L, Jung A. The structure and function of endophilin proteins. *Cell Biochem Biophys* July 2011;**60**(3):137–54.

32. Khelfaoui M, Pavlowsky A, Powell AD, Valnegri P, Cheong KW, Blandin Y, et al. Inhibition of RhoA pathway rescues the endocytosis defects in Oligophrenin1 mouse model of mental retardation. *Hum Mol Genet* July 15, 2009;**18**(14):2575–83.

33. Nakano-Kobayashi A, Kasri NN, Newey SE, Van Aelst L. The Rho-linked mental retardation protein OPHN1 controls synaptic vesicle endocytosis via endophilin A1. *Curr Biol* July 14, 2009;**19**(13):1133–9.

34. Khelfaoui M, Gambino F, Houbaert X, Ragazzon B, Muller C, Carta M, et al. Lack of the presynaptic RhoGAP protein oligophrenin1 leads to cognitive disabilities through dysregulation of the cAMP/PKA signalling pathway. *Philos Trans R Soc Lond B Biol Sci* January 5, 2014;**369**(1633):20130160.

35. Valnegri P, Khelfaoui M, Dorseuil O, Bassani S, Lagneaux C, Gianfelice A, et al. A circadian clock in hippocampus is regulated by interaction between oligophrenin-1 and Rev-erbalpha. *Nat Neurosci* October 2011;**14**(10):1293–301.

36. Maaskant M, van de Wouw E, van Wijck R, Evenhuis HM, Echteld MA. Circadian sleep-wake rhythm of older adults with intellectual disabilities. *Res Dev Disabil* April 2013;**34**(4):1144–51.

37. Kutsche K, Yntema H, Brandt A, Jantke I, Nothwang HG, Orth U, et al. Mutations in ARHGEF6, encoding a guanine nucleotide exchange factor for Rho GTPases, in patients with X-linked mental retardation. *Nat Genet* October 2000;**26**(2):247–50.

38. Bagrodia S, Bailey D, Lenard Z, Hart M, Guan JL, Premont RT, et al. A tyrosine-phosphorylated protein that binds to an important regulatory region on the cool family of p21-activated kinase-binding proteins. *J Biol Chem* August 6, 1999;**274**(32):22393–400.

39. Feng Q, Albeck JG, Cerione RA, Yang W. Regulation of the Cool/Pix proteins: key binding partners of the Cdc42/Rac targets, the p21-activated kinases. *J Biol Chem* February 15, 2002;**277**(7):5644–50.

40. Meyer MA. Highly expressed genes within hippocampal sector CA1: Implications for the physiology of memory. *Neurol Int* April 22, 2014;**6**(2):5388.

41. Ramakers GJ, Wolfer D, Rosenberger G, Kuchenbecker K, Kreienkamp HJ, Prange-Kiel J, et al. Dysregulation of Rho GTPases in the alphaPix/Arhgef6 mouse model of X-linked intellectual disability is paralleled by impaired structural and synaptic plasticity and cognitive deficits. *Hum Mol Genet* January 15, 2012;**21**(2):268–86.

42. Node-Langlois R, Muller D, Boda B. Sequential implication of the mental retardation proteins ARHGEF6 and PAK3 in spine morphogenesis. *J Cell Sci* December 1, 2006;**119**(Pt 23):4986–93.

43. Boda B, Alberi S, Nikonenko I, Node-Langlois R, Jourdain P, Moosmayer M, et al. The mental retardation protein PAK3 contributes to synapse formation and plasticity in hippocampus. *J Neurosci* December 1, 2004;**24**(48):10816–25.

44. Manser E, Chong C, Zhao ZS, Leung T, Michael G, Hall C, et al. Molecular cloning of a new member of the p21-Cdc42/Rac-activated kinase (PAK) family. *J Biol Chem* October 20, 1995;**270**(42):25070–8.

45. Bagrodia S, Derijard B, Davis RJ, Cerione RA. Cdc42 and PAK-mediated signaling leads to Jun kinase and p38 mitogen-activated protein kinase activation. *J Biol Chem* November 24, 1995;**270**(47):27995–8.

46. Zhao ZS, Manser E. PAK and other Rho-associated kinases—effectors with surprisingly diverse mechanisms of regulation. *Biochem J* March 1, 2005;**386**(Pt 2):201–14.

47. Thevenot E, Moreau AW, Rousseau V, Combeau G, Domenichini F, Jacquet C, et al. p21-Activated kinase 3 (PAK3) protein regulates synaptic transmission through its interaction with the Nck2/Grb4 protein adaptor. *J Biol Chem* November 18, 2011;**286**(46):40044–59.

48. Kreis P, Thevenot E, Rousseau V, Boda B, Muller D, Barnier JV. The p21-activated kinase 3 implicated in mental retardation regulates spine morphogenesis through a Cdc42-dependent pathway. *J Biol Chem* July 20, 2007;**282**(29):21497–506.

49. Kreis P, Rousseau V, Thevenot E, Combeau G, Barnier JV. The four mammalian splice variants encoded by the p21-activated kinase 3 gene have different biological properties. *J Neurochem* August 2008;**106**(3):1184–97.

50. Burbelo PD, Kozak CA, Finegold AA, Hall A, Pirone DM. Cloning, central nervous system expression and chromosomal mapping of the mouse PAK-1 and PAK-3 genes. *Gene* May 31, 1999; **232**(2):209–15.

51. Allen KM, Gleeson JG, Bagrodia S, Partington MW, MacMillan JC, Cerione RA, et al. PAK3 mutation in nonsyndromic X-linked mental retardation. *Nat Genet* September 1998;**20**(1):25–30.

52. Bienvenu T, des Portes V, McDonell N, Carrie A, Zemni R, Couvert P, et al. Missense mutation in PAK3, R67C, causes X-linked nonspecific mental retardation. *Am J Med Genet* August 14, 2000;**93**(4):294–8.

53. Gedeon AK, Nelson J, Gecz J, Mulley JC. X-linked mild nonsyndromic mental retardation with neuropsychiatric problems and the missense mutation A365E in PAK3. *Am J Med Genet Part A* August 1, 2003;**120A**(4):509–17.

54. Peippo M, Koivisto AM, Sarkamo T, Sipponen M, von Koskull H, Ylisaukko-oja T, et al. PAK3 related mental disability: further characterization of the phenotype. *Am J Med Genet Part A* October 15, 2007;**143A**(20):2406–16.

55. Magini P, Pippucci T, Tsai IC, Coppola S, Stellacci E, Bartoletti-Stella A, et al. A mutation in PAK3 with a dual molecular effect deregulates the RAS/MAPK pathway and drives an X-linked syndromic phenotype. *Hum Mol Genet* July 1, 2014;**23**(13):3607–17.

56. Rejeb I, Saillour Y, Castelnau L, Julien C, Bienvenu T, Taga P, et al. A novel splice mutation in PAK3 gene underlying mental retardation with neuropsychiatric features. *Eur J Hum Genet* November 2008;**16**(11):1358–63.

57. Donnelly AJ, Partington MW, Ryan AK, Mulley JC. Regional localisation of two non-specific X-linked mental retardation genes (MRX30 and MRX31). *Am J Med Genet* July 12, 1996;**64**(1):113–20.

58. des Portes V, Soufir N, Carrie A, Billuart P, Bienvenu T, Vinet MC, et al. Gene for nonspecific X-linked mental retardation (MRX 47) is located in Xq22.3-q24. *Am J Med Genet* October 31, 1997;**72**(3): 324–8.

59. De Roo M, Klauser P, Muller D. LTP promotes a selective long-term stabilization and clustering of dendritic spines. *PLoS Biol* September 9, 2008;**6**(9):e219.

60. Dubos A, Combeau G, Bernardinelli Y, Barnier JV, Hartley O, Gaertner H, et al. Alteration of synaptic network dynamics by the intellectual disability protein PAK3. *J Neurosci* January 11, 2012;**32**(2):519–27.

61. Meng J, Meng Y, Hanna A, Janus C, Jia Z. Abnormal long-lasting synaptic plasticity and cognition in mice lacking the mental retardation gene Pak3. *J Neurosci* July 13, 2005;**25**(28):6641–50.

62. Combeau G, Kreis P, Domenichini F, Amar M, Fossier P, Rousseau V, et al. The p21-activated kinase PAK3 forms heterodimers with PAK1 in brain implementing trans-regulation of PAK3 activity. *J Biol Chem* August 31, 2012;**287**(36):30084–96.

63. Boda B, Jourdain L, Muller D. Distinct, but compensatory roles of PAK1 and PAK3 in spine morphogenesis. *Hippocampus* 2008;**18**(9): 857–61.

64. Huang W, Zhou Z, Asrar S, Henkelman M, Xie W, Jia Z. p21-Activated kinases 1 and 3 control brain size through coordinating neuronal complexity and synaptic properties. *Mol Cell Biol* February 2011;**31**(3):388–403.

65. Kandel ER. The molecular biology of memory storage: a dialogue between genes and synapses. *Science* November 2, 2001;**294**(5544): 1030–8.

66. Hayashi ML, Choi SY, Rao BS, Jung HY, Lee HK, Zhang D, et al. Altered cortical synaptic morphology and impaired memory consolidation in forebrain- specific dominant-negative PAK transgenic mice. *Neuron* June 10, 2004;**42**(5):773–87.

67. Ma QL, Yang F, Frautschy SA, Cole GM. PAK in Alzheimer disease, Huntington disease and X-linked mental retardation. *Cell Logist* April 1, 2012;**2**(2):117–25.

68. Hayashi ML, Rao BS, Seo JS, Choi HS, Dolan BM, Choi SY, et al. Inhibition of p21-activated kinase rescues symptoms of fragile X syndrome in mice. *Proc Natl Acad Sci USA* July 3, 2007;**104**(27): 11489–94.

69. Dolan BM, Duron SG, Campbell DA, Vollrath B, Shankaranarayana Rao BS, Ko HY, et al. Rescue of fragile X syndrome phenotypes in Fmr1 KO mice by the small-molecule PAK inhibitor FRAX486. *Proc Natl Acad Sci USA* April 2, 2013; **110**(14):5671–6.

70. Shimojima K, Sugawara M, Shichiji M, Mukaida S, Takayama R, Imai K, et al. Loss-of-function mutation of collybistin is responsible for X-linked mental retardation associated with epilepsy. *J Hum Genet* August 2011;**56**(8):561–5.

71. Reid T, Bathoorn A, Ahmadian MR, Collard JG. Identification and characterization of hPEM-2, a guanine nucleotide exchange factor specific for Cdc42. *J Biol Chem* November 19, 1999;**274**(47): 33587–93.

72. Marco EJ, Abidi FE, Bristow J, Dean WB, Cotter P, Jeremy RJ, et al. ARHGEF9 disruption in a female patient is associated with X linked mental retardation and sensory hyperarousal. *J Med Genet* February 2008;**45**(2):100–5.

73. Lesca G, Till M, Labalme A, Vallee D, Hugonenq C, Philip N, et al. De novo Xq11.11 microdeletion including ARHGEF9 in a boy with mental retardation, epilepsy, macrosomia, and dysmorphic features. *Am J Med Genet Part A* July 2011;**155A**(7):1706–11.

74. Harvey K, Duguid IC, Alldred MJ, Beatty SE, Ward H, Keep NH, et al. The GDP-GTP exchange factor collybistin: an essential determinant of neuronal gephyrin clustering. *J Neurosci* June 23, 2004; **24**(25):5816–26.

75. Kalscheuer VM, Musante L, Fang C, Hoffmann K, Fuchs C, Carta E, et al. A balanced chromosomal translocation disrupting ARHGEF9 is associated with epilepsy, anxiety, aggression, and mental retardation. *Hum Mutat* January 2009;**30**(1):61–8.

76. Kneussel M, Engelkamp D, Betz H. Distribution of transcripts for the brain-specific GDP/GTP exchange factor collybistin in the developing mouse brain. *Eur J Neurosci* February 2001;**13**(3): 487–92.

77. Kins S, Betz H, Kirsch J. Collybistin, a newly identified brain-specific GEF, induces submembrane clustering of gephyrin. *Nat Neurosci* January 2000;**3**(1):22–9.

78. Grosskreutz Y, Hermann A, Kins S, Fuhrmann JC, Betz H, Kneussel M. Identification of a gephyrin-binding motif in the GDP/GTP exchange factor collybistin. *Biol Chem* October 2001; **382**(10):1455–62.

79. Tretter V, Kerschner B, Milenkovic I, Ramsden SL, Ramerstorfer J, Saiepour L, et al. Molecular basis of the gamma-aminobutyric acid A receptor alpha3 subunit interaction with the clustering protein gephyrin. *J Biol Chem* October 28, 2011;**286**(43):37702–11.

80. Kowalczyk S, Winkelmann A, Smolinsky B, Forstera B, Neundorf I, Schwarz G, et al. Direct binding of GABAA receptor beta2 and beta3 subunits to gephyrin. *Eur J Neurosci* February 2013;**37**(4):544–54.

81. Yu W, Jiang M, Miralles CP, Li RW, Chen G, de Blas AL. Gephyrin clustering is required for the stability of GABAergic synapses. *Mol Cell Neurosci* December 2007;**36**(4):484–500.

82. Patrizi A, Scelfo B, Viltono L, Briatore F, Fukaya M, Watanabe M, et al. Synapse formation and clustering of neuroligin-2 in the absence of GABAA receptors. *Proc Natl Acad Sci USA* September 2, 2008;**105**(35):13151–6.

83. Meyer G, Kirsch J, Betz H, Langosch D. Identification of a gephyrin binding motif on the glycine receptor beta subunit. *Neuron* September 1995;**15**(3):563–72.

84. Patrizi A, Viltono L, Frola E, Harvey K, Harvey RJ, Sassoe-Pognetto M. Selective localization of collybistin at a subset of inhibitory synapses in brain circuits. *J Comp Neurol* January 1, 2012;**520**(1):130–41.

85. Kuhse J, Kalbouneh H, Schlicksupp A, Mukusch S, Nawrotzki R, Kirsch J. Phosphorylation of gephyrin in hippocampal neurons by cyclin-dependent kinase CDK5 at Ser-270 is dependent on collybistin. *J Biol Chem* September 7, 2012;**287**(37):30952–66.

86. Poulopoulos A, Aramuni G, Meyer G, Soykan T, Hoon M, Papadopoulos T, et al. Neuroligin 2 drives postsynaptic assembly at perisomatic inhibitory synapses through gephyrin and collybistin. *Neuron* September 10, 2009;**63**(5):628–42.

87. Hoon M, Soykan T, Falkenburger B, Hammer M, Patrizi A, Schmidt KF, et al. Neuroligin-4 is localized to glycinergic postsynapses and regulates inhibition in the retina. *Proc Natl Acad Sci USA* February 15, 2011;**108**(7):3053–8.

88. Saiepour L, Fuchs C, Patrizi A, Sassoe-Pognetto M, Harvey RJ, Harvey K. Complex role of collybistin and gephyrin in GABAA receptor clustering. *J Biol Chem* September 17, 2010;**285**(38):29623–31.

89. Bang ML, Owczarek S. A matter of balance: role of neurexin and neuroligin at the synapse. *Neurochem Res* June 2013;**38**(6):1174–89.

90. Soykan T, Schneeberger D, Tria G, Buechner C, Bader N, Svergun D, et al. A conformational switch in collybistin determines the differentiation of inhibitory postsynapses. *EMBO J* September 17, 2014;**33**(18):2113–33.

91. Jedlicka P, Hoon M, Papadopoulos T, Vlachos A, Winkels R, Poulopoulos A, et al. Increased dentate gyrus excitability in neuroligin-2-deficient mice in vivo. *Cereb Cortex* February 2011;**21**(2):357–67.

92. Panzanelli P, Gunn BG, Schlatter MC, Benke D, Tyagarajan SK, Scheiffele P, et al. Distinct mechanisms regulate GABAA receptor and gephyrin clustering at perisomatic and axo-axonic synapses on CA1 pyramidal cells. *J Physiol* October 15, 2011;**589**(Pt 20):4959–80.

93. Reddy-Alla S, Schmitt B, Birkenfeld J, Eulenburg V, Dutertre S, Bohringer C, et al. PH-domain-driven targeting of collybistin but not Cdc42 activation is required for synaptic gephyrin clustering. *Eur J Neurosci* April 2010;**31**(7):1173–84.

94. Tyagarajan SK, Ghosh H, Harvey K, Fritschy JM. Collybistin splice variants differentially interact with gephyrin and Cdc42 to regulate gephyrin clustering at GABAergic synapses. *J Cell Sci* August 15, 2011;**124**(Pt 16):2786–96.

95. Mayer S, Kumar R, Jaiswal M, Soykan T, Ahmadian MR, Brose N, et al. Collybistin activation by GTP-TC10 enhances postsynaptic gephyrin clustering and hippocampal GABAergic neurotransmission. *Proc Natl Acad Sci USA* December 17, 2013;**110**(51):20795–800.

96. Stenmark H. Rab GTPases as coordinators of vesicle traffic. *Nat Rev Mol Cell Biol* August 2009;**10**(8):513–25.

97. Ng EL, Tang BL. Rab GTPases and their roles in brain neurons and glia. *Brain Res Rev* June 2008;**58**(1):236–46.

98. Cheng H, Ma Y, Ni X, Jiang M, Guo L, Ying K, et al. Isolation and characterization of a human novel RAB (RAB39B) gene. *Cytogenet Genome Res* 2002;**97**(1–2):72–5.

99. Oldak M, Sciezynska A, Mlynarski W, Borowiec M, Ruszkowska E, Szulborski K, et al. Evidence against RAB40AL being the locus for Martin-Probst X-linked deafness-intellectual disability syndrome. *Hum Mutat* October 2014;**35**(10):1171–4.

100. Giannandrea M, Bianchi V, Mignogna ML, Sirri A, Carrabino S, D'Elia E, et al. Mutations in the small GTPase gene RAB39B are responsible for X-linked mental retardation associated with autism, epilepsy, and macrocephaly. *Am J Hum Genet* February 12, 2010;**86**(2):185–95.

101. Vanmarsenille L, Giannandrea M, Fieremans N, Verbeeck J, Belet S, Raynaud M, et al. Increased dosage of RAB39B affects neuronal development and could explain the cognitive impairment in male patients with distal Xq28 copy number gains. *Hum Mutat* March 2014;**35**(3):377–83.

102. Andersen EF, Baldwin EE, Ellingwood S, Smith R, Lamb AN. Xq28 duplication overlapping the int22h-1/int22h-2 region and including RAB39B and CLIC2 in a family with intellectual and developmental disability. *Am J Med Genet Part A* July 2014;**164A**(7):1795–801.

103. Wilson GR, Sim JC, McLean C, Giannandrea M, Galea CA, Riseley JR, et al. Mutations in RAB39B cause X-linked intellectual disability and early-onset Parkinson disease with alpha-synuclein pathology. *Am J Hum Genet* December 4, 2014;**95**(6):729–35.

104. Bellucci A, Zaltieri M, Navarria L, Grigoletto J, Missale C, Spano P. From alpha-synuclein to synaptic dysfunctions: new insights into the pathophysiology of Parkinson's disease. *Brain Res* October 2, 2012;**1476**:183–202.

105. Erdman RA, Maltese WA. Different Rab GTPases associate preferentially with alpha or beta GDP-dissociation inhibitors. *Biochem Biophys Res Commun* March 23, 2001;**282**(1):4–9.

106. D'Adamo P, Menegon A, Lo Nigro C, Grasso M, Gulisano M, Tamanini F, et al. Mutations in GDI1 are responsible for X-linked non-specific mental retardation. *Nat Genet* June 1998;**19**(2):134–9.

107. Strobl-Wildemann G, Kalscheuer VM, Hu H, Wrogemann K, Ropers HH, Tzschach A. Novel GDI1 mutation in a large family with nonsyndromic X-linked intellectual disability. *Am J Med Genet Part A* December 2011;**155A**(12):3067–70.

108. Pinto D, Delaby E, Merico D, Barbosa M, Merikangas A, Klei L, et al. Convergence of genes and cellular pathways dysregulated in autism spectrum disorders. *Am J Hum Genet* May 1, 2014;**94**(5):677–94.

109. D'Adamo P, Welzl H, Papadimitriou S, Raffaele di Barletta M, Tiveron C, Tatangelo L, et al. Deletion of the mental retardation gene Gdi1 impairs associative memory and alters social behavior in mice. *Hum Mol Genet* October 1, 2002;**11**(21):2567–80.

110. Bianchi V, Gambino F, Muzio L, Toniolo D, Humeau Y, D'Adamo P. Forebrain deletion of alphaGDI in adult mice worsens the pre-synaptic deficit at cortico-lateral amygdala synaptic connections. *PLoS One* 2012;**7**(1):e29763.

111. Bachner D, Sedlacek Z, Korn B, Hameister H, Poustka A. Expression patterns of two human genes coding for different rab GDP-dissociation inhibitors (GDIs), extremely conserved proteins involved in cellular transport. *Hum Mol Genet* April 1995;**4**(4):701–8.

112. Bianchi V, Farisello P, Baldelli P, Meskenaite V, Milanese M, Vecellio M, et al. Cognitive impairment in Gdi1-deficient mice is associated with altered synaptic vesicle pools and short-term synaptic plasticity, and can be corrected by appropriate learning training. *Hum Mol Genet* January 1, 2009;**18**(1):105–17.

113. Takai Y, Sasaki T, Shirataki H, Nakanishi H. Rab3A small GTP-binding protein in Ca(2+)-dependent exocytosis. *Genes Cells* July 1996;**1**(7):615–32.

114. D'Adamo P, Wolfer DP, Kopp C, Tobler I, Toniolo D, Lipp HP. Mice deficient for the synaptic vesicle protein Rab3a show impaired spatial reversal learning and increased explorative activity but none of the behavioral changes shown by mice deficient for the Rab3a regulator Gdi1. *Eur J Neurosci* April 2004;**19**(7):1895–905.

115. Mohrmann K, Gerez L, Oorschot V, Klumperman J, van der Sluijs P. Rab4 function in membrane recycling from early endosomes depends on a membrane to cytoplasm cycle. *J Biol Chem* August 30, 2002;**277**(35):32029–35.

116. Fischer von Mollard G, Stahl B, Li C, Sudhof TC, Jahn R. Rab proteins in regulated exocytosis. *Trends Biochem Sci* April 1994;**19**(4):164–8.

117. Bonanomi D, Benfenati F, Valtorta F. Protein sorting in the synaptic vesicle life cycle. *Prog Neurobiol* November 2006;**80**(4):177–217.

118. Wucherpfennig T, Wilsch-Brauninger M, Gonzalez-Gaitan M. Role of Drosophila Rab5 during endosomal trafficking at the synapse and evoked neurotransmitter release. *J Cell Biol* May 12, 2003; **161**(3):609–24.

119. Smith SM, Renden R, von Gersdorff H. Synaptic vesicle endocytosis: fast and slow modes of membrane retrieval. *Trends Neurosci* November 2008;**31**(11):559–68.

120. Voglmaier SM, Kam K, Yang H, Fortin DL, Hua Z, Nicoll RA, et al. Distinct endocytic pathways control the rate and extent of synaptic vesicle protein recycling. *Neuron* July 6, 2006;**51**(1):71–84.

121. Chater TE, Goda Y. The role of AMPA receptors in postsynaptic mechanisms of synaptic plasticity. *Front Cell Neurosci* 2014;**8**:401.

122. Gan Q, Salussolia CL, Wollmuth LP. Assembly of AMPA receptors: mechanisms and regulation. *J Physiol* January 1, 2015; **593**(1):39–48.

123. Shepherd JD, Huganir RL. The cell biology of synaptic plasticity: AMPA receptor trafficking. *Annu Rev Cell Dev Biol* 2007;**23**:613–43.

124. Lu W, Roche KW. Posttranslational regulation of AMPA receptor trafficking and function. *Curr Opin Neurobiol* June 2012;**22**(3): 470–9.

125. Huganir RL, Nicoll RA. AMPARs and synaptic plasticity: the last 25 years. *Neuron* October 30, 2013;**80**(3):704–17.

126. Bassani S, Folci A, Zapata J, Passafaro M. AMPAR trafficking in synapse maturation and plasticity. *Cell Mol Life Sci* December 2013;**70**(23):4411–30.

127. Gecz J, Barnett S, Liu J, Hollway G, Donnelly A, Eyre H, et al. Characterization of the human glutamate receptor subunit 3 gene (GRIA3), a candidate for bipolar disorder and nonspecific X-linked mental retardation. *Genomics* December 15, 1999;**62**(3):356–68.

128. Chiyonobu T, Hayashi S, Kobayashi K, Morimoto M, Miyanomae Y, Nishimura A, et al. Partial tandem duplication of GRIA3 in a male with mental retardation. *Am J Med Genet Part A* July 1, 2007;**143A**(13):1448–55.

129. Wu Y, Arai AC, Rumbaugh G, Srivastava AK, Turner G, Hayashi T, et al. Mutations in ionotropic AMPA receptor 3 alter channel properties and are associated with moderate cognitive impairment in humans. *Proc Natl Acad Sci USA* November 13, 2007;**104**(46):18163–8.

130. Bonnet C, Leheup B, Beri M, Philippe C, Gregoire MJ, Jonveaux P. Aberrant GRIA3 transcripts with multi-exon duplications in a family with X-linked mental retardation. *Am J Med Genet Part A* June 2009;**149A**(6):1280–9.

131. Bonnet C, Masurel-Paulet A, Khan AA, Beri-Dexheimer M, Callier P, Mugneret F, et al. Exploring the potential role of disease-causing mutation in a gene desert: duplication of noncoding elements 5′ of GRIA3 is associated with GRIA3 silencing and X-linked intellectual disability. *Hum Mutat* February 2012;**33**(2):355–8.

132. Philippe A, Malan V, Jacquemont ML, Boddaert N, Bonnefont JP, Odent S, et al. Xq25 duplications encompassing GRIA3 and STAG2 genes in two families convey recognizable X-linked intellectual disability with distinctive facial appearance. *Am J Med Genet Part A* June 2013;**161A**(6):1370–5.

133. Philips AK, Siren A, Avela K, Somer M, Peippo M, Ahvenainen M, et al. X-exome sequencing in Finnish families with intellectual disability—four novel mutations and two novel syndromic phenotypes. *Orphanet J Rare Dis* 2014;**9**:49.

134. Adamczyk A, Mejias R, Takamiya K, Yocum J, Krasnova IN, Calderon J, et al. GluA3-deficiency in mice is associated with increased social and aggressive behavior and elevated dopamine in striatum. *Behav Brain Res* April 1, 2012;**229**(1):265–72.

135. Zamanillo D, Sprengel R, Hvalby O, Jensen V, Burnashev N, Rozov A, et al. Importance of AMPA receptors for hippocampal synaptic plasticity but not for spatial learning. *Science* June 11, 1999;**284**(5421):1805–11.

136. Meng Y, Zhang Y, Jia Z. Synaptic transmission and plasticity in the absence of AMPA glutamate receptor GluR2 and GluR3. *Neuron* July 3, 2003;**39**(1):163–76.

137. Toyoda H, Wu LJ, Zhao MG, Xu H, Jia Z, Zhuo M. Long-term depression requires postsynaptic AMPA GluR2 receptor in adult mouse cingulate cortex. *J Cell Physiol* May 2007;**211**(2): 336–43.

138. Steenland HW, Kim SS, Zhuo M. GluR3 subunit regulates sleep, breathing and seizure generation. *Eur J Neurosci* March 2008; **27**(5):1166–73.

139. Boucheix C, Rubinstein E. Tetraspanins. *Cell Mol Life Sci* August 2001;**58**(9):1189–205.

140. Hemler ME. Targeting of tetraspanin proteins—potential benefits and strategies. *Nat Rev Drug Discov* September 2008;**7**(9):747–58.

141. Berditchevski F. Complexes of tetraspanins with integrins: more than meets the eye. *J Cell Sci* December 2001;**114**(Pt 23): 4143–51.

142. Yanez-Mo M, Barreiro O, Gordon-Alonso M, Sala-Valdes M, Sanchez-Madrid F. Tetraspanin-enriched microdomains: a functional unit in cell plasma membranes. *Trends Cell Biol* September 2009;**19**(9):434–46.

143. Maecker HT, Todd SC, Levy S. The tetraspanin superfamily: molecular facilitators. *FASEB J* May 1997;**11**(6):428–42.

144. Hemler ME. Tetraspanin functions and associated microdomains. *Nat Rev Mol Cell Biol* October 2005;**6**(10):801–11.

145. Holinski-Feder E, Chahrockh-Zadeh S, Rittinger O, Jedele KB, Gasteiger M, Lenski C, et al. Nonsyndromic X-linked mental retardation: mapping of MRX58 to the pericentromeric region. *Am J Med Genet* September 10, 1999;**86**(2):102–6.

146. Zemni R, Bienvenu T, Vinet MC, Sefiani A, Carrie A, Billuart P, et al. A new gene involved in X-linked mental retardation identified by analysis of an X;2 balanced translocation. *Nat Genet* February 2000;**24**(2):167–70.

147. Abidi FE, Holinski-Feder E, Rittinger O, Kooy F, Lubs HA, Stevenson RE, et al. A novel 2 bp deletion in the TM4SF2 gene is associated with MRX58. *J Med Genet* June 2002;**39**(6):430–3.

148. Gomot M, Ronce N, Dessay S, Zemni R, Ayrault AD, Moizard MP, et al. TM4SF2 gene involvement reconsidered in an XLMR family after neuropsychological assessment. *Am J Med Genet* November 1, 2002;**112**(4):400–4.

149. De Vos B, Frints S, Borghgraef M, Fryns JP. Cognitive and behavioral characteristics in 4 affected males of a family with nonspecific X-linked mental retardation and TM4 SF2-gene mutation. *Genet Couns* 2002;**13**(2):191–4.

150. Maranduba CM, Sa Moreira E, Muller Orabona G, Pavanello RC, Vianna-Morgante AM, Passos-Bueno MR. Does the P172H mutation at the TM4SF2 gene cause X-linked mental retardation? *Am J Med Genet Part A* February 1, 2004;**124A**(4):413–5.

151. Noor A, Gianakopoulos PJ, Fernandez B, Marshall CR, Szatmari P, Roberts W, et al. Copy number variation analysis and sequencing of the X-linked mental retardation gene TSPAN7/TM4SF2 in patients with autism spectrum disorder. *Psychiatr Genet* June 2009;**19**(3):154–5.

152. Piton A, Gauthier J, Hamdan FF, Lafreniere RG, Yang Y, Henrion E, et al. Systematic resequencing of X-chromosome synaptic genes in autism spectrum disorder and schizophrenia. *Mol Psychiatry* August 2011;**16**(8):867–80.

153. Bassani S, Cingolani LA, Valnegri P, Folci A, Zapata J, Gianfelice A, et al. The X-linked intellectual disability protein TSPAN7 regulates excitatory synapse development and AMPAR trafficking. *Neuron* March 22, 2012;**73**(6):1143–58.

154. Perez JL, Khatri L, Chang C, Srivastava S, Osten P, Ziff EB. PICK1 targets activated protein kinase Calpha to AMPA receptor clusters in spines of hippocampal neurons and reduces surface levels of the AMPA-type glutamate receptor subunit 2. *J Neurosci* August 1, 2001;**21**(15):5417–28.

155. Hoskins R, Hajnal AF, Harp SA, Kim SK. The *C. elegans* vulval induction gene lin-2 encodes a member of the MAGUK family of cell junction proteins. *Development* January 1996;**122**(1): 97–111.

156. Hata Y, Butz S, Sudhof TC. CASK: a novel dlg/PSD95 homolog with an N-terminal calmodulin-dependent protein kinase domain identified by interaction with neurexins. *J Neurosci* April 15, 1996;**16**(8):2488–94.

157. Montgomery JM, Zamorano PL, Garner CC. MAGUKs in synapse assembly and function: an emerging view. *Cell Mol Life Sci* April 2004;**61**(7–8):911–29.

158. Moog U, Uyanik G, Kutsche K. CASK-related disorders. In: Pagon RA, Adam MP, Ardinger HH, Bird TD, Dolan CR, Fong CT, et al., editors. *GeneReviews®. Seattle (WA)*; 1993.

159. Gillespie JM, Hodge JJ. CASK regulates CaMKII autophosphorylation in neuronal growth, calcium signaling, and learning. *Front Mol Neurosci* 2013;**6**:27.

160. Hsueh YP, Yang FC, Kharazia V, Naisbitt S, Cohen AR, Weinberg RJ, et al. Direct interaction of CASK/LIN-2 and syndecan heparan sulfate proteoglycan and their overlapping distribution in neuronal synapses. *J Cell Biol* July 13, 1998;**142**(1): 139–51.

161. Zheng CY, Seabold GK, Horak M, Petralia RS. MAGUKs, synaptic development, and synaptic plasticity. *Neuroscientist* October 2011;**17**(5):493–512.

162. Butz S, Okamoto M, Sudhof TC. A tripartite protein complex with the potential to couple synaptic vesicle exocytosis to cell adhesion in brain. *Cell* September 18, 1998;**94**(6):773–82.

163. Tabuchi K, Biederer T, Butz S, Sudhof TC. CASK participates in alternative tripartite complexes in which Mint 1 competes for binding with caskin 1, a novel CASK-binding protein. *J Neurosci* June 1, 2002;**22**(11):4264–73.

164. Maximov A, Sudhof TC, Bezprozvanny I. Association of neuronal calcium channels with modular adaptor proteins. *J Biol Chem* August 27, 1999;**274**(35):24453–6.

165. Fairless R, Masius H, Rohlmann A, Heupel K, Ahmad M, Reissner C, et al. Polarized targeting of neurexins to synapses is regulated by their C-terminal sequences. *J Neurosci* November 26, 2008;**28**(48):12969–81.

166. Setou M, Nakagawa T, Seog DH, Hirokawa N. Kinesin superfamily motor protein KIF17 and mLin-10 in NMDA receptor-containing vesicle transport. *Science* June 9, 2000;**288**(5472): 1796–802.

167. Lin EI, Jeyifous O, Green WN. CASK regulates SAP97 conformation and its interactions with AMPA and NMDA receptors. *J Neurosci* July 17, 2013;**33**(29):12067–76.

168. Jeyifous O, Waites CL, Specht CG, Fujisawa S, Schubert M, Lin EI, et al. SAP97 and CASK mediate sorting of NMDA receptors through a previously unknown secretory pathway. *Nat Neurosci* August 2009;**12**(8):1011–9.

169. Hsueh YP, Wang TF, Yang FC, Sheng M. Nuclear translocation and transcription regulation by the membrane-associated guanylate kinase CASK/LIN-2. *Nature* March 16, 2000;**404**(6775): 298–302.

170. Wang TF, Ding CN, Wang GS, Luo SC, Lin YL, Ruan Y, et al. Identification of Tbr-1/CASK complex target genes in neurons. *J Neurochem* December 2004;**91**(6):1483–92.

171. Hsueh YP. Calcium/calmodulin-dependent serine protein kinase and mental retardation. *Ann Neurol* October 2009;**66**(4):438–43.

172. Najm J, Horn D, Wimplinger I, Golden JA, Chizhikov VV, Sudi J, et al. Mutations of CASK cause an X-linked brain malformation phenotype with microcephaly and hypoplasia of the brainstem and cerebellum. *Nat Genet* September 2008;**40**(9):1065–7.

173. Chao HW, Hong CJ, Huang TN, Lin YL, Hsueh YP. SUMOylation of the MAGUK protein CASK regulates dendritic spinogenesis. *J Cell Biol* July 14, 2008;**182**(1):141–55.

174. Samuels BA, Hsueh YP, Shu T, Liang H, Tseng HC, Hong CJ, et al. Cdk5 promotes synaptogenesis by regulating the subcellular distribution of the MAGUK family member CASK. *Neuron* December 6, 2007;**56**(5):823–37.

175. Huang TN, Chang HP, Hsueh YP. CASK phosphorylation by PKA regulates the protein-protein interactions of CASK and expression of the NMDAR2b gene. *J Neurochem* March 2010;**112**(6):1562–73.

176. Atasoy D, Schoch S, Ho A, Nadasy KA, Liu X, Zhang W, et al. Deletion of CASK in mice is lethal and impairs synaptic function. *Proc Natl Acad Sci USA* February 13, 2007;**104**(7):2525–30.

177. Watkins RJ, Patil R, Goult BT, Thomas MG, Gottlob I, Shackleton S. A novel interaction between FRMD7 and CASK: evidence for a causal role in idiopathic infantile nystagmus. *Hum Mol Genet* May 15, 2013;**22**(10):2105–18.

178. Makino K, Kuwahara H, Masuko N, Nishiyama Y, Morisaki T, Sasaki J, et al. Cloning and characterization of NE-dlg: a novel human homolog of the Drosophila discs large (dlg) tumor suppressor protein interacts with the APC protein. *Oncogene* May 22, 1997; **14**(20):2425–33.

179. Sans N, Petralia RS, Wang YX, Blahos 2nd J, Hell JW, Wenthold RJ. A developmental change in NMDA receptor-associated proteins at hippocampal synapses. *J Neurosci* February 1, 2000;**20**(3): 1260–71.

180. van Zundert B, Yoshii A, Constantine-Paton M. Receptor compartmentalization and trafficking at glutamate synapses: a developmental proposal. *Trends Neurosci* July 2004;**27**(7):428–37.

181. Petralia RS, Sans N, Wang YX, Wenthold RJ. Ontogeny of postsynaptic density proteins at glutamatergic synapses. *Mol Cell Neurosci* July 2005;**29**(3):436–52.

182. Washbourne P, Liu XB, Jones EG, McAllister AK. Cycling of NMDA receptors during trafficking in neurons before synapse formation. *J Neurosci* September 22, 2004;**24**(38):8253–64.

183. Washbourne P, Bennett JE, McAllister AK. Rapid recruitment of NMDA receptor transport packets to nascent synapses. *Nat Neurosci* August 2002;**5**(8):751–9.

184. Muller BM, Kistner U, Kindler S, Chung WJ, Kuhlendahl S, Fenster SD, et al. SAP102, a novel postsynaptic protein that interacts with NMDA receptor complexes in vivo. *Neuron* August 1996;**17**(2):255–65.

185. Sans N, Wang PY, Du Q, Petralia RS, Wang YX, Nakka S, et al. mPins modulates PSD-95 and SAP102 trafficking and influences NMDA receptor surface expression. *Nat Cell Biol* December 2005;**7**(12):1179–90.

186. Zheng CY, Petralia RS, Wang YX, Kachar B, Wenthold RJ. SAP102 is a highly mobile MAGUK in spines. *J Neurosci* March 31, 2010; **30**(13):4757–66.

187. Chen BS, Gray JA, Sanz-Clemente A, Wei Z, Thomas EV, Nicoll RA, et al. SAP102 mediates synaptic clearance of NMDA receptors. *Cell Rep* November 29, 2012;**2**(5):1120–8.

188. Yoshii A, Sheng MH, Constantine-Paton M. Eye opening induces a rapid dendritic localization of PSD-95 in central visual neurons. *Proc Natl Acad Sci USA* February 4, 2003;**100**(3):1334–9.

189. Masuko N, Makino K, Kuwahara H, Fukunaga K, Sudo T, Araki N, et al. Interaction of NE-dlg/SAP102, a neuronal and endocrine tissue-specific membrane-associated guanylate kinase protein, with calmodulin and PSD-95/SAP90. A possible regulatory role in molecular clustering at synaptic sites. *J Biol Chem* February 26, 1999;**274**(9):5782–90.

190. McGee AW, Dakoji SR, Olsen O, Bredt DS, Lim WA, Prehoda KE. Structure of the SH3-guanylate kinase module from PSD-95 suggests a mechanism for regulated assembly of MAGUK scaffolding proteins. *Mol Cell* December 2001;**8**(6):1291–301.

191. Bonnet SA, Akad DS, Samaddar T, Liu Y, Huang X, Dong Y, et al. Synaptic state-dependent functional interplay between postsynaptic density-95 and synapse-associated protein 102. *J Neurosci* August 14, 2013;**33**(33):13398–409.

192. Dakoji S, Tomita S, Karimzadegan S, Nicoll RA, Bredt DS. Interaction of transmembrane AMPA receptor regulatory proteins with multiple membrane associated guanylate kinases. *Neuropharmacology* November 2003;**45**(6):849–56.

193. Cuthbert PC, Stanford LE, Coba MP, Ainge JA, Fink AE, Opazo P, et al. Synapse-associated protein 102/dlgh3 couples the NMDA receptor to specific plasticity pathways and learning strategies. *J Neurosci* March 7, 2007;**27**(10):2673–82.

194. Murata Y, Constantine-Paton M. Postsynaptic density scaffold SAP102 regulates cortical synapse development through EphB and PAK signaling pathway. *J Neurosci* March 13, 2013;**33**(11): 5040–52.

195. Tarpey P, Parnau J, Blow M, Woffendin H, Bignell G, Cox C, et al. Mutations in the DLG3 gene cause nonsyndromic X-linked mental retardation. *Am J Hum Genet* August 2004; **75**(2):318–24.

196. Meyer G, Varoqueaux F, Neeb A, Oschlies M, Brose N. The complexity of PDZ domain-mediated interactions at glutamatergic synapses: a case study on neuroligin. *Neuropharmacology* October 2004;**47**(5):724–33.

197. Lauks J, Klemmer P, Farzana F, Karupothula R, Zalm R, Cooke NE, et al. Synapse associated protein 102 (SAP102) binds the C-terminal part of the scaffolding protein neurobeachin. *PloS One* 2012;**7**(6):e39420.

198. Garcia EP, Mehta S, Blair LA, Wells DG, Shang J, Fukushima T, et al. SAP90 binds and clusters kainate receptors causing incomplete desensitization. *Neuron* October 1998;**21**(4):727–39.

199. Thurner P, Gsandtner I, Kudlacek O, Choquet D, Nanoff C, Freissmuth M, et al. A two-state model for the diffusion of the A2A adenosine receptor in hippocampal neurons: agonist-induced switch to slow mobility is modified by synapse-associated protein 102 (SAP102). *J Biol Chem* March 28, 2014; **289**(13):9263–74.

200. Jahn R, Schiebler W, Ouimet C, Greengard PA. 38,000-dalton membrane protein (p38) present in synaptic vesicles. *Proc Natl Acad Sci USA* June 1985;**82**(12):4137–41.

201. Wiedenmann B, Franke WW. Identification and localization of synaptophysin, an integral membrane glycoprotein of Mr 38,000 characteristic of presynaptic vesicles. *Cell* July 1985;**41**(3): 1017–28.

202. Navone F, Jahn R, Di Gioia G, Stukenbrok H, Greengard P, De Camilli P. Protein p38: an integral membrane protein specific for small vesicles of neurons and neuroendocrine cells. *J Cell Biol* December 1986;**103**(6 Pt 1):2511–27.

203. Takamori S, Holt M, Stenius K, Lemke EA, Gronborg M, Riedel D, et al. Molecular anatomy of a trafficking organelle. *Cell* November 17, 2006;**127**(4):831–46.

204. Arthur CP, Stowell MH. Structure of synaptophysin: a hexameric MARVEL-domain channel protein. *Structure* June 2007;**15**(6): 707–14.

205. Rehm H, Wiedenmann B, Betz H. Molecular characterization of synaptophysin, a major calcium-binding protein of the synaptic vesicle membrane. *EMBO J* March 1986;**5**(3):535–41.

206. Thomas L, Hartung K, Langosch D, Rehm H, Bamberg E, Franke WW, et al. Identification of synaptophysin as a hexameric channel protein of the synaptic vesicle membrane. *Science* November 18, 1988;**242**(4881):1050–3.

207. Johnston PA, Sudhof TC. The multisubunit structure of synaptophysin. Relationship between disulfide bonding and homo-oligomerization. *J Biol Chem* May 25, 1990;**265**(15):8869–73.

208. Gincel D, Shoshan-Barmatz V. The synaptic vesicle protein synaptophysin: purification and characterization of its channel activity. *Biophysical J* December 2002;**83**(6):3223–9.

209. Valtorta F, Pennuto M, Bonanomi D, Benfenati F. Synaptophysin: leading actor or walk-on role in synaptic vesicle exocytosis? *BioEssays* April 2004;**26**(4):445–53.

210. Thiele C, Hannah MJ, Fahrenholz F, Huttner WB. Cholesterol binds to synaptophysin and is required for biogenesis of synaptic vesicles. *Nat Cell Biol* January 2000;**2**(1):42–9.

211. Rizzoli SO. Synaptic vesicle recycling: steps and principles. *EMBO J* April 16, 2014;**33**(8):788–822.

212. Regnier-Vigouroux A, Tooze SA, Huttner WB. Newly synthesized synaptophysin is transported to synaptic-like microvesicles via constitutive secretory vesicles and the plasma membrane. *EMBO J* December 1991;**10**(12):3589–601.

213. Leube RE. The topogenic fate of the polytopic transmembrane proteins, synaptophysin and connexin, is determined by their membrane-spanning domains. *J Cell Sci* March 1995;**108**(Pt 3): 883–94.

214. Leube RE, Wiedenmann B, Franke WW. Topogenesis and sorting of synaptophysin: synthesis of a synaptic vesicle protein from a gene transfected into nonneuroendocrine cells. *Cell* November 3, 1989;**59**(3):433–46.

215. Pennuto M, Bonanomi D, Benfenati F, Valtorta F. Synaptophysin I controls the targeting of VAMP2/synaptobrevin II to synaptic vesicles. *Mol Biol Cell* December 2003;**14**(12):4909–19.

216. Siddiqui TJ, Vites O, Stein A, Heintzmann R, Jahn R, Fasshauer D. Determinants of synaptobrevin regulation in membranes. *Mol Biol Cell* June 2007;**18**(6):2037–46.

217. Pennuto M, Dunlap D, Contestabile A, Benfenati F, Valtorta F. Fluorescence resonance energy transfer detection of synaptophysin I and vesicle-associated membrane protein 2 interactions during exocytosis from single live synapses. *Mol Biol Cell* August 2002;**13**(8):2706–17.

218. Heuser JE, Reese TS, Dennis MJ, Jan Y, Jan L, Evans L. Synaptic vesicle exocytosis captured by quick freezing and correlated with quantal transmitter release. *J Cell Biol* May 1979;**81**(2): 275–300.

219. Heuser JE, Reese TS. Structural changes after transmitter release at the frog neuromuscular junction. *J Cell Biol* March 1981;**88**(3): 564–80.

220. Miller TM, Heuser JE. Endocytosis of synaptic vesicle membrane at the frog neuromuscular junction. *J Cell Biol* February 1984;**98**(2): 685–98.

221. Valtorta F, Fesce R, Grohovaz F, Haimann C, Hurlbut WP, Iezzi N, et al. Neurotransmitter release and synaptic vesicle recycling. *Neuroscience* 1990;**35**(3):477–89.

222. Fesce R, Grohovaz F, Valtorta F, Meldolesi J. Neurotransmitter release: fusion or 'kiss-and-run'? *Trends Cell Biol* January 1994; **4**(1):1–4.

223. Valtorta F, Meldolesi J, Fesce R. Synaptic vesicles: is kissing a matter of competence? *Trends Cell Biol* August 2001;**11**(8):324–8.

224. Kwon SE, Chapman ER. Synaptophysin regulates the kinetics of synaptic vesicle endocytosis in central neurons. *Neuron* June 9, 2011;**70**(5):847–54.

225. Daly C, Sugimori M, Moreira JE, Ziff EB, Llinas R. Synaptophysin regulates clathrin-independent endocytosis of synaptic vesicles. *Proc Natl Acad Sci USA* May 23, 2000;**97**(11):6120–5.

226. Daly C, Ziff EB. Ca2+-dependent formation of a dynamin-synaptophysin complex: potential role in synaptic vesicle endocytosis. *J Biol Chem* March 15, 2002;**277**(11):9010–5.

227. Horikawa HP, Kneussel M, El Far O, Betz H. Interaction of synaptophysin with the AP-1 adaptor protein gamma-adaptin. *Mol Cell Neurosci* November 2002;**21**(3):454–62.

228. Tarpey PS, Smith R, Pleasance E, Whibley A, Edkins S, Hardy C, et al. A systematic, large-scale resequencing screen of X-chromosome coding exons in mental retardation. *Nat Genet* May 2009;**41**(5):535–43.

229. Janz R, Sudhof TC, Hammer RE, Unni V, Siegelbaum SA, Bolshakov VY. Essential roles in synaptic plasticity for synaptogyrin I and synaptophysin I. *Neuron* November 1999;**24**(3): 687–700.

II. FUNCTION OF MUTATED GENES IN INTELLECTUAL DISABILITY (ID) AND AUTISM

230. Schmitt U, Tanimoto N, Seeliger M, Schaeffel F, Leube RE. Detection of behavioral alterations and learning deficits in mice lacking synaptophysin. *Neuroscience* August 18, 2009;**162**(2):234—43.

231. Gordon SL, Leube RE, Cousin MA. Synaptophysin is required for synaptobrevin retrieval during synaptic vesicle endocytosis. *J Neurosci* September 28, 2011;**31**(39):14032—6.

232. Gordon SL, Cousin MA. X-linked intellectual disability-associated mutations in synaptophysin disrupt synaptobrevin II retrieval. *J Neurosci* August 21, 2013;**33**(34):13695—700.

233. McMahon HT, Bolshakov VY, Janz R, Hammer RE, Siegelbaum SA, Sudhof TC. Synaptophysin, a major synaptic vesicle protein, is not essential for neurotransmitter release. *Proc Natl Acad Sci USA* May 14, 1996;**93**(10):4760—4.

10

SHANK Mutations in Intellectual Disability and Autism Spectrum Disorder

Michael J. Schmeisser[1,2], Chiara Verpelli[3,4]

[1]Institute for Anatomy and Cell Biology, Ulm University, Ulm, Germany; [2]Department of Neurology, Ulm University, Ulm, Germany; [3]CNR Neuroscience Institute, Milan, Italy; [4]Department of Medical Biotechnology and Translational Medicine, University of Milan, Milan, Italy

SHANK MUTATIONS AND HUMAN NEURODEVELOPMENTAL DISORDERS

SHANK1 deletions, which are caused by de novo copy number variations, were found in seven patients with high functional autism.[1] Four males were from a multigenerational family that carries inherited deletions of 63.8 kb, eliminating exons 1–20 of *SHANK1*. Interestingly, two females in the same family carry the deletion with no clinical symptoms. In the same study, an unrelated male with a de novo deletion at the same locus exhibited high functional autism without intellectual disability (ID). These results suggest that *SHANK1* deletions cause high functional autism in males, whereas tentatively, similar deletions result in no such phenotype in females. This suggests some type of linkage between *SHANK1* mutations and sex. Although samples sizes are still small, no *SHANK1* duplications have yet been found in any ASD patient.

SHANK2 mutations are associated with autism spectrum disorder (ASD), moderate ID, developmental delay, and mild motor deficits. Initially, three penetrant de novo mutations and seven rare inherited variants in *SHANK2* have been detected in patients with ASD and/or ID.[2] Other independent studies reported further *SHANK2* mutations.[3–8] However, no *SHANK2* duplications have yet been found in patients.

The *SHANK3* gene has been most extensively studied because it is the main gene associated with neuropsychiatric symptoms of patients with Phelan McDermid syndrome (PMS).[9–11] The syndrome is characterized by a significant expressive language delay, ID, hypotonia, minor craniofacial dysmorphisms, increased tolerance to pain, epilepsy, and autism-like features.[12] Translocations, encompassing the last two exons of *SHANK3* and parts of *ACR*, have been observed in a patient with a PMS-like phenotype, which further indicates the role of *SHANK3* in this syndrome.[13] Interestingly, the typical phenotypic variability in PMS-patients is also present in patients carrying *SHANK3* de novo or truncating mutations.[14] In general, *SHANK3* is strongly involved in the pathogenesis of ASD, and *SHANK3* truncating mutations are associated with moderate to profound ID. Since the initial identification of de novo mutations, interstitial and terminal deletions of SHANK3,[15] mutations in this gene have been identified in various studies on ASD and/or ID patients.[14–27] Unlike SHANK1 and SHANK2, SHANK3 duplications have been observed in patients with neuropsychiatric conditions. For example, one PMS-patient carrying a 22q13 deletion has a brother who exhibits a reciprocal 22qter duplication and is affected by Asperger syndrome,[15] an ASD variant. In addition, the sister of a boy with a SHANK3 deletion and ASD has a reciprocal SHANK3 duplication associated with a clinical diagnosis of attention-deficit hyperactivity disorder.[16] Furthermore, increased levels of SHANK3 gene methylation were found in a cohort of patients with ASD. These results suggest that epigenetic dysregulation of SHANK3 gene may also contribute to ASD pathogenesis.[28]

Leblond et al. performed a large meta-analysis on SHANK mutations in ASD confirming that mutations in SHANK1 were detected in 0.04% of ASD patients all with normal intelligence quotient, whereas mutations in SHANK2 were found in 0.17% of ASD patients associated with mild to moderate ID and mutations in SHANK3 were identified in 0.69% of ASD patients displaying moderate to severe/profound ID.[14] These results imply that mutations in SHANK1, SHANK2, or SHANK3 have varying impacts on brain physiology and function.

Moreover, there is increasing evidence to suggest a SHANK-related genetic and biological overlap between ASD and schizophrenia (SCZ). In a study that analyzed 199 patients with a diagnosis of SCZ, an association was demonstrated between the SHANK1 promoter variant rs3818280 and a deficiency of working memory.[29] In addition, rare SHANK2 missense variants[30] and two de novo mutations in SHANK3[31] were found while analyzing cohorts of patients affected by SCZ.

In the past few years, a number of studies have also demonstrated that a variety of genetic alterations can sustain broad susceptibility to both autistic and epileptic manifestations.[32] In particular, data indicate that SHANK genes are involved in both of these pathologies. For example, a large 22q13 deletion containing SHANK3 was found in a patient with rolandic epilepsia and slow-wave sleep syndrome (CSWSS)[33] and more recently, a large de novo 19q13 deletion encompassing SHANK1 was also found in a patient with CSWSS.[34]

SHANK EXPRESSION

Shank (or ProSAP) proteins, encoded by Shank1, Shank2, and Shank3 in rodents and located in the postsynaptic density (PSD) of glutamatergic synapses,

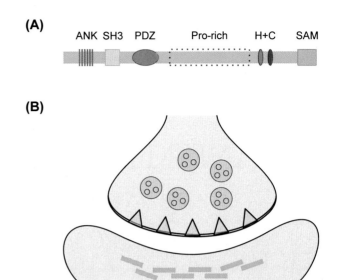

FIGURE 1 (A) Schematic overview of the domain composition of full-length Shank. ANK, ankyrin repeats; SH3, Src homology 3 domain; PDZ, PSD95/Dlg1/ZO1 domain; Pro-rich, proline-rich region; H + C, Homer and Cortactin binding sites; SAM, sterile alpha motif domain. (B) Schematic presentation of the postsynaptic Shank platform at the excitatory synapse. (A, B): Shank is marked with orange. *Adapted from Schmeisser.[80]*

comprise five conserved protein–protein interaction domains in sequence: 5-6 N-terminal ankyrin repeats (ANK), a Src homology 3 domain (SH3), a PDZ domain, a proline-rich region (Pro), Homer and Cortactin binding sites (H + C), and a sterile alpha motif domain (SAM) at the very C-terminus (Figure 1). The three Shank genes code for several messenger ribonucleic acid (mRNA) splice variants that generate several protein isoforms, including full-length Shank proteins, which are large proteins of approximately 180–230 kDa. With these domains Shank proteins interact with more than 30 synaptic proteins including other scaffold molecules, glutamatergic receptors, and cytoskeletal proteins.[35–38] In addition, Shank molecules self-associate via their SAM domain in the presence of Zn^{2+}; in particular Zn^{2+} acts specifically on Shank2 and Shank3 and regulates the formation of a huge postsynaptic molecular assembly platform for other PSD proteins.[37,39]

Shank1 is composed of 23 exons coding for four different isoforms.[40] Shank2 is composed of 25 exons also coding for four different isoforms.[38,41,42] Shank3 is composed of 22 exons coding for an extensive number of mRNA and protein isoforms derived from multiple intragenic promoters and alternatively spliced coding exons.[28,43,44] In the 5′ promoter of Shank3, five CpG islands are present, which display a brain region–specific deoxyribonucleic acid methylation pattern causing tissue-specific expression of Shank3.[45–47] These different isoforms are thought to be expressed in a cell-type, developmental and activity-dependent manner and were shown to have different effects on spine number and morphology.[44] Regarding their subcellular location, mRNAs coding for Shank proteins are widely expressed close to synapses in the mammalian brain with significant regional differences.[48]

The three *Shank* genes appear to be coexpressed in most principal neurons in areas such as cerebral cortex and hippocampus. *Shank1* mRNA is strongly present in brain, especially in neurons of the cortex and hippocampus, and in cerebellar Purkinje cells, whereas low levels of *Shank1* mRNA are also present in the striatum.[48,49] Among the three family members, *Shank1* mRNA is the most abundant transcript in the neuropil of the rat hippocampus, followed by *Shank3* and then *Shank2* mRNA. All three transcripts are more enriched in the neuropil than in the somata, which indicates that local translation is an essential source of Shank proteins at synapse.[50] Furthermore, translation of dendritic *Shank1* mRNA is controlled by fragile X mental retardation protein (FMRP).[51,52] *Shank2* mRNA is strongly expressed in the brain and at lower levels in the kidney and liver.[40,53] In particular, *Shank2* mRNA is present in neurons of the cortex, hippocampus and striatum, whereas in the cerebellum, it is selectively expressed only in Purkinje cells.[41,48,49,54] *Shank3* mRNA is highly expressed in the brain, heart, and spleen.[40] In the brain, *Shank3* mRNA expression overlaps with *Shank2* mRNA distribution except for the hippocampus, where it is predominantly found in CA3 neurons, and in the cerebellum, where *Shank3* expression is restricted to granule cells.[48,49,54]

On a subcellular level, Shank proteins are differently located in the PSD, and modification of their distribution has a critical role in structural changes of spine morphology during synaptic activity. Assembly of Shank1 at the synapse needs the formation of a complex with GKAP and PSD-95.[55] Under basal conditions, Shank1 is diffused in the body of spines, whereas Shank2 is more concentrated closer to the PSD. After depolarization there is a strong increase of Shank1 on the tip of the spines that is reverted within 30 min.[56] These data corroborate the hypothesis that Shank2 and Shank3 are core elements of the PSD protein complex whereas Shank1 is more involved in plastic changes of spines. Shank proteins are also differently incorporated into the PSD during neuronal development.[40,41] In particular Shank2 is one of the first proteins that appears in the developing PSD, followed by Shank3, with Shank1 being incorporated only later.[37] These data suggest that Shank2 and Shank3 are critical for the initial assembly and stability of immature synapses whereas Shank1 has a major role in synapse maturation.[37,57] Further studies show that synaptic targeting of Shank2 and Shank3 is mediated via their C-terminal SAM

domains,[58] whereas Shank1 is targeted to the synapse by its PDZ domain.[57] This highlights the fact that Shank1 also has different biological properties during synapse formation compared with Shank2 and Shank3.

SHANK FUNCTION

As already outlined, Shank proteins are large scaffold proteins predominantly found in the brain and specifically located in the PSD, where they exhibit a variety of synaptic functions. The most prominent is the formation of molecular assembly platforms, which interconnect major synaptic proteins with each other.[59] Via their domains, Shanks interact with many signaling and scaffolding molecules and proteins associated with the cytoskeleton. In particular, they interact with *N*-methyl-D-aspartate (NMDA)-type glutamate receptors (via GKAP/SAPAP and SAP90/PSD-95),[54,60] metabotropic glutamate receptors (via Homer/VESL),[61] and α-amino-3-hydroxy-5-methyl-4-isoxazolepropionic acid (AMPA)-type glutamate receptors (via glutamate receptor interacting protein and/or via direct PDZ domain interaction).[35,62] They also interact with the actin-based cytoskeleton via cortactin[53] α-fodrin,[63] or Abp1.[64] Together with Homer proteins, they form a mesh-like matrix structure that serves as an assembly platform for other proteins residing within the postsynaptic density.[65] Thus, Shank proteins are considered master scaffolding molecules of the PSD and are essential for the structural integrity of dendritic spines and functionally involved in dynamic changes of spine morphology.

Overexpressed Shank1 in rat hippocampal neurons, for example, causes enlargement of dendritic spines mediated by the PDZ domain and the Homer binding site.[57] The Shank1–Homer1b complex further interacts with mGluR1/5 and IP3R, establishing the best condition for intracellular calcium release associated with ERK phosphorylation, an essential molecular pathway for proper spine maturation.[66] In line with this, the increased Shank1 levels found in PSD fractions obtained from FMRP-deficient mice[52] could be interpreted as a molecular response to counteract the abnormal development of thin and elongated spines in the absence of FMRP. Overexpressed Shank2 in rat hippocampal neurons accumulates at synapses and causes spine enlargement. In turn, reduction of endogenous Shank2 significantly decreases spine volume, which suggests that Shank2 is also essential for spine maturation.[67] Interestingly, a SHANK2 variant based on a truncating mutation identified in a patient with ASD (R462X) does not accumulate at synapses of primary neurons and is not able to induce the formation of normal spines and synapses either in vitro or in vivo.[67] This example leads us to consider that the effects of truncating *SHANK2* mutations on neuronal cell biology might strongly be related to ASD pathology. The functional synaptic role of Shank3 has been corroborated by in vitro studies showing that Shank3 is crucial to maintaining the functional integrity of dendritic spines and that its expression is sufficient to induce spine formation in cerebellar aspiny neurons.[68] Several de novo truncating mutations in *SHANK3* found in patients affected by ASD and/or ID have been studied in vitro using overexpressed mutant Shank3 proteins mimicking these mutations. These studies provide evidence that truncated Shank3 is unable to localize efficiently to synapses and to regulate synapse morphology and function properly.[27,69–71]

SHANK MUTANT MICE

To study Shank function and the consequences of *Shank* mutations in vivo, several *Shank* mutant mouse models have been generated to date. For *Shank1*, one mutant line is available in which exons 14 and 15 encoding the PDZ domain of Shank1 are targeted leading to a loss of all known murine Shank1 isoforms.[72] For *Shank2*, two mutant lines are available: one in which exons 6 and 7 are targeted[73] and one in which only exon 7 is targeted.[74] Both targeted regions encode the PDZ domain of Shank2 and both models are devoid of all known Shank2 isoforms.[73,74] For *Shank3*, eight mutant lines are available, six of which are based on a deletion strategy, one disrupting exon 21, the most frequent site for human *SHANK3* mutations, and one of which is an overexpression model. Among the deletion lines, there are three independently generated models in which the genetic region encoding the N-terminal Ankyrin repeats domain is targeted: exons 4–7,[49] exons 4–9,[43,75] and exon 9,[76] respectively. Moreover, there is one model with a disruption of exon 11 encoding the SH3 domain[74] and one with a disruption of exons 13–16 encoding the PDZ domain.[49] Because of the transcriptional complexity of *Shank3*, none of these Shank3 deletion lines is lacking all known Shank3 isoforms; that is, in each of these mutants, an individual set of Shank3 isoforms is still expressed. The exon 21 model disrupts the *Shank3* sequence encoding the proline-rich region near the Homer binding domain,[77] resulting in the expression of C-terminally truncated Shank3 variants, and the Shank3 overexpression model is based on a modified BAC clone containing a sequence encoding for enhanced green fluorescent protein–tagged mouse Shank3, leading to approximately 50% more total Shank3 protein.[78]

Mutations in either *SHANK* gene can lead to several different neuropsychiatric conditions, but predominantly to ASD.[79] This is why behavioral characterization

of *Shank* mutant mice is primarily focused on the core features of ASD such as social interaction deficits and repetitive patterns of behavior, as well as frequent comorbidities.[38] *Shank* mutants should further help identify the neuroanatomical and molecular origin of these behavioral phenotypes to develop future treatment options for Shankopathies or possibly for ASD in general.[80]

As outlined, only one *Shank1* mutant line has been generated so far and was introduced by Morgan Sheng's laboratory in 2008.[72] With respect to autistic-like behavior at the adult stage, no deficits in social interaction have yet been reported in this line[81]; increased self-grooming appears only in a social context and digging is not elevated, but strongly reduced.[82] Interestingly, communication is markedly impaired: Compared with controls, *Shank1* mutant pups emitted fewer isolation-induced ultrasonic vocalizations (USVs) and the temporal organization of call sequences was decreased.[83,84] In addition, adult male *Shank1* mutants showed reduced scent marking behavior, and social modulation of USVs in response to female urine was not present.[83] Hypoactivity, motor coordination deficits, increased anxiety, impaired contextual fear learning, and enhanced acquisition, but impaired retention of spatial memory are additional behavioral features of adult *Shank1* mutants.[72,81] On the morphological level, only glutamatergic synapses in the hippocampal CA1 stratum radiatum of adult *Shank1* mutants have been evaluated so far. CA1 spine density is slightly reduced, and to some extent, the remaining spines are smaller, as is the thickness of the PSD.[72] Schaffer collateral CA3–CA1 physiology in juvenile *Shank1* mutants further revealed reduced basal synaptic transmission by extracellular recording of field excitatory postsynaptic potentials and reduced frequency of miniature excitatory postsynaptic currents (mEPSCs).[72] In contrast to these investigations in CA1, the molecular consequences of Shank1 deletion were evaluated in biochemically purified PSDs from whole forebrain of adult animals and revealed reduced levels of the direct Shank interactors Homer and GKAP.[72]

Two *Shank2* mutant lines are currently available, independently generated by the laboratories of Tobias Boeckers (*Shank2*^{ex7})[74] and Eunjoon Kim (*Shank2*$^{ex6+7}$).[73] Although the paradigms used to characterize these two *Shank2* mutant lines were not the same, similar autistic-like behavioral traits could be observed in both models: Adult *Shank2*$^{ex7-/-}$ and *Shank2*$^{ex6+7-/-}$ mutants show moderate abnormalities in social interaction, increased self-grooming (depending on sex and paradigm), and repetitive jumping (the latter behavior was observed but remains unpublished for *Shank2*$^{ex7-/-}$). However, both lines do not show elevated, but rather, strongly reduced digging behavior.[73,74] Moderate communication deficits are further present in both *Shank2*$^{ex7-/-}$ and *Shank2*$^{ex6+7-/-}$ adult mutants,[73,74,85] as well as in $Shank2^{ex7-/-}$ pups.[74,85] Importantly, hyperactivity is one of the strongest behavioral phenotypes in both $Shank2^{ex7-/-}$ and $Shank2^{ex6+7-/-}$ adult mutants and can already be observed in heterozygotes. In addition, mutants of both lines show increased anxiety.[73,74] Spatial memory and nesting behavior are also impaired but have only been analyzed in adult $Shank2^{ex6+7-/-}$ mutants (similar results were obtained but remain unpublished for $Shank2^{ex7-/-}$)[73]; hind limb clasping was only observed and evaluated in adult $Shank2^{ex7-/-}$ mutants.[74] Only glutamatergic synapses in the adult hippocampal CA1 stratum radiatum have been morphologically evaluated in both $Shank2^{ex7-/-}$ and $Shank2^{ex6+7-/-}$ mutants. Except for a slight reduction in dendritic spine density in $Shank2^{ex7-/-}$ mutants, no marked changes were detectable. However, only a limited amount of morphological parameters have been assessed.[73,74] Schaffer collateral CA3-CA1 physiology in juvenile $Shank2^{ex7-/-}$ and $Shank2^{ex6+7-/-}$ mutants revealed conflicting results, though: $Shank2^{ex7-/-}$ mutants exhibit reduced basal synaptic transmission, reduced frequency of mEPSCs, an increased NMDA/AMPA ratio, and enhanced longterm potentiation (LTP).[74] In contrast, $Shank2^{ex6+7-/-}$ mutants exhibit no change in basal synaptic transmission or mEPSC frequency, a decreased NMDA/AMPA ratio, and reduced LTP.[73] It still needs to be clarified whether these paradoxical results are related to the slightly different genetic targeting strategies or to the different protocols used for the electrophysiological measurements in the different laboratories. Molecular effects of Shank2 deletion were analyzed in whole brain from each mutant line and in individual brain regions from $Shank2^{ex7-/-}$ mutants at both the juvenile and adult stages.[73,74] A largely overlapping phenomenon is upregulation of the main NMDAR subunit GluN1, both in $Shank2^{ex7-/-}$ and $Shank2^{ex6+7-/-}$ mutants. Synaptic upregulation of Shank3 was evaluated and observed only in $Shank2^{ex7-/-}$ mutants, and reduced NMDAR signaling only in $Shank2^{ex6+7-/-}$ mutants.[73,74] Interventional studies have been performed only in $Shank2^{ex6+7-/-}$ mutants.[73] Direct NMDAR stimulation with D-cycloserine and indirect NMDAR stimulation with a positive allosteric modulator of mGluR5 called CDPPB are both sufficient to normalize NMDAR function and signaling and significantly ameliorate social impairments in $Shank2^{ex6+7-/-}$ mutants.[73] Importantly, these pharmacological rescue experiments not only corroborate that NMDAR function/signaling is reduced in $Shank2^{ex6+7-/-}$ mutants, they might also open up novel strategies possibly to ameliorate ASD-associated social interaction deficits in humans with *SHANK2* deletions/mutations.

As mentioned, six loss-of-Shank3-function models have been generated with a deletion strategy to obtain knockout animals: one $Shank3^{ex4-9J}$ by Joseph Buxbaum,[75] another $Shank3^{ex4-9B}$ with a slightly different targeting strategy by Yong-hui Jiang,[43] a $Shank3^{ex9}$ by Eunjoon Kim,[76] a $Shank3^{ex11}$ by Tobias Boeckers,[74] and both a $Shank3^{ex4-7}$ and a $Shank3^{ex13-16}$ by Guoping Feng.[49] Another $Shank3$ mutant line was introduced by the laboratory of Craig Powell.[77] It is based on the disruption of exon 21, the most frequent site of *SHANK3* mutations in humans,[14] and results in a C-terminal truncation of Shank3; therefore, it is called $Shank3^{\Delta C/\Delta C}$. Several reasons may account for the phenotypic variability among these seven Shank3 mutant lines: first is all of the different gene targeting strategies and the presence of an individual set of remaining Shank3 isoforms in each model, but also the genotype of the mice analyzed, their genetic background (for heterozygous and homozygous mutants of the $Shank3^{ex4-9B}$ line, strong strain effects on behavioral phenotypes were absent, as shown by Drapeau et al.[86]), age and sex, analysis of different brain regions, and the application of different protocols for analysis. This is why we will focus on the discussion of robust major phenotypes among the models, as follows. Autistic-like behaviors were thus far assessed in all loss-of-Shank3-function models except for $Shank3^{ex11}$ mice (for a summary of the behavioral findings in each mutant line see Table 1). The strongest phenotypes observed among the different lines are impaired social interaction, increased repetitive behavior, impaired cognitive functions, and motor coordination deficits (marked as bold + italic in Table 1). Moreover, individual lines also exhibit communication deficits, increased anxiety, cognitive impairments, hypoactivity, or increased pain sensitivity.[43,49,74,75,76,77,86-88] An interesting behavioral aspect was raised by Kouser et al., who suggested an avoidance phenotype toward inanimate objects in $Shank3^{\Delta C/\Delta C}$ mice.[77] With respect to morphology, adult hippocampal CA1 neurons were evaluated in $Shank3^{ex4-9-/-J}$, $Shank3^{ex11-/-}$, and $Shank3^{\Delta C/\Delta C}$ mutants. Interestingly, morphological alterations are subtle if at all observable. The only findings are slightly reduced spine density and increased spine length in juvenile $Shank3^{ex4-9-/-J}$ mutants at 4 weeks of age and slightly reduced spine length, but normal spine density in adult animals of the same line.[43] In both, $Shank3^{ex11-/-}$ and $Shank3^{\Delta C/\Delta C}$ mutants, no morphological phenotypes could be observed in CA1.[74,77] In $Shank3^{ex13-16-/-}$ mutants, medium spiny neurons of the dorsolateral striatum were evaluated instead of CA1 pyramidal neurons, and morphological alterations are more pronounced: increased complexity of the dendritic tree, reduced spine density, increased spine neck width, as well as shorter and thinner PSDs, in addition to increased striatal volume in general.[49] Taken together, these findings indicate brain region and/or neuronal subtype-specific morphological alterations in the Shank3 mutant brain. Synapse physiology in juveniles was obtained from all lines except for $Shank3^{ex11-/-}$ mice. One strongly

TABLE 1   Summary of behavioral phenotypes in loss-of-Shank3-function mouse lines

	Shank3$^{ex4-7-/-}$	Shank3$^{ex4-9+/-B}$	Shank3$^{ex4-9-/-B}$	Shank3$^{ex4-9-/-J}$	Shank3$^{ex9-/-}$	Shank3$^{ex13-16-/-}$	Shank3$^{\Delta C/\Delta C}$
Social interaction	*Impaired*	*Impaired*	*Impaired*	*Impaired*	Unaltered	*Impaired*	*Impaired*
Repetitive behaviors	Not investigated	*Increased*	*Increased*	*Increased*	Unaltered	*Increased*	*Increased*
Communication	Not investigated	*Impaired*	Unaltered	*Impaired*	Unaltered	Not investigated	Unaltered
Anxiety	Unaltered	Unaltered	Unaltered	Not investigated	Not investigated	*Increased*	Unaltered
Cognitive functions	Not investigated	Unaltered	*Impaired*	*Impaired*	*Impaired*	Unaltered	*Impaired*
Motor coordination	Not investigated	*Impaired*	*Impaired*	*Impaired*	Not investigated	Unaltered	*Impaired*
Locomotion	Not investigated	Unaltered	Unaltered	*Hypoactivity*	Unaltered	Unaltered	*Hypoactivity*
Pain sensitivity	Not investigated	Unaltered	Unaltered	Not investigated	Not investigated	Not investigated	*Increased*

Behavioral phenotypes are marked in bold + italic.

overlapping phenomenon is decreased LTP at CA3-CA1 synapses, as found in Shank3$^{ex4-9+/-B}$, Shank3$^{ex4-9-/-B}$, Shank3$^{ex4-9-/-J}$, and Shank3$^{\Delta C/\Delta C}$ mutants. These data imply impaired synaptic plasticity independent of the underlying Shank3 mutation.[43,75,77,87] However, LTP is unchanged in Shank3$^{ex9-/-}$ mutants and has not yet been assessed in Shank3$^{ex4-7-/-}$ or Shank3$^{ex13-16-/-}$ mice.[49,76] Regarding basal synaptic transmission, results were more diverse: At CA3-CA1 synapses, a decrease was observed in Shank3$^{ex4-9+/-B}$, Shank3$^{ex4-9-/-B}$, Shank3$^{ex9-/-}$, and Shank3$^{\Delta C/\Delta C}$, but not in Shank3$^{ex4-9-/-J}$ or Shank3$^{ex13-16-/-}$ mutants.[43,49,75–77,87,88] In turn, basal synaptic transmission is indeed decreased at corticostriatal synapses in both Shank3$^{ex4-7-/-}$ and Shank3$^{ex13-16-/-}$ mutants.[49] These observations repeatedly point toward the brain region and/or neuronal subtype-specificity in the Shank3 mutant brain. This is strongly supported by data obtained on miniature inhibitory postsynaptic currents in Shank3$^{ex9-/-}$ mutants that are increased in CA1 and decreased in mPFC pyramidal neurons, which indicate region-specific excitatory/inhibitory (E/I) imbalances.[76] An E/I imbalance with a shift toward excitation was further observed in the insular cortex of adult Shank3$^{ex13-16-/-}$ mice.[89] On the molecular level, a major overlapping phenotype among various Shank3 mutants is the reduction of AMPA receptor subunits at synapses[43,49,74,75] and of Homer1b/c and specific NMDA receptor subunits in Shank3$^{ex4-9-/-J}$ and Shank3$^{ex13-16-/-}$ mutants, respectively.[43,49] However, none of these phenomena can be seen in Shank3$^{\Delta C/\Delta C}$ animals; these mutants only show strong upregulation of mGluR5 in synaptic fractions.[77] In Shank3$^{ex4-9-/-J}$ mice, both decreased synaptic AMPA receptor subunits and decreased LTP might be explained by the impairment in activity-dependent redistribution of GluA1, as found

in primary hippocampal neurons from this mutant line.[43] Interventional studies have been performed only in Shank3$^{ex4-9+/-B}$ mice to date.[75] The strongest and most robust synaptic phenotypes of this line, decreased LTP and basal synaptic transmission at CA3-CA1 Schaffer collateral synapses, were chosen and used as a readout after systemic treatment of these mutants with either an active peptide derivate of insulin-like growth factor (IGF)1, (1–3)IGF1, or full-length IGF1. Intriguingly, both neurotrophic agents are able to reverse these physiological deficits. In addition, full-length IGF1 is also able to restore the motor coordination deficits of mutant animals.[88] Although the exact molecular actions of IGF1 in Shank3$^{ex4-9+/-B}$ mice still have to be elucidated, this substance might be a promising compound for translational treatment studies in Shank3 mutants and other ASD mouse models, especially because targeting the IGF-1 pathway has already proven successful in antagonizing synaptic and behavioral phenotypes in a mouse model of Rett syndrome.[90–92]

Because some individuals with neuropsychiatric conditions have duplication of SHANK3, Huda Zoghbi's laboratory generated and characterized Shank3-overexpressing mutants with approximately 50% more total Shank3 protein.[78] Behaviorally, these animals show manic-like behavior including hyperactivity with an increased sensitivity to amphetamine, abnormal circadian rhythms, and hyperphagia. Impairment in social interaction and subtle communication deficits could also be identified, but no increase in repetitive behaviors is observed.[78] Morphologically, spine density is increased in the CA1 stratum radiatum and physiological analyses show hyperexcitability discharges and electrographic seizures in several brain regions including CA1, the dentate gyrus, and the frontal cortex.

The latter findings are corroborated by the delineation of an E/I imbalance shifted toward excitation in mutant primary hippocampal neurons, including an increased density of excitatory and a decreased density of inhibitory presynaptic terminals.[78] Regarding molecular alterations, F-actin levels are increased at excitatory synapses in mutant primary hippocampal neurons, most probably owing to enhanced interaction of Shank3 with the Arp2/3 complex, an initiator of actin nucleation and branching. Further interesting findings are the redistribution of the actin-related protein profilin2 from inhibitory to excitatory synapses and decreased levels of the actin-related protein mena at inhibitory synapses in mutant primary hippocampal neurons. Taken together, these molecular findings are in line with these morphological and physiological observations.[78] The manic-like behavior in Shank3-overexpressing mice is not antagonized by systemic application of lithium, a standard mood-stabilizing drug for the treatment of affective disorders in humans. However, systemic treatment with valproate, another mood-stabilizer and anticonvulsant, is able to reverse the hyperactivity and the frequency of epileptiform spikes.[78]

HUMAN IN VITRO MODELING OF SHANK MUTATIONS

Human induced pluripotent stem cells (hiPSCs) represent a new tool to study synaptic defects and signaling pathways involved in the pathogenesis of ASD and ID. They can be obtained from human fibroblasts or keratinocytes by overexpression of specific genes[93,94] and further be differentiated into neurons and glial cells.[95–97] In light of all of the discrepancies found in different *Shank* mutant mice, hiPSCs may represent a good model to better understand the complex molecular roles that human SHANK proteins have in neuronal function. Considering the large number of *SHANK* variants detected in ASD and/or ID patients thus far and the heterogeneity in terms of deletion size found in PMS, hiPSCs promise major advances in the study of specific *SHANK* mutations. Because hiPSCs retain the entire genetic profile of individual ASD patients, specific differences and/or similarities among patients could be evaluated in future studies. In differentiated neurons from hiPSCs of PMS patients, reduced SHANK3 protein expression and synaptic transmission defects specific for excitatory neurons have already been identified. Similar to what has also been shown in $Shank3^{ex4-9+/-B}$ mice,[88] these defects can be restored by application of IGF1.[98] This study illustrates the potential of hiPSCs as a model to study human SHANK protein functions, which may open the way for development of an hiPSC library that could be used to

detect and clarify synaptic defects resulting from individual *SHANK* mutations. In a personalized medicine approach, this could lead to the desired development and screening of novel drugs that may modulate or even normalize SHANK expression and/or function not only in cell culture but possibly in affected patients as well.

CONCLUSIONS

ASD and ID are serious conditions that greatly affect and limit the quality of life for those who experience them, both the affected patients and their families. With the discovery of *SHANK* mutations and their significant connection to neurodevelopmental pathologies, research on the specific role and function of SHANK proteins has been rapidly promoted from the analysis of basic molecular properties to rodent and human model systems. In the past decade, both molecular studies and the generation and basic characterization of several *Shank* mutant mice have contributed to a much better understanding of Shank in synaptic function. However, there remains an urgent need to fully characterize and better compare the available *Shank* mutant lines for behavioral, circuit-specific and molecular alterations, to identify the origin of common and different phenotypes, especially because growing evidence implicates mutation-specific alterations in each mutant line and each affected patient alike. In the near future, we therefore have to perform even more careful and detailed analyses of clinical features in patients with different *SHANK* mutations than we do now, to try to mimic exactly the same mutations in mouse and hiPSC models and use them to distinguish individual behavioral, circuit-specific, and molecular features. A pilot study including nine PMS children showed that 3 months of IGF1 treatment was associated with significant improvement in both social impairment and restrictive behaviors.[99] However, this is the only evidence for a possible indirect and general therapeutic approach for patients with *SHANK* mutations. Ultimately, it will be essential to create a detailed Shankopathy-related genetic and molecular framework upon which researchers will discover novel molecular pathways and novel approaches in the development of therapeutic treatments to ameliorate or even reverse the symptoms, and thus to increase the quality of life for both affected patients and families.

Acknowledgments

This work was supported by Baustein 3.2 L.SBN.0081 of Ulm University (to M.J.S.) and by the Fondazione CARIPLO project 2013-0879 (to C.V.) Foundation Jérôme Lejeune (to C.V.).

References

1. Sato D, Lionel AC, Leblond CS, et al. SHANK1 deletions in males with autism spectrum disorder. *Am J Hum Genet* 2012;**90**(5):879–87.

2. Berkel S, Marshall CR, Weiss B, et al. Mutations in the SHANK2 synaptic scaffolding gene in autism spectrum disorder and mental retardation. *Nat Genet* 2010;**42**(6):489–91.

3. Pinto D, Pagnamenta AT, Klei L, et al. Functional impact of global rare copy number variation in autism spectrum disorders. *Nature* 2010;**466**(7304):368–72.

4. Wischmeijer A, Magini P, Giorda R, et al. Olfactory receptor-related duplicons mediate a microdeletion at 11q13.2q13.4 associated with a syndromic phenotype. *Mol Syndromol* 2011;**1**(4):176–84.

5. Leblond CS, Heinrich J, Delorme R, et al. Genetic and functional analyses of SHANK2 mutations suggest a multiple hit model of autism spectrum disorders. *PLoS Genet* 2012;**8**(2):e1002521.

6. Chilian B, Abdollahpour H, Bierhals T, et al. Dysfunction of SHANK2 and CHRNA7 in a patient with intellectual disability and language impairment supports genetic epistasis of the two loci. *Clin Genet* 2013;**84**(6):560–5.

7. Schluth-Bolard C, Labalme A, Cordier MP, et al. Breakpoint mapping by next generation sequencing reveals causative gene disruption in patients carrying apparently balanced chromosome rearrangements with intellectual deficiency and/or congenital malformations. *J Med Genet* 2013;**50**(3):144–50.

8. Sanders SJ, Murtha MT, Gupta AR, et al. De novo mutations revealed by whole-exome sequencing are strongly associated with autism. *Nature* 2012;**485**(7397):237–41.

9. Phelan MC, Rogers RC, Saul RA, et al. 22q13 deletion syndrome. *Am J Med Genet* 2001;**101**(2):91–9.

10. Bonaglia MC, Giorda R, Borgatti R, et al. Disruption of the ProSAP2 gene in a t(12;22)(q24.1;q13.3) is associated with the 22q13.3 deletion syndrome. *Am J Hum Genet* 2001;**69**(2):261–8.

11. Bonaglia MC, Giorda R, Mani E, et al. Identification of a recurrent breakpoint within the SHANK3 gene in the 22q13.3 deletion syndrome. *J Med Genet* 2006;**43**(10):822–8.

12. Phelan K, McDermid HE. The 22q13.3 deletion syndrome (Phelan-McDermid syndrome). *Mol Syndromol* 2012;**2**(3–5):186–201.

13. Misceo D, Rødningen OK, Barøy T, et al. A translocation between Xq21.33 and 22q13.33 causes an intragenic SHANK3 deletion in a woman with Phelan-McDermid syndrome and hypergonadotropic hypogonadism. *Am J Med Genet A* 2011;**155A**(2):403–8.

14. Leblond CS, Nava C, Polge A, et al. Meta-analysis of SHANK mutations in autism spectrum disorders: a gradient of severity in cognitive impairments. *PLoS Genet* 2014;**10**(9):e1004580.

15. Durand CM, Betancur C, Boeckers TM, et al. Mutations in the gene encoding the synaptic scaffolding protein SHANK3 are associated with autism spectrum disorders. *Nat Genet* 2007;**39**(1):25–7.

16. Moessner R, Marshall CR, Sutcliffe JS, et al. Contribution of SHANK3 mutations to autism spectrum disorder. *Am J Hum Genet* 2007;**81**(6):1289–97.

17. Gauthier J, Spiegelman D, Piton A, et al. Novel de novo SHANK3 mutation in autistic patients. *Am J Med Genet B Neuropsychiatr Genet* 2009;**150B**(3):421–4.

18. Hamdan FF, Gauthier J, Araki Y, et al. Excess of de novo deleterious mutations in genes associated with glutamatergic systems in nonsyndromic intellectual disability. *Am J Hum Genet* 2011;**88**(3):306–16.

19. Kolevzon A, Cai G, Soorya L, et al. Analysis of a purported SHANK3 mutation in a boy with autism: clinical impact of rare variant research in neurodevelopmental disabilities. *Brain Res* 2011;**1380**:98–105.

20. Schaaf CP, Sabo A, Sakai Y, et al. Oligogenic heterozygosity in individuals with high-functioning autism spectrum disorders. *Hum Mol Genet* 2011;**20**(17):3366–75.

21. Waga C, Okamoto N, Ondo Y, et al. Novel variants of the SHANK3 gene in Japanese autistic patients with severe delayed speech development. *Psychiatr Genet* 2011;**21**(4):208–11.

22. Boccuto L, Lauri M, Sarasua SM, et al. Prevalence of SHANK3 variants in patients with different subtypes of autism spectrum disorders. *Eur J Hum Genet* 2013;**21**(3):310–6.

23. Liu Y, Du Y, Liu W, Yang C, Wang H, Gong X. Lack of association between NLGN3, NLGN4, SHANK2 and SHANK3 gene variants and autism spectrum disorder in a Chinese population. *PLoS One* 2013;**8**(2):e56639.

24. Soorya L, Kolevzon A, Zweifach J, et al. Prospective investigation of autism and genotype-phenotype correlations in 22q13 deletion syndrome and SHANK3 deficiency. *Mol Autism* 2013;**4**(1):18.

25. Nemirovsky SI, Córdoba M, Zaiat JJ, et al. Whole genome sequencing reveals a de novo SHANK3 mutation in familial autism spectrum disorder. *PLoS One* 2015;**10**(2):e0116358.

26. Hara M, Ohba C, Yamashita Y, Saitsu H, Matsumoto N, Matsuishi T. De novo SHANK3 mutation causes Rett syndrome-like phenotype in a female patient. *Am J Med Genet A* 2015;**167**(7):1593–6.

27. Cochoy DM, Kolevzon A, Kajiwara Y, et al. Phenotypic and functional analysis of SHANK3 stop mutations identified in individuals with ASD and/or ID. *Mol Autism* 2015;**6**:23.

28. Zhu L, Wang X, Li XL, et al. Epigenetic dysregulation of SHANK3 in brain tissues from individuals with autism spectrum disorders. *Hum Mol Genet* 2014;**23**(6):1563–78.

29. Lennertz L, Wagner M, Wölwer W, et al. A promoter variant of SHANK1 affects auditory working memory in schizophrenia patients and in subjects clinically at risk for psychosis. *Eur Arch Psychiatry Clin Neurosci* 2012;**262**(2):117–24.

30. Peykov S, Berkel S, Schoen M, et al. Identification and functional characterization of rare SHANK2 variants in schizophrenia. *Mol Psychiatry* 2015;**20**(12):1487–8. http://dx.doi.org/10.1038/mp.2014.172.

31. Gauthier J, Champagne N, Lafrenière RG, et al. De novo mutations in the gene encoding the synaptic scaffolding protein SHANK3 in patients ascertained for schizophrenia. *Proc Natl Acad Sci USA* 2010;**107**(17):7863–8.

32. Allen AS, Berkovic SF, Cossette P, et al. De novo mutations in epileptic encephalopathies. *Nature* 2013;**501**(7466):217–21.

33. Lesca G, Rudolf G, Labalme A, et al. Epileptic encephalopathies of the Landau-Kleffner and continuous spike and waves during slow-wave sleep types: genomic dissection makes the link with autism. *Epilepsia* 2012;**53**(9):1526–38.

34. Dimassi S, Labalme A, Lesca G, et al. A subset of genomic alterations detected in rolandic epilepsies contains candidate or known epilepsy genes including GRIN2A and PRRT2. *Epilepsia* 2014;**55**(2):370–8.

35. Sheng M, Kim E. The Shank family of scaffold proteins. *J Cell Sci* 2000;**113**(Pt 11):1851–6.

36. Grabrucker AM, Schmeisser MJ, Schoen M, Boeckers TM. Postsynaptic ProSAP/Shank scaffolds in the cross-hair of synaptopathies. *Trends Cell Biol* 2011;**21**(10):594–603.

37. Grabrucker AM, Knight MJ, Proepper C, et al. Concerted action of zinc and ProSAP/Shank in synaptogenesis and synapse maturation. *EMBO J* 2011;**30**(3):569–81.

38. Jiang YH, Ehlers MD. Modeling autism by SHANK gene mutations in mice. *Neuron* 2013;**78**(1):8–27.

39. Baron MK, Boeckers TM, Vaida B, et al. An architectural framework that may lie at the core of the postsynaptic density. *Science* 2006;**311**(5760):531–5.

40. Lim S, Naisbitt S, Yoon J, et al. Characterization of the Shank family of synaptic proteins. Multiple genes, alternative splicing, and differential expression in brain and development. *J Biol Chem* 1999;**274**:29510–8.

41. Boeckers TM, Kreutz MR, Winter C, et al. Proline-rich synapse-associated protein-1/cortactin binding protein 1 (ProSAP1/CortBP1) is a PDZ-domain protein highly enriched in the postsynaptic density. *J Neurosci* 1999;**19**(15):6506–18.

42. Boeckers TM, Bockmann J, Kreutz MR, Gundelfinger ED. ProSAP/Shank proteins – a family of higher order organizing molecules of the postsynaptic density with an emerging role in human neurological disease. *J Neurochem* 2002;**81**(5):903–10.

43. Wang X, McCoy PA, Rodriguiz RM, et al. Synaptic dysfunction and abnormal behaviors in mice lacking major isoforms of Shank3. *Hum Mol Genet* 2011;**20**(15):3093–108.

44. Wang X, Xu Q, Bey AL, Lee Y, Jiang YH. Transcriptional and functional complexity of Shank3 provides a molecular framework to understand the phenotypic heterogeneity of SHANK3 causing autism and Shank3 mutant mice. *Mol Autism* 2014;**5**:30.

45. Ching TT, Maunakea AK, Jun P, et al. Epigenome analyses using BAC microarrays identify evolutionary conservation of tissue-specific methylation of SHANK3. *Nat Genet* 2005;**37**(6):645–51.

46. Beri S, Tonna N, Menozzi G, Bonaglia MC, Sala C, Giorda R. DNA methylation regulates tissue-specific expression of Shank3. *J Neurochem* 2007;**101**(5):1380–91.

47. Maunakea AK, Nagarajan RP, Bilenky M, et al. Conserved role of intragenic DNA methylation in regulating alternative promoters. *Nature* 2010;**466**(7303):253–7.

48. Bockers TM, Segger-Junius M, Iglauer P, et al. Differential expression and dendritic transcript localization of Shank family members: identification of a dendritic targeting element in the 3′ untranslated region of Shank1 mRNA. *Mol Cell Neurosci* 2004;**26**(1):182–90.

49. Peça J, Feliciano C, Ting JT, et al. Shank3 mutant mice display autistic-like behaviours and striatal dysfunction. *Nature* 2011;**472**(7344):437–42.

50. Epstein I, Tushev G, Will TJ, Vlatkovic I, Cajigas IJ, Schuman EM. Alternative polyadenylation and differential expression of Shank mRNAs in the synaptic neuropil. *Philos Trans R Soc Lond B Biol Sci* 2014;**369**(1633):20130137.

51. Darnell JC, Jensen KB, Jin P, Brown V, Warren ST, Darnell RB. Fragile X mental retardation protein targets G quartet mRNAs important for neuronal function. *Cell* 2001;**107**(4):489–99.

52. Schütt J, Falley K, Richter D, Kreienkamp HJ, Kindler S. Fragile X mental retardation protein regulates the levels of scaffold proteins and glutamate receptors in postsynaptic densities. *J Biol Chem* 2009;**284**(38):25479–87.

53. Du Y, Weed SA, Xiong W-C, Marshall TD, Parsons JT. Identification of a novel cortactin SH3 domain-binding protein and its localization to growth cones of cultured neurons. *Mol Cell Biol* 1998;**18**(10):5838–51.

54. Boeckers TM, winter C, Smalla KH, et al. Proline-rich synapse-associated proteins ProSAP1 and ProSAP2 interact with synaptic proteins of the SAPAP/GKAP family. *Biochem Biophys Res Commun* 1999;**264**(1):247–52.

55. Romorini S, Piccoli G, Jiang M, et al. A functional role of postsynaptic density-95-guanylate kinase-associated protein complex in regulating shank assembly and stability to synapses. *J Neurosci* 2004;**24**(42):9391–404.

56. Tao-Cheng JH, Dosemeci A, Gallant PE, Smith C, Reese T. Activity induced changes in the distribution of Shanks at hippocampal synapses. *Neuroscience* 2010;**168**(1):11–7.

57. Sala C, Piech V, Wilson NR, Passafaro M, Liu GS, Sheng M. Regulation of dendritic spine morphology and synaptic function by Shank and Homer. *Neuron* 2001;**31**(1):115–30.

58. Boeckers TM, Liedtke T, Spilker C, et al. C-terminal synaptic targeting elements for postsynaptic density proteins ProSAP1/Shank2 and ProSAP2/Shank3. *J Neurochem* 2005;**92**(3):519–24.

59. Kreienkamp HJ. Scaffolding proteins at the postsynaptic density: shank as the architectural framework. *Handb Exp Pharmacol* 2008;(186):365–80.

60. Naisbitt S, Kim E, Tu JC, et al. Shank, a novel family of postsynaptic density proteins that binds to the NMDA receptor/PSD-95/GKAP complex and cortactin. *Neuron* 1999;**23**(3):569–82.

61. Tu JC, Xiao B, Naisbitt S, et al. Coupling of mGluR/Homer and PSD-95 complexes by the Shank family of postsynaptic density proteins. *Neuron* 1999;**23**(3):583–92.

62. Uchino S, Wada H, Honda S, et al. Direct interaction of post-synaptic density-95/Dlg/ZO-1 domain-containing synaptic molecule Shank3 with GluR1 alpha-amino-3-hydroxy-5-methyl-4-isoxazole propionic acid receptor. *J Neurochem* 2006;**97**(4):1203–14.

63. Bockers TM, Mameza MG, Kreutz MR, et al. Synaptic scaffolding proteins in rat brain. Ankyrin repeats of the multidomain Shank protein family interact with the cytoskeletal protein alpha-fodrin. *J Biol Chem* 2001;**276**(43):40104–12.

64. Qualmann B, Boeckers TM, Jeromin M, Gundelfinger ED, Kessels MM. Linkage of the actin cytoskeleton to the postsynaptic density via direct interactions of Abp1 with the ProSAP/Shank family. *J Neurosci* 2004;**24**(10):2481–95.

65. Hayashi MK, Tang C, Verpelli C, et al. The postsynaptic density proteins Homer and Shank form a polymeric network structure. *Cell* 2009;**137**(1):159–71.

66. Sala C, Roussignol G, Meldolesi J, Fagni L. Key role of the postsynaptic density scaffold proteins Shank and Homer in the functional architecture of Ca2+ homeostasis at dendritic spines in hippocampal neurons. *J Neurosci* 2005;**25**(18):4587–92.

67. Berkel S, Tang W, Treviño M, et al. Inherited and de novo SHANK2 variants associated with autism spectrum disorder impair neuronal morphogenesis and physiology. *Hum Mol Genet* 2012;**21**(2):344–57.

68. Roussignol G, Ango F, Romorini S, et al. Shank expression is sufficient to induce functional dendritic spine synapses in aspiny neurons. *J Neurosci* 2005;**25**(14):3560–70.

69. Durand CM, Perroy J, Loll F, et al. SHANK3 mutations identified in autism lead to modification of dendritic spine morphology via an actin-dependent mechanism. *Mol Psychiatry* 2012;**17**(1):71–84.

70. Verpelli C, Dvoretskova E, Vicidomini C, et al. Importance of Shank3 protein in regulating metabotropic glutamate receptor 5 (mGluR5) expression and signaling at synapses. *J Biol Chem* 2011;**286**(40):34839–50.

71. Arons MH, Thynne CJ, Grabrucker AM, et al. Autism-associated mutations in ProSAP2/Shank3 impair synaptic transmission and neurexin-neuroligin-mediated transsynaptic signaling. *J Neurosci* 2012;**32**(43):14966–78.

72. Hung AY, Futai K, Sala C, et al. Smaller dendritic spines, weaker synaptic transmission, but enhanced spatial learning in mice lacking Shank1. *J Neurosci* 2008;**28**(7):1697–708.

73. Won H, Lee HR, Gee HY, et al. Autistic-like social behaviour in Shank2-mutant mice improved by restoring NMDA receptor function. *Nature* 2012;**486**(7402):261–5.

74. Schmeisser MJ, Ey E, Wegener S, et al. Autistic-like behaviours in mice lacking ProSAP1/Shank2. *Nature* 2012;**486**(7402):256–60.

75. Bozdagi O, Sakurai T, Papapetrou D, et al. Haploinsufficiency of the autism-associated Shank3 gene leads to deficits in synaptic function, social interaction, and social communication. *Mol Autism* 2010;**1**(1):15.

76. Lee J, Chung C, Ha S, et al. Shank3-mutant mice lacking exon 9 show altered excitation/inhibition balance, enhanced rearing, and spatial memory deficit. *Front Cell Neurosci* 2015;**9**:94.

77. Kouser M, Speed HE, Dewey CM, et al. Loss of predominant Shank3 isoforms results in hippocampus-dependent impairments in behavior and synaptic transmission. *J Neurosci* 2013;**33**(47):18448–68.

78. Han K, Holder JL, Schaaf CP, et al. SHANK3 overexpression causes manic-like behaviour with unique pharmacogenetic properties. *Nature* 2013;**503**(7474):72−7.

79. Guilmatre A, Huguet G, Delorme R, Bourgeron T. The emerging role of SHANK genes in neuropsychiatric disorders. *Dev Neurobiol* 2014;**74**(2):113−22.

80. Schmeisser MJ. Translational neurobiology in Shank mutant mice − model systems for neuropsychiatric disorders. *Ann Anat* 2015; **200**:115−7.

81. Silverman JL, Turner SM, Barkan CL, et al. Sociability and motor functions in Shank1 mutant mice. *Brain Res* 2011;**1380**:120−37.

82. Sungur A, Vörckel KJ, Schwarting RK, Wöhr M. Repetitive behaviors in the Shank1 knockout mouse model for autism spectrum disorder: developmental aspects and effects of social context. *J Neurosci Methods* 2014;**234**:92−100.

83. Wöhr M, Roullet FI, Hung AY, Sheng M, Crawley JN. Communication impairments in mice lacking Shank1: reduced levels of ultrasonic vocalizations and scent marking behavior. *PLoS One* 2011; **6**(6):e20631.

84. Wöhr M. Ultrasonic vocalizations in Shank mouse models for autism spectrum disorders: detailed spectrographic analyses and developmental profiles. *Neurosci Biobehav Rev* 2014;**43**:199−212.

85. Ey E, Torquet N, Le Sourd AM, et al. The Autism ProSAP1/Shank2 mouse model displays quantitative and structural abnormalities in ultrasonic vocalisations. *Behav Brain Res* 2013;**256**:677−89.

86. Drapeau E, Dorr NP, Elder GA, Buxbaum JD. Absence of strong strain effects in behavioral analyses of Shank3-deficient mice. *Dis Model Mech* 2014;**7**(6):667−81.

87. Yang M, Bozdagi O, Scattoni ML, et al. Reduced excitatory neurotransmission and mild autism-relevant phenotypes in adolescent Shank3 null mutant mice. *J Neurosci* 2012;**32**(19):6525−41.

88. Bozdagi O, Tavassoli T, Buxbaum JD. Insulin-like growth factor-1 rescues synaptic and motor deficits in a mouse model of autism and developmental delay. *Mol Autism* 2013;**4**(1):9.

89. Gogolla N, Takesian AE, Feng G, Fagiolini M, Hensch TK. Sensory integration in mouse insular cortex reflects GABA circuit maturation. *Neuron* 2014;**83**(4):894−905.

90. Tropea D, Giacometti E, Wilson NR, et al. Partial reversal of Rett Syndrome-like symptoms in MeCP2 mutant mice. *Proc Natl Acad Sci USA* 2009;**106**(6):2029−34.

91. Castro J, Garcia RI, Kwok S, et al. Functional recovery with recombinant human IGF1 treatment in a mouse model of Rett Syndrome. *Proc Natl Acad Sci USA* 2014;**111**(27):9941−6.

92. Mellios N, Woodson J, Garcia RI, et al. β2-Adrenergic receptor agonist ameliorates phenotypes and corrects microRNA-mediated IGF1 deficits in a mouse model of Rett syndrome. *Proc Natl Acad Sci USA* 2014;**111**(27):9947−52.

93. Farra N, Zhang WB, Pasceri P, Eubanks JH, Salter MW, Ellis J. Rett syndrome induced pluripotent stem cell-derived neurons reveal novel neurophysiological alterations. *Mol Psychiatry* 2012;**17**(12): 1261−71.

94. Takahashi K, Yamanaka S. Induction of pluripotent stem cells from mouse embryonic and adult fibroblast cultures by defined factors. *Cell* 2006;**126**(4):663−76.

95. Marchetto MC, Carromeu C, Acab A, et al. A model for neural development and treatment of Rett syndrome using human induced pluripotent stem cells. *Cell* 2010;**143**(4):527−39.

96. Stockmann M, Linta L, Föhr KJ, et al. Developmental and functional nature of human iPSC derived motoneurons. *Stem Cell Rev* 2013;**9**(4):475−92.

97. Verpelli C, Carlessi L, Bechi G, et al. Comparative neuronal differentiation of self-renewing neural progenitor cell lines obtained from human induced pluripotent stem cells. *Front Cell Neurosci* 2013;**7**:175.

98. Shcheglovitov A, Shcheglovitova O, Yazawa M, et al. SHANK3 and IGF1 restore synaptic deficits in neurons from 22q13 deletion syndrome patients. *Nature* 2013;**503**(7475):267−71.

99. Kolevzon A, Bush L, Wang AT, et al. A pilot controlled trial of insulin-like growth factor-1 in children with Phelan-McDermid syndrome. *Mol Autism* 2014;**5**(1):54.

11

Mutations in Synaptic Adhesion Molecules

Jaewon Ko[1], Caterina Montani[2,3], Eunjoon Kim[4,5], Carlo Sala[2,3]

[1]Department of Biochemistry, College of Life Science & Biotechnology, Yonsei University, Seoul, South Korea;
[2]CNR Neuroscience Institute, Milan, Italy; [3]Department of Medical Biotechnology and Translational Medicine,
University of Milan, Milan, Italy; [4]Center for Synaptic Brain Dysfunctions, Institute for Basic Science (IBS), Daejeon,
South Korea; [5]Department of Biological Sciences, Korea Advanced Institute of Science and Technology (KAIST),
Daejeon, South Korea

INTRODUCTION

Synaptic cell adhesion molecules (SCAMs) in the brain enable pre- and postsynaptic recognition and are responsible for mechanical stabilization of synaptic contacts, as well as for synapse organization through assembling signaling molecules, neurotransmitter receptors, and the actin cytoskeleton. Several studies clearly showed that SCAMs are involved not just in physical adhesion but can control synapse formation, regulate dendritic spine morphology, and modify synaptic receptor function in an activity-dependent manner.[1–19]

The full array of proteins responsible for specific synaptic adhesion in the nervous system has been largely determined and includes cadherins, immunoglobulin-containing cell adhesion molecules (Ig-CAMs), neurexins and neuroligins, ephrins and Eph receptors, SynCAMs and IgLONs that belong to Ig-CAMs, protein tyrosine phosphatase (PTP) family, and interleukin-1 receptor accessory protein-like 1 (IL1RAPL1), leucine-rich repeat-containing CAMs such as netrin-G ligands (NGLs), leucine-rich repeat transmembrane neuronal (LRRTMs) Slit- and NTRK-like family (Slitrks), and synaptic adhesion-like molecules.[1–7,20,21]

Each of these SCAMs differs in terms of homo/heterophilic adhesion, calcium sensitivity, and synaptic/extrasynaptic localization and is thought to act in different processes, such as recognition of specific target domains within a neuron, synaptic differentiation, synaptic stability, and synaptic plasticity. A strong correlation between neurodevelopmental disorders and mutations in neurexins/neuroligins and PTPδ/IL1RAPL1 families of genes has been well-identified. In this chapter, we provide an overview about the most recent data on how these mutated SCAM families might pathologically influence diverse pre- and postsynaptic functions. Furthermore, we focus on studies that have started to shed light on the molecular interactions by which these mammalian SCAMs shape the developing synapse and determine the molecular organization of the mature synaptic contact.

MUTATIONS IN THE NEUREXIN/ NEUROLIGIN COMPLEX

Neurexin/Neuroligin Complex and Function

The neuroligins (NLGNs) form a family of postsynaptic cell adhesion proteins that interact trans-synaptically with the presynaptic neurexins (NRXNs) family in a Ca^{2+}-dependent manner. Indeed ultrastructural and functional studies indicate postsynaptic localization of NLGNs, whereas NRXNs are found on both sides of synaptic membrane[1,22,23] (Figure 1).

All four neuroligin genes (NLGN1–4) and three neurexin genes (NRXN1–3) are widely expressed in mammalian brains. The neurexin genes can generate, by alternative promoter choice, two transcripts for each NRXN gene (α-NRXN and β-NRXN) and, by alternative splicing at six canonical splicing sites, more than 1000 neurexins isoforms, the functions of which have been studied.[24,25]

The extracellular domain of α-NRXNs contains six laminin/neurexin/sex hormone-binding globulin-domains (LNS-domains) organized into modules separated by three epidermal growth factor—like domains, whereas the β-NRXNs contain only one LNS domain.

In humans there are five NLGNs genes, one more than other mammalian species that have only three or four genes.[26,27] Both NLGN3 and NLGN4 gene are localized to the human X chromosome whereas the NLGN4 gene is complemented on the Y chromosome by a similar NLGN5. For an unknown reason, the sequence of the mouse NLGN4 homolog is much lower than NLGN4 in other species.[27]

Also, for NLGNs genes several isoforms can be generated by alternative splicing at two sites in the extracellular domain.[24,25]

Interestingly, the alternative splicing of NRXNs and NLGNs determines binding to different partners and defines something similar to an adhesive code.[28–31] For example, NLGN1, B isoform, containing the B insert, is a master switch that determines binding to NRXNs isoforms. Specifically, NLGN1B selectively binds only β isoforms of NRXNs whereas NLGN1 (ΔB) binds to both α- and β-NRXNs.[29,32] Synaptic activity might also regulate the alternative splicing of NRXNs and functionally mediate trans-synaptic ligand switching among different partners.[33]

Both α- and β-NRXNs can also bind the leucine-rich repeat transmembrane protein LRRTM2, another postsynaptic SCAM.[34,35]

The C-terminal intracellular tail of both NLGNs and NRXNs bear a PDZ binding motif that allows NLGNs

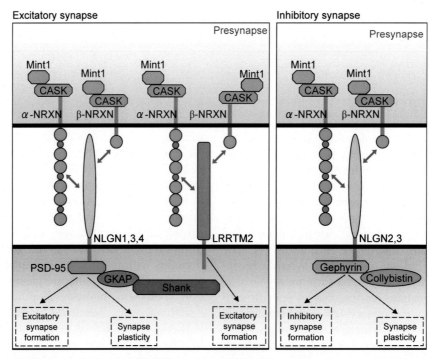

FIGURE 1   The drawing depicts a schematic representation of the NLGN—NRXN complexes and putative synaptic functions at excitatory and inhibitory synapses.

to bind the PDZ3 domains of PSD-95 whereas NRXNs interacts with proteins of the synaptic release machinery, including Mint1 and calcium/calmodulin-dependent serine protein kinase.[31,36,37]

Several experimental data indicate that NRXNs and NLGNs interactions have a role during the formation of synapse. The first evidence showed that, using an artificial synapse-formation assay, NLGNs were able to trigger presynaptic development in contacting axons when presented alone on the surface of nonneuronal cells.[38] In addition, NRXNs can induce the differentiation of GABAergic and glutamatergic postsynaptic specializations when expressed on the surface of nonneuronal cells co-cultured with primary neurons.[39]

A number of other articles demonstrated that in cultured neurons, overexpression of either NLGN1 or NLGN2 induces the formation of excitatory and inhibitory synapses[30,31,39,40] via the modulation of the scaffold proteins PSD-95 (or other intracellular proteins[41]) and gephyrin, respectively.[42–47] Similarly LRRTM2 induces the formation of excitatory synapses via extracellular interaction with NRXN1.[34,35]

On the contrary, knockdown of all NLGNs results in a decrease in the density of both excitatory and inhibitory synapses, although this is not confirmed in all studies.[41,48–50]

Other data showed that overexpression of β-NRXNs or addition of recombinant β-NRXN to cell cultures is able to reduce surface $GABA_A\alpha1R$ expression and prevent the normal developmental increase in GABAergic transmission without decreasing the synapse number.[51] However these effects seem not to be mediated via interactions with NLGNs, but to result from direct extracellular interaction of β-NRXNs with $GABA_A\alpha1R$.[51]

Despite the strong and clear data obtained in vitro, manipulation of the expression of NRXNs and NLGNs in vivo argues against their synaptogenic activity.

Mice deleted of all NLGNs or all α-NRXNs die after birth, not because of the absence of synapses but instead because of alteration synaptic transmission.[52,53]

For example, in the triple-NLGN knockout (KO) in mice, both GABAergic/glycinergic and glutamatergic transmission are functionally impaired, but the general synaptic density is maintained.[52]

Deletion of all α-NRXNs induces a twofold reduction in the density of inhibitory synapses whereas the number of excitatory synapses is not changed; however, the presynaptic release of synaptic vesicles is altered, which indicates a role for α-NRXNs in regulating the maturation of presynaptic terminals.[53]

The difference between in vitro and in vivo experiments can be explained by genetic compensation in vivo by other synaptic CAMs, or by the fact that synapses formed in dissociated neuronal cultures can be more easily manipulated by acute and transient gene overexpression of deletion. However a report showed that whereas the global loss of NLGN1 does not result in reduced synaptogenesis, a sparse NLGN1 knockdown induced by in utero electroporation of specific ribonucleic acid interference (RNAi) for NLGN1 leads to a dramatic loss of synapses.[54] Thus, the defects in synaptogenesis are observed in NLGN1-deficient neurons only if neighboring neurons express NLGN1, which indicates that there is possible competition among neurons and synapses for the bringing to presynaptic NRXN.

NRXNs/NLGNs Complex at the Glutamatergic and GABAergic Synapse

In addition to its role in synapse formation, the NRXNs/NLGNs complex seems important in regulating the functional maturation and plasticity of both excitatory and inhibitory synapses.

For example, the perturbation of NRXNs–NLGNs interaction prevents activity-dependent surface delivery of the GluA1 AMPA receptor.[55]

The NLGN3 proteins are localized to both inhibitory and excitatory synapses, depending on the neuron subtype analyzed.[56–58] For example, NLGN3 in the molecular layer of the cerebellum is primarily detected at excitatory synapses whereas in the inner granular layer, it is present at both glutamatergic and GABAergic synapses.[58] Overexpression of NLGN3 in hippocampal neuronal cultures increases AMPA receptor-mediated but not NMDA receptor-mediated currents, which indicates that NLGN3 may have a role in the maturation and unsilencing of glutamatergic synapses.[41]

On the contrary, NLGN1, but not NLGN2 or NLGN3, regulates the abundance of NMDA receptors at the postsynaptic membrane via direct interaction of the extracellular domain of the glutamate NMDA receptor GluN1 subunit.[59]

Thus, at mature synapses, NLGN1 is important for the regulation of NMDA receptor-mediated synaptic responses,[49,50,60] because silencing of NLGN1 in the adult brain reduces NMDA receptor-mediated currents in the hippocampus[60] and inhibits the expression of long-term potentiation (LTP) in the amygdala.[50]

In cultured hippocampal neurons, chemical stimulation that induces either LTP or long-term depression leads to a corresponding membrane accumulation or endocytosis of NGLN1/3, which occurs in a microtubule- and dynein-dependent manner.[61] Again, in cultured rat cortical neurons, NLGN3 is associated with and is able to activate Epac2, a protein kinase A–independent cAMP target and Rap-GEF. Epac2 activation, likely by D1–D5 G protein–coupled receptors, induces spine shrinkage, increases spine motility, removes synaptic GluA2/3, and depresses excitatory transmission, whereas its inhibition promotes spine enlargement and stabilization.[62] Synaptic activity can also activate $Ca^{(2+)}$/calmodulin kinase II (CaMKII) that robustly phosphorylates the intracellular domain of NLGN1 and induces its localization to excitatory synapses.[63]

Finally, NLGN1 but not NLGN3 is necessary for LTP in young CA1 in hippocampus, and this requirement persists into adulthood in the dentate gyrus.[64] This peculiar function of NLGN1 depends on its extracellular domain containing the B site splice insertion important for specific binding with neurexin.[64]

The NRXN–NLGN complex is also important for regulating maturation of the presynaptic compartment, as demonstrated by the finding that the postsynaptic complex of PSD-95 and NLGNs can modulate the release probability of transmitter vesicles at synapses and presynaptic short-term plasticity in the hippocampus.[65,66]

Using both α-NRXN–deficient and transgenically rescued mice, it has been demonstrated that changes in synaptic properties induced by NRXNs result from selective alterations in N- and P/Q-type VDCC-mediated currents,[67] which suggests involvement of α-NRXN in the regulation of presynaptic Ca^{2+} influx via these channels.

Thus, as activity-dependent[33,68] retrograde factors, NRXNs and NLGNs may induce modification of neuronal excitability and synaptic transmission, functions directly related to the processing and storage of information in the nervous system.

It has been clearly demonstrated that NLGN2 is specifically implicated in recruitment of the postsynaptic scaffold proteins of the inhibitory synapses. Indeed, the intracellular C-terminal domain of NLGN2 interacts with gephyrin and collybistin, key scaffold components of the inhibitory postsynaptic membrane.[47,48,69]

Gephyrin is important for the postsynaptic localization of both glycine and GABA_A receptors, whereas activated collybistin recruits gephyrin to the postsynaptic membrane.

Thus, NLGN2 activates collybistin via binding with gephyrin and induces the clustering of inhibitory GABA receptors. The deletion of NLGN2 in mice therefore causes loss of postsynaptic formation at inhibitory synapses[47] and the reduction of inhibitory synaptic responses.[68]

Some in vitro data also suggest that NRXN isoforms have distinct roles in the development and maturation of brain inhibitory synapses,[33,69,70] because α-NRXN is primarily expressed by GABAergic synapses whereas β-NRXNs localize to both excitatory and inhibitory synapses.[30,71]

Thus, all of the in vitro and in vivo data suggest that NRXNs and NLGNs function as molecular switches that regulate excitatory–inhibitory balance in the brain.

During brain development and synapse formation, these SCAMs might be one of the molecular elements that control the formation of a correct excitatory–inhibitory balance by contributing to either the formation or maturation of the synapses.

Similarly, in the adult brain, both NRXNs and NLGNs might be involved in regulating excitation–inhibition balance during activity-dependent synapse plasticity. Thus, not surprisingly, mutations in the gene that codifies for either NRXNs and NLGNs contribute to dysregulation of this crucial balance that has a major role in autism spectrum disorders (ASDs), schizophrenia, and other neurodevelopmental disorders.

Mutations of NRXN and NLGN Human Gene

Mutations in the human genes encoding *Nrxn1*, *Nlgn1*, *Nlgn3*, and *Nlgn4* have been identified in individuals with autism and other neurodevelopmental diseases. For the *Nrxn1* gene, seven point mutations, two distinct translocations, and four different large-scale deletions have been identified.[72–78]

Truncating mutations in both *Nrxn1* and *Nrxn2* genes have also been identified in ASD and schizophrenia.[79]

In the *Nlgn4* gene, at least 10 different mutations have been observed (two frame shifts, five missense mutations, and three internal deletions), whereas for *Nlgn3*, a single point mutation has been identified (the R451C substitution).[80–84] Also, deletions of X-chromosomal deoxyribonucleic acid (DNA) that includes the *Nlgn4* gene were detected in patients affected by ASD.[73,85–87]

Mutations in the *Nrxn1α* gene have also been found in individuals affected by pure schizophrenia[88,89] whereas some *Nrxn3* alterations have been linked to different types of addiction.[90,91] Rare point mutations of the *Nlgn2* gene associated with schizophrenia have been also described by Sun et al.[92]

Thus, dysfunctions in synaptic adhesion molecules seem to be characterized by the manifestation of a continuum of neuronal disabilities that include autism, intellectual disability (ID), and schizophrenia.[93]

The association between NLGNs gene mutation and autism has been also confirmed by the observation that some autism-like phenotypes have been found in *Nlgn1*, *Nlgn3*, and *Nlgn4* mutant mice.[26,94–97]

All of these studies indicate that single mutations or deletion of one of the *Nlgn* or *Nrxn* genes do not perturb the overall synapse structure and formation, which suggests that these proteins are implicated in building the synapses but also that small changes in their functions induce important changes in the neural network leading to cognitive impairments.

Most mutations associated with ASDs that have been identified basically disrupt NLGN expression. However, a number of point mutations in NRXN and NLGN genes also have been found to be associated with ID and ASD and induce loss-of-function or gain-of-function effects.

One of these point mutation, the R451C substitution in *Nlgn3* gene, was identified in ASD patients,[98] and when reproduced in vitro, alters trafficking of NLGN3, leading to retention of the protein in the endoplasmic reticulum.[94,99]

Mice carrying this mutation display deficits in social interactions, increased synaptic inhibition in the somatosensory cortex, and, surprisingly, increased AMPA receptor-mediated excitatory synaptic transmission in the hippocampus.[95,98] A similar point mutation introduced to NLGN1 dramatically increased NMDA receptor currents in hippocampal neurons in vitro.[100]

In the *Nlgn4* gene, the point mutation (R704C) that is localized to the cytoplasmic region close to the transmembrane domain has been identified associated with autism.[80]

The function of this mutation was tested in the context of NLGN3, where it dramatically impaired synapse function[101] by causing a major decrease in AMPA receptor-mediated synaptic transmission in hippocampal pyramidal neurons without interfering with both NMDA and GABA receptor-mediated synaptic transmission. Thus, most of the NLGN mutations associated with neurodevelopmental disease may manifest phenotypic effects through the change in the excitation—inhibition correct ratio. However, it important to know in which brain area these synaptic and circuit alterations occur.

For example, it has been suggested that NLGN1 is required for the amygdala-related storage of associative fear memory, which indicates that the functions of NLGN1 in the amygdala might be linked to autism-related emotional and social behaviors.[50]

Most mutations identified in the *Nrxn1* and *Nrxn3* genes were associated with schizophrenia, but the functional consequences for synapse of these mutations have not been fully clarified.[1,16] However, it is possible to hypnotize that, based on the importance of NRXNs for presynaptic vesicle release and PSD assembly in both excitatory[53,102,103] and inhibitory synapses,[71] NRXN protein alteration may also induce an imbalance in the excitatory—inhibitory ratio during development and the dysregulation of activity-dependent synapse development and plasticity.

All NLGNs have a large extracellular catalytically inactive acetylcholinesterase-homologous domain[104,105] that mediates the homo- and heterodimerization of NLGN required for its function but not for binding with NRXN.[31,47,106]

Specific metalloproteases can process the extracellular domain of NRXNs, generating a secreted form of NRXN and a membrane-tethered C-terminal fragment, which subsequently becomes a substrate for the presenilin/γ—secretase complex.[107,108] Thus, presenilin can regulate NRXN/NLGN1 accumulation at synaptic terminals, which indicates that alteration of this process can contribute to altered synaptic function in familiar Alzheimer disease.

NLGN1 and NLGN3 also undergo proteolytic cleavage.[109–111] N-Methyl-D-aspartate receptor activation can induce the cleavage of NLGN1 and cause destabilization of NRXN1β. The cleavage of NLGN3 is affected in glioblastoma proliferation because the extracellular domain released by activated neurons can trigger a receptor-mediated proliferative pathway in glial cells.[111]

Along this line, it has been shown that NLGN1 can regulate neurite formation, and this effect depends on interaction with NRXN1β and fibroblast grown factor receptor 1 (FGFR1).[112] Indeed there is a strong sequence similarity between NRXN1β and FGF8, which suggests that the FGFR1 binding site on NRXN1 is similar to the FGFR binding site on FGF8 and that alteration of NRXN1 interaction with FGFR might lead to superactivation of FGF signaling observed in some forms of autism.[112]

In conclusion, genetic and functional data indicate that mutations in one of the multiple members of NLGN and NRXN are always associated with major neurodevelopmental disorders and that all of these molecules have an important role in regulating synapse structure and function.

MUTATIONS IN PTPδ/IL1RAPL1 COMPLEX

IL1RAPL1 Protein Complex and Function

Interleukin-1 receptor accessory protein-like 1 (IL1RAPL1) is a transmembrane protein of 696 amino acids that belongs to a new Toll/IL-1 receptor family and shares 52% homology with the IL-1 receptor accessory protein (IL-1RAcP). Interleukin-1 receptor accessory protein-like 1 is structurally formed by three extracellular immunoglobulin (Ig)-like domains, a transmembrane domain, an intracellular Toll/IL-1R homology domain (TIR domain), and a unique c-terminal tail. The *Il1rapl1* gene extends for 1.3 Mbases on chromosome X in the Xp22.1−21.3 region.[113] *Il1rapl1* cDNA is composed of 11 exons, for a total 3.6 kb.

Another member of this class is IL1RAPL1 homologue, IL1RAPL2 (or TIGIRR-1, 3 Ig domain-containing IL-1 receptor-related) that shares 63% amino acid identity with IL1RAPL1.[114]

Interleukin-1 receptor accessory protein-like 1 transcript is expressed at a low level in fetal and adult brain; the first detectable transcript in mouse brain is at embryonic day (E)10.5, with an increased level at E12.5 that remains the same in adult life. The high level of expression of IL1RAPL1 in brain areas involved in memory development, such as hippocampus, dentate gyrus, and entorhinal cortex, suggests that this gene may have a specialized role in physiological processes underlying memory and learning abilities.[113,115] It is also highly expressed in mouse olfactory bulb and tubercle, which may be correlated with the evolutionary trend implicating the predominant role of olfactory perception in behavioral development in lower mammals.[113] In the amygdaloid complex, expression spans all excitatory (basolateral amygdala) and inhibitory (intercalated cells and central amygdala) regions homogeneously.[116]

Analysis of the other tissues reveal the transcription of IL1RAPL1 in heart, ovary, and skin, and a lesser level of expression in tonsil, fetal liver, prostate, testis, small intestine, placenta, and colon. Expression was not detected in spleen, lymph node, thymus, bone marrow, leukocytes, lung, liver, skeletal muscle, kidney, or pancreas.[114] Interleukin-1 receptor accessory protein-like 1 messenger ribonucleic acid (mRNA) and protein expression is low compared with that of VGLUT1 or GAD67,[116] which indicates that in general, IL1RAPL1 is considered a low-abundant protein in the brain.

However, the level of IL1RAPL expression was significantly upregulated after kainite treatment and LTP induction, suggesting a possible role for this gene in activity-dependent brain plasticity.[117]

Immunocytochemical staining with anti-IL1RAPL1 antibody shows that endogenous protein clusters are distributed in the dendrites of cultured cortical neurons and partially overlapped with postsynaptic Shank1 clusters[118]; meanwhile, overexpression of IL1RAPL1 increases staining signals of excitatory postsynaptic protein PSD-95 and Shank2.[118,119] A comparison of Shank and synaptophysin (a marker of presynaptic compartment) cluster signals underlines predominant postsynaptic localization of IL1RAPL1.[118] Moreover, there is a high level of colocalization between IL1RAPL1 and PSD-95; instead, it is only partial with VGAT (a marker of inhibitory synapse), so IL1RAPL1 is mostly localized in excitatory synapses in the postsynaptic membrane.[118]

In contrast to other members of the Toll/IL-1 receptor family, IL1RAPL1 has 150 additional and unique amino acids at the C-terminus, which interact with neuronal calcium sensor-1,[120] regulating N-type voltage-gated calcium channel activity in PC12 cells and in neurons; this indicates that IL1RAPL1 protein is also partially localized at the presynaptic membrane.[121]

Stable expression of IL1RAPL1 in PC12 cells induces specific silencing of N-type voltage-gated calcium channel (NVGCC) activity, which explains the secretion deficit observed in these cells. Importantly, this modulation of VGCC activity is mediated by NCS-1. Indeed, specific loss-of-function of N-VGCC was observed in PC12 cells overexpressing NCS-1 and total recovery of N-VGCC activity was obtained by downregulation of NCS-1 in IL1RAPL1-overexpressing cells. Because both proteins are highly expressed in neurons, these results suggest that IL1RAPL1 regulates N-VGCC and/or NCS-1–dependent synaptic and neuronal activities.[121]

However, in vitro, IL1RAPL1 has a major role in presynaptic differentiation and dendritic spine formation and stabilization in cortical and hippocampal neurons. Synthetic RNA against IL1RAPL1 can reduce the number of dendritic protrusions in neuron culture,[119] and IL1RAPL1 overexpression in neurons increases VGLUT1 (an excitatory presynaptic marker) staining and dendritic spine number.[118,122] Furthermore, the increase in synapse number is associated with an increase in miniature excitatory postsynaptic potential (mEPSC) frequency.[118]

Pavlowsky et al.[118] showed that the first and second PDZ domains of PSD-95 bind to the C-terminal tail of IL1RAPL1 that contains a putative PDZ binding motif. Using gain- and loss-of-function experiments in neurons, it was demonstrated that IL1RAPL1 regulates the synaptic localization of PSD-95 by controlling c-Jun terminal kinase (JNK) activity and PSD-95 phosphorylation.[118]

Interleukin-1 receptor accessory protein-like 1 overexpression in hippocampal primary cultured neurons increases spine density without affecting morphology.[118,122] This effect requires both extracellular and intracellular domains of IL1RAPL1 and does not depend on PSD-95 interaction.[118,122] The extracellular domain is sufficient to increase excitatory presynaptic compartment recruitment (intensity level of VGLUT1 staining).[122]

Indeed, multiple interactors are needed to induce spine formation: The TIR domain can recruit a synaptic RhoGAP, RhoGAP2; meanwhile, the extracellular domain can bind to receptor tyrosine phosphatase δ (PTPδ), a member of LAR-RPTP family, which suggests a role of IL1RAPL1 as a synaptic cell adhesion protein.[119,122]

Thus, the extracellular domain of IL1RAPL1 induces excitatory synapse formation by binding particular splice variants of PTPδ[119,123] localized at the pre synaptic terminal (Figure 2).[122]

Blocking IL1RAPL1–PTPδ interaction abolished Rho-GAP2 recruitment at excitatory synapses, which suggests that IL1RAPL1 is involved in a novel trans-synaptic signaling pathway that regulates excitatory synapse and dendritic spine formation.[7,122]

However, it has not been shown definitively whether dendritic recruitment of IL1RAPL1 by PTPδ is sufficient

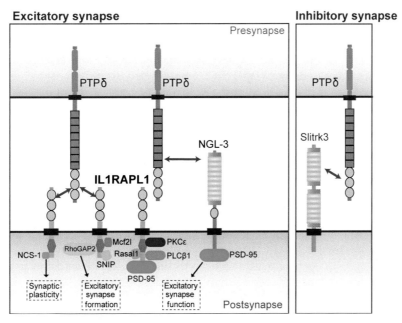

FIGURE 2   The drawing depicts a schematic representation of the IL1RAPL1—PTPδ complexes and putative synaptic functions at excitatory and inhibitory synapses.

to recruit postsynaptic proteins, for example, by direct aggregation of IL1RAPL1 on dendrites. This probability is supported by the finding that a soluble IL1RAPL1 ectodomain inhibits postsynaptic differentiation by PTPδ.[119]

All of these findings suggest that the IL1RAPL1 complex, similar to the neuroligin—neurexin complex, regulates trans-synaptic signaling that induces excitatory synapse and dendritic spine formation in brain.

It was been discovered through affinity chromatography that a new partner of IL1RAPL1, Mcf2-like (Mcf2l), a Rho guanine nucleotide exchange factor (GEF), activates RhoA and Cdc42, and binds to TIR domain of IL1RAPL1. RhoA and Rac1 are implicated in the cytoskeletal dynamics that induce the structural change of excitatory spines. Actin cytoskeletal dynamics are regulated by RhoA-dependent activation of Rho-associated protein kinase (ROCK).[124]

Knockdown of endogenous Mcf2l and treatment with an inhibitor of ROCK partially suppressed IL1RAPL1--induced excitatory synapse formation of cortical neurons, which suggests that IL1RAPL1 controls spine formation of cortical neurons through the Mcf2l-RhoA--ROCK signaling pathway, as well.[124]

Furthermore, the expression of IL1RAPL1 affected the turnover of AMPA receptor subunits and the Mcf2l--RhoA-ROCK signaling pathway acts downstream of IL1RAPL1 in excitatory synapse stabilization.[124] One process important in maintaining synaptic strength and in stabilization of recently formed synapses is the constitutive replacement of synaptic GluA1 by GluA2/3 (AMPAR subunits).[125] This process takes up to 20 h.

Overexpression of IL1RAPL1 for 2—3 days in cortical neurons leads to the replacement of newly inserted AMPA receptor compositions through the Mcf2l-RhoA-ROCK signaling pathway. In summary, IL1RAPL1, through the Mcf2l-RhoA-ROCK signaling pathway, regulates the formation and stabilization of glutamatergic synapses between cortical neurons.[124]

In vivo, the role of *Il1rapl1b*, an ortholog of IL1RAPL1, was analyzed in olfactory sensory neurons of zebrafish. Antisense morpholino oligonucleotide against *il1rapl1b* suppressed both synaptic vesicle accumulation and axon terminal remodeling. Consistently, overexpression of *Il1rapl1b* stimulated synaptic vesicle accumulation. Swapping the carboxyl-terminal domain of *Il1rapl1b* with that of mouse IL-1 receptor accessory protein abolished the stimulatory effect. On the other hand, a substitution mutation in the TIR domain suppressed the morphological remodeling of axon terminals. Thus, regulation of synaptic vesicle accumulation and subsequent morphological remodeling by Il1rapl1b appeared to be mediated by distinct domains.[126]

Loss of IL1RAPL1 in KO mice leads to a slight but significant reduction of spine density in the cortex[127] and in the CA1 region of hippocampus[118]; meanwhile, the architecture of this contact is unchanged (spine shape and presynaptic and postsynaptic structure).[118] Functionally, the reduction in excitatory synapse number results in a small, insignificant reduction in mEPSC and LTP impairment only with a paradigm of theta burst stimulation (LTP for high-frequency stimulation is comparable to wild-type [WT] mice).[118] Data from behavioral studies demonstrated that *Il1rapl1* KO male mice are impaired in spatial memory and cued fear memory formation.[116] In addition, the acquisition and retention of spatial reference memory, spatial working memory, and long-term fear memories are also altered in KO mice.[128] Social interaction is increased in *Il1rapl1* KO mice and their motor coordination is improved, but motor learning ability is comparable with WT mice.[128] Finally, *Il1rapl1* KO mice show enhanced locomotor activity and reduced anxiety-like behavior.[128]

Abnormalities in the formation and function of cerebellar circuitry potentially contribute to cognitive deficits in humans. The absence of IL1RAPL1 causes transient disinhibition of deep cerebellar nuclei neurons; upstream, in the cerebellar cortex, developmental perturbations have been also found in the activity level of molecular layer interneurons. Thus, IL1RAPL1 exerts a key function during cerebellar development in establishing local excitation–inhibition balance.[129] More than 90% of autistic patients exhibit cerebellar abnormalities[130]; thus, this results provide additional insight into physiological defects in patients.

Mutations of *IL1RAPL1* Human Gene

Different mutations in the *IL1RAPL1* gene have been discovered in members of families with ID and ASD.

First, Carriè et al. identified a patient with a C–A transition in exon 11 that changes the codon codifying tyrosine (TAC) to a stop codon (TAA) (Y459X), resulting in a protein lacking part of the TIR domain and all of the C-terminal tail.[113]

In another family, three males with ID and an intelligence quotient IQ <70 have a truncated form of protein that lacks the last 210 amino acids in the cytoplasmic domain because of a mutation G1460A in exon 10 of the gene resulting in a substitution trp487stop (W487X).[131] Moreover, in three brothers with an IQ of 55, hyperactivity, attention deficit, auto-aggressivity, and dysmorphism have been discovered to carry a truncated form of IL1RAPL1 caused by a deletion in exon 11.[132] Another mutation (7 nucleotide deletion c.1730delTACTCTT) in exon 9 causes a frame shift at Ile367 with a premature stop codon (TGA) 6 codons downstream (p.Ile367SerfsX6), resulting in a truncated protein that lacks a part of the transmembrane domain as well as the entire cytoplasmic domain; this deletion produces a truncated IL1RAPL1 protein unable to reach the cell surface.[130] In another family, a frame shift mutation (A28EfsX15) results in the exclusion of exons 3, 4, 5, 6, and 7.[130] Patients with the last two described mutations are affected by both ID and ASD.[130]

Another deletion in the extracellular domain (exons 2, 3, 4, 5, and 6 of the gene) was described by Nawara et al. (2008) and Franek at al. (2011).[133,134] The patients have hyperactivity ID, aggressivity,[133] low IQ, and

dysmorphism.[134] The same research group discovered in two male brothers a deletion in exons 1–5; interestingly, the patients have ID but are not autistic.[134]

Deletions of exons coding for the extracellular regions have been found in two German patients from two different unrelated families and share low IQ and psychomotor development delay. One has exon 2 deleted; in the other, the deletion starts 245,454 base pairs (bp) after exon 2 and ends 117,424 bp after exon 5.[135]

An Italian patient with ID, ASD, and an epilepsy episode has a 285-kb deletion in chromosome Xp21.3–21.2, with breakpoints lying in *IL1RAPL1* gene exon 3.[136]

An inversion in chromosome X has also been identified, inv(X)(p21.3q27.1),[137] and a complex deletion-inversion that leads to a loss of a number of genes and to the creation of a fusion protein between IL1RAPL1 and dystrophin.[138]

Duplication can also lead to pathology: A 15.5-Mb duplication (Xp11.4-p21.3 region containing 41 genes including *IDX*, *IL1RAPL1*, and *TSPAN7*) can lead to ID, which suggests the importance of the correct dosage of protein.[139]

Deletions involving the *IL1RAPL1* gene are summarized in Ramos-Brossier et al.[140]

Most of the described mutations includes large deletions and most involve the first few exons coding for the extracellular domain of IL1RAPL1 protein. Some authors suggest that because of the frequent incidence of genomic rearrangements, such as pericentromeric inversions, this region must be particularly prone to recombination.[133,134,137,140]

In summary, most of the mutations described lead to the absence of IL1RAPL1 production or to a small or truncated form of the protein, which can result in the loss of some protein–protein interactions because of the lack of interacting regions or loss of correct protein localization in the synapse.[113,120,130–141]

Mutations and deletions of the *IL1RAPL1* gene are related to different phenotypes (even in the same family and in patients with the same mutation), including different severity of ID, association with ASD, and other physical features. Moreover, the phenotype of carrier females is interesting: Although they largely have normal cognitive skills, some display mild cognitive impairment or learning difficulties, likely attributable to different X-inactivation patterns.[131]

Il1rapl1 KO Mice as Animal Model for ID and ASD

The learning deficiencies and memory declines observed in *Il1rapl1* KO mice mimic the symptoms of ID children with *IL1RAPL1* mutations.[128] Children with deletions and mutation in the *IL1RAPL1* gene have a delay in the onset of walking capacity and speech and need specific intensive education programs.[134–136,142] In line with the *IL1RAPL1* gene being associated with ASD[130,132,143] *Il1rapl1* KO mice have stereotyped behaviors[128] and reduced behavioral flexibility, displaying poor performance in the reversal task of the T-maze left–right discrimination test but not in the Barnes maze test.[128] However, in the rotarod test, *Il1rapl1* KO mice perform better than WT mice,[128] which may be attributable to the stereotypic behaviors of *Il1rapl1* KO mice. Indeed, better performance in the repetitive test of motor coordination was also reported for mutant mice exhibiting autistic behavior.[144,145] Intriguingly, the social interaction of *Il1rapl1* KO mice is increased in one-chamber and Crawley's three-chamber social interaction tests,[128] whereas vocal communication of *il1rapl1* KO mice are comparable to those of WT mice.[128]

Locomotor activity is also enhanced in *Il1rapl1* KO mice,[128] reminiscent of the hyperactivity reported for ID patients with mutations in the *IL1RAPL1* gene.[133–136] Finally, *Il1rapl1* KO mice demonstrate a clear deficit in fear memories[116,128,146] and reduced anxiety.[128]

These studies with mutant mice reveal that the ablation of IL1RAPL1 affects diverse brain functions including learning, memory, behavioral flexibility, locomotor activity, and anxiety.[118,128,146]

A decrease in spine density in *Il1rapl1* mutant mice will cause excitation and inhibition imbalances in many brain circuits, because IL1RAPL1 is widely expressed in the brain.[113,116,146] Thus, it is reasonable that multiple brain functions are affected by the *Il1rapl1* mutation.[128]

For instance, altered E/I balance at the hippocampus-basolateral amygdala projections leads to a deficit in contextual memory expression rather than memory formation, which suggests that cognitive disability in humans may result from the deficiency of synapses involved at different steps of the cognitive process, including memory restitution and behavioral expression.[146]

Further investigation of the molecular mechanism of IL1RAPL1-mediated excitatory synapse formation would identify potential drug targets and *Il1rapl1* KO mice will be useful to assess possible new treatments.[128]

Protein Tyrosine Phosphatase δ in Regulation of IL1RAPL1-Dependent Synapse Formation

Protein tyrosine phosphatase δ is a member of the leukocyte common antigen-related (LAR)-RPTP family,[147,148] a subfamily of receptor PTP (RPTP) type IIa, localized on synaptic membrane with a role in axon outgrowth and guidance.[149–152] Protein tyrosine phosphatase σ and LAR are the other vertebrate members of

the LAR-RPTP family.[153,154] LAR-RPTPs, encoded by three independent genes, are about 65% identical in aa sequence and share a similar domain structure[155,156] LAR-RPTPs have three Ig-like domains and eight fibronectin III (FNIII) domains in the extracellular domain (ECD), which suggests a role of LAR-RPTPs in cell–cell and cell–matrix interactions and therefore in synaptic adhesion and synapse organization. The intracellular region contains two PTP domains. The membrane-proximal phosphatase domain (D1) is catalytically active, whereas the other domain (D2) is catalytically inactive and is involved in protein–protein interactions.[155,157–159] LAR-RPTPs can interlink distinct tyrosine phosphorylation signaling pathways, mostly by dephosphorylating elements of these pathways. For example, there is an interaction between PTPσ D1 domain and PTPδ D2 domain that has a negative regulatory function.[160]

LAR-RPTPs expressed in the brain regulate the formation of trans-synaptic protein complexes at both excitatory and inhibitory synapses, contributing to the three following aspects of synapse development. One is to mediate cell–cell adhesion at synapses: For instance, the full-length extracellular domain of PTPδ functions as a ligand to promote cell adhesion, neurite outgrowth, and axon guidance.[157,161,162] The second is to mediate presynaptic differentiation through local recruitment of synaptic vesicles and release and recycling machinery (a form of retrograde synaptogenic signaling triggered by the binding of the postsynaptic partner to axonal RPTPs). The third is to trigger postsynaptic differentiation through local recruitment of neurotransmitter receptors, scaffolds, and signaling proteins (a form of anterograde synaptogenic signaling triggered by the binding of presynaptic RPTPs to dendritic binding partners).[6,18]

In situ hybridization of mouse brain slices revealed that PTPδ mRNA is present in diverse brain regions.[147,163–165] Protein tyrosine phosphatase δ mRNA, together with LAR and PTPσ mRNA, displays overlapping and differential distribution patterns in the brain. For example, PTPδ mRNA is more abundant than the others in the reticular thalamic area, cortical layer 4, hippocampal CA2 region, and the mitral cell layer of the olfactory bulb, whereas it is less abundant in the internal granule layer of the olfactory bulb and the septal area.

Structurally, LAR-RPTPs undergo proteolytic processing that generates an extracellular subunit that remains noncovalently bound to the transmembrane region of the protein.[6,161] Proteolytic cleavage of PTPδ takes place at a site in the ECD located near the membrane, and the two cleaved products (150 and 85 kDa; E and P subunits) from a longer form (220 kDa) and are detected on the cell surface as a noncovalently associated complex.[166]

Immunoblotting with the antibody that was raised against the D1 domain of LAR but recognizes all three

LAR-RPTPs showed that LAR-RPTP proteins are widely expressed in different regions of the rat central nervous system and at higher levels in postnatal day (P)7 brain than in adult (P45) brain, consistent with mRNA expression data.[150] The approximately 85-kDa band of the LAR-RPTP protein shows the biochemical fractionation pattern expected for an integral membrane protein. LAR-RPTP is enriched in postsynaptic density (PSD) fractions, although to a lesser extent than PSD-95. At 7 days in vitro, LAR-RPTPs show fine punctate immunostaining in cell bodies and dendrites of cultured hippocampal neurons and only partial colocalization with PSD-95 or with bassoon, a presynaptic active zone protein.[150] With neuronal maturation, an increasing fraction of LAR puncta becomes synaptically localized and an increasing percentage of synapses show detectable LAR staining. These immunocytochemical and biochemical findings are consistent with LAR-RPTPs being enriched at excitatory synapses but more widely distributed in neurons than PSD-95.

Neurons expressing any single LAR-RPTP RNA interference (RNAi), or any combination of them, show a lower density of dendritic spines and PSD-95 puncta than did vector-transfected cells. The LAR-RPTP RNAi—transfected neurons also show a substantial decrease in the surface staining intensity of the GluA2 subunit of AMPA receptors.[150] These results indicate that LAR-RPTPs are important in developing and maintaining excitatory synapses.

LAR-RPTPs bind to multiple postsynaptic ligands to mediate various trans-synaptic complexes: netrin-G ligand-3 (NGL-3),[165,167] neurotrophin receptor tropomyosin-related kinase C (TrkC),[168] IL1RAPL1,[119,122] interleukin-1 receptor accessory protein (IL1RAcP),[127] and Slit and NTRK-like family (Slitrks).[169,170] Netrin-G ligand-3 binds to LAR, PTPσ, and PTPδ through its first two FNIII domains, whereas all others bind to the Ig domain region of LAR-RPTPs. In addition, LAR-RPTPs bind to postsynaptic partners in an isoform-specific manner. For instance, all three LAR-RPTPs bind to NGL-3, TrkC binds selectively to PTPσ, and IL1RAPL1 selectively to PTPδ, IL1RAcP to LAR, PTPσ, and PTPδ, and Slitrks selectively to PTPδ and PTPσ (Figure 2).[169,170]

The Slitrk family consists of six brain-specific transmembrane proteins (Slitrk1—6) that are able to induce presynaptic differentiation. All Slitrks can interact with PTPδ.[168] Intriguingly, Slitrk3 induces inhibitory, but not excitatory, presynaptic differentiation.[169,170] Knockdown of distinct LAR-RPTP members in cultured neurons co-cultured with Slitrk-expressing cells produces specific phenotypes: knockdown of PTPσ abolishes the activity of Slitrk1 and Slitrk2 in triggering excitatory presynaptic differentiation, whereas knockdown of PTPδ compromises the activity of Slitrk1—3 in inducing inhibitory presynaptic differentiation.[169,170] It remains to be

determined how PTPδ governs synapse organization in distinct synapse types.[6]

Vertebrate LAR-RPTPs possess multiple splice sites mini exons (me), called meA, meB, meC, and meD.[119,148,166] The meA and meB peptides of LAR-RPTPs are particularly important for modulating interactions with their ligands: The meA is predicted to affect the length of a loop region between the D and E β-strands of the second Ig-like domain, whereas the meB is predicted to affect the spacing between the second and third Ig-like domains. This feature is crucial to regulate the binding-affinity.[119,166]

The PTPδ isoform that contains inserts at both meA and meB sites, a major brain isoform of PTPδ, binds to all Slitrks, IL1RAPL1, and IL1RacP, probably with different binding affinities. Because the meA and meB splice inserts of PTPδ control its binding to IL1RAPL1 and IL1RAcP differentially, it is possible that differential splicing of PTPδ in GABAergic versus glutamatergic axons contributes to selectivity in partner binding and function. Such a mechanism is reminiscent of the role of alternative splicing in neurexins in terms of controlling binding to various postsynaptic ligands.[16]

However, more complicated mechanisms involving axon-selective co-receptors or suppressors to regulate specificity of interactions cannot be ruled out.[171]

Intracellularly, the D2 domain of PTPδ, which is catalytically inactive, interacts with diverse cytoplasmic proteins, including liprin-α, MIM-B, Trio, and Ena/Vasp.[6,172] Liprin-α is an adaptor protein that links PTPδ to diverse presynaptic active zone proteins, including RIM, ELKS, GIT1, and CASK. Liprin-α is not a substrate of PTPδ and is likely to bring phosphotyrosine proteins close to the proximity of the catalytically active D1 domain. MIM-B, Trio, and Ena/Vasp are known to regulate the actin cytoskeleton at presynaptic nerve terminals. These mechanisms may contribute to the presynaptic development induced by presynaptic PTPδ clustering.

In vivo functions of PTPδ have been explored by mouse genetic approaches. Protein tyrosine phosphatase δ-deficient mice are semi-lethal owing to insufficient food intake.[164] They also exhibit impaired learning and memory in the Morris water maze, T-maze, and radial arm maze tasks. In addition, PTPδ-deficient hippocampal synapses display enhanced long-term potentiation (LTP) and paired-pulse facilitation. Therefore, it seems that PTPδ is important for hippocampal LTP and learning and memory, and that hippocampal LTP does not necessarily promotes spatial learning and memory. In addition, double deletion of PTPδ and PTPσ has been shown to impair motor axon targeting,[173] which suggests that the two proteins are functionally redundant.

Interestingly, PTPδ is associated with diverse neurological and psychiatric disorders in humans. Mutations in the chromosomal locus of the PTPδ gene (9p24.3—p23) have been associated with restless legs syndrome,[174,175] ASD,[176] attention-deficit hyperactivity disorder,[177] and bipolar disorder and schizophrenia.[89] However, little is known about how PTPδ deletion leads to these dysfunctions.

CONCLUSIONS

It has been well-demonstrated that in humans, deletions or mutations in some of the family of genes that codify for synaptic adhesion molecules such as neurexins—neuroligins and PTPδ—IL1RAPL1 are associated with several cognitive disorders, including ASD, ID, and schizophrenia. Although an increasing number of mutations and affected patients will be described in the near future, the development and functional characterization of in vitro and in vivo models that mimics the mutations will help develop new possible pharmacological or genetic treatments. The challenge will be to identify therapeutic targets for the multiple and diverse synaptic and neuronal alterations induced by mutations of these synaptic adhesion molecules.

Acknowledgments

This work was supported by Comitato Telethon Fondazione Onlus (grants GGP13187 and GGP11095 (to C.S.)); Fondazione CARIPLO project 2012-0593 (to C.S.); and the Yonsei University Future-leading Research Initiative of 2014 (to J.K.).

References

1. Südhof TC. Neuroligins and neurexins link synaptic function to cognitive disease. *Nature* 2008;**455**(7215):903—11.
2. Woo J, Kwon SK, Kim E. The NGL family of leucine-rich repeat-containing synaptic adhesion molecules. *Mol Cell Neurosci* 2009;**42**(1):1—10.
3. Nam J, Mah W, Kim E. The SALM/Lrfn family of leucine-rich repeat-containing cell adhesion molecules. *Semin Cell Dev Biol* 2011;**22**(5):492—8.
4. Bukalo O, Dityatev A. Synaptic cell adhesion molecules. *Adv Exp Med Biol* 2012;**970**:97—128.
5. Reissner C, Runkel F, Missler M. Neurexins. *Genome Biol* 2013;**14**(9):213.
6. Um JW, Ko J. LAR-RPTPs: synaptic adhesion molecules that shape synapse development. *Trends Cell Biol* 2013;**23**(10):465—75.
7. Sala C, Segal M. Dendritic spines: the locus of structural and functional plasticity. *Physiol Rev* 2014;**94**(1):141—88.
8. Yamagata M, Sanes JR, Weiner JA. Synaptic adhesion molecules. *Curr Opin Cell Biol* 2003;**15**(5):621—32.
9. Dalva MB, McClelland AC, Kayser MS. Cell adhesion molecules: signalling functions at the synapse. *Nat Rev Neurosci* 2007;**8**(3):206—20.
10. Valnegri P, Sala C, Passafaro M. Synaptic dysfunction and intellectual disability. *Adv Exp Med Biol* 2012;**970**:433—49.
11. Biederer T, Stagi M. Signaling by synaptogenic molecules. *Curr Opin Neurobiol* 2008;**18**(3):261—9.
12. Shen K, Scheiffele P. Genetics and cell biology of building specific synaptic connectivity. *Annu Rev Neurosci* 2010;**33**:473—507.
13. de Wit J, Hong W, Luo L, Ghosh A. Role of leucine-rich repeat proteins in the development and function of neural circuits. *Annu Rev Cell Dev Biol* 2011;**27**:697—729.
14. Yuzaki M. Cbln1 and its family proteins in synapse formation and maintenance. *Curr Opin Neurobiol* 2011;**21**(2):215—20.
15. Krueger DD, Tuffy LP, Papadopoulos T, Brose N. The role of neurexins and neuroligins in the formation, maturation, and function of vertebrate synapses. *Curr Opin Neurobiol* 2012;**22**(3):412—22.
16. Missler M, Südhof TC, Biederer T. Synaptic cell adhesion. *Cold Spring Harb Perspect Biol* 2012;**4**(4):a005694.
17. Song YS, Kim E. Presynaptic proteoglycans: sweet organizers of synapse development. *Neuron* 2013;**79**(4):609—11.
18. Takahashi H, Craig AM. Protein tyrosine phosphatases PTPδ, PTPσ, and LAR: presynaptic hubs for synapse organization. *Trends Neurosci* 2013;**36**(9):522—34.
19. de Wit J, Ghosh A. Control of neural circuit formation by leucine-rich repeat proteins. *Trends Neurosci* 2014;**37**(10):539—50.
20. Bang ML, Owczarek S. A matter of balance: role of neurexin and neuroligin at the synapse. *Neurochem Res* 2013;**38**(6):1174—89.
21. Ko J. The leucine-rich repeat superfamily of synaptic adhesion molecules: LRRTMs and Slitrks. *Mol Cells* 2012;**34**(4):335—40.
22. Tallafuss A, Constable JR, Washbourne P. Organization of central synapses by adhesion molecules. *Eur J Neurosci* 2010;**32**(2):198—206.
23. Taniguchi H, Gollan L, Scholl FG, et al. Silencing of neuroligin function by postsynaptic neurexins. *J Neurosci* 2007;**27**(11):2815—24.
24. Schreiner D, Nguyen TM, Russo G, et al. Targeted combinatorial alternative splicing generates brain region-specific repertoires of neurexins. *Neuron* 2014;**84**(2):386—98.
25. Treutlein B, Gokce O, Quake SR, Südhof TC. Cartography of neurexin alternative splicing mapped by single-molecule long-read mRNA sequencing. *Proc Natl Acad Sci USA* 2014;**111**(13):E1291—9.
26. Blundell J, Blaiss CA, Etherton MR, et al. Neuroligin-1 deletion results in impaired spatial memory and increased repetitive behavior. *J Neurosci* 2010;**30**(6):2115—29.
27. Bolliger MF, Pei J, Maxeiner S, Boucard AA, Grishin NV, Sudhof TC. Unusually rapid evolution of neuroligin-4 in mice. *Proc Natl Acad Sci USA* 2008;**105**(17):6421—6.
28. Graf ER, Kang Y, Hauner AM, Craig AM. Structure function and splice site analysis of the synaptogenic activity of the neurexin-1 beta LNS domain. *J Neurosci* 2006;**26**(16):4256—65.
29. Boucard AA, Chubykin AA, Comoletti D, Taylor P, Sudhof TC. A splice code for trans-synaptic cell adhesion mediated by binding of neuroligin 1 to alpha- and beta-neurexins. *Neuron* 2005;**48**(2):229—36.
30. Chih B, Gollan L, Scheiffele P. Alternative splicing controls selective trans-synaptic interactions of the neuroligin-neurexin complex. *Neuron* 2006;**51**(2):171—8.
31. Dean C, Scholl FG, Choih J, et al. Neurexin mediates the assembly of presynaptic terminals. *Nat Neurosci* 2003;**6**(7):708—16.
32. Koehnke J, Katsamba PS, Ahlsen G, et al. Splice form dependence of beta-neurexin/neuroligin binding interactions. *Neuron* 2010;**67**(1):61—74.
33. Iijima T, Wu K, Witte H, et al. SAM68 regulates neuronal activity-dependent alternative splicing of neurexin-1. *Cell* 2011;**147**(7):1601—14.
34. de Wit J, Sylwestrak E, O'Sullivan ML, et al. LRRTM2 interacts with Neurexin1 and regulates excitatory synapse formation. *Neuron* 2009;**64**(6):799—806.
35. Ko J, Fuccillo MV, Malenka RC, Südhof TC. LRRTM2 functions as a neurexin ligand in promoting excitatory synapse formation. *Neuron* 2009;**64**(6):791—8.

36. Irie M, Hata Y, Takeuchi M, et al. Binding of neuroligins to PSD-95. *Science* 1997;**277**:1511–5.

37. Dean C, Dresbach T. Neuroligins and neurexins: linking cell adhesion, synapse formation and cognitive function. *Trends Neurosci* 2006;**29**(1):21–9.

38. Scheiffele P, Fan J, Choih J, Fetter R, Serafini T. Neuroligin expressed in nonneuronal cells triggers presynaptic development in contacting axons. *Cell* 2000;**101**(6):657–69.

39. Graf ER, Zhang X, Jin SX, Linhoff MW, Craig AM. Neurexins induce differentiation of GABA and glutamate postsynaptic specializations via neuroligins. *Cell* 2004;**119**(7):1013–26.

40. Levinson JN, Chéry N, Huang K, et al. Neuroligins mediate excitatory and inhibitory synapse formation: involvement of PSD-95 and neurexin-1beta in neuroligin-induced synaptic specificity. *J Biol Chem* 2005;**280**(17):17312–9.

41. Shipman SL, Schnell E, Hirai T, Chen BS, Roche KW, Nicoll RA. Functional dependence of neuroligin on a new non-PDZ intracellular domain. *Nat Neurosci* 2011;**14**(6):718–26.

42. Levinson JN, El-Husseini A. Building excitatory and inhibitory synapses: balancing neuroligin partnerships. *Neuron* 2005;**48**(2):171–4.

43. Prange O, Wong TP, Gerrow K, Wang YT, El-Husseini A. A balance between excitatory and inhibitory synapses is controlled by PSD-95 and neuroligin. *Proc Natl Acad Sci USA* 2004;**101**(38):13915–20.

44. Varley ZK, Pizzarelli R, Antonelli R, et al. Gephyrin regulates GABAergic and glutamatergic synaptic transmission in hippocampal cell cultures. *J Biol Chem* 2011;**286**(23):20942–51.

45. Gerrow K, Romorini S, Nabi SM, Colicos MA, Sala C, El-Husseini A. A preformed complex of postsynaptic proteins is involved in excitatory synapse development. *Neuron* 2006;**49**(4):547–62.

46. Lise MF, El-Husseini A. The neuroligin and neurexin families: from structure to function at the synapse. *CMLS* 2006;**63**(16):1833–49.

47. Poulopoulos A, Aramuni G, Meyer G, et al. Neuroligin 2 drives postsynaptic assembly at perisomatic inhibitory synapses through gephyrin and collybistin. *Neuron* 2009;**63**(5):628–42.

48. Chih B, Engelman H, Scheiffele P. Control of excitatory and inhibitory synapse formation by neuroligins. *Science* 2005;**307**(5713):1324–8.

49. Kim J, Jung SY, Lee YK, et al. Neuroligin-1 is required for normal expression of LTP and associative fear memory in the amygdala of adult animals. *Proc Natl Acad Sci USA* 2008;**105**(26):9087–92.

50. Jung SY, Kim J, Kwon OB, et al. Input-specific synaptic plasticity in the amygdala is regulated by neuroligin-1 via postsynaptic NMDA receptors. *Proc Natl Acad Sci USA* 2010;**107**(10):4710–5.

51. Zhang C, Atasoy D, Arac D, et al. Neurexins physically and functionally interact with GABA(A) receptors. *Neuron* 2010;**66**(3):403–16.

52. Varoqueaux F, Aramuni G, Rawson RL, et al. Neuroligins determine synapse maturation and function. *Neuron* 2006;**51**(6):741–54.

53. Missler M, Zhang W, Rohlmann A, et al. Alpha-neurexins couple Ca^{2+} channels to synaptic vesicle exocytosis. *Nature* 2003;**423**(6943):939–48.

54. Kwon HB, Kozorovitskiy Y, Oh WJ, et al. Neuroligin-1-dependent competition regulates cortical synaptogenesis and synapse number. *Nature Neurosci* 2012;**15**(12):1667–74.

55. Mondin M, Labrousse V, Hosy E, et al. Neurexin-neuroligin adhesions capture surface-diffusing AMPA receptors through PSD-95 scaffolds. *J Neurosci* 2011;**31**(38):13500–15.

56. Levinson JN, Li R, Kang R, Moukhles H, El-Husseini A, Bamji SX. Postsynaptic scaffolding molecules modulate the localization of neuroligins. *Neuroscience* 2010;**165**(3):782–93.

57. Budreck EC, Scheiffele P. Neuroligin-3 is a neuronal adhesion protein at GABAergic and glutamatergic synapses. *Eur J Neurosci* 2007;**26**(7):1738–48.

58. Baudouin SJ, Gaudias J, Gerharz S, et al. Shared synaptic pathophysiology in syndromic and nonsyndromic rodent models of autism. *Science* 2012;**338**(6103):128–32.

59. Budreck EC, Kwon OB, Jung JH, et al. Neuroligin-1 controls synaptic abundance of NMDA-type glutamate receptors through extracellular coupling. *Proc Natl Acad Sci USA* 2013;**110**(2):725–30.

60. Soler-Llavina GJ, Fuccillo MV, Ko J, Sudhof TC, Malenka RC. The neurexin ligands, neuroligins and leucine-rich repeat transmembrane proteins, perform convergent and divergent synaptic functions in vivo. *Proc Natl Acad Sci USA* 2011;**108**(40):16502–9.

61. Schapitz IU, Behrend B, Pechmann Y, et al. Neuroligin 1 is dynamically exchanged at postsynaptic sites. *J Neurosci* 2010;**30**(38):12733–44.

62. Woolfrey KM, Srivastava DP, Photowala H, et al. Epac2 induces synapse remodeling and depression and its disease-associated forms alter spines. *Nat Neurosci* 2009;**12**(10):1275–84.

63. Bemben MA, Shipman SL, Hirai T, et al. CaMKII phosphorylation of neuroligin-1 regulates excitatory synapses. *Nat Neurosci* 2014;**17**(1):56–64.

64. Shipman SL, Nicoll RA. A subtype-specific function for the extracellular domain of neuroligin 1 in hippocampal LTP. *Neuron* 2012;**76**(2):309–16.

65. Futai K, Kim MJ, Hashikawa T, Scheiffele P, Sheng M, Hayashi Y. Retrograde modulation of presynaptic release probability through signaling mediated by PSD-95-neuroligin. *Nature Neurosci* 2007;**10**(2):186–95.

66. Stan A, Pielarski KN, Brigadski T, et al. Essential cooperation of N-cadherin and neuroligin-1 in the transsynaptic control of vesicle accumulation. *Proc Natl Acad Sci USA* 2010;**107**(24):11116–21.

67. Zhang W, Rohlmann A, Sargsyan V, et al. Extracellular domains of alpha-neurexins participate in regulating synaptic transmission by selectively affecting N- and P/Q-type Ca^{2+} channels. *J Neurosci* 2005;**25**(17):4330–42.

68. Chubykin AA, Atasoy D, Etherton MR, et al. Activity-dependent validation of excitatory versus inhibitory synapses by neuroligin-1 versus neuroligin-2. *Neuron* 2007;**54**(6):919–31.

69. Fu Z, Vicini S. Neuroligin-2 accelerates GABAergic synapse maturation in cerebellar granule cells. *Mol Cell Neurosci* 2009;**42**(1):45–55.

70. Ko J, Soler-Llavina GJ, Fuccillo MV, Malenka RC, Sudhof TC. Neuroligins/LRRTMs prevent activity- and Ca^{2+}/calmodulin-dependent synapse elimination in cultured neurons. *J Cell Biol* 2011;**194**(2):323–34.

71. Kang Y, Zhang X, Dobie F, Wu H, Craig AM. Induction of GABAergic postsynaptic differentiation by alpha-neurexins. *J Biol Chem* 2008;**283**(4):2323–34.

72. Feng J, Schroer R, Yan J, et al. High frequency of neurexin 1beta signal peptide structural variants in patients with autism. *Neurosci Lett* 2006;**409**(1):10–3.

73. Marshall CR, Noor A, Vincent JB, et al. Structural variation of chromosomes in autism spectrum disorder. *Am J Hum Genet* 2008;**82**(2):477–88.

74. Szatmari P, Paterson AD, Zwaigenbaum L, et al. Mapping autism risk loci using genetic linkage and chromosomal rearrangements. *Nat Genet* 2007;**39**(3):319–28.

75. Kim HG, Kishikawa S, Higgins AW, et al. Disruption of neurexin 1 associated with autism spectrum disorder. *Am J Hum Genet* 2008;**82**(1):199–207.

76. Yan J, Noltner K, Feng J, et al. Neurexin 1alpha structural variants associated with autism. *Neurosci Lett* 2008;**438**(3):368–70.

77. Zahir FR, Baross A, Delaney AD, et al. A patient with vertebral, cognitive and behavioural abnormalities and a de novo deletion of NRXN1alpha. *J Med Genet* 2008;**45**(4):239–43.

78. Bishop DV, Scerif G. Klinefelter syndrome as a window on the aetiology of language and communication impairments in children: the neuroligin-neurexin hypothesis. *Acta Paediatr* 2011;**100**(6):903–7.

79. Gauthier J, Siddiqui TJ, Huashan P, et al. Truncating mutations in NRXN2 and NRXN1 in autism spectrum disorders and schizophrenia. *Human Genet* 2011;**130**(4):563–73.

80. Jamain S, Quach H, Betancur C, et al. Mutations of the X-linked genes encoding neuroligins NLGN3 and NLGN4 are associated with autism. *Nat Genet* 2003;**34**(1):27–9.

81. Laumonnier F, Bonnet-Brilhault F, Gomot M, et al. X-linked mental retardation and autism are associated with a mutation in the NLGN4 gene, a member of the neuroligin family. *Am J Hum Genet* 2004;**74**(3):552–7.

82. Yan Y, Yang D, Zarnowska ED, et al. Directed differentiation of dopaminergic neuronal subtypes from human embryonic stem cells. *Stem Cells* 2005;**23**(6):781–90.

83. Yan J, Feng J, Schroer R, et al. Analysis of the neuroligin 4Y gene in patients with autism. *Psychiatr Genet* 2008;**18**(4):204–7.

84. Talebizadeh Z, Lam DY, Theodoro MF, Bittel DC, Lushington GH, Butler MG. Novel splice isoforms for NLGN3 and NLGN4 with possible implications in autism. *J Med Genet* 2006;**43**(5):e21.

85. Chocholska S, Rossier E, Barbi G, Kehrer-Sawatzki H. Molecular cytogenetic analysis of a familial interstitial deletion Xp22.2-22.3 with a highly variable phenotype in female carriers. *Am J Med Genet A* 2006;**140**(6):604–10.

86. Lawson-Yuen A, Saldivar JS, Sommer S, Picker J. Familial deletion within NLGN4 associated with autism and Tourette syndrome. *Eur J Hum Genet* 2008;**16**(5):614–8.

87. Macarov M, Zeigler M, Newman JP, et al. Deletions of VCX-A and NLGN4: a variable phenotype including normal intellect. *J Intellect Disabil Res* 2007;**51**(Pt 5):329–33.

88. Kirov G, Gumus D, Chen W, et al. Comparative genome hybridization suggests a role for NRXN1 and APBA2 in schizophrenia. *Hum Mol Genet* 2008;**17**(3):458–65.

89. Walsh T, McClellan JM, McCarthy SE, et al. Rare structural variants disrupt multiple genes in neurodevelopmental pathways in schizophrenia. *Science* 2008;**320**(5875):539–43.

90. Hishimoto A, Liu QR, Drgon T, et al. Neurexin 3 polymorphisms are associated with alcohol dependence and altered expression of specific isoforms. *Hum Mol Genet* 2007;**16**(23):2880–91.

91. Lachman HM, Fann CS, Bartzis M, et al. Genomewide suggestive linkage of opioid dependence to chromosome 14q. *Hum Mol Genet* 2007;**16**(11):1327–34.

92. Sun C, Cheng MC, Qin R, et al. Identification and functional characterization of rare mutations of the neuroligin-2 gene (NLGN2) associated with schizophrenia. *Hum Mol Genet* 2011;**20**(15):3042–51.

93. Morrow EM, Yoo SY, Flavell SW, et al. Identifying autism loci and genes by tracing recent shared ancestry. *Science* 2008;**321**(5886):218–23.

94. Comoletti D, De Jaco A, Jennings LL, et al. The Arg451Cys-neuroligin-3 mutation associated with autism reveals a defect in protein processing. *J Neurosci* 2004;**24**(20):4889–93.

95. Tabuchi K, Blundell J, Etherton MR, et al. A neuroligin-3 mutation implicated in autism increases inhibitory synaptic transmission in mice. *Science* 2007;**318**(5847):71–6.

96. Jamain S, Radyushkin K, Hammerschmidt K, et al. Reduced social interaction and ultrasonic communication in a mouse model of monogenic heritable autism. *Proc Natl Acad Sci USA* 2008;**105**(5):1710–5.

97. Rothwell PE, Fuccillo MV, Maxeiner S, et al. Autism-associated neuroligin-3 mutations commonly impair striatal circuits to boost repetitive behaviors. *Cell* 2014;**158**(1):198–212.

98. Etherton M, Földy C, Sharma M, et al. Autism-linked neuroligin-3 R451C mutation differentially alters hippocampal and cortical synaptic function. *Proc Natl Acad Sci USA* 2011;**108**(33):13764–9.

99. Chih B, Afridi SK, Clark L, Scheiffele P. Disorder-associated mutations lead to functional inactivation of neuroligins. *Human Mol Genet* 2004;**13**(14):1471–7.

100. Khosravani H, Altier C, Zamponi GW, Colicos MA. The Arg473Cys-neuroligin-1 mutation modulates NMDA mediated synaptic transmission and receptor distribution in hippocampal neurons. *FEBS Lett* 2005;**579**(29):6587–94.

101. Etherton MR, Tabuchi K, Sharma M, Ko J, Sudhof TC. An autism-associated point mutation in the neuroligin cytoplasmic tail selectively impairs AMPA receptor-mediated synaptic transmission in hippocampus. *EMBO J* 2011;**30**(14):2908–19.

102. Nam CI, Chen L. Postsynaptic assembly induced by neurexin-neuroligin interaction and neurotransmitter. *Proc Natl Acad Sci USA* 2005;**102**(17):6137–42.

103. Heine M, Thoumine O, Mondin M, Tessier B, Giannone G, Choquet D. Activity-independent and subunit-specific recruitment of functional AMPA receptors at neurexin/neuroligin contacts. *Proc Natl Acad Sci USA* 2008;**105**(52):20947–52.

104. Arac D, Boucard AA, Ozkan E, et al. Structures of neuroligin-1 and the neuroligin-1/neurexin-1 beta complex reveal specific protein-protein and protein-Ca^{2+} interactions. *Neuron* 2007;**56**(6):992–1003.

105. Chen X, Liu H, Shim AH, Focia PJ, He X. Structural basis for synaptic adhesion mediated by neuroligin-neurexin interactions. *Nat Struct Mol Biol* 2008;**15**(1):50–6.

106. Comoletti D, Flynn R, Jennings LL, et al. Characterization of the interaction of a recombinant soluble neuroligin-1 with neurexin-1beta. *J Biol Chem* 2003;**278**(50):50497–505.

107. Saura CA, Servián-Morilla E, Scholl FG. Presenilin/γ-secretase regulates neurexin processing at synapses. *PLoS One* 2011;**6**(4):e19430.

108. Bot N, Schweizer C, Ben Halima S, Fraering PC. Processing of the synaptic cell adhesion molecule neurexin-3beta by Alzheimer disease alpha- and gamma-secretases. *J Biol Chem* 2011;**286**(4):2762–73.

109. Suzuki K, Hayashi Y, Nakahara S, et al. Activity-dependent proteolytic cleavage of neuroligin-1. *Neuron* 2012;**76**(2):410–22.

110. Peixoto RT, Kunz PA, Kwon H, et al. Transsynaptic signaling by activity-dependent cleavage of neuroligin-1. *Neuron* 2012;**76**(2):396–409.

111. Venkatesh HS, Johung TB, Caretti V, et al. Neuronal Activity Promotes Glioma Growth through Neuroligin-3 Secretion. *Cell* 2015;**161**(4):803–16.

112. Gjørlund MD, Nielsen J, Pankratova S, et al. Neuroligin-1 induces neurite outgrowth through interaction with neurexin-1β and activation of fibroblast growth factor receptor-1. *FASEB J* 2012;**26**(10):4174–86.

113. Carrie A, Jun L, Bienvenu T, et al. A new member of the IL-1 receptor family highly expressed in hippocampus and involved in X-linked mental retardation. *Nat Genet* 1999;**23**(1):25–31.

114. Born TL, Smith DE, Garka KE, Renshaw BR, Bertles JS, Sims JE. Identification and characterization of two members of a novel class of the interleukin-1 receptor (IL-1R) family. Delineation of a new class of IL-1R-related proteins based on signaling. *J Biol Chem* 2000;**275**(52):41528.

115. Gao X, Xi G, Niu Y, et al. A study on the correlation between IL1RAPL1 and human cognitive ability. *Neurosci Lett* 2008;**438**(2):163–7.

116. Houbaert X, Zhang CL, Gambino F, et al. Target-specific vulnerability of excitatory synapses leads to deficits in associative memory in a model of intellectual disorder. *J Neurosci* 2013;33(34):13805—19.

117. Boda B, Mas C, Muller D. Activity-dependent regulation of genes implicated in X-linked non-specific mental retardation. *Neuroscience* 2002;114(1):13—7.

118. Pavlowsky A, Gianfelice A, Pallotto M, et al. A postsynaptic signaling pathway that may account for the cognitive defect due to IL1RAPL1 mutation. *Curr Biol* 2010;20(2):103—15.

119. Yoshida T, Yasumura M, Uemura T, et al. IL-1 receptor accessory protein-like 1 associated with mental retardation and autism mediates synapse formation by trans-synaptic interaction with protein tyrosine phosphatase {delta}. *J Neurosci* 2011;31(38):13485—99.

120. Bahi N, Friocourt G, Carrie A, et al. IL1 receptor accessory protein like, a protein involved in X-linked mental retardation, interacts with Neuronal Calcium Sensor-1 and regulates exocytosis. *Hum Mol Genet* 2003;12(12):1415—25.

121. Gambino F, Pavlowsky A, Béglé A, et al. IL1-receptor accessory protein-like 1 (IL1RAPL1), a protein involved in cognitive functions, regulates N-type Ca^{2+}-channel and neurite elongation. *Proc Natl Acad Sci USA* 2007;104(21):9063—8.

122. Valnegri P, Montrasio C, Brambilla D, Ko J, Passafaro M, Sala C. The X-linked intellectual disability protein IL1RAPL1 regulates excitatory synapse formation by binding PTP delta and RhoGAP2. *Hum Mol Genet* 2011;20(24):4797—809.

123. Yamagata A, Yoshida T, Sato Y, et al. Mechanisms of splicing-dependent trans-synaptic adhesion by PTPδ-IL1RAPL1/IL-1RAcP for synaptic differentiation. *Nat Commun* 2015;6:6926.

124. Hayashi T, Yoshida T, Ra M, Taguchi R, Mishina M. IL1RAPL1 associated with mental retardation and autism regulates the formation and stabilization of glutamatergic synapses of cortical neurons through RhoA signaling pathway. *PLoS One* 2013;8(6):e66254.

125. Granger AJ, Shi Y, Lu W, Cerpas M, Nicoll RA. LTP requires a reserve pool of glutamate receptors independent of subunit type. *Nature* 2013;493(7433):495—500.

126. Yoshida T, Mishina M. Zebrafish orthologue of mental retardation protein IL1RAPL1 regulates presynaptic differentiation. *Mol Cell Neurosci* 2008;39(2):218—28.

127. Yoshida T, Shiroshima T, Lee SJ, et al. Interleukin-1 receptor accessory protein organizes neuronal synaptogenesis as a cell adhesion molecule. *J Neurosci* 2012;32(8):2588—600.

128. Yasumura M, Yoshida T, Yamazaki M, et al. IL1RAPL1 knockout mice show spine density decrease, learning deficiency, hyperactivity and reduced anxiety-like behaviours. *Sci Rep* 2014;4:6613.

129. Gambino F, Kneib M, Pavlowsky A, et al. IL1RAPL1 controls inhibitory networks during cerebellar development in mice. *Eur J Neurosci* 2009;30(8):1476—86.

130. Piton A, Michaud JL, Peng H, et al. Mutations in the calcium-related gene IL1RAPL1 are associated with autism. *Hum Mol Genet* 2008;17(24):3965—74.

131. Tabolacci E, Pomponi MG, Pietrobono R, Terracciano A, Chiurazzi P, Neri G. A truncating mutation in the IL1RAPL1 gene is responsible for X-linked mental retardation in the MRX21 family. *Am J Med Genet A* 2006;140(5):482—7.

132. Youngs EL, Henkhaus R, Hellings JA, Butler MG. IL1RAPL1 gene deletion as a cause of X-linked intellectual disability and dysmorphic features. *Eur J Med Genet* 2011;55.

133. Nawara M, Klapecki J, Borg K, et al. Novel mutation of IL1RAPL1 gene in a nonspecific X-linked mental retardation (MRX) family. *Am J Med Genet A* 2008;146A(24):3167—72.

134. Franek KJ, Butler J, Johnson J, et al. Deletion of the immunoglobulin domain of IL1RAPL1 results in nonsyndromic X-linked intellectual disability associated with behavioral problems and mild dysmorphism. *Am J Med Genet A* 2011;155A(5):1109—14.

135. Behnecke A, Hinderhofer K, Bartsch O, et al. Intragenic deletions of IL1RAPL1: report of two cases and review of the literature. *Am J Med Genet A* 2011;155A(2):372—9.

136. Barone C, Bianca S, Luciano D, Di Benedetto D, Vinci M, Fichera M. Intragenic ILRAPL1 deletion in a male patient with intellectual disability, mild dysmorphic signs, deafness, and behavioral problems. *Am J Med Genet A* 2013;161A(6):1381—5.

137. Leprêtre F, Delannoy V, Froguel P, Vasseur F, Montpellier C. Dissection of an inverted X(p21.3q27.1) chromosome associated with mental retardation. *Cytogenet Genome Res* 2003;101(2):124—9.

138. Wheway JM, Yau SC, Nihalani V, et al. A complex deletion-inversion-deletion event results in a chimeric IL1RAPL1-dystrophin transcript and a contiguous gene deletion syndrome. *J Med Genet* 2003;40(2):127—31.

139. Froyen G, Van Esch H, Bauters M, et al. Detection of genomic copy number changes in patients with idiopathic mental retardation by high-resolution X-array-CGH: important role for increased gene dosage of XLMR genes. *Hum Mutat* 2007;28(10):1034—42.

140. Ramos-Brossier M, Montani C, Lebrun N, et al. Novel IL1RAPL1 mutations associated with intellectual disability impair synaptogenesis. *Hum Mol Genet* 2015;24(4):1106—18.

141. Koh JW, Kang SY, Kim GH, Yoo HW, Yu J. Central precocious puberty in a patient with X-linked adrenal hypoplasia congenita and Xp21 contiguous gene deletion syndrome. *Ann Pediatr Endocrinol Metab* 2013;18(2):90—4.

142. Yasumura M, Uemura T, Yamasaki M, Sakimura K, Watanabe M, Mishina M. Role of the internal Shank-binding segment of glutamate receptor delta2 in synaptic localization and cerebellar functions. *Neurosci Lett* 2008;433(2):146—51.

143. Bhat SS, Ladd S, Grass F, et al. Disruption of the IL1RAPL1 gene associated with a pericentromeric inversion of the X chromosome in a patient with mental retardation and autism. *Clin Genet* 2008;73(1):94—6.

144. Kwon CH, Luikart BW, Powell CM, et al. Pten regulates neuronal arborization and social interaction in mice. *Neuron* 2006;50(3):377—88.

145. Nakatani J, Tamada K, Hatanaka F, et al. Abnormal behavior in a chromosome-engineered mouse model for human 15q11-13 duplication seen in autism. *Cell* 2009;137(7):1235—46.

146. Zhang CL, Houbaert X, Lepleux M, et al. The hippocampo-amygdala control of contextual fear expression is affected in a model of intellectual disability. *Brain Struct Funct* 2014;220.

147. Mizuno K, Hasegawa K, Katagiri T, Ogimoto M, Ichikawa T, Yakura H. MPTP delta, a putative murine homolog of HPTP delta, is expressed in specialized regions of the brain and in the B-cell lineage. *Mol Cell Biol* 1993;13(9):5513—23.

148. Mizuno K, Hasegawa K, Ogimoto M, Katagiri T, Yakura H. Developmental regulation of gene expression for the MPTP delta isoforms in the central nervous system and the immune system. *FEBS Lett* 1994;355(3):223—8.

149. Yang T, Yin W, Derevyanny VD, Moore LA, Longo FM. Identification of an ectodomain within the LAR protein tyrosine phosphatase receptor that binds homophilically and activates signalling pathways promoting neurite outgrowth. *Eur J Neurosci* 2005;22(9):2159—70.

150. Dunah AW, Hueske E, Wyszynski M, et al. LAR receptor protein tyrosine phosphatases in the development and maintenance of excitatory synapses. *Nat Neurosci* 2005;8(4):458—67.

151. Sajnani G, Aricescu AR, Jones EY, Gallagher J, Alete D, Stoker A. PTPsigma promotes retinal neurite outgrowth non-cell-autonomously. *J Neurobiol* 2005;**65**(1):59–71.

152. Johnson KG, Van Vactor D. Receptor protein tyrosine phosphatases in nervous system development. *Physiol Rev* 2003;**83**(1): 1–24.

153. Streuli M, Krueger NX, Hall LR, Schlossman SF, Saito H. A new member of the immunoglobulin superfamily that has a cytoplasmic region homologous to the leukocyte common antigen. *J Exp Med* 1988;**168**(5):1523–30.

154. Yan H, Grossman A, Wang H, et al. A novel receptor tyrosine phosphatase-sigma that is highly expressed in the nervous system. *J Biol Chem* 1993;**268**(33):24880–6.

155. Pulido R, Serra-Pagès C, Tang M, Streuli M. The LAR/PTPd/PTPs subfamily of transmembrane protein-tyrosine-phosphatases: multiple human LAR,PTPd, and PTPs isoforms are expressed in a tissue-specific manner and associate with the LAR-interacting protein LIP.1. *Proc Natl Acad Sci USA* 1995;**92**:11686–90.

156. Brady-Kalnay SM, Tonks NK. Protein tyrosine phosphatases as adhesion receptors. *Curr Opin Cell Biol* 1995;**7**(5):650–7.

157. Gonzalez-Brito MR, Bixby JL. Differential activities in adhesion and neurite growth of fibronectin type III repeats in the PTP-delta extracellular domain. *Int J Dev Neurosci* 2006;**24**(7):425–9.

158. Blanchetot C, Tertoolen LG, Overvoorde J, den Hertog J. Intra- and intermolecular interactions between intracellular domains of receptor protein-tyrosine phosphatases. *J Biol Chem* 2002;**277**(49):47263–9.

159. Wallace MJ, Fladd C, Batt J, Rotin D. The second catalytic domain of protein tyrosine phosphatase delta (PTP delta) binds to and inhibits the first catalytic domain of PTP sigma. *Mol Cell Biol* 1998;**18**(5):2608–16.

160. Steward O, Wallace CS, Lyford GL, Worley PF. Synaptic activation causes the mRNA for the IEG arc to localize selectively near activated postsynaptic sites on dendrites. *Neuron* 1998;**21**(4):741–51.

161. Wang J, Bixby JL. Receptor tyrosine phosphatase-delta is a homophilic, neurite-promoting cell adhesion molecular for CNS neurons. *Mol Cell Neurosci* 1999;**14**(4–5):370–84.

162. Sun QL, Wang J, Bookman RJ, Bixby JL. Growth cone steering by receptor tyrosine phosphatase delta defines a distinct class of guidance cue. *Mol Cell Neurosci* 2000;**16**(5):686–95.

163. Schaapveld RQ, Schepens JT, Bachner D, et al. Developmental expression of the cell adhesion molecule-like protein tyrosine phosphatases LAR, RPTPdelta and RPTPsigma in the mouse. *Mech Dev* 1998;**77**(1):59–62.

164. Uetani N, Kato K, Ogura H, et al. Impaired learning with enhanced hippocampal long-term potentiation in PTPdelta-deficient mice. *EMBO J* 2000;**19**(12):2775–85.

165. Kwon SK, Woo J, Kim SY, Kim H, Kim E. Trans-synaptic adhesions between netrin-G ligand-3 (NGL-3) and receptor tyrosine phosphatases LAR, protein-tyrosine phosphatase delta (PTPdelta), and PTPsigma via specific domains regulate excitatory synapse formation. *J Biol Chem* 2010;**285**(18):13966–78.

166. Pulido R, Krueger NX, Serra-Pagès C, Saito H, Streuli M. Molecular characterization of the human transmembrane protein-tyrosine phosphatase delta. Evidence for tissue-specific expression of alternative human transmembrane protein-tyrosine phosphatase delta isoforms. *J Biol Chem* 1995;**270**(12):6722–8.

167. Woo J, Kwon SK, Choi S, et al. Trans-synaptic adhesion between NGL-3 and LAR regulates the formation of excitatory synapses. *Nat Neurosci* 2009;**12**(4):428–37.

168. Takahashi H, Arstikaitis P, Prasad T, et al. Postsynaptic TrkC and presynaptic PTPσ function as a bidirectional excitatory synaptic organizing complex. *Neuron* 2011;**69**(2):287–303.

169. Takahashi H, Katayama K, Sohya K, et al. Selective control of inhibitory synapse development by Slitrk3-PTPδ trans-synaptic interaction. *Nat Neurosci* 2012;**15**(3):389–98. S381–2.

170. Yim YS, Kwon Y, Nam J, et al. Slitrks control excitatory and inhibitory synapse formation with LAR receptor protein tyrosine phosphatases. *Proc Natl Acad Sci USA* 2013;**110**(10):4057–62.

171. Lee K, Kim Y, Lee SJ, et al. MDGAs interact selectively with neuroligin-2 but not other neuroligins to regulate inhibitory synapse development. *Proc Natl Acad Sci USA* 2013;**110**(1):336–41.

172. Woodings JA, Sharp SJ, Machesky LM. MIM-B, a putative metastasis suppressor protein, binds to actin and to protein tyrosine phosphatase delta. *Biochem J* 2003;**371**(Pt 2):463–71.

173. Uetani N, Chagnon MJ, Kennedy TE, Iwakura Y, Tremblay ML. Mammalian motoneuron axon targeting requires receptor protein tyrosine phosphatases sigma and delta. *J Neurosci* 2006;**26**(22): 5872–80.

174. Schormair B, Kemlink D, Roeske D, et al. PTPRD (protein tyrosine phosphatase receptor type delta) is associated with restless legs syndrome. *Nat Genet* 2008;**40**(8):946–8.

175. Yang Q, Li L, Yang R, et al. Family-based and population-based association studies validate PTPRD as a risk factor for restless legs syndrome. *Mov Disord* 2011;**26**(3):516–9.

176. Pinto D, Pagnamenta AT, Klei L, et al. Functional impact of global rare copy number variation in autism spectrum disorders. *Nature* 2010;**466**(7304):368–72.

177. Elia J, Gai X, Xie HM, et al. Rare structural variants found in attention-deficit hyperactivity disorder are preferentially associated with neurodevelopmental genes. *Mol Psychiatry* 2010;**15**(6): 637–46.

12

CNTNAP2 Mutations in Autism

Olga Peñagarikano

Department of Pharmacology, School of Medicine,
University of the Basque Country, Leioa, Spain

CONTACTIN-ASSOCIATED PROTEIN-LIKE 2 AS AN AUTISM RISK GENE

Autism spectrum disorder (ASD) comprises a group of developmental disabilities characterized by impaired social interaction and communication accompanied by repetitive and stereotyped behaviors and restricted interests.[1] Other symptoms frequently associated with ASD are intellectual disability, epilepsy, hyperactivity, and sleep, sensory, and gastrointestinal abnormalities.[2] Therefore, the final individual clinical phenotype among ASD patients can vary dramatically. The genetic contribution to ASD became apparent with the realization that patients with certain syndromes caused by a single gene (e.g., fragile X syndrome) showed higher than expected co-occurrence with autistic characteristics (i.e., syndromic autism). Whole-genome linkage and association studies helped to identify loci and variants positively associated with the disorder. These studies revealed extraordinary heterogeneity in the genetic basis of ASD; to date, no major gene has been identified as responsible for the disorder, but rather, hundreds of risk genes with either rare variants with large effect or common variants with small effect have been identified.[3] Thus, it is not surprising that the fundamental structural, neuropathological,

and molecular pathways affected in ASD have not been conclusively identified.[4] However, despite this genetic heterogeneity, a thorough understanding of the biological pathways affected by these genes could provide a unifying mechanism for autism pathophysiology, because each of these risk genes likely affects the development and function of brain circuits that mediate social behavior and communication, even at different levels. One of the most replicated genes as contributing to ASD, which is supported by both common and rare variation, is contactin associated protein-like 2 (*CNTNAP2*). A summary of *CNTNAP2* variation as it relates to ASD can be found in Table 1.

The first suggestion of the involvement of the *CNTNAP2* gene in neurodevelopmental disorders came from a rare patient said to have Tourette syndrome, obsessive compulsive disorder, intellectual disability, and language dysfunction.[5] This patient carried a heterozygous translocation disrupting the coding region of *CNTNAP2*, although this chromosomal translocation likely also disrupted the normal expression of genes located elsewhere in the genome. Since then, several patients with ASD-related symptoms have been reported to carry a chromosomal rearrangement in the *CNTNAP2* chromosomal region[6-9]; however, the

TABLE 1   Autism Spectrum Disorder—Related Phenotypes Associated With Genetic Variation in *CNTNAP2*

Genetic Change		Location	Phenotype	Refs.
709delG		Exon 22	ASD Epilepsy Hyperactivity Language regression	72
G731S I869T R1119H D1129H I1253T T1278I		Exon 14 Exon 17 Exon 20 Exon 21 Exon 23 Exon 24	ASD	20
H275R		Exon 6	ASD	23
CNV (deletion)		Promoter	ASD	31
rs7794745	Major allele T	Intron 2	ASD	19
rs2710102	Major allele C	Intron 13	Age at first word in ASD	22
			Nonword repetition in SLI	28,32
			Expressive language abilities in SLI	28
			Receptive language abilities in SLI	
	Minor allele T	Intron 13	Nonword repetition in dyslexia	27
			Selective mutism	39
			Social anxiety	
rs851715	Major allele A	Intron 13	Nonword repetition in SLI	32
rs759178	Major allele G			
rs1922892	Major allele T			
rs2538991	Major allele C			
rs2538976	Major allele G			
rs10246256	Major allele T	Intron 13	Nonword repetition in SLI	28,32
			Expressive language abilities in SLI	28
			Receptive language abilities in SLI	
rs2710117	Major allele A	Intron 14	Nonword repetition in SLI	28,32
			Expressive language abilities in SLI	28
			Receptive language abilities in SLI	
rs17236239	Minor allele G	Intron 13	Nonword repetition in SLI	28,32
			Expressive language abilities in SLI	
			Receptive language abilities in SLI	28
			Age at first phrase in ASD	26
rs1718101			Age at first phrase in ASD	26
rs4431523	Minor allele G	Intron 13	Receptive language abilities in SLI	32
rs34712024		Promoter	ASD	35
rs71781329		Promoter	Language development in ASD	35
Complex chromosomal rearrangement		7q32.1-7q35	Language delay ASD	6
CNV (deletion)		7q34-7q36.2 Several genes	Language delay Epilepsy Intellectual disability	8
CNV (deletion)		7q33-q35 Several genes Exons 1—3 *CNTNAP2*	Stuttering	30

causality of *CNTNAP2* is confounded by these long rearrangements.

In 2006, a homozygous single base deletion in exon 22 of *CNTNAP2* (3709delG) was identified in an Older Amish family with a syndromic form of ASD called cortical dysplasia-focal epilepsy (CDFE) syndrome (MIM 610042).[10] This deletion led to a premature stop codon in the protein encoded by the gene (I1253X), which was predicted to be nonfunctional. Patients were homozygous for the mutation and inherited it from heterozygous unaffected parents. The recessive nature of the syndrome, with a Mendelian inheritance pattern, strongly indicates loss of function of the CNTNAP2 protein as the cause of the disorder. In fact, Falivelli and collaborators[11] have shown that this mutation causes the protein to be secreted to the extracellular matrix instead of staying at the membrane as its original form (see the discussion on protein function below). Clinically, patients with CDFE syndrome were reported to develop normally until intractable focal seizures began in early childhood (1–9 years old), after which language regression, hyperactivity, impulsive and aggressive behavior, and intellectual disability developed in all children. In addition, about two-thirds of the patients fulfilled the diagnostic criteria for ASD diagnosis, which makes CDFE one of the disorders with the highest penetrance for ASD. Several of the patients with CDFE syndrome underwent resective surgery for epilepsy (although they all had a recurrence of seizures between 6 and 15 months after surgery) and neuropathological analysis of brain tissue showed evidence of abnormalities in neuronal migration, as had been presumed from the evidence of cortical dysplasia showed by magnetic resonance imaging (MRI) analysis.[10] This report was the first to provide strong causal evidence for the *CNTNAP2* gene in ASD, and the fact that patients showed deficits in neuronal migration opened a new role for *CNTNAP2* in development of the brain, because the only known function of CNTNAP2 until this study was published was related to myelination,[12] which takes place postnatally.

The most severe symptoms presented by patients with CDFE syndrome were intractable epileptic seizures. The prevalence of epilepsy in children with autism has been estimated to be around 30% and there seems to be a bimodal peak in the onset of epilepsy, which is usually either during early infancy (below 5 years of age) or during adolescence. In addition, the risk of presenting epilepsy is higher if the subject presents with intellectual disability.[13,14] The fact that these disorders co-occur together in a higher than expected manner suggests a common underlying neurobiology. In fact, epileptiform electroencephalogram abnormalities are common in autism regardless of the presence of clinical epilepsy per se.[15] However, it is not known to what extent the presence of epilepsy or epileptiform activity contributes to behavioral and cognitive deterioration. An emerging hypothesis is that autism, epilepsy, and intellectual disability arise from similar network dysfunction, which accounts for their convergence. Malformations of cortical development and organization, as in the case of neuronal migration abnormalities seen with *CNTNAP2* mutations, are a common cause of intractable epilepsy[16] and would certainly affect cortical function, which could lead to the behavioral phenotype seen in ASD. Another possible common neurobiological pathway involves the development of interneuron circuits,[17] which, although not investigated in CDFE patients, was observed in mice lacking the *Cntnap2* gene,[18] as will be described subsequently.

In 2008, three studies published in the *American Journal of Human Genetics* provided additional evidence for the association of different rare and common variants in *CNTNAP2* with ASD. (1) Arking et al.[19] identified a common polymorphism (rs7794745) in *CNTNAP2* significantly associated with autism susceptibility. (2) Bakkaloglu et al.[20] comprehensively resequenced the coding regions of *CNTNAP2* in hundreds of ASD patients and controls and identified a total of 27 nonsynonymous changes; 13 were rare and unique to patients, eight of which were predicted to be deleterious by bioinformatic approaches and/or altered residues conserved across species. Interestingly, one variant at a highly conserved position, I869T, was inherited by four affected children in three unrelated families but was not found in 4010 control chromosomes, a statistically significant enrichment. Another variant, D1129H was present in monozygotic twins, both affected with autism. Their father, who carried the same mutation, did not have an autism diagnosis. Both of these variants have been shown to be arrested to different extent in the endoplasmic reticulum.[11] (3) Alarcon and colleagues, who had previously identified a language quantitative trait locus on chromosome 7q35,[21] were the first to show that a variant in *CNTNAP2* (rs2710102) was associated with the language endophenotype *age at first word* in ASD.[22] A growing number of reports have subsequently linked common and rare variation in this gene with an increased risk of autism or autism-related endophenotypes, including a severe de novo mutation (H275R) identified by exome resequencing.[23] Endophenotypes are measurable components of a phenotype that help establish a link between a disorder and a genotype. They are helpful in psychiatric diseases because the diagnosis is deconstructed, allowing for a more simple and successful genetic analysis.[24] This approach assumes that distinct factors control normal variation in each ASD-related behavioral domain and that ASD emerges as a convergence of abnormalities in all of them.[25] Endophenotype analysis has led to the identification of *CNTNAP2* as having a major role in language development in ASD and other language related disorders. For example, Anney and collaborators[26] identified two new variants (rs1718101, rs17236239) linked to the endophenotype *age at first phrase* in autism. In addition, the same variant identified by Alarcon et al. as linked to the endophenotype *age at first word* in autism (rs2710102), has been linked to the endophenotype *nonsense-word repetition*, a task that requires reproducing a pronounceable but meaningless word in response to a spoken model, in developmental dyslexia, although in this case the association was driven by the opposite allele.[27] Several other variants nearby rs2710102, which cluster in intron 13, have been associated with the same endophenotype, *nonsense-word repetition*, in subjects with specific language impairment.[28] Interestingly, some of these variants (rs2710102, rs759178, rs17236239, and rs2538976) have been associated with early language development in a large screen of a phenotypically normal population.[29] This finding is consistent with the notion that genetic risk variants are likely to affect individual differences in cognition and behavior in the general population and supports the idea

that ASD emerges as the extreme of a continuum of normal behavioral variation.[25] Additional complex chromosomal rearrangements and large deletions affecting *CNTNAP2* (in addition to other genes) have been reported in other language-related deficits such as language delay[6,8] and stuttering.[30] Thus, common and rare variants were shown to be associated with either ASD or a related endophenotype (Figure 1). However, in contrast to the CDFE mutation, in which the disorder is transmitted in a Mendelian autosomal recessive manner, the pathogenicity of most of these variants is uncertain and their effect on protein function or gene expression remains to be elucidated. Most of the common variants associated with language endophenotypes in ASD and specific language impairment cluster in a narrow intronic region between exons 13 and 14 and are likely to be in linkage disequilibrium with the causal variant, rather than causal themselves. The rare variants identified are heterozygous and inherited from an apparently unaffected parent. Therefore, even in the case of nonsynonymous coding changes that are predicted to be deleterious, the variant must be viewed as a risk factor rather than causal. Thus, variation on the other *CNTNAP2* allele, or other transgenetic, epigenetic, or environmental factors, must

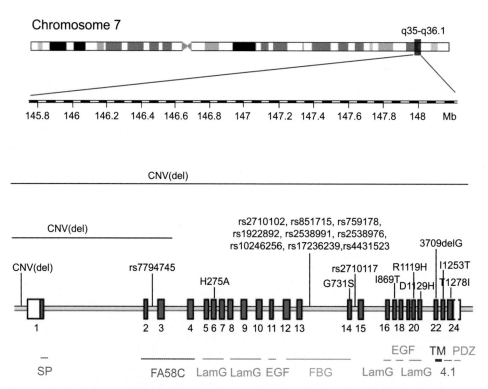

FIGURE 1   **Schematic representation of the location of the mutations and variants found within *CNTNAP2* associated with neurodevelopmental disorders.** The *CNTNAP2* gene spans 2.3 Mb on chromosome 7. Exons are presented as numbered dark blue boxes and introns as a light blue line. Variants associated with disease are indicated. The protein structural domains encoded by the specific exons are presented at the bottom. SP, signal peptide; FA58C, coagulation factor 5/8C terminal domain; LamG, laminin G; EGF, epidermal growth factor; FBG, fibrinogen-like domain; TM, transmembrane domain; 4.1, protein 4.1B binding domain; PDZ, PSD95/DlgA/ZO-1 homology protein–protein interaction domain. *Adapted from Peñagarikano and Geschwind.* Trends Mol Med *2012; 18(3): 156–163. Reprinted with permission from Elsevier.*

also be considered. De novo variations in regulatory regions of *CNTNAP2*, which result in altered functional levels of the protein, have also been identified.[31] The *CNTNAP2* gene contains a regulatory element directly bound by the transcription factor forkhead box P2 (*FOXP2*).[32] Interestingly, disruptions of FOXP2 cause developmental speech and language disorder,[33,34] which suggests that these genes are involved in a circuitry related to human language. Chiochetti and collaborators[35] sequenced the 5′ promoter of the *CNTNAP2* gene in ASD trios to study potential variation that could affect gene expression. They found an association of variant rs34712024 with ASD and rs71781329 with language development. These variants were predicted to alter transcription factor binding sites. These results led to the conclusion that a reduced level of CNTNAP2 during neuronal development increases liability for ASD. Maekawa and colleagues[36] tested the expression of nine putative autism candidate genes in scalp hair follicles of an ASD sample and found decreased CNTNAP2 expression in the autism cohort compared with control subjects, and concluded that scalp hair follicles could be a beneficial genetic biomarker resource for brain diseases, supporting the role of downregulation of CNTNAP2 in ASD risk.

As presented above for *CNTNAP2* variants, the genetic contribution to ASD should be viewed as their effect on the development and function of neuronal circuits mediating social cognition and language (Figure 2). As more patients have been identified, it has become apparent that individuals with mutations in *CNTNAP2* show a combination of four main features to different degrees: autistic characteristics, seizures, language impairment, and intellectual disability.[37] From the perspective of genes affecting circuits and ultimately behavior, it should not be surprising that the association of *CNTNAP2* variants with the language endophenotype is not specific. Studies have suggested that these same variants are also associated with social behavior endophenotypes such as sociability and social inhibition in normal and autistic populations[38] and selective mutism (e.g., failure to speak in one or more social settings despite speaking normally in other settings) in social anxiety disorder.[39] Such a pleiotropic effect is not surprising for a gene whose loss of function leads to the abnormal development of frontal–striatal brain circuits that are involved in many behavioral and cognitive processes (see the subsequent discussion on gene function). The availability of new brain imaging techniques is helping to determine what brain areas are affected by these genetic variants and how the latter affect brain function.

UNRAVELING *CNTNAP2* FUNCTION THROUGH NEUROIMAGING

Noninvasive human brain imaging allows assessment of the brain in vivo and is currently one of the few ways to investigate functional genotype–phenotype associations in human brain. By studying humans with genetic variants that have been shown to confer risk to ASD, we can gain insight into gene function. Structural MRI, despite its limitations (often small sample sizes and difficulty to have a completely matched control sample) has provided solid evidence of alterations in brain structures and functions associated with many psychiatric disorders. Tan and colleagues[40] investigated variation in white and gray matter morphology in normal individuals carrying a single nucleotide polymorphism in the *CNTNAP2* gene (rs7794745) that had been previously reported to confer risk to ASD.[19] The authors found that despite the absence of behavioral abnormalities, subjects homozygous for the risk allele showed significant cerebral morphological variation, including reductions in gray and white matter volume in several regions that have already been implicated in ASD (cerebellum, fusiform gyrus, and occipital and frontal cortices), which suggests that this polymorphism could disrupt fronto-occipital connections. In a similar manner, Dennis et al.[41] found altered structural brain connectivity in normal subjects homozygous for the risk allele for variant rs2710102, which had previously been associated with the endophenotype *age at first word* in ASD.[22] Using functional neuroimaging (fMRI), Whalley and collaborators[42] found that healthy

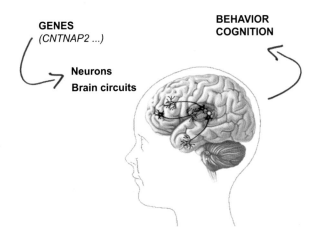

FIGURE 2 Schematic representation of the location of the mutations and variants found within *CNTNAP2* associated with neurodevelopmental disorders. CNTNAP2 is expressed in brain regions important for social cognition, language, and implicit learning such as the frontal cortex (pink), the anterior temporal cortex (blue), and the basal ganglia (green). Its contribution to the clinical phenotype is seen as an influence on the development and function of these brain circuits. *Adapted from Peñagarikano and Geschwind. Trends Mol Med 2012; 18(3): 156–163. Reprinted with permission from Elsevier.*

individuals carrying the risk alleles for both rs2710102 and rs7794745 showed significant increases in activation in the right inferior frontal gyrus (Broca's area homologue) and right middle temporal cortex during a sentence completion task. In a similar manner, Scott-Van Zeeland et al.[43] demonstrated through fMRI that the variant rs2710102 leads to abnormal frontal lobe functional brain connectivity in human subjects. The authors found that the medial prefrontal cortex (mPFC) showed genotype based differential activity during implicit learning tasks known to engage fronto-striatal circuits, a region previously shown to have enriched CNTNAP2 expression.[44] The mPFC is part of a network that is generally more active during resting baseline than during a task that requires externally directed attention.[45] Risk allele carriers showed a smaller reduction in activity upon requiring attention. To investigate whether this genetic risk allele modulates functional interactions between mPFC and more posterior cortical regions, irrespective of the functional demands of the task, the authors performed functional connectivity analysis and found that nonrisk individuals had greater long-range anterior-posterior connectivity, whereas risk allele carriers had increased local connectivity.[43] It has been shown that weakening of local and strengthening of long-range connectivity are natural steps in brain maturation,[46] which could indicate more immature connectivity patterns in CNTNAP2 risk allele carriers.

These studies provide a mechanistic link between specific genetic risk for ASD and empirical data implicating brain anatomy and function and are consistent with emerging theories of a potential unifying abnormality in ASD pathophysiology that implicate abnormal neural connectivity.[47] The heterogeneity in the genetics and neurobiology of ASD (e.g., genes involved in different neurological processes converge in the behavioral phenotype) has led to the proposal that ASD is a developmental disconnection syndrome.[48] The organization of neuronal circuits during brain development requires the precise and timed action of different biological mechanisms, including neuronal development and migration, dendritic maturation, axon path finding, and synapse formation. Abnormalities at any of these levels could lead to the disconnection of brain areas important for higher-order cognitive function. Among the different brain structures, the cerebral cortex has been attributed to have a key role in cognitive and emotional processes, including social behavior and language. Formation of the cerebral neocortex, the largest region of the cortex composed of six distinct layers, can be divided into three main steps: neuronal proliferation, migration, and organization of the cortical layers.[49] During and after migrating into their proper layers, the neurons in each layer extend processes to establish synaptic connections with other neurons

within the cortex as well as with subcortical structures, and create functional neuronal circuits that will allow the processing of cognitive and emotional information. Some of these subcortical structures, such as the basal ganglia and amygdala, have also been implicated in ASD. Therefore, the precise development and functioning (e.g., synaptic activity) of these circuits is required for proper functioning of the circuit, and disruption of any of these steps could lead to the abnormal behavioral outcome seen in ASD. Because disconnectivity related to the CNTNAP2 genotype is independent of diagnosis,[43] disconnectivity is likely a risk factor for ASD but is not itself sufficient for the disorder.

CNTNAP2 GENE FUNCTION

Taken together, the genetics and imaging data suggest that CNTNAP2 has an important role in neurocognitive development, but to understand how CNTNAP2 contributes to both normal development and to the disorder it is important to understand the function of the product it encodes. The CNTNAP2 protein was originally identified in 1999 in rodents as a new member of the neurexin superfamily, and specifically as the mammalian homolog of Drosophila melanogaster's neurexin IV.[12] Neurexins are cell adhesion molecules (CAMs), a group of proteins that mediate cell—cell interactions in the nervous system, which are key for synapse formation and maintenance. This critical process involves the timely coordination of different biological processes such as axonal growth and path finding, assembly of protein complexes, pruning, and maturation.[50] Interestingly, many CAMs have been found to be mutated in ASD, which suggests that the development and/or maintenance of synaptic contacts is a critical factor in ASD pathophysiology[51] (see also Chapter 11). Among these are the neurexin family of presynaptic CAMs; their postsynaptic partners, the neuroligins; the SHANK family of postsynaptic scaffolding proteins, which have an important role in anchoring CAMs and other molecules to the actin cytoskeleton; and contactin and contactin-associated proteins, which are CAMs essential for different axonal and dendritic molecular organizations. Mutations in any of these proteins could lead to abnormal circuit wiring and altered information processing.

Neurexins are presynaptic transmembrane proteins that were first discovered as receptors for alpha-latrotoxin, a toxin found in black widow spiders that binds presynaptic receptors and induce massive neurotransmitter release.[52] A few years later, neuroligins, the postsynaptic transmembrane proteins that interact with neurexins, were discovered.[53] In humans, there are three neurexin genes (NRXN1 through

NRXN3). The neurexin−neuroligin trans-synaptic complex is believed to be important for synaptic development and function.

Contactin associated proteins (CNTNAPs) are also transmembrane CAMs that resemble neurexins, but their function is believed to be restricted to outside the synapse, particularly to neuron−glia interactions in myelinated axons. In humans, there are five *CNTNAP* genes (*CNTNAP1* through *CNTNAP5*). Contactin-associated protein 1 (*CNTNAP1*) receives its name from its interaction with contactin, which is essential for the generation of the axo−glial junction, whereas the rest of the family members do not interact with contactin but are named *contactin-associated protein-like* after their resemblance to CNTNAP1, and have different roles in the neuron−glia junction.[54]

The human *CNTNAP2* gene spans approximately 2.3 Mb at chromosomal region 7q35-q36.1, encompassing almost 1.5% of chromosome 7 and is thought to be the largest gene in the genome. It contains 24 exons and the 9.9-kb full-length messenger ribonucleic acid (mRNA) codes for a protein of 1331 amino acids and a molecular mass of 148 KDa.[55] The *CNTNAP2* gene is expressed mainly in brain and spinal cord, although low levels of expression can be found in ovary and prostate, but not in other tissues at appreciable levels, including peripheral blood cells. Within the brain, its expression pattern based on mRNA in situ hybridization is fairly remarkable, appearing to mark a cortico-striato-thalamic circuit that is involved in diverse higher-order cognitive functions.[22,44] In the cerebral cortex, it shows a pattern of striking enrichment in anterior areas during development, which appears to be preserved in adulthood,[22,44] including especially strong expression in frontal and prefrontal cortical areas. In addition, genome-wide microarray studies of regional gene expression in human fetal brains identified *CNTNAP2* as enriched in perisylvian language-related association cortex.[44]

Regarding its function, CNTNAP2 was originally reported to have a role in neuron−glia interactions and clustering of K^+ channels at the juxtaparanodal region of the nodes of Ranvier.[12,56] The specialization of subcellular domains (i.e., nodes, paranodes, and juxtaparanodes) within this structure, to which different sets of ion channels are localized, permits a rapid and efficient propagation of action potentials in myelinated axons.[54] At a molecular level, CNTNAP2 is a single-pass transmembrane protein with a long extracellular region characterized by the presence of protein−protein interaction domains such as laminin G, EGF repeats, and discoidin-like domains and a short cytoplasmic region characterized by a PDZ domain interacting site.[12] The cytoplasmic region is necessary for the clustering of K^+ channels at juxtaparanodes, although it seems not to

require the PDZ interacting domain.[57] The extracellular region forms a neuron−glia cell adhesion complex with contactin 2 (TAG-1), which seems to be necessary for the proper localization of K^+ channels in this structure.[56] In addition to the nodes of Ranvier, CNTNAP2 has also been shown to associate with K^+ channels in the distal region of the axon initial segment of pyramidal cells, which is a critical region for the generation of action potentials and for the control of pyramidal cell activity,[58] although CNTNAP2 is not necessary for K^+ channel clustering in this region of the cell[59] as it is in myelinated axons. The functional relevance of the presence of CNTNAP2 in myelinated axons, however, remains unclear because no defects in myelination or in electrophysiological properties of nerve conduction have been reported in mice deficient for the *Cntnap2* gene,[56] as will be discussed later. In addition, the fact that the gene is expressed embryonically[12,22,44] and myelination takes place postnatally, together with the increasing number of reports that link the gene to ASD, suggest an additional role for CNTNAP2 in early brain development. Its developmental role is further supported by the imaging and pathology data in patients with CDFE syndrome, as previously described.[10]

It is also possible that CNTNAP2 has other roles as related to neuron−glia interaction in addition to the clustering of K^+ channels in myelinated axons. Although glial cells were originally thought to be connective tissue that glues and holds neuronal circuits together, they are now known to have important roles in the remodeling and functioning of neuronal networks.[60] Therefore, it is reasonable to consider that disruption of neuron−glia interactions could be a factor contributing to ASD. In support of this, neuropathological studies of ASD brains have found to be reactive astrocytosis and gliosis in the cerebellum and neocortex of ASD patients. Although astrocyte activation and reactive gliosis are generally accepted to have many protective effects, they might become detrimental if not resolved in time, which contributes to the pathogenesis of neurological disorders.[61] Changes in microglial morphology and gene expression have also been associated with neurodevelopmental disorders, including ASD.[62] However, it remains unknown whether these changes are a primary cause or a secondary consequence of neuronal deficits (see also Chapter 5).

CNTNAP2 IN ANIMAL MODELS

Animal models are an essential tool when studying gene function in neuropsychiatric disorders and for the development of targeted treatments. *Cntnap2* function has been studied in two main animal models. The zebra finch (*Taeniopygia guttata*) is an ideal model to study language development because its learned vocal communication through auditory guided vocal imitation is well-characterized[63] and learned vocal communication is a prerequisite for language development. The expression of *Cntnap2* in zebra finch brain is enhanced in key song control nuclei.[64,65] Importantly, this enhancement was observed only in males, as would be expected based on the sexual dimorphism of neural circuitry and vocal learning in this species, in which only males learn to sign as a courtship behavior.[66] The expression of *Foxp2* in zebra finch brain includes Area X, the striatal region dedicated to song learning,[67] and knockdown of *Foxp2* in Area X during song learning leads to inaccurate and incomplete reproduction of the tutor's song.[68] Because FOXP2 is a transcription factor, its role in shaping vocal learning most likely depends on its ability to timely regulate expression of its targets (e.g., *Cntnap2* among others). In fact, *Foxp2* expression levels have been reported to be dynamic based on the amount of vocal learning required, and is highly expressed in learning juvenile zebra finches and decreasing as a result of learned singing activity in both juvenile and adults when learning is not required and songs become more stereotyped.[68–70] Although *Cntnap2* regulation by *Foxp2* has not been confirmed in the zebra finch, their punctuate expression in song brain areas suggests this is a strong possibility worth further investigation.

Although evolutionarily separated from humans 70 million years ago, as mammals, mice (*Mus musculus*) have similar neurobiological characteristics and allow us to study the behavioral deficits associated with ASD, to some extent: social interaction, vocal communication, restricted interests, and repetitive behavior.[71] The study of mouse models that recapitulate the human behavioral symptoms can help us understand the effects of these genes in ASD development. When a recessive mutation (suggesting loss of function) was reported on this gene as causing CDFE syndrome with a high penetrance of ASD,[72] we characterized a mouse knockout for the *Cntnap2* gene[56] in relation to autism. When establishing an animal model of a psychiatric disorder, three different levels of validity should be studied: construct validity (derived from an underlying cause of the disease), face validity (reflects key aspects of the human symptoms), and predictive validity (responds to treatments that are effective in the human disease). Remarkably, we found that the *Cntnap2* knockout mouse shows validity at the three levels: (1) the cause of the disease is loss of function of the *Cntnap2* gene, similar to CDFE patients; (2) it demonstrates striking parallels to the core behavioral features of ASD (they show reduced vocal communication, repetitive and restrictive behaviors, and abnormal social interactions) and they show hyperactivity and epileptic seizures, both features described in

CDFE patients[72]; and (3) they respond to autism-directed pharmacological treatment in a similar way as do humans. The main characteristics of this model are described in Figure 3.

In addition to the behavioral deficits, neuropathologically, *Cntnap2* mutant mice have defects in the migration of cortical projection neurons, as was observed in human patients with CDFE syndrome.[72] Defects in neuronal migration during brain development have been reported to cause epilepsy, intellectual disability, and other neurodevelopmental disorders.[73] In addition to neuronal migration abnormalities, the *Cntnap2* mouse model has a reduction in the number of GABAergic interneurons. This interneuron phenotype has been observed in other mouse models of ASD[4] and added a new perspective to *CNTNAP2* function because to date, the study of the functional role of the gene had been restricted to excitatory pyramidal cells, as indicated by its role in myelination. The finding of reduced interneurons in this and other animal models of ASD opens up the possibility that the behavioral phenotype

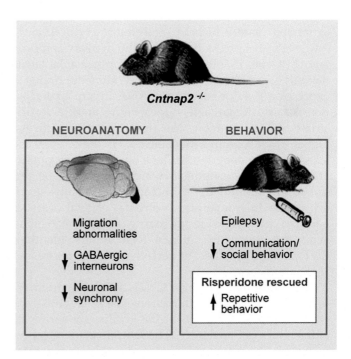

FIGURE 3 **Schematic representation of characterization of the Cntnap2 knockout mouse as a mouse model of ASD.** *Cntnap2* mice have deficits in the core ASD behavioral domains, as well as hyperactivity and epileptic seizures, as have been reported in humans with *CNTNAP2* mutations. Neuropathological and physiological analyses of these mice before the onset of seizures reveal neuronal migration abnormalities, reduced number of interneurons, and abnormal neuronal network activity. In addition, treatment with the FDA-approved drug risperidone ameliorates the targeted repetitive behaviors. These data demonstrate a functional role for CNTNAP2 in brain development and provide a new tool for mechanistic and therapeutic research in ASD. *From Peñagarikano et al. Cell 2011; 147: 235–246. Graphical abstract; with permission.*

observed in ASD is at least in part caused by an excitatory/inhibitory imbalance that has been proposed to be a primary event in ASD pathophysiology[74] and is supported by studies in mice in which altering the neocortical excitation/inhibition balance leads to deficits in social behavior and information processing.[75] Furthermore, GABAergic interneurons have been shown to regulate neuronal synchrony,[76] which we also found to be altered in the Cntnap2 mouse model,[18] and there is increasing evidence of abnormal neuronal synchrony in ASD.[77] Taken together, these data suggest that a disorganized neuronal circuitry, as defined by abnormal neuronal migration and reduced GABAergic interneurons, could cause alterations in information processing in this model. A new function has been added to CNTNAP2 in shaping neuronal networks. Using primary cultures of mouse cortical neurons, Anderson et al.[78] showed that RNA interference-mediated knockdown of CNTNAP2 causes decreased dendritic arborization and abnormal spine development, which indicates a normal role for CNTNAP2 in promoting outgrowth and connectivity. As a consequence, the authors detected a global decline in both excitatory and inhibitory synapse numbers and a decrease in synaptic transmission. Therefore, these data add to the new role of CNTNAP2 in developing neurons that is essential for neural circuit assembly.

With the aim of finding a common neuroanatomical phenotype that describes ASD, Ellegood and collaborators[79] performed a thorough MRI study in 26 mouse models of ASD, including Cntnap2 mutants. This approach provides information not only about the individual models, but also leads to a better understanding of what structures are affected in autism and possibly to increased diagnostic specificity, thus allowing for more targeted treatment, because no single treatment or diagnostic biomarker is likely to exist for ASD as a whole, and it is predicted that only a subset of patients will respond to any individual treatment. Overall, the authors found three separate circuits to be affected in these models: a cortex to basal ganglia loop likely implicated in repetitive behaviors, executive function, and communication; a more dispersed set of brain regions involved in social recognition and autonomic regulation; and a third cluster localized in the cerebellum, which has repeatedly been shown to be affected in autism.[4] The Cntnap2 model clustered with other mouse models of ASD, including 16p11, BALB/c, Gtf2i, Mecp2, and Slc6A4, which showed that a mixture of size increases and decreases with the frontal and parietotemporal lobes decreased in size and the cerebellum increased in size.

One of the ultimate goals of developing animal models of neuropsychiatric diseases is to be able to test pharmacological interventions. In autism, current pharmacotherapy is used to reduce stereotypic behaviors and noncore-associated phenotypes such as irritability and hyperactivity; currently, there is no pharmacological treatment to improve social deficits. Treatment of Cntnap2 mice with risperidone, one of the few drugs approved by the Food and Drug Administration (FDA) for autism treatment, rescues their increased repetitive behavior and hyperactivity but does not improve their social behavior, which is similar to what is seen in human patients. On the one hand, this indicates that this model could be good for testing pharmacological treatments; on the other, this model might help elucidate the different pathways and circuitries responsible for the social and repetitive behavior deficits in ASD.

Focusing on social behavior, we performed an in vivo drug screen in Cntnap2 mutant mice and found that short-term administration of the neuropeptide oxytocin (OXT) improved social deficits.[80] The OXT system is a key mediator of social behavior in mammals, including humans, in many contexts such as maternal behavior, mother–infant bonding, social memory/recognition, and pair bonding[81] (see also Chapter 16). Mice with a genetically altered OXT system—such as knockout mice for the OXT gene, the OXT receptor (OXTR) gene, or CD38 (cluster of differentiation 38), a gene involved in OXT release—all show social deficits that are restored upon OXT administration,[82] and OXT is required for the rewarding properties of social stimuli in mice.[83] In addition, OXT administration improves sociability in inbred mouse strains with naturally occurring lower levels of sociability such as BALB/cByJ and C58/J.[84] Thus, there is growing exploration of OXT's potential for therapeutic efficacy in ASD. A key issue is whether there are actual deficits in this system in some forms of ASD because identifying which patients could potentially benefit the most from OXT treatment is critical. We found a decrease in the number of OXT-immunoreactive neurons in the paraventricular nucleus (PVN) of the hypothalamus in mutant mice and an overall decrease in brain OXT levels.[80] The precise molecular mechanisms of these effects of Cntnap2 deletion on the OXT system is not known. One possibility is that as a cell adhesion molecule, CNTNAP2 affects OXT neuron function through its well-established role in neuron–glia interaction.[56] CNTNAP2 is expressed in OXT neurons, whose development and function depend on dynamic neuron–glia interactions.[85] Alternatively, CNTNAP2 could be involved in the structural development of OXT neurons and therefore affect their functioning, as has been shown for cortical neurons.[78]

The mechanism by which OXT exerts its behavioral effects in this mouse model deserves further study. Neuropeptides such as OXT contribute to network activity by modulating the effect of classical excitatory and inhibitory neurotransmitters. Owen et al.[86] showed that OXT stimulates fast-spiking parvalbumin interneuron activity, modulating circuit signal-to-noise ratio and improving information processing. As stated before, interneurons, and specifically the parvalbumin subtype, have a critical role in regulating network activity[76] and their dysfunction has been implicated in ASD. We previously found that the *Cntnap2* mouse model shows deficits in GABAergic interneurons, and OXT receptor null mice have fewer GABAergic synapses.[87] Therefore, it is possible that OXT compensates for GABAergic deficits in this mouse model. Although GABA is inhibitory in adult brain, it is excitatory during fetal and early postnatal periods, owing to elevated intracellular chloride concentrations, and OXT has been shown to be involved in its perinatal excitatory to inhibitory shift by reducing intracellular chloride levels.[88] Tyzio et al.[89] found that this process is altered in the *Fmr1* knockout model, a model for fragile X syndrome, which also has a reduced number of GABAergic interneurons[90]; preliminary results in the *Fmr1* model suggest reduced OXT immunoreactivity in the PVN.[91] Thus, studies have begun to investigate intranasal OXT effects in fragile X syndrome and have found an improvement in eye gaze frequency during a social task, which suggests that OXT could be a potential treatment for social anxiety in this syndrome.[92] These results suggests that studying OXT in other defined genetic forms of ASD would be valuable because a key goal remains to discern which forms of ASD show direct or indirect dysregulation of this system, because we suspect that these patients are the most likely to benefit from treatment with OXT (see Chapter 16 for more information on OXT and ASD).

In conclusion, because the understanding of *CNTNAP2* function previously focused primarily on postnatal development, these studies set a new direction for investigating its role during development and in the formation and function of neuronal circuits. In addition, although ASD is a complex neurodevelopmental disorder of which only about 10–15% is due to single gene mutations, the studies described throughout this chapter on *CNTNAP2* support the integrative use of animal models and human studies of a single gene causing ASD to understand its pathophysiology and develop targeted treatments.

Acknowledgments

I would like to thank all of my colleagues and collaborators who dedicated their work to studying the genetic contribution of *CNTNAP2* to ASD, because they have made this work possible. OP is supported by NARSAD Young Investigator Grant 23663.

References

1. APA. *Diagnostic and statistical manual of mental disorders*. 5th ed. Washington, DC: American Psychiatric Association (American Psychiatric Publishing); 2013.

2. Geschwind DH. Advances in autism. *Annu Rev Med* 2009;**60**:367.

3. Abrahams BS, Geschwind DH. Advances in autism genetics: on the threshold of a new neurobiology. *Nat Rev Genet* 2008;**9**:341.

4. Peñagarikano O, Chen JA, Belgard TG, Swarup V, Geschwind DH. The emerging picture of autism spectrum disorders: genetics and pathology. *Annu Rev Pathol Mech Dis* 2015;**10**.

5. Verkerk AJ, et al. CNTNAP2 is disrupted in a family with Gilles de la Tourette syndrome and obsessive compulsive disorder. *Genomics* 2003;**82**:1.

6. Poot M, et al. Disruption of CNTNAP2 and additional structural genome changes in a boy with speech delay and autism spectrum disorder. *Neurogenetics* 2010;**11**:81.

7. Rossi E, et al. A 12Mb deletion at 7q33-q35 associated with autism spectrum disorders and primary amenorrhea. *Eur J Med Genet* November–December 2008;**51**:631.

8. Sehested LT, et al. Deletion of 7q34-q36.2 in two siblings with mental retardation, language delay, primary amenorrhea, and dysmorphic features. *Am J Med Genet A* December 2010;**152A**:3115.

9. Al-Murrani A, Ashton F, Aftimos S, George AM, Love DR. Amino-terminal microdeletion within the CNTNAP2 gene associated with variable expressivity of speech delay. *Case Rep Genet* 2012;**2012**:172408.

10. Strauss KA, et al. Recessive symptomatic focal epilepsy and mutant contactin-associated protein-like 2. *N. Engl J Med* 2006;**354**:1370.

11. Falivelli G, et al. Inherited genetic variants in autism-related CNTNAP2 show perturbed trafficking and ATF6 activation. *Hum Mol Genet* November 1, 2012;**21**:4761.

12. Poliak S, et al. Caspr2, a new member of the neurexin superfamily, is localized at the juxtaparanodes of myelinated axons and associates with K^+ channels. *Neuron* 1999;**24**:1037.

13. Rossi PG, Parmeggiani A, Bach V, Santucci M, Visconti P. EEG features and epilepsy in patients with autism. *Brain Dev* May–June, 1995;**17**:169.

14. Volkmar FR, Nelson DS. Seizure disorders in autism. *J Am Acad Child Adolesc Psychiatry* January 1990;**29**:127.

15. Trauner DA. Behavioral correlates of epileptiform abnormalities in autism. *Epilepsy Behav* November 5, 2014;**47**.

16. Guerrini R, Dobyns WB, Barkovich AJ. Abnormal development of the human cerebral cortex: genetics, functional consequences and treatment options. *Trends Neurosci* March 2008;**31**:154.

17. Chu J, Anderson SA. Development of cortical interneurons. *Neuropsychopharmacology* January 2015;**40**:16.

18. Peñagarikano O, et al. Absence of CNTNAP2 leads to epilepsy, neuronal migration abnormalities and core autism-related deficits. *Cell* 2011;**147**.

19. Arking DE, et al. A common genetic variant in the neurexin superfamily member CNTNAP2 increases familial risk of autism. *Am J Hum Genet* 2008;**82**:160.

20. Bakkaloglu B, et al. Molecular cytogenetic analysis and resequencing of contactin associated protein-like 2 in autism spectrum disorders. *Am J Hum Genet* 2008;**82**:165.

21. Alarcón M, et al. Evidence for a language quantitative trait locus on chromosome 7q in multiplex autism families. *Am J Hum Genet* 2002;**70**:60.

22. Alarcón M, et al. Linkage, association, and gene-expression analyses identify CNTNAP2 as an autism-susceptibility gene. *Am J Hum Genet* 2008;**82**:150.

23. O'Roak BJ, et al. Exome sequencing in sporadic autism spectrum disorders identifies severe de novo mutations. *Nat Genet* 2011;**46**:585.

24. Gottesman II, Gould TD. The endophenotype concept in psychiatry: etymology and strategic intentions. *Am J Psychiatry* April 2003;**160**:636.

25. Geschwind DH. Autism: many genes, common pathways? *Cell* October 31, 2008;**135**:391.

26. Anney R, et al. Individual common variants exert weak effects on the risk for autism spectrum disorderspi. *Hum Mol Genet* November 1, 2012;**21**:4781.

27. Peter B, et al. Replication of CNTNAP2 association with nonword repetition and support for FOXP2 association with timed reading and motor activities in a dyslexia family sample. *J Neurodev Disord* 2011;**3**:39.

28. Newbury DF, et al. Investigation of dyslexia and SLI risk variants in reading- and language-impaired subjects. *Behav Genet* 2011;**41**:90.

29. Whitehouse AJ, Bishop DV, Ang QW, Pennell CE, Fisher SE. CNTNAP2 variants affect early language development in the general population. *Genes Brain Behav* June 2011;**10**:451.

30. Petrin AL, et al. Identification of a microdeletion at the 7q33-q35 disrupting the CNTNAP2 gene in a Brazilian stuttering case. *Am J Med Genet Part A* December 2010;**152A**:3164.

31. Nord AS, et al. Reduced transcript expression of genes affected by inherited and de novo CNVs in autism. *Eur J Hum Genet* 2011;**19**:727.

32. Vernes SC, et al. A functional genetic link between distinct developmental language disorders. *N Engl J Med* 2008;**359**:2337.

33. Lai CS, Fisher SE, Hurst JA, Vargha-Khadem F, Monaco AP. A forkhead-domain gene is mutated in a severe speech and language disorder. *Nature* 2001;**413**:519.

34. MacDermot KD, et al. Identification of FOXP2 truncation as a novel cause of developmental speech and language deficits. *Am J Hum Genet* 2005;**76**:1074.

35. Chiocchetti AG, et al. Variants of the CNTNAP2 5′ promoter as risk factors for autism spectrum disorders: a genetic and functional approach. *Mol Psychiatry* September 16, 2014;**20**.

36. Maekawa M, et al. Utility of scalp hair follicles as a novel source of biomarker genes for psychiatric illnesses. *Biol Psychiatry* September 11, 2014;**78**.

37. Rodenas-Cuadrado P, Ho J, Vernes SC. Shining a light on CNTNAP2: complex functions to complex disorders. *Eur J Hum Genet* February 2014;**22**:171.

38. Steer CD, Golding J, Bolton PF. Traits contributing to the autistic spectrum. *PLoS One* 2010;**5**:e12633.

39. Stein MB, et al. A common genetic variant in the neurexin superfamily member CNTNAP2 is associated with increased risk for selective mutism and social anxiety-related traits. *Biol Psychiatry* 2011;**69**:825.

40. Tan GC, Doke TF, Ashburner J, Wood NW, Frackowiak RS. Normal variation in fronto-occipital circuitry and cerebellar structure with an autism-associated polymorphism of CNTNAP2. *Neuroimage* 2010;**53**:1030.

41. Dennis EL, et al. Altered structural brain connectivity in healthy carriers of the autism risk gene, CNTNAP2. *Brain Connect* 2011;**1**:447.

42. Whalley HC, et al. Genetic variation in CNTNAP2 alters brain function during linguistic processing in healthy individuals. *Am J Med Genet B Neuropsychiatr Genet* December 2011;**156B**:941.

43. Scott-Van Zeeland AA, et al. Altered functional connectivity in frontal lobe circuits is associated with variation in the autism risk gene CNTNAP2. *Sci Transl Med* 2010;**2**:56.

44. Abrahams BS, et al. Genome-wide analyses of human perisylvian cerebral cortical patterning. *Proc Natl Acad Sci USA* 2007;**104**:17849.

45. Raichle ME, et al. A default mode of brain function. *Proc Natl Acad Sci USA* 2001;**98**:676.

46. Dosenbach NU, et al. Prediction of individual brain maturity using fMRI. *Science* 2010;**329**:1358.

47. Belmonte MK, et al. Autism and abnormal development of brain connectivity. *J Neurosci* 2004;**24**:9228.

48. Geschwind DH, Levitt P. Autism spectrum disorders: developmental disconnection syndromes. *Curr Opin Neurobiol* 2007;**17**:103.

49. Rubenstein JL. Annual research review: development of the cerebral cortex: implications for neurodevelopmental disorders. *J Child Psychol Psychiatry Allied Discip* April 2011;**52**:339.

50. Harris KM. Structure, development, and plasticity of dendritic spines. *Curr Opin Neurobiol* June 1999;**9**:343.

51. Zoghbi HY. Postnatal neurodevelopmental disorders: meeting at the synapse? *Science* October 31, 2003;**302**:826.

52. Ushkaryov YA, Petrenko AG, Geppert M, Südhof TC. Neurexins: synaptic cell surface proteins related to the alpha-latrotoxin receptor and laminin. *Science* 1992;**257**:50.

53. Ichtchenko K, et al. Neuroligin 1: a splice site-specific ligand for beta-neurexins. *Cell* 1995;**81**:435.

54. Poliak S, Peles E. The local differentiation of myelinated axons at nodes of Ranvier. *Nat Rev Neurosci* 2003;**4**:968.

55. Nakabayashi K, Scherer SW. The human contactin-associated protein-like 2 gene (CNTNAP2) spans over 2 Mb of DNA at chromosome 7q35. *Genomics* 2001;**73**:108.

56. Poliak S, et al. Juxtaparanodal clustering of Shaker-like K$^+$ channels in myelinated axons depends on Caspr2 and TAG-1. *J Cell Biol* September 15, 2003;**162**:1149.

57. Horresh I, et al. Multiple molecular interactions determine the clustering of Caspr2 and Kv1 channels in myelinated axons. *J Neurosci* 2008;**28**:14213.

58. Inda MC, DeFelipe J, Muñoz A. Voltage-gated ion channels in the axon initial segment of human cortical pyramidal cells and their relationship with chandelier cells. *Natl Acad Sci USA* 2006;**103**:2920.

59. Ogawa Y, et al. Postsynaptic density-93 clusters Kv1 channels at axon initial segments independently of Caspr2. *J Neurosci* 2008;**28**:5731.

60. Verkhratsky A. Physiology of neuronal-glial networking. *Neurochem Int* November 2010;**57**:332.

61. Pekny M, Wilhelmsson U, Pekna M. The dual role of astrocyte activation and reactive gliosis. *Neurosci Lett* April 17, 2014;**565**:30.

62. Frick LR, Williams K, Pittenger C. Microglial dysregulation in psychiatric disease. *Clin Dev Immunol* 2013;**2013**:608654.

63. Williams H. Birdsong and singing behavior. *Ann NY Acad Sci* June 2004;**1016**:1.

64. Panaitof SC, Abrahams BS, Dong H, Geschwind DH, White SA. Language-related Cntnap2 gene is differentially expressed in sexually dimorphic song nuclei essential for vocal learning in songbirds. *J Comp Neurol* 2010;**518**:1995.

65. Condro MC, White SA. Distribution of language-related Cntnap2 protein in neural circuits critical for vocal learning. *J Comp Neurol* January 1, 2014;**522**:169.

66. Nottebohm F, Arnold AP. Sexual dimorphism in vocal control areas of the songbird brain. *Science* 1976;**194**:211.

67. Teramitsu I, Kudo LC, London SE, Geschwind DH, White SA. Parallel FoxP1 and FoxP2 expression in songbird and human brain predicts functional interaction. *J Neurosci* March 31, 2004;**24**:3152.

68. Haesler S, et al. Incomplete and inaccurate vocal imitation after knockdown of FoxP2 in songbird basal ganglia nucleus Area X. *PLoS Biol* December 2007;**5**:e321.

69. Teramitsu I, White SA. FoxP2 regulation during undirected singing in adult songbirds. *J Neurosci* July 12, 2006;**26**:7390.

70. Teramitsu I, Poopatanapong A, Torrisi S, White SA. Striatal FoxP2 is actively regulated during songbird sensorimotor learning. *PLoS One* 2010;**5**:e8548.

71. Crawley JN. Behavioral phenotyping strategies for mutant mice. *Neuron* 2008;**57**:809.

72. Strauss KA, et al. *N. Engl J Med* 2006;**354**:1370−7.

73. Guerrini R, et al. Variable epilepsy phenotypes associated with a familial intragenic deletion of the SCN1A gene. *Epilepsia* December 2010;**51**:2474.

74. Rubenstein JL, Merzenich MM. Model of autism: increased ratio of excitation/inhibition in key neural systems. *Genes Brain Behav* 2003;**2**:255.

75. Yizhar O, et al. Neocortical excitation/inhibition balance in information processing and social dysfunction. *Nature* September 8, 2011;**477**:171.

76. Sohal VS, Zhang F, Yizhar O, Deisseroth K. Parvalbumin neurons and gamma rhythms enhance cortical circuit performance. *Nature* June 4, 2009;**459**:698.

77. Uhlhaas PJ, Singer W. Neural synchrony in brain disorders: relevance for cognitive dysfunctions and pathophysiology. *Neuron* October 5, 2006;**52**:155.

78. Anderson GR, et al. Candidate autism gene screen identifies critical role for cell-adhesion molecule CASPR2 in dendritic arborization and spine development. *Proc Natl Acad Sci USA* October 30, 2012;**109**:18120.

79. Ellegood J, et al. Clustering autism: using neuroanatomical differences in 26 mouse models to gain insight into the heterogeneity. *Mol Psychiatry* September 9, 2014;**20**.

80. Penagarikano O, et al. Oxytocin modulates social behavior in the Cntnap2 mouse model of ASD. *Sci Transl Med* January 2015;**7**:271.

81. McCall C, Singer T. The animal and human neuroendocrinology of social cognition, motivation and behavior. *Nat Neurosci* May 2012;**15**:681.

82. Modi ME, Young LJ. The oxytocin system in drug discovery for autism: animal models and novel therapeutic strategies. *Horm Behav* March 2012;**61**:340.

83. Dolen G, Darvishzadeh A, Huang KW, Malenka RC. Social reward requires coordinated activity of nucleus accumbens oxytocin and serotonin. *Nature* September 12, 2013;**501**:179.

84. Teng BL, et al. Prosocial effects of oxytocin in two mouse models of autism spectrum disorders. *Neuropharmacology* September 2013;**72**:187.

85. Theodosis DT, Schachner M, Neumann ID. Oxytocin neuron activation in NCAM-deficient mice: anatomical and functional consequences. *Eur J Neurosci* December 2004;**20**:3270.

86. Owen SF, et al. Oxytocin enhances hippocampal spike transmission by modulating fast-spiking interneurons. *Nature* August 22, 2013;**500**:458.

87. Sala M, et al. Pharmacologic rescue of impaired cognitive flexibility, social deficits, increased aggression, and seizure susceptibility in oxytocin receptor null mice: a neurobehavioral model of autism. *Biol Psychiatry* May 1, 2011;**69**:875.

88. Tyzio R, et al. Maternal oxytocin triggers a transient inhibitory switch in GABA signaling in the fetal brain during delivery. *Science* December 15, 2006;**314**:1788.

89. Tyzio R, et al. Oxytocin-mediated GABA inhibition during delivery attenuates autism pathogenesis in rodent offspring. *Science* February 7, 2014;**343**:675.

90. Selby L, Zhang C, Sun QQ. Major defects in neocortical GABAergic inhibitory circuits in mice lacking the fragile X mental retardation protein. *Neurosci Lett* February 2, 2007;**412**:227.

91. Francis SM, et al. Oxytocin and vasopressin systems in genetic syndromes and neurodevelopmental disorders. *Brain Res* January 22, 2014;**1580**.

92. Hall SS, Lightbody AA, McCarthy BE, Parker KJ, Reiss AL. Effects of intranasal oxytocin on social anxiety in males with fragile X syndrome. *Psychoneuroendocrinology* April 2012;**37**:509.

CHAPTER

13

Planar Cell Polarity Gene Mutations in Autism Spectrum Disorder, Intellectual Disabilities, and Related Deletion/Duplication Syndromes

Nathalie Sans[1,2], Jérôme Ezan[1,2],
Maité M. Moreau[1,2], Mireille Montcouquiol[1,2]

[1]INSERM, Neurocentre Magendie U1215, Bordeaux, France; [2]University of Bordeaux, Bordeaux, France

INTRODUCTION

The adult mammalian brain is the site of cognitive and emotional processing, and its structure and functions are the ultimate result of numerous complex, coordinated developmental mechanisms. Because many genetic factors have a role during the prenatal, perinatal and postnatal developmental periods, specific genetic vulnerability will affect proper brain development and increase susceptibility to mental disorders or intellectual disabilities (IDs) of neurodevelopmental origin.[1,2] The European Brain Council estimated that each year, almost 40% of the European Union population experiences some sort of mental disorder, and neurodevelopmental pathologies account for a sizable part of them. These is therefore, one of the most important challenges for future therapy in coming years.[3]

During development, disruption of proliferation, migration, polarity, guidance, branching, or synaptogenesis can affect the shape, size, organization, or connectivity of the brain. Patients with disruptions in these fundamental mechanisms typically will exhibit developmental delay and can also develop more serious neurodevelopmental disorders ranging from mild to severe IDs, with or without autism spectrum disorder (ASD) and/or seizures and epilepsy, depending on the severity of the brain malformation. For instance, the balance between proliferation and differentiation has been suggested as an explanation for the differences in brain size.[4] In the worst cases, patients with primary microcephaly (reduced brain size) have IDs. Improper neuronal migration also results in a wide range of diseases including lissencephaly (smooth brain surface) and cortical dysplasia/heterotopia (neurons mislocalization), which will eventually lead to neurobehavioral disorders such as ASD (see chapter 4).[5] Defects in synaptic connections or in mechanisms involved in synaptic plasticity will also lead to these neurodevelopmental disorders. Interestingly, there is mounting evidence that neurodevelopmental and neuropsychiatric disorders share molecular pathways.[6]

The purpose of this review is to emphasize the significance of one of these pathways, planar cell polarity (PCP) signaling, in vertebrate brain development. We will examine how disruption of its components affects neurodevelopmental processes, which in turn might cause ASD/ID and related pathologies.

THE PCP PATHWAY: FROM INVERTEBRATES TO HUMANS, FROM EPITHELIUM TO NEURON

Most, if not all, cell types and tissues exhibit several aspects of polarization, and the vertebrate brain is no exception. The concept of cell polarity is perhaps best exemplified in epithelial tissues, where in addition to the ubiquitous cellular asymmetry seen along the apical—basolateral axis, many tissues and organs are polarized within the plane of the epithelium. Another type of polarity, PCP, in epithelia can be defined as the coordinated and uniform orientation/polarization of cells or appendages of cells (such a cilia, stereocilia, or hair) within the plane of a tissue.[7] Pioneering genetic and molecular studies in *Drosophila* provided the first model to unravel PCP and its components.[8,9] In *Drosophila*, the initial definition of PCP referred to the specific and coordinated orientation of structures perpendicular to the axis of the epithelium. The most studied of these structures is the actin-rich hair (or trichrome) covering the wings of the animals, whose coordinated orientation within the plane of the epidermis defines the axis of PCP (proximal—distal) along the epithelium. Another well-studied structure, the ommatidia (photoreceptors) of the eye of the animals, operates rotation within the epithelium during its differentiation.[10] Except for one study,[11] there is consensus that in these examples of classical PCP in *Drosophila*, the Wnt family of proteins takes no part.[12,13] This specific type of polarity is controlled by a variety of signaling cassettes, as indicated later in this review, and core PCP signaling in this case is composed upstream of six core PCP proteins, namely frizzled (fzd), vang, flamingo, dishevelled (dvl), diego, and prickle, the mutation of any of these leads to disruption of PCP.

In vertebrates, and notably *Xenopus* and zebrafish, disruption of core PCP genes leads to a different type of phenotype, namely a convergent-extension (CE) phenotype, in which the absence of core PCP genes impairs the collective and coordinated migration of cells (in various axis) and leads to severe disruption of the extension of the anteroposterior axis of the animal. Such disruption results in shorter animals, a phenotype whose cellular basis shares some common traits with the craniorachischisis phenotype observed in mammals with core PCP mutations. The CE phenotype in vertebrates is not specific to core PCP genes; this phenotype is observed as a consequence of the mutation of a large number of genes, many of them in relation to the regulation of cell adhesion or the cytoskeleton.[14] Contrary to *Drosophila*, the mutation (or in most cases, downregulation) of members of the Wnt family leads to this CE phenotype, opening the door to a much larger definition of PCP genes in vertebrates compared with invertebrates. At this point, it is safer to refer to PCP signaling rather than PCP, as in *Drosophila*.

Work from our laboratory revealed that classical PCP signaling is conserved in mammals.[15–18] The inner ear epithelia (cochlear and vestibular epithelia) were the original tissue models used in these studies to identify PCP phenotypes in mammals and validate the conservation of function of most core PCP genes from invertebrates. In these tissues, the PCP phenotype is similar in essence to what is observed in epithelial *Drosophila* wing cells. Building on these seminal studies and on the phenotype, a growing number of genes were labeled PCP genes in mammals. We named some of them PCP-associated proteins, based on their weaker PCP phenotype than the classical core PCP genes when mutated (including some with no original PCP function in invertebrates). However, some of these studies should be regarded with caution, because many of these so-called PCP genes mutations lead to a weak PCP cochlear phenotype that could well be interpreted as a delay in maturation or patterning of the tissue.[18] The localization of PCP proteins in the same subcellular domains as adhesion molecules could lead to an indirect adhesion-dependent phenotype.

Obviously, craniorachischisis (see subsequent discussion) is also the major phenotype common to all core PCP genes mutation in mammals (Table 1). Thus, it is fair to make a distinction between genes whose mutations lead to a major phenotype in both the inner ear and the neural tube and other genes whose mutations lead to a phenotype in one or the other of the tissues with various gradients of severity (Table 2). When looking for human consequences of PCP signaling disruption, it should also be kept in mind that these important genes will have a major phenotype when mutated and may never be identified because of embryonic lethality. On the other hand, one can expect subtler and less dramatic mutations to occur and allow survival, but then it might be harder to define in terms of phenotype. Other important questions to address in mammals, and notably in humans, are: Can we define a common phenotype or a specific readout of PCP disruption at the anatomical level? And even more challenging, what, if any, are the specific cognitive deficits that can be linked to early disruption of PCP signaling?

Because PCP signaling is involved in a large number of cellular processes (asymmetric cell division, migration, axonal guidance, collective cell migration, synaptogenesis, synaptic plasticity, etc.), and because PCP genes have multiple orthologs in mammals compared with invertebrates, we need to start to disentangle the specific cellular processes each gene may control. As a prerequisite, the use of conditional mutants (at various stages of development and in adults) is a necessary step to carefully analyze the anatomical and functional consequences of the disruption of each of these genes.

MORE THAN ONE PATHWAY

PCP is believed to rely on at least three key functional molecular modules of asymmetrically distributed proteins in epithelial tissues, which constitute the PCP signaling pathways: the core PCP module and its associated downstream proteins, the Fat-Ds module, and the $G\alpha i/mPins$ module.[18,19] These molecular asymmetries may be transient during development, and therefore are not always observed. This does not preclude the PCP pathway from signaling efficiently, and PCP proteins may localize in various subcellular compartments (not necessarily asymmetrically) in nonepithelial cells such as neurons and/or glial cells. This review will essentially describe the relevance of the two first modules: the core PCP and Fat-Ds, in ASD/ID and related disorders.

The Core PCP Module

The core PCP signaling cascade was initially characterized in *Drosophila*, where it refers to the polarization of epithelial cells along the horizontal plane of the epithelium, orthogonal to the apicobasal axis.[20] It depends on the asymmetrical distribution of a group of six specific proteins at the membrane of epithelial cells and is conserved in mammals (Figure 1).[21,22] Thus, the core PCP signaling cascade is composed of three transmembrane proteins called Van Gogh/strabismus (vang/stbm), flamingo/starry night (fmi/stan), frizzled (fz) and their mammalian orthologs including several members including Van Gogh-like 1 and 2 (Vangl1/2), cadherin/epidermal growth factor (EGF)/laminin G (LAG) seven-pass G-type receptors 1, 2, and 3 (Celsr1/2/3), and Frizzled 1/2/3/6 (Fz1/2/3/6). The three others are cytosolic proteins Dishevelled (Dsh), Prickle, and Diego (Dgo), whose mammalian orthologs are Dishevelled 1, 2, and 3 (Dvl1/2/3), Prickle1 and 2 (Pk1/2), and Diversin/Ankrd6.[18] Their mutations lead to the most severe form of neural tube defects (NTDs) in mouse, called craniorachischisis (Table 1). Wnt proteins were not clearly involved, likely owing to redundancy, but they might act mainly through their interaction with Frizzled receptors in vertebrate PCP establishment, but also in *Drosophila*.[11] Although activated by Wnt ligands in some contexts, PCP signaling (alternatively called the Wnt noncanonical PCP) pathway, does not implicate β-catenin. The implication of the Wnt canonical pathway in neuropsychiatric disorders has been reviewed elsewhere and will not be the subject of this chapter.[23–25] When noncanonical Wnt ligands (such as Wnt5a or Wnt11) bind Fz receptor, the cytoplasmic scaffold protein Dishevelled is activated

TABLE 1　Core PCP Signaling Components and Mouse Phenotypes

Proteins	Experimental Model	Ear Phenotype	NTD Phenotype	Others Phenotype	References
Celsr1	Spin cycle (Scy) mutant mice	Inner ear hair cell orientation defects, defective convergent extension, deaf	Severe NTD; SB; CR	Failure of eyelid closure	70
	Crash (Crsh) mutant mice	Inner ear hair cell orientation defects, defective convergent extension, deaf	Severe NTD; SB; CR	Failure of eyelid closure; Lung morphogenesis defects	70,306
Celsr2	Celsr2−/− mice	—	—	Hydrocephalus, impaired cilia function	307
Celsr2/3	Celsr2/3 mutant mice	—	—	Lethal hydrocephalus, defect ciliogenesis	307
Celsr3	Celsr3 mutant mice	—	—	Homozygote died after birth, defects in several major axonal tracts at postnatal day (P)0	81,88
	Celsr3/Foxg1 mutant mice	—	—	Defects in corticothalamic, thalamocortical and subcerebral axons	88
	Celsr3/Dlx5/6 mutant mice	—	—	Defects in corticothalamic, thalamocortical and subcerebral axons	88
	Celsr3/Emx1 mutant mice	—	—	Defect in cortical spinal tract	88
Diego-Ankrd6 (Diversin)	Xenopus	—	—	Ciliary functions	308
	Ankrd6−/−; Vangl2lp/+ knockout mice	PCP defects in inner ear sensory organ	—		181
	Mice: Retroviral vector encoding shRNA into adult mice SVZ	—	—	Decreased proliferation of neuroblasts during migration	309
Dvl1	Dvl1 Null mutant mice	—	—	Abnormal social behavior and sensorimotor gating, but no changes in acquisition of spatial learning in water maze test	113,114
	Dvl1-ΔPDZ overexpression in Nucleus Accumbens	—	—	Increased susceptibility to chronic social defeat stress and induced prodepression-like effects	310
Dvl2	Dvl2−/− mice	—	(2–3%) have incomplete thoracic NTD with exencephaly	Death at birth with defect in cardiac neural crest development mild abnormalities of vertebral bodies and ribs	311,312
	Dvl2−/−;Lp/+	Stereocilia misorientation			313
Dvl1/2	Dvl1/2 double homozygote mutant	Disruption of uniform stereociliary bundle orientation	CR, NTD, SB	Somite defects with aberrant somite patterning	311,313

Gene	Model			Phenotype	Ref
Dvl3	Dvl3 mutant		—	Death at birth with heart defects	314
	Dvl2/3 double homozygote mutant	Cochlear abnormalities	CR	Lethal owing to severe gastrulation defects	315
Dvl	Triple KO mice for Dvls (Dvl TKOhGFAP-Cre)		—	Hydrocephaly	310
	Pharmacological inhibitor of DVL in mice		—	Increased susceptibility to chronic social defeat stress and induced prodepression-like affects	310
Fzd3	Fzd3$^{-/-}$ and conditional mutant mice		Incomplete closure of neural tube (NT)	Curled tail and flexed hind limbs, enlarged lateral ventricles, severe defects in several major axon tracts within central nervous system forebrain regions associated with somatosensory deficiencies	82,122,123,316
			—	Hypermethylation of Fzd3 increased congenital hydrocephalus risk	317
Fzd4	Fzd4$^{-/-}$ mutant mice		—	Growth of retinal capillaries, development of esophagus, survival of cerebellar neurons, and maintenance of vasculature within cochlea	318,319
Fzd5	Fzd5 conditional mutant mice		—	Fz5 is required for yolk sac and placental angiogenesis and for Paneth cell maturation in intestinal crypts	320,321
Fzd6	Fzd6$^{-/-}$ mutant mice		—	Altered hair patterns	121
Fzd3/6	Fzd3$^{-/-}$; Fzd6$^{-/-}$	Defects in orientation of hair bundles and cristae	NTD, CR	Death within minutes of birth, curled tail, unfused eyelids	124
Fzd9	Mouse hippocampus frizzled 9-null mice		—	Williams syndrome-like: Increased apoptotic cell death and increased precursor proliferation during hippocampal development, severe deficits on tests of visuospatial learning/memory	383
Prickle1	Deletion of mpk1 gene in mice		—	Embryonic lethal at e6.5	323
	Prickle1 +/− mice		—	Seizure phenotype	190
Prickle1&2	Mice tissue and Neuro2a cells		—	Regulate positive neurite formation during brain development	324
Prickle2	Prickle2 mutant mice		—	Altered social interactions, learning abnormalities and behavioral inflexibility	384
			—	Robinow syndrome: Developed shorter stature, and craniofacial defects with wide spaced eyes, flat nose, short snout, prominent forehead,	325

Continued

II. FUNCTION OF MUTATED GENES IN INTELLECTUAL DISABILITY (ID) AND AUTISM

TABLE 1 Core PCP Signaling Components and Mouse Phenotypes—cont'd

Proteins	Experimental Model	Ear Phenotype	NTD Phenotype	Others Phenotype	References
				abnormal appearance of eyelid and eyelashes, and fused mandibular incisors	
				Abnormal morphology and motility in motile cilia of ependyma	326
	Prickle2$^{+/-}$ and $^{-/-}$ mice	—	—	Seizure phenotype	190
	Mouse hippocampal neurons and slices			↓dentritic branching, synapse number and PSD size; ↓ frequency and size of spontaneous mEPSCs	384
Vangl1	Looptail mice Lpp1		Failure of NT closure		327,328,15,329
Vangl2	Looptail (Lp/Lp)	Inner ear hair cell orientation defects in both inner and outer hair cells	CR, NTD, SB		15,162,330
	Looptail (Lp/Lp)			Commissural axon growth cone guidance	331
	Looptail (Lp/Lp)			Cell proliferation and fate determination	73
	Looptail (Lp/Lp)			Polarized cell movements such as convergence and extension movements during gastrulation	330,332–335
	Looptail (Lp/Lp)			FBM neuron migration	333,336–338
	Looptail (Lp/Lp)			Wound repair defects	339
	Looptail (Lp/Lp)			Defect in reproductive tract development	340
	Looptail (Lp/Lp)			Tumor cell migration	341–343
	Looptail (Lp/Lp)			Defect in hair follicle development	344
	Looptail (Lp/Lp) and Vangl2$^{\Delta/\Delta}$			Misorientation of cilia in many tissues and organs	307,345,346,16,347
	Looptail (Lp/Lp)			Development and defects branching morphogenesis in kidney and in lung architecture	306,348
	Lp/+ Crc/+	Inner ear hair cell orientation defects in both inner and outer hair cells			15

NTD, neural tube defect; CR, craniorachischisis; SB, spina bifida; Nac, nucleus accumbens.

TABLE 2   PCP-Related Signaling Components and Mouse Phenotypes

Proteins	Experimental Model	Ear Phenotype	NTD Phenotype	Others Phenotype	References
Daam1	Daam1-deficient mice		NTD	Embryonic and neonatal lethality with multiple cardiac defects, defect heart morphogenesis, embryos develop ocular defects (anophthalmia or microphthalmia)	349,350
Dact1	Dact1⁻/⁻ mice		NTD, SB	Partial neonatal lethality, abnormal embryogenesis, short tail, blind-ended colons, and abnormal reproductive/renal/urinary/vertebrae/cardiovascular system	39,351,352
	Cultured hippocampal neurons			Abnormal dendritic spine morphology, synapse morphology and miniature excitatory postsynaptic current	39
Diaph3	Diap3-overexpressing mice	Progressive hearing loss, abnormal inner hair cell stereociliary bundle and synaptic ribbon morphology, decreased inner hair cell stereocilia number		Early mortality owing to cardiac defects Abnormal cardiovascular system morphology	353
Dlg1 (Sap-97)	Dlgh1 null mice	Abnormal arrangement of hair cells in the organ of Corti accompanied by disorganized arrangement of hair cell rows		Neonatal lethality, abnormal renal/kidney/urinary system and bone formation, impaired smooth muscle contractility, cardiovascular defect, respiratory distress, and cyanosis	239,354
Dlg3 (Sap-102)	SAP102 KO mice			Alterations in spatial learning, locomotor activation, LTP, and spike-timing-dependent plasticity	355
	Dlg3 KO mice			Forebrain deletion, posterior truncation, and failure to initiate embryo turning	356
Mapk3 (Erk1)	16p11.2 mice model			Partial postnatal lethality, hyperactivity, stereotypic behavior, impaired hearing, abnormal response to novel object, abnormal striatum, hypothalamus, cortex and corpus callosum morphology, decreased body size	357,358
	ERK1⁻/⁻ mice			Hyperactivity, altered synaptic plasticity, enhancement of striatal-mediated learning and memory	359
Mapk1 (Erk2)	Erk2 cKO mice			Abnormal proliferation of neural stem cells in the ventricular zone during embryonic development	
	Erk2⁻/⁻ mice Erk2 knockdown mice			Lethality of Erk2⁻/⁻ mice and semilethality of Erk2⁻/⁺ mice. Impaired long-term memory	360

Continued

II. FUNCTION OF MUTATED GENES IN INTELLECTUAL DISABILITY (ID) AND AUTISM

TABLE 2　PCP-Related Signaling Components and Mouse Phenotypes—cont'd

Proteins	Experimental Model	Ear Phenotype	NTD Phenotype	Others Phenotype	References
	Erk2 brain cKO mice			Anomalies in multiple aspects of social behaviors related to facets of autism-spectrum disorders, decreased anxiety-related behaviors and impaired long-term memory	361
Erk1/2	BTBR mice model			Ras/Raf/ERK1/2 signaling to be upregulated in the brain	362
	Erk1$^{-/-}$, Erk2 brain cKO mice			Neonatally lethal, histological defects in the brain associated with abnormal neurogenesis phenotype	363
Inversin	inv/inv mutant mice			Hair patterning defects	184,364–367
				Multiorgan defects including renal cysts, altered left-right laterality, hepatobiliary duct and kidneys abnormalities	
				Cardiopulmonary and liver malformations	
Jnk1/Mapk8	JK1$^{\Delta NES}$ mice			Reduced body weight, protected from obesity-associated hepatic steatosis and adipose tissue inflammation	368
				Abnormal epidermis, metabolism, cardiac muscle contractility and immune system	369
Jnk1/2	Jnk1$^{-/-}$;Jnk2$^{-/-}$		NTD, exencephaly	Died during midgestation with dilated heart, abnormal neural tube development, dysregulated developmental apoptosis and brain abnormalities	370,371
	Jnk1$^{-/+}$;Jnk2$^{-/-}$		25% fetuses display exencephaly	Partial postnatal lethality, abnormal eye, lung, intestine, kidney morphology, abnormal hair follicle development	370,372
	Jnk1$^{-/+}$;Jnk2$^{-/-}$			Developmental defects in the eye	370
Jnk2	Jnk2$^{-/-}$			Partial postnatal lethality	373
				Improved motor function	
Jnk3/Mapk10	Jnk3$^{-/-}$ hippocampal neurons and mice			Resistance to kainic acid—induced seizures and apoptosis	371,373,374
				Improved motor function	
Nhs	Xcat mouse model			Abnormal lens morphology, cataract	375
Ror2	Ror2$^{-/-}$	abnormal middle ear ossicle morphology		Complete neonatal lethality, abnormal embryo size, skeleton and cranium	376,377

II. FUNCTION OF MUTATED GENES IN INTELLECTUAL DISABILITY (ID) AND AUTISM

Gene	Model	Cellular phenotype		Phenotype	References
	Ror2^W749FLAG/W749FLAG			morphology, blood homeostasis, limb, tail, respiratory system morphology, heart development, and limb formation Postnatal model for Robinow syndrome, reduced body mass, skeletal and craniofacial defects, brachydactyly, reduced fertility	378
Scrib1	Mouse/rat hippocampal neurons and slices			↓ βPIX, PAK, GIT, CaMKII; ↑ Rac1-GTP; ↑ c-Fos activity; ↑ ERK1/2 phosphorylation; impaired activity-dependent actin polymerization; ↑ synaptic pruning; altered basal neuronal morphology; ↓ basal synaptic transmission; ↓ impaired LTP, NMDA trafficking	71,108,159,224
	Scrib1^crc/+ mice			Enhanced learning and memory; impaired social behavior	70,379
	Crc/Crc	Misorientation of hair bundles in cochlear outer hair cells, defects in stereociliary polarization	NTD, CR		15,67,69
Sec24	Sec24bY613 mutants	Smaller cochlea and deficits in orientation of both outer and inner hair cells	Open TD, CR	Complete lethality, deficits in convergent extension, failure of eyelid fusion and abnormal size, abnormal arrangement of outflow tract vessels	255,256
Smurf2	Smurf1^−/−;Smurf2^−/− mice			Convergent extension defects, gastrulation defects	259
	Smurf1^−/−;Smurf2^+/− or Smurf1^+/−;Smurf2^−/− mice	Misorientation and disorganization of sensory hair cells	NTD25% NTD, exencephaly, SB	Looped tail	
Wnt2	Wnt2b cKO mice			Decreased size of olfactory bulb	380
Wnt4	Wnt4^−/− mice			Died after birth, impaired development of kidney, pituitary gland, and female reproductive system	381
Wnt5a	Wnt5a^−/− mice	Reduced outgrowth of external ear		Mutants die perinatally, exhibit caudal truncation with shortened anterior –posterior axis, truncation of the snout, tongue and mandible, short limbs, which lack digits, absent genital tubercle and lung abnormalities	382
Wnt11	Wnt11^−/− mice	Complete neonatal lethality, smaller kidneys, defect in ureteric branching			256,383

NTD, neural tube defect; CR, craniorachischisis; SB, spina bifida.

II. FUNCTION OF MUTATED GENES IN INTELLECTUAL DISABILITY (ID) AND AUTISM

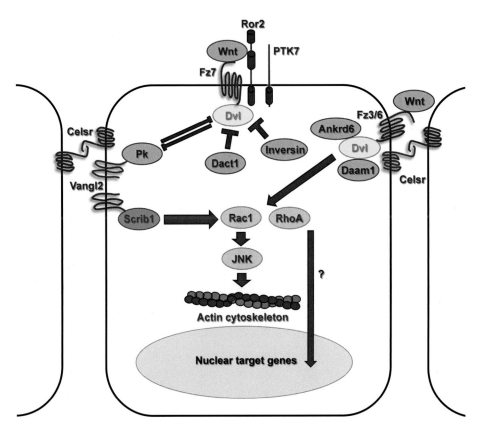

FIGURE 1　**Schematic representation of core PCP signaling (also called Wnt noncanonical PCP pathway).** Description of the main proteins of the signaling pathway is provided in the text. Core PCP proteins are composed of six proteins including three transmembrane proteins called Vangl, Frizzled (Fz), and Celsr, and three cytosolic proteins called Prickle (Pk), Dishevelled (Dvl), and Diego/Ankrd6. These proteins are modulated or associated with protein partners that ultimately lead to cytoskeletal rearrangements. To date, no regulation of transcriptional target in mammals has been evidenced after activation of the core PCP signaling. Arrows indicate activation; blunted arrows indicate inhibition.

by its recruitment to the plasma membrane. The receptor tyrosine kinase Ror2 can associate with Fz7 and Vangl2 and act as a coreceptor for Wnt5a to mediate PCP signaling (Figure 1).[26,27] As originally described in *Drosophila* and *Xenopus* animal models, Dvl regulates multiple aspects of cytoskeleton rearrangements, thereby controlling cell movements and polarity pathways.[28,29] Planar cell polarity signaling is also regulated in mammals through this scaffold protein at multiple levels.[30,31] For instance, Dvl signals through Daam1 and RhoA but also through Rac1 to activate JNK. The cytoplasmic tail of Vang recruits Prickle to plasma membrane, where it binds to Dvl and antagonizes Dvl recruitment by Fz, whereas Diego competes with Pk for Dvl binding.[32–34] Other core regulators of PCP include atypical cadherins Celsr1/3.[35] Beside the core PCP genes, various groups reported that additional PCP-associated genes had similar PCP roles in mammals. Among these genes, *Dlg*, *Scrib1*, and *Dact1* are particularly relevant to this chapter. Scrib was originally characterized as a tumor suppressor in *Drosophila* that forms a polarity complex with Dlg and Lgl[36] and

investigations from our laboratory have led to its identification as a cytosolic partner of Vangl2 critical for PCP establishment.[15,16] Dact1 (also called Dapper/Frodo) was identified as a Dvl-interacting protein regulator of Wnt canonical signaling[37,38] but also PCP through genetic and biochemical interaction with Vangl2.[39] It also negatively regulates Dvl by promoting its degradation through autophagy machinery.[40–42] Importantly, DACT1 mutations in human have been found in NTDs.[43]

The Fat-Dachsous Module (Integrating PCP and Hippo Signaling Pathways)

Establishment of cell and tissue polarity in *Drosophila* is also driven by a second module of proteins including the atypical cadherins Fat (Ft) and Dachsous (Ds) and the Golgi-resident Four-jointed protein (Fj) (Figure 2). Fat and Ds are able to form opposite heterodimers at neighboring cell membranes, whereas the Fj kinase controls their graded expression and is ultimately

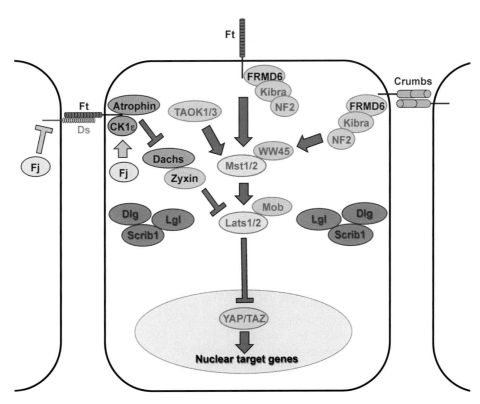

FIGURE 2 **Schematic representation of Fat-Dachsous module (integrating PCP and Hippo signaling pathways).** Description of the main proteins of the signaling pathway is provided in the text. Fat (Ft) controls PCP signaling by recruiting atrophin and CK1 but molecular mechanisms up-/downstream remain unclear (probably owing to the large molecular size of these proteins, which are difficult to handle at the molecular biology/biochemical level). In parallel, Ft also regulate the core Hippo signaling proteins (highlighted in green), either through Dachs or the FRMD6/Kibra/NF2 complex. YAP and TAZ are regulators triggering the transcription of nuclear target genes promoting cell proliferation and inhibiting apoptosis. Arrows indicate activation; blunted arrows indicate inhibition.

responsible for the downstream polarization of Dachs, an atypical myosin. Polarization of Dachs is critical for orientation of cell division and tissue elongation.[44] Dachsous binds to Fat directly and negatively regulates its activity.[45] Fat regulates PCP at least in part by binding the transcriptional corepressor Atrophin[46] and CK1.[47] The functional relationship of this group to the core PCP group remains an open question. It has long been suggested that the Fat/Ds signaling cassette acts in parallel or upstream of the core PCP module and reinforces correct PCP establishment through their independent parallel inputs, but evidence shows that the core PCP module, through Prickle, may also affect Fat/Ds-induced polarization.[48,49] Importantly, this pathway is conserved in vertebrates, with four Fat orthologs (Fat1−4) and two Ds orthologs (Dchs1−2). It controls tissue organization, growth, and polarization[50,51] in various tissues, including the brain.[52] The cytoplasmic tail of Fat appears to intersect not only with the core PCP signaling but also with tissue growth through the Hippo pathway.[53,54] Hippo signaling is a conserved pathway that controls organ size by regulating cell proliferation and apoptosis,[55] and contributes to cancer

development when mutated.[56] The core Hippo pathway was also originally described using genetic studies in the *Drosophila* model. It is composed of a kinase cascade in which Mst1/2 (ortholog of *Drosophila* Hpo) kinases and WW45 (Sav in *Drosophila*) form a complex to phosphorylate and activate Lats1/2 (ortholog of *Drosophila* Wts) (Figure 2). In turn, the transcription co-activators YAP and TAZ, two major downstream effectors of the Hippo pathway, are phosphorylated by Lats1/2, sequestered in the cytoplasm, and eventually degraded through the ubiquitin/proteasome system. In the absence of YAP/TAZ phosphorylation, these proteins translocate into the nucleus and interact with TEAD1-4 (ortholog of *Drosophila* Sd) and other transcription factors to induce expression of genes that promote cell proliferation and inhibit apoptosis.[57] The exact nature of extracellular signals and membrane receptors regulating the Hippo pathway remains elusive. During cell contact inhibition, Fat has appeared as a potential interesting candidate. Through Dachs inhibition, Fat may have an inhibitory effect on YAP/TAZ functions by relieving Lats1/2 degradation induced by Zyxin (Figure 2).[58] Mst1/2 and Lats1/2 are activated at multiple levels including upstream molecules such as the complex Frmd6 (ortholog of *Drosophila* Expanded), Kibra and NF2 (ortholog of *Drosophila* Merlin), and Crumbs, which promote membrane association of the kinases, therefore enhancing their potential. Finally, the Hippo pathway may also intersect with PCP signaling through Scrib1, which acts as a scaffold for several Hippo pathway components.[59] Loss of Scrib1 disrupts the inhibitory association of TAZ with the core Hippo kinases Mst and Lats.[60]

PLANAR CELL POLARITY AND THE BRAIN

All core PCP gene orthologs are expressed during brain development in mouse[61,62] and even in adult. However, specific profiles of expression of PCP proteins during development or in adult tissue (e.g., cortex, hippocampus, cerebellum) are almost nonexistent.[63] The importance of PCP signaling in brain morphogenesis and connectivity is attested to by one of the major phenotypes common to all core PCP genes mutants, craniorachischisis, which is the most severe form of NTDs (Table 1).[64,65] Craniorachischisis is a congenital malformation of the nervous system that affects 1/1000 children in human, and whose molecular bases are still poorly known (see subsequent discussion).

Initial observations of this phenotype are largely based on an analysis of the brain of various spontaneous mouse mutants for PCP genes, including the Looptail (Vangl2$^{LP/LP}$ mice mutated for vangl2 on S464N), the Circletail (Scrib1$^{Crc/Crc}$ animals mutated for scribble, truncation of the protein after PDZ2), and the Crasher mice (Celsr1$^{Crsh/Crsh}$, animals mutated for the protocadherin Celsr1).[66] At birth, the structures of the brain of these mutants are always severely damaged with, typically, a large mass of forebrain tissue present at the anterior surface of the brain, and a global reduction in the size of the brain, including the hippocampus and also of the layers of the neocortex (when sufficiently preserved).[67−71] To date, the severity of the phenotypes (and early lethality) have prevented clear and thorough analysis of the specific role of PCP genes in the development of the brain, let alone the eventual impact on later cognitive functions, but they suggest disruption of pivotal developmental mechanisms such as cell division and migration. There is a plethora of studies demonstrating the role of PCP molecules in oriented cell division in invertebrates, vertebrates, and mammals, notably in the orientation and regulation of the dynamics of the spindle of division.[72,73] Any cortical dysgenesis observed in a PCP mutant could depend partly on the disruption of such a mechanism.

Regarding migration, PCP signaling has been involved in a vast array of developmental processes controlling tissue organization in vertebrates,[74,75] many of which rely on the control of cell movement or its directionality. On the other hand, studies identifying similar phenotypes in the mammalian central nervous system are scarce. Yet, proper regulation of neuronal migration is crucial to establish the shape of the brain, and the intricate neural architecture of the six-layered mammalian neocortex is one of the best model systems to study embryonic neuronal migration in mammalian brain. The normal layered structure of the tissue depends on the ability of neural stem cells to differentiate into neurons and migrate into the correct cortical layers. In human, mutations in genes controlling these processes have severe consequences for cortical development, leading to intractable epilepsy, mental retardation, schizophrenia, dyslexia, and autism.[76−80]

Proteins of the Fat family (Fat1−4) are good candidates to control neuronal migration in the neocortex, as well as members of the Celsr family (Celsr1−3). These two families are composed of large and atypical cadherins, with long extracellular domains allowing homophilic interactions in trans (between cells), for cell adhesion and/or cell communication. On the one hand, analysis of the murine neocortex of full knockout (KO) mutants for Fat4 failed to reveal a strong migratory phenotype, but downregulation of the proteins via small hairpin ribonucleic acid (shRNA) supports a role for the protein in this process.[52] On the other hand, mutation of Celsr3 affects tangential and radial interneuron migration in the mouse forebrain.[35] Connectivity of the brain, including axonal extension and guidance, is the second important developmental process that is affected by PCP gene mutations. The impact on dendritic development is addressed later in this chapter, but links between axonal guidance and PCP signaling are now firmly established, with different specificity among genes. Regarding axonal guidance in mammals, the clearest examples are members of the Celsr family (flamingo or starry-night in invertebrates), and most notably, Celsr3. Celsr3 is a major player in axonal guidance, via homophilic as well as heterophilic interactions. Celsr3 mutant mice have defects in several major axonal tracts, including commissural spinal cord axons, thalamocortical, corticofugal, and subcerebral axons, and the development of some commissures is defective.[81] The other core PCP gene whose mutation leads to a similar and clear guidance phenotype is Frizzled 3, one member of the Frizzled family.[81,82] Both Celsr3 and Fz3 mutants have nearly identical phenotypes, which suggests that these proteins function together in a common axon guidance mechanism. Of note, the Hippo pathway could also be involved. Nf2 and Yap have emerged as regulators of callosal axonal navigation.[83]

For all of other PCP genes, we know little in mammals and even for the few about we know, the molecular bases still have to be clearly deciphered.

PLANAR CELL POLARITY SIGNALING, DENDRITIC DEVELOPMENT, SYNAPTOGENESIS, AND SYNAPTIC PLASTICITY

In addition to their role in axonal guidance, PCP proteins have been shown to modulate dendritic extension and branching. Neurons elaborate complex dendritic arbors with primary, secondary, tertiary, and more branches in a highly specific manner, and their proper arborization are crucial for neuronal function, neuronal networks, and subsequent neuronal communication. Indeed, abnormal dendritic development correlates with autism, IDs, and other developmental disorders.[84,85] In *Drosophila*, the large atypical cadherin Flamingo/Celsr is required to control the extension and/or guidance of dendrites of multiple types of neurons during neural development, something later confirmed in cultures using RNA interference and in conditional KO mouse brain.[86–89] Wnt proteins and their receptors, the Frizzled receptors, have also been involved in this process. Wnt2, Wnt5a, and Wnt7a promote dendrite arborization in the hippocampus.[90–92] However, Wnt5a seems to have no effect on growth in cell cortical culture and it has an inhibitory effect in the absence of Ryk, which suggests that Ryk may act to repress Wnt5a/Frizzled-mediated growth inhibition in these cortical neurons.[93] Ror2 interacts with Frizzled[94] and the knockdown of Ror1 or Ror2 in culture decreased branching and length of neurites.[95] Vangl2, which can also interact with the Frizzled receptors in *cis*[16] also affects dendritic branching and complexity. Using knockdown of Vangl2 in culture, Ohtsuka and collaborators showed that loss of Vangl2 decreased the development of dendrites.[96] Interestingly, a previous study using *Dishevelled-1* mutant mice showed that the loss of Dishevelled-1 results in poor dendritic development.[90] This was also the case in Dact1, Fjx1, and Prickle2 mutants.[97–99] Using the *circletail* mutant mouse (Scrib1[crc]), which expresses a spontaneous truncation of Scrib1 after its second PDZ domain,[100] we showed that Scrib1 participates in the proper maturation of the dendritic tree of CA1 pyramidal cells. Homozygote Scrib1[crc/crc] mice die at birth, whereas heterozygote Scrib1[crc/+] mice have a 50% ubiquitous reduction in the level of the full-length Scrib1.[71] In Scrib1[crc/+] mice, CA1 hippocampal neurons have the characteristic morphology of CA1 pyramidal neurons with an apical dendrite and three to five basal dendrites. However, we showed that Scrib1[crc] mutation leads to an overgrowth of the basal dendritic arborization whereas apical dendrites have normal length but increased intersections/branching only in their distal portion.[71] Only half of the full-length Scrib1 is present with a truncated form of Scrib1, which might have a dominant negative role in mutants. Thus, it will be necessary to check in a full KO model whether the phenotype is conserved. Nevertheless, all of these are consistent with a role of PCP proteins in controlling the dynamics of the cytoskeleton in various tissues and species.

Coordination between the presynaptic and the postsynaptic sites and synaptogenesis are the last step in establishing neuronal connectivity. At excitatory synapses, the head of a dendritic spine is a characterized structure as opposed to the axonal presynaptic bouton. A strong relationship exists between the structure and function of these spines, which are definitively associated with a broad variety of psychiatric and neurologic disorders.[101,102] We have shown that Scrib1 is also implicated in synaptogenesis. Indeed, the number of spines is reduced in CA1 pyramidal cells of Scrib1[crc/+] mice, but the remaining ones are larger, on average.[71] These observations were recapitulated in vitro by manipulating Scrib1 levels in hippocampal neurons. Our electrophysiological analysis in hippocampal slices also revealed weakened synaptic strength and defects in synaptic plasticity in Scrib1[crc/+] hippocampal neurons. Dvl1 mutant mice also exhibit significant deficits in spine number.[103] To date, the role of the different Celsr or Fzd expressed in CA1 neurons or the role of Vangl2 upstream of Scrib1 on synaptic components is unclear. Using, Foxg1[cre]-Celsr3 and Dlx[cre]-Celsr3 mutants, Zhou and collaborators showed that the density of dendritic spines also significantly decreased and that LTP was affected in both mutants.[104] Many Fzd receptors are expressed in hippocampal neurons. Knockdown of Fzd5 has been shown to block the ability of Wnt7a to stimulate synaptogenesis.[105] Yoshioka et al. showed that Vangl1 and Vangl2 were expressed in adult rat neurons, where they are tightly associated with the postsynaptic density (PSD) fraction.[106] Using Golgi's method in Vangl2 *looptail* mice or shRNA in culture, it was shown that dendritic spine density was decreased in the absence of Vangl2.[96,107] Prickle2, another postsynaptic core PCP component, inhibits an N-cadherin—Vangl2 interaction that is required for normal spine formation.[107] This study confirmed the role of Prickle2 in neuronal function described by Bassuk and collaborators, who showed that Prickle2[−/−] dendrites have fewer spines and that the loss of Prickle2 alters the PSD and decreases basal synaptic activity.[99] We also found that in the Scrib1[crc/+], the composition of PSD was altered.[71] This phenotype was associated with mislocalization of the Rac signaling pathway downstream of Scrib1. Interestingly, GluN2A and GluA1 were less abundant in the PSD of Scrib1$^{crc/+}$ compared with wild-type mice (Piguel, Moreau and Sans, unpublished). These defects were linked to postsynaptic deficits that are consistent with Scrib1 regulating glutamate receptor trafficking.[108] The non-canonical tyrosine kinase-like orphan receptor Ror2, which is a co-receptor for Wnt5a, also regulates synaptic NMDAR-mediated currents.[109] Ror2 has been shown to activate the noncanonical signaling pathway, involving Dvl and JNK/c-Jun (AP-1), which are essential for cell polarity and migration,[110] and to inhibit the β-catenin–dependent signaling pathway.[111] Other PCP proteins are found at synapses, although their role is not clearly defined.[95,112] Thus, PCP signaling is involved in the regulation of glutamate receptors, which are the key components of glutamatergic synapses involved in modulating synaptic transmission, synaptic plasticity, and more integrated brain function.

Finally, the cortical and hippocampal networks participate in cognitive and emotional processes, among other. Wynshaw-Boris and collaborators were the first to show that Dvl KO mice had behavioral impairments. In 1997, they showed that Dvl1-deficient mice exhibited reduced social interactions and deficit in sensorimotor gating[113] but no defect in social memory task.[114] In 2010, we showed that Scrib1-deficient mice exhibit enhanced learning and memory abilities and impaired social behavior, two features relevant to ASD. After these studies, other behavioral tests showed that Foxg1^{cre}-Celsr3 and Dlx^{cre}-Celsr3 mutants were hyperactive and were impaired in the Morris water maze.[104] Abnormal behavior was also found in Prickle2 KO mice, including altered social interaction, learning abnormalities, and behavioral inflexibility.[99] All of these studies and others point to an important role for PCP proteins and signaling in hippocampal maturation, connectivity, and function.

PLANAR CELL POLARITY SIGNALING AND HUMAN GENETICS

Deletions and mutations in PCP genes have been linked, directly or indirectly, to neurodevelopmental pathologies affecting many body systems. The main neurodevelopmental pathology involving PCP genes is probably NTD, in which neural tube closure is compromised, but PCP signaling defects also affect sensory systems (hearing, balance, and vision), skeletal development, tissue homeostasis (polycystic kidney disease), the lungs or reproductive system, and even the cardiovascular system.[64,115–120] More will probably be identified, but in the past 2 decades, an increasing amount of studies have linked PCP proteins to developmental delay, IDs, or ASD and related deletion syndromes, which we review here.

Core PCP Mutations Associated with ASD/IDs

The FRIZZLED/WNT cassette

The Frizzled receptors (Fzd) seven transmembrane proteins with an extracellular N-terminal domain containing a highly conserved cysteine-rich domain and a variable-length C-terminal tail. Originally, Fzd6 was shown to control hair patterning in mammals.[121] Later, Fzd3 and Fzd6 were shown to be involved in axonal growth during development.[122,123] In 2006, Nathans and collaborators found using double KO that Fzd3/6 were also involved in PCP signaling in neural tube closure as well as in the cochlea, and that they were partially interchangeable.[124,125] Interestingly, Fzd1, Fzd2, and Fzd7 have also been involved in convergent extension and closure and are highly redundant.[126,127] These receptors clearly have independent functions in the canonical and noncanonical PCP pathway. So has Fzd4, which can activate both the canonical Wnt signaling pathway and the noncanonical Rho pathway.[128,129]

The *FZD3* gene is positioned in chromosomic region *8p* [*8p21.1*], which is a potential hub for developmental neuropsychiatric disorders such as schizophrenia and autism.[130] FZD3 stands for Frizzled class receptor 3 (FZD3), also known as Frizzled Family Receptor 3 or Fz3 (666 aa; 76 kDa). Fzd3 interacts with Vangl2 and regulates PCP in the cochlea.[16] Single nucleotide mutations in the *FZD3* gene showed strong correlations with schizophrenia in the Japanese[131] and Chinese populations.[132–134] Numerous rearrangements in 8p have been associated with mild autism or IDs. A 6-year-old girl with partial trisomy 8p(21–23) with autism associated with mild dysmorphic features and moderate learning disability was reported by Papanikolaou et al. in 2006.[135] Several *8p23.1-p11.1* duplications encompassing the *FDZ3* gene have been found in patients with agenesis of the corpus callosum, developmental delay, and IDs.[136] So far, no specific mutations in *FZD3* have been associated with ASD or IDs, but we found in the Decipher database (https://decipher.sanger.ac.uk) an individual with obesity and delayed speech and language development, with a 0.18-megabase (Mb) gain encompassing *FZD3* and *EXTL3* genes (ID 279,976).

The *FZD4* gene is located on chromosome 11 [*11q14.2-q21*]. FZD4 stands for Frizzled class receptor 4 (FZD4), also known as Fz4; EVR1; FEVR; Fz-4; FzE4; GPCR; hFz4; CD344; FZD4S, a member of the frizzled gene family. FDZ4 is a seven-transmembrane domain receptor (537 aa; 59 kDa) with a cysteine-rich domain (CRD) in the N-terminal extracellular region able to bind Wnt protein, two cysteine residues in the second and third extracellular loops, two extracellular N-linked glycosylation sites, and a C-terminal PDZ-binding motif. In 2002, *FZD4* was found to be associated with familial exudative vitreoretinopathy (EVR), which is a hereditary ocular disorder characterized by a failure of peripheral retinal vascularization.[137] Using high-density whole-genome oligonucleotide array comparative genomic hybridization, Pober and collaborators defined a 35-Mb interstitial deletion of 11q14.1-q23.2 containing the FZD4 gene and a 1-Mb deletion of 16q22.3-q23.1 in an EVR patient with multiple abnormalities including growth retardation, facial anomalies, cleft palate, and minor digital anomalies.[138] They also analyzed different patients and found that deletions of the FZD4 gene located within the telomeric segment account for dysmorphic craniofacial features, growth and mental retardation, and mild digital anomalies.[138] Several mutations on the FZD4 gene are known to cause inherited as well as sporadic FEVR, and some can be accompanied by IDs.[139]

The **FZD5 gene** is located on chromosome 2 [*2q33.3-q34*]. FZD5 stands for Frizzled class receptor 5 (FZD5), also known as Fz5; C2orf31, fz-5, Frizzled 5, fzE5, Frizzled Family Receptor 5, seven-transmembrane receptor Frizzled-5, Chromosome 2 Open Reading Frame 31, HFZ5, hFz53, a member of the frizzled gene family. FDZ5 is a seven-transmembrane domain receptor (585 aa; 64 kDa) with a cysteine-rich domain (CRD) in the N-terminal extracellular region and a C-terminal intracellular region. The noncanonical Wnt5A is able to bind the human FZD5 receptor, which is an important paralog of FZD3.[140] In 2014, Butler and collaborators reported a 42-year-old man with developmental defects and a large *2q33.1-q34* deletion that contains, among others, the FZD5 gene.[141] A similar deletion in *2q33.3-q34* was previously found in an autistic male with dysmorphic features.[142]

The **FRZ9 gene** (initially called FZD3) is located on chromosome 7 [*7q11.23*]. FZD9 stands for Frizzled class receptor 9 (FZD9), also known as Frizzled (*Drosophila*) homolog 9, seven-transmembrane spanning receptor 9, Frizzled homolog 9 (*Drosophila*), and is a member of the frizzled gene family. FDZ9 is a seven-transmembrane domain receptor (591 aa; 64 kDa) with a cysteine-rich domain (CRD) in the N-terminal extracellular region and a C-terminal PDZ-binding motif. FDZ9 has not been directly implicated in the PCP pathway, but activation of FZD9 inhibits the β-catenin pathway and regulates osteoblast function via noncanonical Wnt-signaling pathways.[143] Indeed, FZD3 is an important paralog of FZD9. The FZD9 gene has been associated with Williams syndrome because it is located within the Williams syndrome common deletion region of chromosome 7.[144,145] Children affected by this syndrome have similar characteristic facial features and most have cardiovascular problems, developmental delay, learning disabilities,

and attention deficit disorder.[146] This region is also involved in 7q11.23 duplication syndrome and the patient affected often have IDs associated or not with delayed speech and language development, hearing impairment, and macroencephaly or microcephaly (Decipher database).

The WNT proteins are the main ligand of the FZD receptors, but a clear link between a specific WNT and specific receptors involved in PCP has not yet been identified. Three major WNTs are considered to be non-canonical WNT ligands: WNT4, WNT5A, and WNT11. WNT2 will be also considered here as a known ligand of FZD2 or FZD9.

The **WNT2 gene** is localized on chromosome 7 [*7q31.2*]. WNT2 stands for wingless-type MMTV integration site family, member 2 (WNT2), also known as INT1L1, Int-1-Related Protein, Secreted Growth Factor-1 is a secreted protein that controls essential developmental processes. WNT2 encodes secreted cysteine-rich putative glycoproteins (360 aa; 40 kDa) that have been involved in cell polarity. The *7q31-q33* region has been linked to autism and was found to be adjacent to a chromosomal breakpoint in an individual with autism region.[147] Sheffield and collaborators were among the first to hypothesize that rare mutations occurring in the WNT2 gene increased susceptibility to autism.[148] In 2010, Kato and collaborators also showed a significant association between WNT2 and autism in a Japanese population.[149] Moreover, a haplotype of WNT2 was significantly associated with ASDs in the Han Chinese population.[150] In 2012, Chiu and collaborators detected an interaction between the WNT2 gene and language development in autistic disorder.[151]

The **WNT2B gene** is localized on chromosome 1 [*1p13.2*]. WNT2B stands for wingless-type MMTV integration site family, member 2B (WNT2B) and is a secreted protein that controls essential developmental processes. WNT2B encodes cysteine-rich putative glyco-proteins (391 aa; 43 kDa) that have been involved in brain, lung, and kidney development. In 2007, using high-resolution comparative genomic hybridization, Bryndorf and collaborators described a girl with severe mental retardation, short stature, and dysmorphic features with an interstitial deletion with breakpoints in band 1p13.1 and 1p21.1 encompassing the WNT2B and NTNG1 genes.[152]

The **WNT5A gene** is located on chromosome 3 [*3p14.3*]. WNT5A stands for wingless-type MMTV integration site family, member 5A (WNT5A), also known as −5A protein, hWNT5A, or protein −5a. WNT5A encodes a cysteine-rich putative glycoprotein (380 aa; 42 kDa), which has typical features of secreted factors with a hydrophobic signal sequence and 21 conserved cysteine residues on which relative spacing is maintained. Missense mutations in the WNT5A gene

II. FUNCTION OF MUTATED GENES IN INTELLECTUAL DISABILITY (ID) AND AUTISM

have been associated with autosomal-dominant Robinow syndrome.[153,154] Up to 20% of patients with Robinow syndrome may have some IDs; their medical conditions often include hearing loss and developmental problems.[155,156] WNT5A interacts with Ror2, which is also involved in Robinow syndrome.[157,158]

The *WNT11* gene is located on chromosome 11 [*11q13.5*]. WNT11 stands for wingless-type MMTV integration site family, member 11 (WNT11), also known as HWNT11 or protein Wnt-11. *WNT11* encodes a cysteine-rich putative glycoprotein (354 aa; 39 kDa) that has been implicated in rare cases of ASD, although this is not yet confirmed.[159]

Van Gogh-Like Genes: VANGL1 *and* VANGL2

The Van Gogh-like 1 and 2 proteins (Vangl) are tetraspanin proteins with intracellular N- and C-terminal domains and a C-terminal PDZ binding domain.[160] Severe NTD in unborn humans has been linked to a mutation in *VANGL2*.[161,162] Importantly, these studies conclude that severe effects of these gene mutations during in utero development probably are incompatible with life and would explain why, to date, no mutation in the *VANGL* genes have been associated with ASD or ID.

The *VANGL1* gene is positioned in the chromosomic region *1p* [*1p13.1-p21*]. VANGL1 stands for Van Gogh-like 1 (VANGL1), a 524 aa tetraspanin protein, with intracellular N- and C-terminal domains[163] involved in general polarity establishment. Mutations of *VANGL1* cause NTD in humans.[164,165] *VANGL1* is also involved in cancer development.[166–168] *1p13.2, 1p13.3* duplications were found to be associated with ASD and the copy number variant (CNV) of interest was later confirmed by an independent method,[159,169] whereas *1p13.2 and 1p13.3* deletion-duplications were found in a family affected by sporadic ASD from the Simons Simplex Collection.[159,170]

The *VANGL2* gene is positioned in the chromosomic region 1q22 [*1q22-q23*]. Van Gogh-like 2 (Vangl2) is a 521 aa tetraspanin protein, with intracellular N- and C-terminal domains,[160] involved in general planar polarity establishment.[15,16] Mutations in *VANGL2* cause NTD in humans[161,162,165,171] and are also involved in cancer development.[172] 1q22 microduplications, encompassing the *VANGL2* gene among others, were found in the Decipher database in individuals with microcephaly, IDs, delayed speech and language development, stereotypic behavior, strabismus, and scoliosis.

DISHEVELLED

Dishevelled 1, 2, and 3 (Dvl1, Dvl2, and Dvl3) also function as key players in Wnt/PCP signaling.[30]

Alignment of family members reveals three conserved domains: a DIX (DishevelledAxin) domain; a PDZ (PSD95-Discs Large-ZO1) domain, which recognizes and binds short motifs at the C-termini of proteins, but may bind other motifs as well; and a DEP (DishevelledEGL10-Pleckstrin) domain, which is conserved among a set of proteins that have in common the ability to regulate various GTPases, including both heterotrimeric G-proteins and Ras-like small GTPases. DishevelledEGL10-Pleckstrin and PDZ domains are involved in PCP signaling. A mutation in the DEP domain impairs both membrane localization and the function of Dsh in PCP signaling, which indicates that translocation is important for function. The first report correlating autism-like features and failure in DVL1 function in PCP establishment was provided by Wynsham-Boris and collaborators, who described abnormal social behavior and sensorimotor gating deficits in mice lacking *Dvl1*.[113] Subsequent studies revealed that disruption of *Dvl* genes can be implicated in several developmental defects.[31]

The *DVL1* gene is localized on chromosome 1 [*1p36.33*]. DVL1 stands for DISHEVELLED 1 (Homologous to *Drosophila* Dsh) (DVL-1), also called segment polarity protein Dishevelled homolog 1 (DSH Homolog 1), which is a cytoplasmic phosphoprotein (695 aa; 75 kDa). The 1p36 deletion is a common terminal deletion syndrome with variable breakpoints from bands 1p36.13 to 1p36.33.[173] The clinical features consist of craniofacial dysmorphism, moderate to severe IDs, delayed growth, hypotonia, seizures, limited speech ability, malformations, hearing deficits, vision impairment, and distinct facial features. The symptoms may vary, depending on the exact location of the deletion. In a study on CNVs, a 1p36 microdeletion was overrepresented in ID cases.[174] De novo frameshift mutations in *DVL1* were also found in several unrelated individuals with Robinow syndrome.[175,176]

The *DVL2* gene is localized on chromosome 17 [*17p13.1*]. DVL2 stands for DISHEVELLED 2 (Homologous to *Drosophila* Dsh) DVL-2, also called segment polarity protein Dishevelled homolog 2 or DSH Homolog 2, which is a cytoplasmic phosphoprotein (736 aa; 79 kDa). DVL2 has been involved in alk-positive anaplastic large cell lymphoma via signaling in the Wnt noncanonical pathways.[177] Several deletions in this region have been described, including a microdeletion in the distal portion of 17p13.1 encompassing *DVL2* in patients with characteristic dysmorphic features, developmental delay, and IDs.[178] Vitkup and collaborators used a network-based functional analysis of rare genetic variants and found *DVL2* among the genes affected by rare de novo CNVs in autism.[179]

The Orthologs of Diego: Ankyrin Repeat Domain 6 (ANKRD6) and INVERSIN

The *ANKRD6* gene is positioned in chromosomic region *6q* [*6q15*]. ANKRD6 stands for Ankyrin Repeat Domain-Containing Protein 6 (ANKRD6) (727 aa; 80 kDa), also known as Diversin or KIAA0957, which is a cytoplasmic ankyrin repeat domain-containing protein with eight N-terminal ankyrin repeats, a central domain, and a C-terminal domain, and which has been found to be a predisposing factor to NTD.[180] Ankrd6 is a core PCP component that interacts with Dvl1 and regulates PCP in the cochlea.[181] 6q15 microduplications, encompassing the *ANKRD6* gene among others, were found in the Decipher database in individuals presenting cognitive impairment (Decipher ID244600), ASD with IDs (Decipher ID251748) or ASD, and delayed speech and language development (Decipher ID4090).

The *INVS* gene is positioned in chromosomic region *9q* [*9q31.1*]. INVS stands for Inversin 1 (INV1) (1065 aa; 118 kDa), also known as Nephrocystin 2, NPHP2, Nephronophthisis 2 (Infantile), INV2, Inversion of Embryo Turning Homolog 2, nephrocystin-2, and NPH2. Invs is a cytoplasmic ankyrin repeat domain-containing protein with two IQ calmodulin-binding domains that can interact with N-cadherin.[182] Inv1 is involved in renal tubular development and function, and in left–right axis determination. Mutations of INVS have been associated with nephronophthisis type 2, a renal disease with extrarenal manifestations including developmental delay and situs inversus[183] in relation to PCP signaling.[184]

PRICKLE homolog: PRICKLE1 and PRICKLE2

The *PRICKLE1* gene is located on chromosome 12 [*12q12*]. PRICKLE1 stands for the homologue of *Drosophila* PRICKLE LIKE1 (PRICKLE1) also named PK1, or REST-INTERACTING LIM DOMAIN PROTEIN (RILP). Prickle1 is an intracellular protein (831 aa; 94 kDa) composed of three N-terminal LIM domains and three C-terminal nuclear localization signals.[185] Prickle1 is required in the PCP pathway that controls convergent extension during gastrulation and neural tube closure and is a potential negative regulator of the WNT/β-catenin signaling pathway.[186] *PRICKLE1* is involved in epilepsy and NTDs.[187–190] Using whole-exome sequencing on 100 ASD individuals from 40 families, two heterozygous and damaging SNVs in *cis* within the *PRICKLE1* gene were reported.[191] In parallel, using a family approach, Bassuk and collaborators recognized *PRICKLE1* as an ASD gene through extensive in vivo and in vitro functional analysis.[192] Geschwind and collaborators used a totally different approach consisting of analyzing transcriptome organization between autistic and normal brain by gene coexpression network analysis and reported significant PRICKLE1 expression differences between frontal and temporal cortex in control and autism samples.[193]

The *PRICKLE2* gene is located on chromosome 3 [*3p14.1*]. PRICKLE2 stands for the homologue of *Drosophila* PRICKLE-LIKE 2 (PRICKLE2), also named PK2 or EPM5. Prickle2 is an intracellular protein (844 aa; 95 kDa) composed of an N-terminal PET domain followed by three LIM domains and a C-terminal prickle homology domain.[185] Prickle2 has been involved in PCP in the vestibular system[194] and is localized to the PSD, where it interacts with PSD-95 and NMDAR.[195] Mutations in PRICKLE2 may underlie the pathogenesis of human spina bifida[196] and also epilepsy and autism. Bassuk and collaborators identified two distinct heterozygous *PRICKLE2* variants (p.E8Q and p.V153I) that were shared by ASD affected siblings and inherited paternally.[99] Notably, *Prickle2* KO mice have social deficits and enhanced spatial memory similar to what we reported for $Scrib1^{crc/+}$ mice.[71,99]

Planar Cell Polarity Effector Genes Mutated in ASD/IDs

In addition to the conserved set of six main core PCP genes originally identified in *Drosophila*, several associated and effector proteins have been identified in the past 15 years. Among these associated/effector families, we can find Daam1, Dact, Diaphanous, NHS, PTK7, Ror1/2, and Scrib1, as shown in Figure 1. From those, only *SCRIB* and *DACT1* have been associated with weaker forms of NTD.[43,197] It was shown that mutations in *SCRIB1* may underlie the pathogenesis of human spina bifida.[198] In that study, Finnell and collaborators found one novel missense mutation in control (p.A1257T) that was predicted to be benign and not to lead to spina bifida.[198]

DAAM1

The *DAAM1* gene is located on chromosome 14 [*14q23.1*]. DAAM1 stands for Dishevelled-Associated Activator of Morphogenesis 1, also known as KIAA0666, which is a widely expressed protein belonging to the diaphanous-related formin family.[199] Daam1 is a cytoplasmic protein (1078 aa; 123 kDa) that contains an N-terminal GTPase-binding domain (GBD), followed by the diaphanous inhibitory domain (DID), a central proline-rich FH1 domain and a more C-terminal FH2 domain, and a diaphanous autoregulatory domain (DAD) at the C terminus.[200] Daam1 is involved in both actin polymerization and microtubule stabilization, and interacts with Dvl and Rho to regulate PCP.[201] Microdeletions at the breakpoints of 14q21.1 (0.8 Mb), 14q23.1 (0.9 Mb) encompassing the *DAAM1* gene and a 1.3 Mb deletion at 16q23.1 were found in a 4-year-old girl with developmental delay, hypotonia, and dysmorphic features.[202] A de novo 14q23.1–q23.3 microdeletion was also found in a male with spherocytosis, congenital heart defect, cryptorchidism, hypoplasia of corpus callosum, epilepsy, and developmental delay who was diagnosed with a neuroblastoma at age 9 months.[203] In 2013, a 265-kb duplication of *DAAM1* was associated with cerebral palsy.[204] Two-thirds of children who have this motor disorder are mildly to severely intellectually impaired, and the disease is often accompanied by disturbances of sensation, perception, communication, autism, and epilepsy, and by secondary musculoskeletal problems. In the Decipher database, several cases with loss of the *DAAM1* gene are reported with phenotypes including IDs (Decipher ID 299,147 and 265,080).

DACT1

The *DACT1* gene is located on chromosome 14 [*14q23.1*]. DACT1 stands for Dapper, Antagonist of b-Catenin (DACT1), also known as DAPPER1, DPR1, FRODO, HDPR1, or THYEX3, which is a protein interacting with DVL that belongs to the Dapper family.[37,38] Dact1 is a cytoplasmic protein (836 aa; 90 kDa) containing seven Dapper homology domains, including a leucine zipper, a serine-rich region, and a PDZ-binding domain that has a role in the canonical and/or noncanonical Wnt signaling pathways through interaction with Dvl and/or Vangl2.[39] *DACT1* has been associated with craniorachischisis.[43] *DACT1* is positioned close to the *DAAM1* gene and thus is deleted in the Decipher ID 265,080, presenting microcephaly and IDs among other symptoms.

DIAPH3

The *DIAPH3* gene is located on chromosome 13 [*13q21.2*]. DIAPH3 stands for Diaphanous-Related Formin 3 (DIAPH3), also known as Auditory Neuropathy, Autosomal Dominant 1 (AUNA 1), DRF3, or DIA2, which belongs to the diaphanous subfamily of formins.[205] Diaph3 is a cytoplasmic protein (1193 aa; 136 kDa) that contains an N-terminal FMNL-DIAPH1-DAAM1 (FDD) domain, followed by a central proline-rich formin domain (FH1) and a C-terminal formin homology domains (FH2), which contains a putative nuclear localization signal.[205] Diaph3 is related to Daam1 and both are involved in actin remodeling and regulation of cell movement and adhesion. *DIAPH3* was first characterized as a gene responsible for AUNA in a United States family.[206,207] The mutation was situated in the 5′ UTR of the human *DIAPH3* gene and

was responsible for the overexpression of DIAPH3. In 2011, an amino-acid substitution at position 614 of the *DIAPH3* gene (Pro614Thr), and a deletion was found in a normally intelligent 13-year-old patient with ASD and mild dysmorphic features.[208] Several cases of duplication or large deletion have been inventoried in the Decipher database associated with ASD with or without IDs.

NHS

The *NHS* gene is located on chromosome X [*Xp22.13*]. NHS stands for Nance-Horan syndrome protein (NHS), also known as Congenital Cataracts and Dental Anomalies Protein, CTRCT40, CXN, or SCML1, a novel regulator of actin remodeling and cell morphology.[209] Nhs is a putative nuclear protein (1651 aa; 179 kDa) containing four conserved nuclear localization signals that have a role during the development of the eyes, teeth, and brain. Nhsl1b, which is related to the human NHS protein, is an effector of PCP signaling that interacts with Scrib1.[210] *NHS* has been associated with Nance-Horan syndrome, which is a rare X-linked condition composed of congenital cataract with microcornea, distinctive dental, evocative facial anomalies, and IDs.[211]

ROR2

The ***ROR2* gene** is positioned in the chromosomic region 9q [*9q22.31*]. ROR2 stands for the Orphan Receptor Tyrosine Kinase-like Receptor 2 (ROR2), a receptor tyrosine kinase also known as BDB, BDB1, or NTRKR2. Ror2 is a large transmembrane glycoprotein that functions as cell surface receptors with in vitro protein kinase activity.[212] Ror2 is involved in PCP by interacting with Fzd3.[4] *ROR2* is also involved in cancer development.[213] A 7.7 Mb deletion on 9q22.1–q22.32a encompassing the *ROR2* and *PTCH* genes was found in a 12-year-old girl with features of basal cell nevus syndrome, pulmonary valve stenosis, and IDs.[214] Previously, mutations in *ROR2* have been found in autosomal recessive Robinow syndrome or dominantly inherited brachydactyly type 1B.[157,158,215,216]

SCRIB

The ***SCRIB* gene** is localized on chromosome 8 [*8q24.3*]. SCRIB stands for SCRIBBLE 1 (SCRIB1), also called SCRB1, KIAA0147, LAP4, KIAA01473, or VARTUL, and belongs to the LAP family of protein that combines both leucine-rich repeats at their N-terminus and one to four PDZ (PSD-95/Dlg/ZO-1) domains in their structure.[36] Scrib1 is a large cytoplasmic protein (1630 aa; 175 kDa), with leucine-reach repeats at its N-terminus, followed by four PDZ domains and an unstructured C-terminal region that has a role in apical–basal polarity. All these domains are involved in protein—protein interactions, which allow Scrib1 to act as a scaffolding protein, linking membrane proteins to intracellular effectors and to the actin cytoskeleton. In human, SCRIB is the target of the human papillomavirus E6 protein, leading to its ubiquitin-mediated degradation.[217] SCRIB has a role as a tumor suppressor involved in several types of cancer,[218–220] just like DLG and LGL, for which SCRIB forms a complex. Montcouquiol and collaborators were the first to show that Scrib1 was involved in PCP signaling in the inner ear,[15] possibly by interacting through a PDZ-PDZBD with the Vangl2/Fzd3 complex.[16] Scrib1 is also known to regulate the size and the shape of dendritic spines through regulating actin dynamics via binding with actin-regulatory molecules such as β-Pix,[71,221] and we have shown that Scrib1 was involved in the post-endocytic trafficking of NMDA receptor subunits, GluN2A and GluN2B.[108] The 8q24.3 region encompassing the SCRIB gene has been associated with ASDs and ADHD (Stam et al., 2009). This region is also subject to deletion or duplication associated with microcephaly, developmental delay, IDs, short stature, and coloboma, craniofacial, cardiac, and renal defects. In 2013, Katsanis and collaborators reported microdeletions on 8q24.3 containing SCRIB, NRBP2, and PUF60 in children presenting microcephaly, craniofacial features and developmental delay.[222] They also found in zebrafish that the knockdown of either Scrib or Puf60 recapitulated some of the phenotypes including the short stature phenotype, and that the knockdown of Scrib, but not Puf60, resulted in coloboma and gross edema. A de novo 2.3-Mb inverted duplication of 8q24.3 was also reported to lead to severe psychomotor mental retardation, ASDs, idiopathic epilepsy, and growth delay. This region contains several genes including GRINA and SCRIB,[223] which we reported to form a complex crucial for GluN2A recycling.[108] We also noticed that several patients in the Decipher database with specific learning disabilities had variable deletions encompassing these two genes. Although not yet confirmed, a large study designed to identify genes with rare CNVs implicated in ASD identified an autistic patient with a 359-kb deleted region in 8q24.3 encompassing five genes, including SCRIB.[159] Moreover, in 2012, Daly and collaborators reported for the first time a de novo missense mutation in the SCRIB1 gene (c.1774C > T, P592S) associated with ASD.[224] Our own results show that Scrib1[crc/+]-deficient mice exhibit enhanced learning and memory abilities and impaired social behavior, two features relevant to ASDs[71] (Moreau and Sans, unpublished), which suggests that Scrib1[crc/+] mice might be a model for studying synaptic dysfunction and human psychiatric disorders (Moreau et al., in preparation). Interestingly, mutant mice for Dvl1 or Prickle2 also display social behavior deficits.[99,113]

Geschwind and collaborators were the first to report differential-splicing events associated with ASD. They used high-throughput RNA sequencing (RNA-Seq) on three autism samples with significant downregulation of A2BP1 and found SCRIB and GRIN1 among the top predicted A2BP1-dependent differential splicing events, again involving the NMDAR-Scrib1 complex in ASD.[193] More recently, in a large neural microexons study, Blencowe and collaborators found misregulations in the SCRIB gene in the brains of individuals with ASD.[225]

Several mutations have also been found in Scrib1-associated proteins such as NOS1AP, β-PIX, GIT, and PAK.[226,227] Bourgeron and collaborators were the first to report nonsynonymous variations within the human NOS1AP gene.[228] ARHGEF7 (β-PIX) and PAK2 have been found to be mutated in ASD patients[179] whereas PAK3 has been associated with nonsyndromic X-linked mental retardation.[229,230]

Associated Proteins Involved in Trafficking of PCP Genes Mutated in ASD/IDs

DLG

Dlg1 and Dlg3 function as new players in PCP signaling. They belong to the membrane-associated guanylate kinase (MAGUK) family of guanylate cyclase. Dlg4/synapse-associated protein-90 (SAP-90)/postsynaptic density-95 (PSD-95) was initially characterized as one of the main protein of the PSD interacting with NMDAR.[231] Several other members were then identified, including Dlg1/SAP-97/hdlg, Dlg2/Chapsyn-110/PSD-93, and Dlg3/SAP-102.[231] These proteins have three PDZ (for PSD-95, Dlg, and ZO-1/Dlg-homologous region) domains, one Src homology 3 domain, and one guanylate kinase-like domain. DLG was originally defined as a tumor suppressor involved in many cancers, but not all the different mammalian homologs might have this function.[232,233] Membrane-associated guanylate kinases have been implicated in the trafficking of receptors to and/or from synapses and/or the anchoring at synapses (for review, see Horak et al.[231]).

The **DLG1 gene** is localized on chromosome 3 [3q29]. DLG1 stands for Drosophila "discs large" tumor suppressor protein, DLG1, also called DLGH1; Synapse-Associated protein 97 (SAP97); and SAP-97; dJ1061C18.1.1, and is the prototype of the MAGUK family. Dlg1 is a cytoplasmic protein (904 aa; 100 kDa) involved in the trafficking of GluA1 and GluN2A subunits of the glutamate receptors.[234–236] In 2003, a Dlg-Stabismus/Vangl2 complex was also involved in vesicle transport to the plasma membrane both in fly and mammalian cells.[237] Two studies in mice showed that *Dlg1* was involved in convergent extension and PCP defects with no clear output in the cochlea.[238,239] However, Dlg1 is clearly involved in oriented cell division, which is another readout of PCP signaling.[240] Several deletions/duplications in the 3q29 region have been described. In the 3q29 microdeletion syndrome, the deleted region is variable and can lead to mental retardation and/or autism disorders, sometime associated with mildly dysmorphic facial features, epilepsy, cerebral palsy, or schizophrenia.[141,241−245] Some rare de novo variants of *DLG1* have also been found to be associated with autism.[179]

The *DLG3* gene is localized on the *chr X* [*Xq13.1*]. DLG3 stands for Synapse-Associated protein 102 (SAP102) *Drosophila* "discs large" tumor suppressor protein, Dlg3, also called Neuroendocrine DLG; NEDLG, which belongs to the MAGUK family. Dlg3 is a cytoplasmic protein (817 aa; 90 kDa) involved in the trafficking of NMDA receptor subunits, GluN2A and GluN2B.[246−248] Lickert and collaborators were the first to show that Dlg3 is involved in PCP signaling in the inner ear and functions with Flattop to position basal bodies and kinocilia.[249,250] In 2004, Tarpey and collaborators were the first to associate *DLG3/SAP102* with X-linked mental retardation.[251] They uncovered mutations in the *DLG3* gene leading to premature stop codon in the coding sequence, leading to a truncated form of the protein in four of 329 families with moderate to severe X-linked mental retardation. Later, a novel splice site mutation (IVS6-1G > A) was identified in several unrelated male with moderate to severe nonsyndromic mental retardation.[252] Two novel splice donor site mutations (c.357 + 1G > C and c.985 + 1G > C) were identified in the *DLG3* gene in unrelated Finnish families affected by X-linked IDs with substantial impairment in cognitive abilities and social and behavioral adaptive skills.[253] It has been shown that the Xq11.1-q21.33 region encompassing *DLG3* is a plausible candidate region for ASD.[254]

SEC24B

The *SEC24B* gene is positioned in chromosomic region *4q* [*4q25*]. SEC24B stands for the SEC24-Related Gene Family, Member B (SEC24B), a component of the COPII complex involved in protein transport from the endoplasmic reticulum. Sec24B (1268 aa; 137 Da) is involved in Vangl2 trafficking.[255,256] Both of these studies revealed that Sec24b homozygous mutant mice exhibit NTD and PCP-related phenotypes in the cochlea. In human, Wang and collaborators discovered a rare missense heterozygous *SEC24B* mutation in NTD patients.[257] In the Decipher database, we found a female patient with moderate IDs with an internal gain of 0.19 in 4:110,433,182-110,619,509 encompassing three genes including *SEC24B*, *CCDC109B*, and *CASP6* (Decipher ID 282,156). Other patients with a larger gain interval also have a cleft mandible and nonmidline cleft lip or ASD with IDs (Decipher ID 250,733 and 274,373, respectively).

SMURF

The *SMURF2* gene is positioned in chromosomic region 17q [*17q23.3-q24.1*]. SMURF2 stands for SMAD Ubiquitination Regulatory Factor 2 (SMURF2), an E3 ubiquitin ligase also known as SMAD Ubiquitination Regulatory Factor 2 or SMAD-Specific E3 Ubiquitin-Protein Ligase 2, belonging to the C2-WW-HECT class.[258] Smurf2 is a HECT domain E3 ubiquitin ligase (748 aa; 86 kDa) that functions in the PCP signaling pathway and targets the core PCP protein Prickle1 for ubiquitin-mediated degradation.[259] In the Decipher database, we found a male patient with an short attention span and specific learning disability with an internal gain of 0.18 in 17:62,464,706-62,645,411 encompassing seven genes including *SMURF2*, *DDX5*, and *CEP95* (Decipher ID 277,450).

Other Downstream Effectors Mutated in ASD/IDs

ERK *Gene*

Scrib1 has been shown to have a role in modulating MAPK signaling[219] and to interact directly with Erk through two well-conserved kinase interaction motif (KIM) docking sites in its C- and N-terminal domain.[260]

The *MAPK3/ERK1* gene is located on chromosome 16 [16p11.2]. MAPK3/ERK1 stands for Mitogen-Activated Protein Kinase 3 (PRKM3), also known as Extracellular Signal-Regulated Kinase 1 (ERK1), p44ERK1, or p44MAPK, a member of the MAP kinase family (379 amino acids; 43 kDa). *MAPK3/ERK1* has been associated with ASD. A chromosomal duplication/deletion of 16p11.2, which includes the *MAPK3* gene encoding ERK1, was found in ASD patients.[261,262] Rare de novo variants in *MAPK3/ERK1* have been found to be associated with ASD.[179]

The *MAPK1/ERK2* gene is located on chromosome 22 [22q11.21-q11.22]. MAPK1/ERK2 stands for Mitogen-Activated Protein Kinase 1 (PRKM1), also known as Extracellular Signal-Regulated Kinase 2 (Erk2) or p42ERK, a member of the MAP kinase family (360 amino acids; 41 kDa). Microdeletions on chromosome 22, which contains the *MAPK1* gene coding for ERK2, were found in a patient with ASD or DiGeorge syndrome associated with velocardiofacial syndrome.[263−265]

JNK *Gene*

In the PCP signaling pathway, activation of JNK may occur downstream of interactions between core PCP molecules.[266,267] In humans, 10 JNK isoforms have been cloned, four of which are produced by alternative splicing of *JNK1* gene; the others derive from the *JNK2* and *JNK3* genes.

The *MAPK10/JNK3* gene is located on chromosome 4 [4q21.3]. MAPK10/JNK3 stands for Mitogen-Activated Protein Kinase 10 (PRKM10), also known as C_Jun Kinase 3 (JNK3) or Stress-Activated Protein Kinase JNK3, a member of the MAP kinase family (464 amino acids; 52 kDa). The *JNK3* gene has been found to be truncated in two unrelated children with IDs and seizures.[268,269]

Fat/Dachsous and Hippo Pathway Mutations Associated with ASD/IDs

The Fat/Dachsous signaling cascade is involved in PCP and cellular proliferation via the Hippo-dependent transcription pathway that involve FRMD1-6, NF2, YAP1, WWC1/2, STK3/4, SAV1, LATS1/2, and MOB1A/1B, the homologs of Expanded, Merlin, Yorkie, Kibra, Hippo, Salvador, Warts, and Mats in *Drosophila*, respectively. The phosphorylation and functional inhibition of YAP1 occur after the binding of Scrib1 to Fat1. Thus, Scrib1 is one of the links that might exist between the Vangl2-dependent PCP signaling pathway and the Fat/Dsh/Hippo pathway.

FAT1

The *FAT1* gene is located on chromosome 4 [4q35.2]. FAT1 stands for FAT1, a large transmembrane protein (4588 aa; 506 kDa), also known as Cadherin-Related Family Member 8, Cadherin Family Member 7, Cadherin ME5, and Cadherin-Related Tumor Suppressor containing 3. Fat1 is a single transmembrane domain protein with extracellular cadherin repeats along with numerous other motifs and a C-terminal cytoplasmic domain containing a PDZ-binding motif.[270] Fat1 is involved in developmental mechanisms and PCP.[271] Several mutations associated with glioblastoma, and colorectal, head, and neck cancer have been reported on *FAT1*.[272,273] In 2006, *FAT1* was associated in affective bipolar disorder in several populations.[274,275] In 2010, *FAT1* was reported as an autism candidate gene. A conventional karyotype analysis and array CGH technology revealed a 4q rare de novo subtelomeric deletion of approximately 6.8 Mb at *4q35.1-35.2* in an 8-year-old autistic boy.[276] The *4q35.2* is prone to genomic rearrangement (Autism Genome Project Consortium 2007[159,223,277,278]). A 12-year-old boy with autism and associated clinical features such as ADHD, OCD, easy bruising, and irregular sleep disturbance was also reported to have a deletion of 1.2 Mb of the long arm of chr4 including *MTNR1A*, the *FAT1* gene, and *F11*.[141,279] More recently, a de novo missense mutation was found in the *FAT1* gene in H3691R (c.11,072A > G) in an autistic patient.[224] In 2014, Pericak-Vanceet and collaborators reported that two obligate carriers (female) in family 17,545 had a history of major depression.[191] They found that *FAT1* had two alterations in this family, and they also discovered a distinct variant in another family. Finally, they also reported that *FAT1* and *ABHD14A* genes carried variants in *cis*.[191]

FAT4

The *FAT4* gene is located on chromosome 4 [4q28.1]. FAT4 stands for FAT atypical cadherin 4 (FATJ; FAT-J; CDHF14; CDHR11; HKLLS2; VMLDS2; and NBLA00548), a large atypical cadherin (4924 aa; 542 KDa) belonging to the protocadherin family that has multiple alternatively spliced transcript variants.[270] Fat4 is a transmembrane domain with a large N-terminal extracellular domain containing a long N-terminal cadherin ectodomain, a flamingo box, three EGF domains, two laminin G domains, a fourth EGF domain, and a C-terminal tail that interacts with several scaffolding and signaling proteins.[280] Fat4 and Dchs1 interact with each other to form an adhesive complex involved in the developing brain and PCP.[271] FAT4 is a tumor suppressor that has been involved in esophageal cancer, lung cancer, pancreatic cancer melanoma, gastric cancer, and breast cancer.[272] *FAT4* has been associated with Van Maldergem syndrome 2 (VMS2) and Hennekam lymphangiectasia-lymphedema syndrome 2 (HKLLS2 [HS]). In 1992, Van Maldergem and collaborators were the first to describe this new syndrome in an 11-year-old girl with IDs, facial abnormalities, and hand malformations.[281] The same clinical findings were also found in a deaf 5-year-old girl.[282] In 2013, the group of Stephen Robertson further characterized the syndrome as an autosomal-recessive disorder with IDs, craniofacial, auditory, renal, skeletal and limb malformations, and a partially penetrant periventricular neuronal heterotopia phenotype and identified biallelic missense and nonsense mutations in the *FAT4* gene in affected individuals from three unrelated families using whole-exome sequencing or targeted Sanger sequencing.[52] Two mutations appear on cysteines involved in disulfide bonds (Cys4159Tyr and Cys4398Phe) and one on Glu2375 (Glu2375Lys) in the cadherin interdomain linker region. In other cases, FAT4 is truncated in or after the cadherin repeats or in the C-terminus lacking the last 143 aa.[52] Homozygous or compound heterozygous mutations in the *FAT4* gene were also found by whole-exome sequencing associated to HS by Alders and collaborators.[283] This syndrome is a genetically heterogeneous disorder characterized by lymphedema, intestinal lymphangiectasia, intellectual deficit, and facial dysmorphism sharing features with VMS. All mutations were found in the N-terminal extracellular cadherin repeats or LAG-like domains.[283]

DCHS1

The *DCHS1* gene is located on chromosome 11 [*11p15.4*]. DCHS1 stands for Dachsous cadherin-related 1 (DCHS1), also named CDH19, CDH25, CDHR6, FIB1, VMLDS1, or Protocadherin 16 (PCDH16). Dchs1 is a large atypical cell adhesion protein (3298 aa; 346 kDa) that belongs to the protocadherin superfamily and is a ligand for Fat4 which is also a protocadherin.[52] Dchs1 and Fat4 interact with each other to form an adhesive complex involved in the developing brain. *DCHS1* has been linked to Van Maldergem Wetzburger Verloes syndrome (VMLDS1 or VM1) with clinical features close to VM2 caused by mutation in the *FAT4* gene. VM1 is an autosomal recessive disorder with multiple clinical features that include IDs associated to typical craniofacial features, auditory malformations resulting in hearing loss, periventricular nodular heterotopia, renal hypoplasia, tracheal anomalies, and skeletal and limb malformations. In 2013, in parallel to the *FAT4* mutations, several homozygous mutations on *DCHS1* were found in unrelated consanguineous families with VM.[52] Three patients, first reported by Mansour et al. (2012),[284] carried a homozygous mutation in the *DCHS1* gene Gly835-to-ter (G835X) substitution in the CR8 domain or a homozygous 1-bp deletion (c.2543delC), resulting in a short protein with 7 N-terminal cadherin repeats.[52] A girl was also identified with a homozygous c.7109A-T transversion in exon 19 (N2370I) in the CR22 domain that is critical for adhesive function of the DCSH1 protein.

FJX1

The *FJX1* gene is located on chromosome 11 [*11p13*]. FJX1 stands for Four Jointed Box 1 (FJX1), also named Putative Secreted Ligand Homologous to Fjx1, Four-Jointed Protein Homolog, or Four-Jointed Box Protein. Fjx1 is a Golgi atypical protein kinase (437 aa; 48 kDa) that is known to phosphorylate serine or threonine residues within the extracellular cadherin domains of Fat and Dachsous.[285] The exact function of FJX1 in humans is not known, but Fjx1 belongs to the PCP pathway and is known to regulate dendrite extension in mice.[98] A 1.155-Mb microdeletion at *11p13* encompassing the *FJX1*, *SLC1A2*, *TRIM44*, and *LDLRAD3* genes was found in a 5.8-year-old Russian patient with IDs, ADHD, speech delay, and hyperdynamia.[286] The symptoms cannot be attributed to *FJX1* only, because the other genes have also been found to be associated with IDs.

NF2

The *NF2* gene is located on chromosome 22 [*22q12.2*]. NF2 stands for Neurofibromin 2 (NF2), also named Merlin or Schwannomin. Nf2 is an intracellular protein (595 aa; 69 kDa) composed of an FERM domain, a flexible coiled-coil region, and a C-terminal hydrophilic tail belonging to the ERM (Ezrin, radixin, moesin) family that interacts with membrane proteins and cytoskeletal components.[287] *Nf2* has two predominant isoforms; alternative splicing also produces several minor isoforms. NF2 is a tumor suppressor and mutations in the *NF2* gene are associated with neurofibromatosis type II (NFII) that is characterized by nervous system and skin tumors, and ocular abnormalities usually appear during adolescence.[287] Nf2 is a potential regulator of the Hippo/SWH (Sav/Wts/Hpo) signaling pathway.[288] In 1992, Gillberg was among the first to subclassify autistic patients according to other medical conditions including neurofibromatosis.[289] Later, several cases were described associating large *22q12* deletions, which encompass the *NF2* gene, and clinical features distinct from neurofibromatosis and including IDs. Bruder and collaborators reported several patients with variable *22q12* deletion including a 9-year-old boy with IDs with no facial dysmorphism, who later developed bilateral vestibular schwannomas; a female with developmental delay, mental retardation, and NFII; and a male with severe mental retardation and bilateral vestibular schwannomas.[290,291] More recently, a 15-year-old girl with IDs, Pierre-Robin sequence (micrognathia and cleft palate), ocular hypertelorism, and bilateral hearing loss also developed severe tumors.[292] More complex *22q12* rearrangements have also been found. For instance, a 2.28-Mb deletion encompassing the *NF2* gene and a 1.61-Mb deletion containing the *MN1* gene were found in a female with cleft palate, an open anterior fontanelle, and developmental delay.[293] Thus, orofacial clefting and IDs with later risks of developing tumors are commonly associated with the *22q12* region involving the *NF2* gene.

YAP1

The *YAP1* gene is located on chromosome 11 [*11q22.1-q22.2*]. YAP1 stands for Yes-Associated Protein 1 (YAP1), also known as YAP, YKI, COB1, YAP2, YAP65, or Yorkie Homolog, an effector of the HIPPO-pathway.[294] Yap1 is a cytoplasmic protein (504 aa; 54 kDa) with a PPxY region, an AKT phosphorylation/14-3-3-binding site, a WW domain, a transcription activation domain, and a C-terminal PDZ-binding motif. Yap1 and Yap2 are the result of alternatively spliced transcript variants of YAP.[295] *YAP1* is a direct oncogenic target in multiple tumor types.[296] In 2014, using exome sequence analysis, Fitzpatrick and collaborators identified two different cosegregating heterozygous nonsense mutations (c.370C > T [p.Arg124*] and c. 1066G > T [p.Glu356*]) in *YAP1* associated with ocular coloboma, with or without hearing impairment, cleft lip/palate, and/or mental retardation.[297] Members of this family have been previously described.[298,299]

PML

The *PML* gene is located on chromosome 15 [*15q22*]. PML stands for Promyelocytic Leukemia (PML), also known as MYL, RNF71, PP8675, and TRIM19, and belongs to the tripartite motif (TRIM) family.[300] Pml is a putative zinc finger protein and potential transcription factor phosphoprotein (882 aa; 97 kDa) that localizes to nuclear bodies. PML stabilizes YAP1 by sumoylation and enhances p73-dependent transcription.[301] The *PML* gene has been implicated in acute promyelocytic leukemia.[112] *PML* has also been linked to autism. A 1-Mb deletion in the *15q22-15q23* region encompassing the *PML* gene was found in a patient with autism, developmental delay, and mild dysmorphism.[302] In this patient, the entire *PML* gene was absent from chromosome 15. Another report mentioned additional copies of different segments of chromosome 15q in an 8-year-old boy diagnosed with autism, along with development delay, seizures, and hypoplastic corpus callosum.[303]

CONCLUSION

The core PCP signaling and associated protein pathway, and the Hippo pathway are conserved pathways that control key mechanisms of development, including cell polarity, tissue organization and shape, cell proliferation and apoptosis, and cell migration, as well as network connection, neuronal plasticity, and higher brain functions. If we follow the hypothesis that aberrant brain connectivity is an important cause of core pathologies such as ASD or IDs, mutations in PCP genes could predict ASD/ID risk, and more generally the risk of developing neurodevelopmental pathologies. Supporting this hypothesis, mutations in some PCP genes such as *DVL2*, *DIAPH3*, *FAT1*, *NF1*, *PRICKLE1* and *PRICKLE2*, *SCRIB1*, and *WNT2* have been reported in ASD patients. Moreover, mutations in genes such as *DLG3*, *FZD9*, *JNK3*, *PAK3*, and *SMURF*, all of which are linked to the PCP pathway, have been reported in ID patients. Other genes such as *DAAM1*, *DACT1*, *DVL1*, *DVL2*, *FAT1*, *FJX1*, *FZD3*, *FZD4*, *FZD9*, *NF2*, *PML*, *ROR2*, *SCRIB1*, *VANGL1*, *VANGL2*, *WNT2B*, and *YAP1*, are located in regions of chromosomes that are subjected to genomic rearrangements such as microdeletions and/or duplications, or even major deletions that lead to multisystemic phenotypes that associate ASD

with/without IDs or seizures but also include hearing impairments, cleft/lip palate, global developmental delay, and short stature, to cite a few. Some conditions include neurofibromatosis or vestibular schwannomas, or different tumors. Indeed, many PCP proteins composing the various PCP pathways also contribute to cancer development when mutated. For example, in humans, *ROR2*,[243] *SCRIB/DLG*,[304] *VANGL1*,[164-166] and *VANGL2*[170] mutations have been associated with several kinds of cancer. Unexpectedly, autism and cancer pathways appear to converge to some extent[305] with several mutated tumor genes, including those involved in PCP signaling, also found involved in ASD or IDs. In the future, studies on these different pathways but also on subnetworks involving the different isoforms found in mammals, as well as links between pathways and downstream effectors, will lead to a better understanding of the mechanisms of action of PCP signaling in higher brain function and diseases. Finally, PCP genes may confer susceptibility to ASD, with and without IDs, through their impact on synapse and glutamate neurotransmission, synaptic LTP, and LTD, which will link them definitively to other biological pathways involved in neurodevelopmental disorders.

Acknowledgments

INSERM, ANR MossyPCP ANR-12-BSV4-0016-01, and ANR SynchAutism ANR-13-SAMA-0012-02, University of Bordeaux and Conseil Régional d'Aquitaine, supported this work. The Montcouquiol/Sans Laboratory is a member of the Labex B.R.A.I.N. (ANR-10-LABX-43). We thank C. Racca for helpful comments and discussion.

References

1. Harrison PJ, et al. Schizophrenia genes, gene expression, and neuropathology: on the matter of their convergence. *Mol Psychiatry* 2005;**10**(1):40—68. image 45.
2. Geschwind DH. Genetics of autism spectrum disorders. *Trends Cogn Sci* 2011;**15**(9):409—16.
3. Wittchen HU, et al. The size and burden of mental disorders and other disorders of the brain in Europe 2010. *Eur Neuropsychopharmacol* 2011;**21**(9):655—79.
4. Lancaster MA, et al. Spindle orientation in mammalian cerebral cortical development. *Curr Opin Neurobiol* 2012;**22**(5):737—46.
5. Evsyukova I, et al. Integrative mechanisms of oriented neuronal migration in the developing brain. *Annu Rev Cell Dev Biol* 2013;**29**:299—353.
6. Cristino AS, et al. Neurodevelopmental and neuropsychiatric disorders represent an interconnected molecular system. *Mol Psychiatry* 2014;**19**(3):294—301.
7. Wallingford JB, et al. Strange as it may seem: the many links between Wnt signaling, planar cell polarity, and cilia. *Genes Dev* 2011;**25**(3):201—13.
8. Adler PN. The frizzled/stan pathway and planar cell polarity in the Drosophila wing. *Curr Top Dev Biol* 2012;**101**:1—31.

9. Singh J, et al. Planar cell polarity signaling: coordination of cellular orientation across tissues. *Wiley Interdiscip Rev Dev Biol* 2012;**1**(4):479–99.

10. Jenny A. Planar cell polarity signaling in the Drosophila eye. *Curr Top Dev Biol* 2010;**93**:189–227.

11. Wu J, et al. Wg and Wnt4 provide long-range directional input to planar cell polarity orientation in Drosophila. *Nat Cell Biol* 2013;**15**(9):1045–55.

12. Lawrence PA, et al. Towards a model of the organisation of planar polarity and pattern in the Drosophila abdomen. *Development* 2002;**129**(11):2749–60.

13. Chen WS, et al. Asymmetric homotypic interactions of the atypical cadherin flamingo mediate intercellular polarity signaling. *Cell* 2008;**133**(6):1093–105.

14. Tada M, et al. Convergent extension: using collective cell migration and cell intercalation to shape embryos. *Development* 2012;**139**(21):3897–904.

15. Montcouquiol M, et al. Identification of Vangl2 and Scrb1 as planar polarity genes in mammals. *Nature* 2003;**423**(6936):173–7.

16. Montcouquiol M, et al. Asymmetric localization of Vangl2 and Fz3 indicate novel mechanisms for planar cell polarity in mammals. *J Neurosci* 2006;**26**(19):5265–75.

17. Giese AP, et al. Gipc1 has a dual role in Vangl2 trafficking and hair bundle integrity in the inner ear. *Development* 2012;**139**(20):3775–85.

18. Ezan J, et al. Revisiting planar cell polarity in the inner ear. *Semin Cell Dev Biol* 2013;**24**(5):499–506.

19. Ezan J, et al. Primary cilium migration depends on G-protein signalling control of subapical cytoskeleton. *Nat Cell Biol* 2013;**15**(9):1107–15.

20. Simons M, et al. Planar cell polarity signaling: from fly development to human disease. *Annu Rev Genet* 2008;**42**:517–40.

21. Montcouquiol M, et al. Noncanonical Wnt signaling and neural polarity. *Annu Rev Neurosci* 2006;**29**:363–86.

22. Sebbagh M, et al. Insight into planar cell polarity. *Exp Cell Res* 2014;**328**(2):284–95.

23. Okerlund ND, et al. Synaptic Wnt signaling-a contributor to major psychiatric disorders? *J Neurodev Disord* 2011;**3**(2):162–74.

24. Kalkman HO. A review of the evidence for the canonical Wnt pathway in autism spectrum disorders. *Mol Autism* 2012;**3**(1):10.

25. Panaccione I, et al. Neurodevelopment in schizophrenia: the role of the wnt pathways. *Curr Neuropharmacol* 2013;**11**(5):535–58.

26. Nishita M, et al. Ror2/Frizzled complex mediates Wnt5a-induced AP-1 activation by regulating Dishevelled polymerization. *Mol Cell Biol* 2010;**30**(14):3610–9.

27. Gao B, et al. Wnt signaling gradients establish planar cell polarity by inducing Vangl2 phosphorylation through Ror2. *Dev Cell* 2011;**20**(2):163–76.

28. Strutt H, et al. Nonautonomous planar polarity patterning in Drosophila: dishevelled-independent functions of frizzled. *Dev Cell* 2002;**3**(6):851–63.

29. Sokol SY. Analysis of Dishevelled signalling pathways during Xenopus development. *Curr Biol* 1996;**6**(11):1456–67.

30. Gao C, et al. Dishevelled: the hub of Wnt signaling. *Cell Signal* 2010;**22**(5):717–27.

31. Wynshaw-Boris A. Dishevelled: in vivo roles of a multifunctional gene family during development. *Curr Top Dev Biol* 2012;**101**:213–35.

32. Jenny A, et al. Diego and Prickle regulate Frizzled planar cell polarity signalling by competing for Dishevelled binding. *Nat Cell Biol* 2005;**7**(7):691–7.

33. Moeller H, et al. Diversin regulates heart formation and gastrulation movements in development. *Proc Natl Acad Sci USA* 2006;**103**(43):15900–5.

34. Tree DR, et al. Prickle mediates feedback amplification to generate asymmetric planar cell polarity signaling. *Cell* 2002;**109**(3):371–81.

35. Boutin C, et al. Celsr1-3 cadherins in PCP and brain development. *Curr Top Dev Biol* 2012;**101**:161–83.

36. Bilder D, et al. Cooperative regulation of cell polarity and growth by Drosophila tumor suppressors. *Science* 2000;**289**(5476):113–6.

37. Cheyette BN, et al. Dapper, a Dishevelled-associated antagonist of beta-catenin and JNK signaling, is required for notochord formation. *Dev Cell* 2002;**2**(4):449–61.

38. Gloy J, et al. Frodo interacts with Dishevelled to transduce Wnt signals. *Nat Cell Biol* 2002;**4**(5):351–7.

39. Suriben R, et al. Posterior malformations in Dact1 mutant mice arise through misregulated Vangl2 at the primitive streak. *Nat Genet* 2009;**41**(9):977–85.

40. Zhang L, et al. Dapper 1 antagonizes Wnt signaling by promoting dishevelled degradation. *J Biol Chem* 2006;**281**(13):8607–12.

41. Ma B, et al. Dapper1 promotes autophagy by enhancing the Beclin1-Vps34-Atg14L complex formation. *Cell Res* 2014;**24**(8):912–24.

42. Ma B, et al. The Wnt signaling antagonist Dapper1 accelerates Dishevelled2 degradation via promoting its ubiquitination and aggregates-induced autophagy. *J Biol Chem* 2015;**290**(19):12346–54.

43. Shi Y, et al. Identification of novel rare mutations of DACT1 in human neural tube defects. *Hum Mutat* 2012;**33**(10):1450–5.

44. Mao Y, et al. Planar polarization of the atypical myosin Dachs orients cell divisions in Drosophila. *Genes Dev* 2011;**25**(2):131–6.

45. Matakatsu H, et al. Interactions between Fat and Dachsous and the regulation of planar cell polarity in the Drosophila wing. *Development* 2004;**131**(15):3785–94.

46. Fanto M, et al. The tumor-suppressor and cell adhesion molecule Fat controls planar polarity via physical interactions with Atrophin, a transcriptional co-repressor. *Development* 2003;**130**(4):763–74.

47. Sopko R, et al. Phosphorylation of the tumor suppressor fat is regulated by its ligand Dachsous and the kinase discs overgrown. *Curr Biol* 2009;**19**(13):1112–7.

48. Matis M, et al. Regulation of PCP by the Fat signaling pathway. *Genes Dev* 2013;**27**(20):2207–20.

49. Merkel M, et al. The balance of prickle/spiny-legs isoforms controls the amount of coupling between core and fat PCP systems. *Curr Biol* 2014;**24**(18):2111–23.

50. Saburi S, et al. Loss of Fat4 disrupts PCP signaling and oriented cell division and leads to cystic kidney disease. *Nat Genet* 2008;**40**(8):1010–5.

51. Saburi S, et al. Functional interactions between Fat family cadherins in tissue morphogenesis and planar polarity. *Development* 2012;**139**(10):1806–20.

52. Cappello S, et al. Mutations in genes encoding the cadherin receptor-ligand pair DCHS1 and FAT4 disrupt cerebral cortical development. *Nat Genet* 2013;**45**(11):1300–8.

53. Matakatsu H, et al. Separating planar cell polarity and Hippo pathway activities of the protocadherins Fat and Dachsous. *Development* 2012;**139**(8):1498–508.

54. Badouel C, et al. SnapShot: the hippo signaling pathway. *Cell* 2011;**145**(3):484–484.e481.

55. Yu FX, et al. The Hippo pathway: regulators and regulations. *Genes Dev* 2013;**27**(4):355–71.

56. Zhao B, et al. The Hippo-YAP pathway in organ size control and tumorigenesis: an updated version. *Genes Dev* 2010;**24**(9):862–74.

57. Zhao B, et al. The Hippo pathway in organ size control, tissue regeneration and stem cell self-renewal. *Nat Cell Biol* 2011;**13**(8):877–83.

58. Rauskolb C, et al. Zyxin links fat signaling to the hippo pathway. *PLoS Biol* 2011;**9**(6):e1000624.

59. Skouloudaki K, et al. Scribble participates in Hippo signaling and is required for normal zebrafish pronephros development. *Proc Natl Acad Sci USA* 2009;**106**(21):8579–84.

60. Cordenonsi M, et al. The Hippo transducer TAZ confers cancer stem cell-related traits on breast cancer cells. *Cell* 2011;**147**(4):759–72.

61. Tissir F, et al. Expression of planar cell polarity genes during development of the mouse CNS. *Eur J Neurosci* 2006;**23**(3):597–607.

62. Rock R, et al. Expression of mouse dchs1, fjx1, and fat-j suggests conservation of the planar cell polarity pathway identified in Drosophila. *Dev Dyn* 2005;**234**(3):747–55.

63. Ying G, et al. The protocadherin gene Celsr3 is required for interneuron migration in the mouse forebrain. *Mol Cell Biol* 2009;**29**(11):3045–61.

64. Juriloff DM, et al. A consideration of the evidence that genetic defects in planar cell polarity contribute to the etiology of human neural tube defects. *Birth Defects Res A Clin Mol Teratol* 2012;**94**(10):824–40.

65. Greene ND, et al. Neural tube defects. *Annu Rev Neurosci* 2014;**37**:221–42.

66. Goodrich LV. The plane facts of PCP in the CNS. *Neuron* 2008;**60**(1):9–16.

67. Rachel RA, et al. Retinal axon misrouting at the optic chiasm in mice with neural tube closure defects. *Genesis* 2000;**27**(1):32–47.

68. Rachel RA, et al. A new allele of Gli3 and a new mutation, circletail (Crc), resulting from a single transgenic experiment. *Genesis* 2002;**33**(2):55–61.

69. Murdoch JN, et al. Circletail, a new mouse mutant with severe neural tube defects: chromosomal localization and interaction with the loop-tail mutation. *Genomics* 2001;**78**(1–2):55–63.

70. Curtin JA, et al. Mutation of Celsr1 disrupts planar polarity of inner ear hair cells and causes severe neural tube defects in the mouse. *Curr Biol* 2003;**13**(13):1129–33.

71. Moreau MM, et al. The planar polarity protein Scribble1 is essential for neuronal plasticity and brain function. *J Neurosci* 2010;**30**(29):9738–52.

72. Wallingford JB. Planar cell polarity and the developmental control of cell behavior in vertebrate embryos. *Annu Rev Cell Dev Biol* 2012;**28**:627–53.

73. Lake BB, et al. Strabismus regulates asymmetric cell divisions and cell fate determination in the mouse brain. *J Cell Biol* 2009;**185**(1):59–66.

74. Gray RS, et al. Planar cell polarity: coordinating morphogenetic cell behaviors with embryonic polarity. *Dev Cell* 2011;**21**(1):120–33.

75. Bayly R, et al. Pointing in the right direction: new developments in the field of planar cell polarity. *Nat Rev Genet* 2011;**12**(6):385–91.

76. Kamiya A, et al. A schizophrenia-associated mutation of DISC1 perturbs cerebral cortex development. *Nat Cell Biol* 2005;**7**(12):1167–78.

77. Galaburda AM, et al. From genes to behavior in developmental dyslexia. *Nat Neurosci* 2006;**9**(10):1213–7.

78. Francis F, et al. Human disorders of cortical development: from past to present. *Eur J Neurosci* 2006;**23**(4):877–93.

79. Pardo CA, et al. The neurobiology of autism. *Brain Pathol* 2007;**17**(4):434–47.

80. Guerrini R, et al. Abnormal development of the human cerebral cortex: genetics, functional consequences and treatment options. *Trends Neurosci* 2008;**31**(3):154–62.

81. Tissir F, et al. Protocadherin Celsr3 is crucial in axonal tract development. *Nat Neurosci* 2005;**8**(4):451–7.

82. Wang Y, et al. Frizzled-3 is required for the development of major fiber tracts in the rostral CNS. *J Neurosci* 2002;**22**(19):8563–73.

83. Lavado A, et al. The tumor suppressor Nf2 regulates corpus callosum development by inhibiting the transcriptional coactivator Yap. *Development* 2014;**141**(21):4182–93.

84. Kulkarni VA, et al. The dendritic tree and brain disorders. *Mol Cell Neurosci* 2012;**50**(1):10–20.

85. Emoto K. Dendrite remodeling in development and disease. *Dev Growth Differ* 2011;**53**(3):277–86.

86. Shima Y, et al. Regulation of dendritic maintenance and growth by a mammalian 7-pass transmembrane cadherin. *Dev Cell* 2004;**7**(2):205–16.

87. Shima Y, et al. Opposing roles in neurite growth control by two seven-pass transmembrane cadherins. *Nat Neurosci* 2007;**10**(8):963–9.

88. Zhou L, et al. Early forebrain wiring: genetic dissection using conditional Celsr3 mutant mice. *Science* 2008;**320**(5878):946–9.

89. Feng J, et al. Planar cell polarity genes, Celsr1-3, in neural development. *Neurosci Bull* 2012;**28**(3):309–15.

90. Rosso SB, et al. Wnt signaling through Dishevelled, Rac and JNK regulates dendritic development. *Nat Neurosci* 2005;**8**(1):34–42.

91. Wayman GA, et al. Activity-dependent dendritic arborization mediated by CaM-kinase I activation and enhanced CREB-dependent transcription of Wnt-2. *Neuron* 2006;**50**(6):897–909.

92. Bian WJ, et al. A novel Wnt5a-Frizzled4 signaling pathway mediates activity-independent dendrite morphogenesis via the distal PDZ motif of Frizzled 4. *Dev Neurobiol* 2014;**75**(8):805–22.

93. Clark CE, et al. Wnt5a induces Ryk-dependent and -independent effects on callosal axon and dendrite growth. *Growth Factors* 2014;**32**(1):11–7.

94. Yamamoto S, et al. Cthrc1 selectively activates the planar cell polarity pathway of Wnt signaling by stabilizing the Wnt-receptor complex. *Dev Cell* 2008;**15**(1):23–36.

95. Paganoni S, et al. Ror1-Ror2 complexes modulate synapse formation in hippocampal neurons. *Neuroscience* 2010;**165**(4):1261–74.

96. Hagiwara A, et al. The planar cell polarity protein Vangl2 bidirectionally regulates dendritic branching in cultured hippocampal neurons. *Mol Brain* 2014;**7**(1):79.

97. Arguello A, et al. Dapper Antagonist of Catenin-1 (Dact1) contributes to dendrite arborization in forebrain cortical interneurons. *Commun Integr Biol* 2013;**6**(6):e26656.

98. Probst B, et al. The rodent Four-jointed ortholog Fjx1 regulates dendrite extension. *Dev Biol* 2007;**312**(1):461–70.

99. Sowers LP, et al. The non-canonical Wnt ligand Wnt5a rescues morphological deficits in Prickle2-deficient hippocampal neurons. *Mol Psychiatry* 2013;**18**(10):1049.

100. Murdoch JN, et al. Disruption of scribble (Scrb1) causes severe neural tube defects in the circletail mouse. *Hum Mol Genet* 2003;**12**(2):87–98.

101. Fiala JC, et al. Dendritic spine pathology: cause or consequence of neurological disorders? *Brain Res Brain Res Rev* 2002;**39**(1):29–54.

102. Sala C, et al. Molecular mechanisms of dendritic spine development and maintenance. *Acta Neurobiol Exp (Wars)* 2008;**68**(2):289–304.

103. Ciani L, et al. Wnt7a signaling promotes dendritic spine growth and synaptic strength through Ca(2)(+)/Calmodulin-dependent protein kinase II. *Proc Natl Acad Sci USA* 2011;**108**(26):10732–7.

104. Feng J, et al. A role for atypical cadherin Celsr3 in hippocampal maturation and connectivity. *J Neurosci* 2012;**32**(40):13729–43.

105. Sahores M, et al. Frizzled-5, a receptor for the synaptic organizer Wnt7a, regulates activity-mediated synaptogenesis. *Development* 2010;**137**(13):2215–25.

106. Yoshioka T, et al. Vangl2, the planar cell polarity protein, is complexed with postsynaptic density protein PSD-95 [corrected]. *FEBS Lett* 2013;**587**(10):1453–9.

107. Nagaoka T, et al. The Wnt/planar cell polarity pathway component Vangl2 induces synapse formation through direct control of N-cadherin. *Cell Rep* 2014;**6**(5):916–27.

108. Piguel NH, et al. Scribble1/AP2 complex coordinates NMDA receptor endocytic recycling. *Cell Rep* 2014;**9**(2):712–27.

109. Cerpa W, et al. RoR2 functions as a noncanonical Wnt receptor that regulates NMDAR-mediated synaptic transmission. *Proc Natl Acad Sci USA* 2015;**112**(15):4797–802.

110. Oishi I, et al. The receptor tyrosine kinase Ror2 is involved in non-canonical Wnt5a/JNK signalling pathway. *Genes Cells* 2003;**8**(7):645–54.

111. Mikels AJ, et al. Purified Wnt5a protein activates or inhibits beta-catenin-TCF signaling depending on receptor context. *PLoS Biol* 2006;**4**(4):e115.

112. Salomoni P, et al. New insights into the role of PML in tumour suppression. *Cell Res* 2008;**18**(6):622–40.

113. Lijam N, et al. Social interaction and sensorimotor gating abnormalities in mice lacking Dvl1. *Cell* 1997;**90**(5):895–905.

114. Long JM, et al. Expanded characterization of the social interaction abnormalities in mice lacking Dvl1. *Genes Brain Behav* 2004;**3**(1):51–62.

115. Yates LL, et al. Planar polarity: A new player in both lung development and disease. *Organogenesis* 2011;**7**(3):209–16.

116. Henderson DJ, et al. Getting to the heart of planar cell polarity signaling. *Birth Defects Res A Clin Mol Teratol* 2011;**91**(6):460–7.

117. Copp AJ, et al. Neural tube defects: recent advances, unsolved questions, and controversies. *Lancet Neurol* 2013;**12**(8):799–810.

118. Papakrivopoulou E, et al. Planar cell polarity and the kidney. *Nephrol Dial Transplant* 2014;**29**(7):1320–6.

119. Wang Y, et al. Wnt and the Wnt signaling pathway in bone development and disease. *Front Biosci (Landmark Ed)* 2014;**19**:379–407.

120. Sadeqzadeh E, et al. Sleeping giants: emerging roles for the fat cadherins in health and disease. *Med Res Rev* 2014;**34**(1):190–221.

121. Guo N, et al. Frizzled6 controls hair patterning in mice. *Proc Natl Acad Sci USA* 2004;**101**(25):9277–81.

122. Wang Y, et al. Axonal growth and guidance defects in Frizzled3 knock-out mice: a comparison of diffusion tensor magnetic resonance imaging, neurofilament staining, and genetically directed cell labeling. *J Neurosci* 2006;**26**(2):355–64.

123. Hua ZL, et al. Frizzled3 is required for the development of multiple axon tracts in the mouse central nervous system. *Proc Natl Acad Sci USA* 2014;**111**(29):E3005–14.

124. Wang Y, et al. The role of Frizzled3 and Frizzled6 in neural tube closure and in the planar polarity of inner-ear sensory hair cells. *J Neurosci* 2006;**26**(8):2147–56.

125. Hua ZL, et al. Partial interchangeability of Fz3 and Fz6 in tissue polarity signaling for epithelial orientation and axon growth and guidance. *Development* 2014;**141**(20):3944–54.

126. Yu H, et al. Frizzled 1 and frizzled 2 genes function in palate, ventricular septum and neural tube closure: general implications for tissue fusion processes. *Development* 2010;**137**(21):3707–17.

127. Yu H, et al. Frizzled 2 and frizzled 7 function redundantly in convergent extension and closure of the ventricular septum and palate: evidence for a network of interacting genes. *Development* 2012;**139**(23):4383–94.

128. Descamps B, et al. Frizzled 4 regulates arterial network organization through noncanonical Wnt/planar cell polarity signaling. *Circ Res* 2012;**110**(1):47–58.

129. Sewduth RN, et al. The ubiquitin ligase PDZRN3 is required for vascular morphogenesis through Wnt/planar cell polarity signalling. *Nat Commun* 2014;**5**:4832.

130. Tabares-Seisdedos R, et al. Chromosome 8p as a potential hub for developmental neuropsychiatric disorders: implications for schizophrenia, autism and cancer. *Mol Psychiatry* 2009;**14**(6):563–89.

131. Katsu T, et al. The human frizzled-3 (FZD3) gene on chromosome 8p21, a receptor gene for Wnt ligands, is associated with the susceptibility to schizophrenia. *Neurosci Lett* 2003;**353**(1):53–6.

132. Yang J, et al. Association study of the human FZD3 locus with schizophrenia. *Biol Psychiatry* 2003;**54**(11):1298–301.

133. Zhang Y, et al. Positive association of the human frizzled 3 (FZD3) gene haplotype with schizophrenia in Chinese Han population. *Am J Med Genet B Neuropsychiatr Genet* 2004;**129B**(1):16–9.

134. Kang C, et al. Association study of the frizzled 3 gene with Chinese Va schizophrenia. *Neurosci Lett* 2011;**505**(2):196–9.

135. Papanikolaou K, et al. A case of partial trisomy of chromosome 8p associated with autism. *J Autism Dev Disord* 2006;**36**(5):705–9.

136. Sajan SA, et al. Both rare and de novo copy number variants are prevalent in agenesis of the corpus callosum but not in cerebellar hypoplasia or polymicrogyria. *PLoS Genet* 2013;**9**(10):e1003823.

137. Robitaille J, et al. Mutant frizzled-4 disrupts retinal angiogenesis in familial exudative vitreoretinopathy. *Nat Genet* 2002;**32**(2):326–30.

138. Li P, et al. Karyotype-phenotype insights from 11q14.1-q23.2 interstitial deletions: FZD4 haploinsufficiency and exudative vitreoretinopathy in a patient with a complex chromosome rearrangement. *Am J Med Genet A* 2006;**140**(24):2721–9.

139. Nallathambi J, et al. Identification of novel FZD4 mutations in Indian patients with familial exudative vitreoretinopathy. *Mol Vis* 2006;**12**:1086–92.

140. He X, et al. A member of the Frizzled protein family mediating axis induction by Wnt-5A. *Science* 1997;**275**(5306):1652–4.

141. Roberts JL, et al. Chromosomal microarray analysis of consecutive individuals with autism spectrum disorders or learning disability presenting for genetic services. *Gene* 2014;**535**(1):70–8.

142. Brandau DT, et al. Autistic and dysmorphic features associated with a submicroscopic 2q33.3-q34 interstitial deletion detected by array comparative genomic hybridization. *Am J Med Genet A* 2008;**146A**(4):521–4.

143. Albers J, et al. Control of bone formation by the serpentine receptor Frizzled-9. *J Cell Biol* 2011;**192**(6):1057–72.

144. Wang YK, et al. A novel human homologue of the Drosophila frizzled wnt receptor gene binds wingless protein and is in the Williams syndrome deletion at 7q11.23. *Hum Mol Genet* 1997;**6**(3):465–72.

145. Merla G, et al. Copy number variants at Williams-Beuren syndrome 7q11.23 region. *Hum Genet* 2010;**128**(1):3–26.

146. Martens MA, et al. Research Review: Williams syndrome: a critical review of the cognitive, behavioral, and neuroanatomical phenotype. *J Child Psychol Psychiatry* 2008;**49**(6):576–608.

147. Ylisaukko-oja T, et al. Search for autism loci by combined analysis of Autism Genetic Resource Exchange and Finnish families. *Ann Neurol* 2006;**59**(1):145–55.

148. Wassink TH, et al. Evidence supporting WNT2 as an autism susceptibility gene. *Am J Med Genet* 2001;**105**(5):406–13.

149. Marui T, et al. Association between autism and variants in the wingless-type MMTV integration site family member 2 (WNT2) gene. *Int J Neuropsychopharmacol* 2010;**13**(4):443–9.

150. Chien YL, et al. Association study of the CNS patterning genes and autism in Han Chinese in Taiwan. *Prog Neuropsychopharmacol Biol Psychiatry* 2011;**35**(6):1512–7.

151. Lin PI, et al. The WNT2 gene polymorphism associated with speech delay inherent to autism. *Res Dev Disabil* 2012;**33**(5):1533–40.

152. Bisgaard AM, et al. Interstitial deletion of the short arm of chromosome 1 (1p13.1p21.1) in a girl with mental retardation, short stature and colobomata. *Clin Dysmorphol* 2007;**16**(2):109–12.

153. Person AD, et al. WNT5A mutations in patients with autosomal dominant Robinow syndrome. *Dev Dyn* 2010;**239**(1):327–37.

154. Roifman M, et al. De novo WNT5A-associated autosomal dominant Robinow syndrome suggests specificity of genotype and phenotype. *Clin Genet* 2015;**87**(1):34–41.

155. Butler MG, et al. Robinow syndrome: report of two patients and review of literature. *Clin Genet* 1987;**31**(2):77–85.

156. Patton MA, et al. Robinow syndrome. *J Med Genet* 2002;**39**(5):305–10.

157. van Bokhoven H, et al. Mutation of the gene encoding the ROR2 tyrosine kinase causes autosomal recessive Robinow syndrome. *Nat Genet* 2000;**25**(4):423–6.

158. Tamhankar PM, et al. Identification of novel ROR2 gene mutations in Indian children with Robinow syndrome. *J Clin Res Pediatr Endocrinol* 2014;**6**(2):79–83.

159. Pinto D, et al. Functional impact of global rare copy number variation in autism spectrum disorders. *Nature* 2010;**466**(7304):368–72.

160. Torban E, et al. An expanding role of Vangl proteins in embryonic development. *Curr Top Dev Biol* 2012;**101**:237–61.

161. Lei YP, et al. VANGL2 mutations in human cranial neural-tube defects. *N Engl J Med* 2010;**362**(23):2232–5.

162. Kibar Z, et al. Contribution of VANGL2 mutations to isolated neural tube defects. *Clin Genet* 2011;**80**(1):76–82.

163. Katoh M. Molecular cloning and characterization of Strabismus 2 (STB2). *Int J Oncol* 2002;**20**(5):993–8.

164. Kibar Z, et al. Novel mutations in VANGL1 in neural tube defects. *Hum Mutat* 2009;**30**(7):E706–15.

165. Iliescu A, et al. Independent mutations at Arg181 and Arg274 of Vangl proteins that are associated with neural tube defects in humans decrease protein stability and impair membrane targeting. *Biochemistry* 2014;**53**(32):5356–64.

166. Ryu HS, et al. KITENIN is associated with tumor progression in human gastric cancer. *Anticancer Res* 2010;**30**(9):3479–86.

167. Lee S, et al. Expression of KITENIN in human colorectal cancer and its relation to tumor behavior and progression. *Pathol Int* 2011;**61**(4):210–20.

168. Yoon TM, et al. Expression of KITENIN and its association with tumor progression in oral squamous cell carcinoma. *Auris Nasus Larynx* 2013;**40**(2):222–6.

169. Pinto D, et al. Convergence of genes and cellular pathways dysregulated in autism spectrum disorders. *Am J Hum Genet* 2014;**94**(5):677–94.

170. Krumm N, et al. Transmission disequilibrium of small CNVs in simplex autism. *Am J Hum Genet* 2013;**93**(4):595–606.

171. Iliescu A, et al. Loss of membrane targeting of Vangl proteins causes neural tube defects. *Biochemistry* 2011;**50**(5):795–804.

172. Piazzi G, et al. Van-Gogh-like 2 antagonises the canonical WNT pathway and is methylated in colorectal cancers. *Br J Cancer* 2013;**108**(8):1750–6.

173. Battaglia A, et al. Further delineation of deletion 1p36 syndrome in 60 patients: a recognizable phenotype and common cause of developmental delay and mental retardation. *Pediatrics* 2008;**121**(2):404–10.

174. Kaminsky EB, et al. An evidence-based approach to establish the functional and clinical significance of copy number variants in intellectual and developmental disabilities. *Genet Med* 2011;**13**(9):777–84.

175. Bunn KJ, et al. Mutations in DVL1 Cause an Osteosclerotic Form of Robinow Syndrome. *Am J Hum Genet* 2015;**96**(4):623–30.

176. White J, et al. DVL1 Frameshift Mutations Clustering in the Penultimate Exon Cause Autosomal-Dominant Robinow Syndrome. *Am J Hum Genet* 2015;**96**(4):612–22.

177. Hegazy SA, et al. Disheveled proteins promote cell growth and tumorigenicity in ALK-positive anaplastic large cell lymphoma. *Cell Signal* 2013;**25**(1):295–307.

178. Zeesman S, et al. Microdeletion in distal 17p13.1: a recognizable phenotype with microcephaly, distinctive facial features, and intellectual disability. *Am J Med Genet A* 2012;**158A**(8):1832–6.

179. Gilman SR, et al. Rare de novo variants associated with autism implicate a large functional network of genes involved in formation and function of synapses. *Neuron* 2011;**70**(5):898–907.

180. Allache R, et al. Genetic studies of ANKRD6 as a molecular switch between Wnt signaling pathways in human neural tube defects. *Birth Defects Res A Clin Mol Teratol* 2015;**103**(1):20–6.

181. Jones C, et al. Ankrd6 is a mammalian functional homolog of Drosophila planar cell polarity gene diego and regulates coordinated cellular orientation in the mouse inner ear. *Dev Biol* 2014;**395**(1):62–72.

182. Nurnberger J, et al. Inversin forms a complex with catenins and N-cadherin in polarized epithelial cells. *Mol Biol Cell* 2002;**13**(9):3096–106.

183. Tory K, et al. Mutations of NPHP2 and NPHP3 in infantile nephronophthisis. *Kidney Int* 2009;**75**(8):839–47.

184. Simons M, et al. Inversin, the gene product mutated in nephronophthisis type II, functions as a molecular switch between Wnt signaling pathways. *Nat Genet* 2005;**37**(5):537–43.

185. Katoh M. Identification and characterization of human PRICKLE1 and PRICKLE2 genes as well as mouse Prickle1 and Prickle2 genes homologous to Drosophila tissue polarity gene prickle. *Int J Mol Med* 2003;**11**(2):249–56.

186. Jenny A, et al. Prickle and Strabismus form a functional complex to generate a correct axis during planar cell polarity signaling. *EMBO J* 2003;**22**(17):4409–20.

187. Bassuk AG, et al. A homozygous mutation in human PRICKLE1 causes an autosomal-recessive progressive myoclonus epilepsy-ataxia syndrome. *Am J Hum Genet* 2008;**83**(5):572–81.

188. Criscuolo C, et al. PRICKLE1 progressive myoclonus epilepsy in Southern Italy. *Mov Disord* 2010;**25**(15):2686–7.

189. Bosoi CM, et al. Identification and characterization of novel rare mutations in the planar cell polarity gene PRICKLE1 in human neural tube defects. *Hum Mutat* 2011;**32**(12):1371–5.

190. Tao H, et al. Mutations in prickle orthologs cause seizures in flies, mice, and humans. *Am J Hum Genet* 2011;**88**(2):138–49.

191. Cukier HN, et al. Exome sequencing of extended families with autism reveals genes shared across neurodevelopmental and neuropsychiatric disorders. *Mol Autism* 2014;**5**(1):1.

192. Paemka L, et al. Seizures are regulated by ubiquitin-specific peptidase 9 X-linked (USP9X), a de-ubiquitinase. *PLoS Genet* 2015;**11**(3):e1005022.

193. Voineagu I, et al. Transcriptomic analysis of autistic brain reveals convergent molecular pathology. *Nature* 2011;**474**(7351):380–4.

194. Deans MR, et al. Asymmetric distribution of prickle-like 2 reveals an early underlying polarization of vestibular sensory epithelia in the inner ear. *J Neurosci* 2007;**27**(12):3139–47.

195. Hida Y, et al. Prickle2 is localized in the postsynaptic density and interacts with PSD-95 and NMDA receptors in the brain. *J Biochem* 2011;**149**(6):693–700.

196. Wen S, et al. Planar cell polarity pathway genes and risk for spina bifida. *Am J Med Genet A* 2010;**152A**(2):299–304.

197. Robinson A, et al. Mutations in the planar cell polarity genes CELSR1 and SCRIB are associated with the severe neural tube defect craniorachischisis. *Hum Mutat* 2012;**33**(2):440–7.

198. Lei Y, et al. Mutations in planar cell polarity gene SCRIB are associated with spina bifida. *PLoS One* 2013;**8**(7):e69262.

199. Habas R, et al. Wnt/Frizzled activation of Rho regulates vertebrate gastrulation and requires a novel Formin homology protein Daam1. *Cell* 2001;**107**(7):843–54.

200. Faix J, et al. Staying in shape with formins. *Dev Cell* 2006;**10**(6):693–706.

201. Ju R, et al. Activation of the planar cell polarity formin DAAM1 leads to inhibition of endothelial cell proliferation, migration, and angiogenesis. *Proc Natl Acad Sci USA* 2010;**107**(15):6906–11.

202. Jiang YH, et al. De novo and complex imbalanced chromosomal rearrangements revealed by array CGH in a patient with an abnormal phenotype and apparently "balanced" paracentric inversion of 14(q21q23). *Am J Med Genet A* 2008;**146A**(15):1986–93.

203. Lehalle D, et al. Multiple congenital anomalies-intellectual disability (MCA-ID) and neuroblastoma in a patient harboring a de novo 14q23.1q23.3 deletion. *Am J Med Genet A* 2014;**164A**(5):1310–7.

204. McMichael G, et al. Rare copy number variation in cerebral palsy. *Eur J Hum Genet* 2014;**22**(1):40–5.

205. Kuhn S, et al. Formins as effector proteins of Rho GTPases. *Small GTPases* 2014;**5**:e29513.

206. Kim TB, et al. A gene responsible for autosomal dominant auditory neuropathy (AUNA1) maps to 13q14-21. *J Med Genet* 2004; **41**(11):872–6.

207. Schoen CJ, et al. Increased activity of Diaphanous homolog 3 (DIAPH3)/diaphanous causes hearing defects in humans with auditory neuropathy and in Drosophila. *Proc Natl Acad Sci USA* 2010;**107**(30):13396–401.

208. Vorstman JA, et al. A double hit implicates DIAPH3 as an autism risk gene. *Mol Psychiatry* 2011;**16**(4):442–51.

209. Brooks SP, et al. The Nance-Horan syndrome protein encodes a functional WAVE homology domain (WHD) and is important for co-ordinating actin remodelling and maintaining cell morphology. *Hum Mol Genet* 2010;**19**(12):2421–32.

210. Walsh GS, et al. Planar polarity pathway and Nance-Horan syndrome-like 1b have essential cell-autonomous functions in neuronal migration. *Development* 2011;**138**(14):3033–42.

211. Burdon KP, et al. Mutations in a novel gene, NHS, cause the pleiotropic effects of Nance-Horan syndrome, including severe congenital cataract, dental anomalies, and mental retardation. *Am J Hum Genet* 2003;**73**(5):1120–30.

212. Masiakowski P, et al. A novel family of cell surface receptors with tyrosine kinase-like domain. *J Biol Chem* 1992;**267**(36):26181–90.

213. Debebe Z, et al. Ror2 as a Therapeutic Target in Cancer. *Pharmacol Ther* 2015;**150**:143–8.

214. Nowakowska B, et al. A girl with deletion 9q22.1-q22.32 including the PTCH and ROR2 genes identified by genome-wide array-CGH. *Am J Med Genet A* 2007;**143A**(16):1885–9.

215. Oldridge M, et al. Dominant mutations in ROR2, encoding an orphan receptor tyrosine kinase, cause brachydactyly type B. *Nat Genet* 2000;**24**(3):275–8.

216. Afzal AR, et al. Recessive Robinow syndrome, allelic to dominant brachydactyly type B, is caused by mutation of ROR2. *Nat Genet* 2000;**25**(4):419–22.

217. Nakagawa S, et al. Human scribble (Vartul) is targeted for ubiquitin-mediated degradation by the high-risk papillomavirus E6 proteins and the E6AP ubiquitin-protein ligase. *Mol Cell Biol* 2000;**20**(21):8244–53.

218. Zhan L, et al. Deregulation of scribble promotes mammary tumorigenesis and reveals a role for cell polarity in carcinoma. *Cell* 2008; **135**(5):865–78.

219. Dow LE, et al. Loss of human Scribble cooperates with H-Ras to promote cell invasion through deregulation of MAPK signalling. *Oncogene* 2008;**27**(46):5988–6001.

220. Elsum IA, et al. Scrib heterozygosity predisposes to lung cancer and cooperates with KRas hyperactivation to accelerate lung cancer progression in vivo. *Oncogene* 2014;**33**(48):5523–33.

221. Audebert S, et al. Mammalian Scribble forms a tight complex with the betaPIX exchange factor. *Curr Biol* 2004;**14**(11):987–95.

222. Dauber A, et al. SCRIB and PUF60 are primary drivers of the multisystemic phenotypes of the 8q24.3 copy-number variant. *Am J Hum Genet* 2013;**93**(5):798–811.

223. Battaglia A, et al. Confirmation of chromosomal microarray as a first-tier clinical diagnostic test for individuals with developmental delay, intellectual disability, autism spectrum disorders and dysmorphic features. *Eur J Paediatr Neurol* 2013;**17**(6):589–99.

224. Neale BM, et al. Patterns and rates of exonic de novo mutations in autism spectrum disorders. *Nature* 2012;**485**(7397):242–5.

225. Irimia M, et al. A highly conserved program of neuronal microexons is misregulated in autistic brains. *Cell* 2014;**159**(7):1511–23.

226. Richier L, et al. NOS1AP associates with Scribble and regulates dendritic spine development. *J Neurosci* 2010;**30**(13):4796–805.

227. Nola S, et al. Scrib regulates PAK activity during the cell migration process. *Hum Mol Genet* 2008;**17**(22):3552–65.

228. Delorme R, et al. Mutation screening of NOS1AP gene in a large sample of psychiatric patients and controls. *BMC Med Genet* 2010;**11**:108.

229. Allen KM, et al. PAK3 mutation in nonsyndromic X-linked mental retardation. *Nat Genet* 1998;**20**(1):25–30.

230. Bienvenu T, et al. Missense mutation in PAK3, R67C, causes X-linked nonspecific mental retardation. *Am J Med Genet* 2000; **93**(4):294–8.

231. Horak M, et al. ER to synapse trafficking of NMDA receptors. *Front Cell Neurosci* 2014;**8**:394.

232. Roberts S, et al. The PDZ protein discs-large (DLG): the 'Jekyll and Hyde' of the epithelial polarity proteins. *FEBS J* 2012;**279**(19): 3549–58.

233. Liu J, et al. DLG5 in cell polarity maintenance and cancer development. *Int J Biol Sci* 2014;**10**(5):543–9.

234. Leonard AS, et al. SAP97 is associated with the alpha-amino-3-hydroxy-5-methylisoxazole-4-propionic acid receptor GluR1 subunit. *J Biol Chem* 1998;**273**(31):19518–24.

235. Sans N, et al. Synapse-associated protein 97 selectively associates with a subset of AMPA receptors early in their biosynthetic pathway. *J Neurosci* 2001;**21**(19):7506–16.

236. Gardoni F, et al. CaMKII-dependent phosphorylation regulates SAP97/NR2A interaction. *J Biol Chem* 2003;**278**(45):44745–52.

237. Lee OK, et al. Discs-Large and Strabismus are functionally linked to plasma membrane formation. *Nat Cell Biol* 2003;**5**(11): 987–93.

238. Rivera C, et al. Requirement for Dlgh-1 in planar cell polarity and skeletogenesis during vertebrate development. *PLoS One* 2013; **8**(1):e54410.

239. Iizuka-Kogo A, et al. Requirement of DLG1 for cardiovascular development and tissue elongation during cochlear, enteric, and skeletal development: possible role in convergent extension. *PLoS One* 2015;**10**(4):e0123965.

240. Saadaoui M, et al. Dlg1 controls planar spindle orientation in the neuroepithelium through direct interaction with LGN. *J Cell Biol* 2014;**206**(6):707–17.

241. Willatt L, et al. 3q29 microdeletion syndrome: clinical and molecular characterization of a new syndrome. *Am J Hum Genet* 2005; **77**(1):154–60.

242. Mulle JG, et al. Microdeletions of 3q29 confer high risk for schizophrenia. *Am J Hum Genet* 2010;**87**(2):229–36.

243. Quintero-Rivera F, et al. Autistic and psychiatric findings associated with the 3q29 microdeletion syndrome: case report and review. *Am J Med Genet A* 2010;**152A**(10):2459–67.

244. Carroll LS, et al. Mutation screening of the 3q29 microdeletion syndrome candidate genes DLG1 and PAK2 in schizophrenia. *Am J Med Genet B Neuropsychiatr Genet* 2011;**156B**(7):844–9.

245. Fernandez-Jaen A, et al. Cerebral palsy, epilepsy, and severe intellectual disability in a patient with 3q29 microduplication syndrome. *Am J Med Genet A* 2014;**164A**(8):2043–7.

246. Muller BM, et al. SAP102, a novel postsynaptic protein that interacts with NMDA receptor complexes in vivo. *Neuron* 1996;**17**(2): 255–65.

247. Sans N, et al. NMDA receptor trafficking through an interaction between PDZ proteins and the exocyst complex. *Nat Cell Biol* 2003;**5**(6):520–30.

248. Sans N, et al. mPins modulates PSD-95 and SAP102 trafficking and influences NMDA receptor surface expression. *Nat Cell Biol* 2005;**7**(12):1179–90.

249. Van Campenhout CA, et al. Dlg3 trafficking and apical tight junction formation is regulated by nedd4 and nedd4-2 e3 ubiquitin ligases. *Dev Cell* 2011;**21**(3):479–91.

250. Gegg M, et al. Flattop regulates basal body docking and positioning in mono- and multiciliated cells. *Elife* 2014;**3**.

251. Tarpey P, et al. Mutations in the DLG3 gene cause nonsyndromic X-linked mental retardation. *Am J Hum Genet* 2004;**75**(2):318–24.

252. Zanni G, et al. A novel mutation in the DLG3 gene encoding the synapse-associated protein 102 (SAP102) causes non-syndromic mental retardation. *Neurogenetics* 2010;**11**(2):251–5.

253. Philips AK, et al. X-exome sequencing in Finnish families with intellectual disability—four novel mutations and two novel syndromic phenotypes. *Orphanet J Rare Dis* 2014;**9**:49.

254. Kantojarvi K, et al. Fine mapping of Xq11.1-q21.33 and mutation screening of RPS6KA6, ZNF711, ACSL4, DLG3, and IL1RAPL2 for autism spectrum disorders (ASD). *Autism Res* 2011;**4**(3):228–33.

255. Merte J, et al. Sec24b selectively sorts Vangl2 to regulate planar cell polarity during neural tube closure. *Nat Cell Biol* 2010;**12**(1):41–6; sup 41–48.

256. Wansleeben C, et al. Planar cell polarity defects and defective Vangl2 trafficking in mutants for the COPII gene Sec24b. *Development* 2010;**137**(7):1067–73.

257. Yang XY, et al. Mutations in the COPII vesicle component gene SEC24B are associated with human neural tube defects. *Hum Mutat* 2013;**34**(8):1094–101.

258. Izzi L, et al. Regulation of the TGFbeta signalling pathway by ubiquitin-mediated degradation. *Oncogene* 2004;**23**(11):2071–8.

259. Narimatsu M, et al. Regulation of planar cell polarity by Smurf ubiquitin ligases. *Cell* 2009;**137**(2):295–307.

260. Nagasaka K, et al. The cell polarity regulator hScrib controls ERK activation through a KIM site-dependent interaction. *Oncogene* 2010;**29**(38):5311–21.

261. Fernandez BA, et al. Phenotypic spectrum associated with de novo and inherited deletions and duplications at 16p11.2 in individuals ascertained for diagnosis of autism spectrum disorder. *J Med Genet* 2010;**47**(3):195–203.

262. Kumar RA, et al. Recurrent 16p11.2 microdeletions in autism. *Hum Mol Genet* 2008;**17**(4):628–38.

263. Saitta SC, et al. Independent de novo 22q11.2 deletions in first cousins with DiGeorge/velocardiofacial syndrome. *Am J Med Genet A* 2004;**124A**(3):313–7.

264. Vorstman JA, et al. The 22q11.2 deletion in children: high rate of autistic disorders and early onset of psychotic symptoms. *J Am Acad Child Adolesc Psychiatry* 2006;**45**(9):1104–13.

265. Mukaddes NM, et al. Autistic disorder and 22q11.2 duplication. *World J Biol Psychiatry* 2007;**8**(2):127–30.

266. Boutros M, et al. Dishevelled activates JNK and discriminates between JNK pathways in planar polarity and wingless signaling. *Cell* 1998;**94**(1):109–18.

267. Warchol ME, et al. Maintained expression of the planar cell polarity molecule Vangl2 and reformation of hair cell orientation in the regenerating inner ear. *J Assoc Res Otolaryngol* 2010;**11**(3):395–406.

268. Shoichet SA, et al. Truncation of the CNS-expressed JNK3 in a patient with a severe developmental epileptic encephalopathy. *Hum Genet* 2006;**118**(5):559–67.

269. Kunde SA, et al. Characterisation of de novo MAPK10/JNK3 truncation mutations associated with cognitive disorders in two unrelated patients. *Hum Genet* 2013;**132**(4):461–71.

270. Katoh Y, et al. Comparative integromics on FAT1, FAT2, FAT3 and FAT4. *Int J Mol Med* 2006;**18**(3):523–8.

271. Sharma P, et al. Regulation of long-range planar cell polarity by Fat-Dachsous signaling. *Development* 2013;**140**(18):3869–81.

272. Katoh M. Function and cancer genomics of FAT family genes (review). *Int J Oncol* 2012;**41**(6):1913–8.

273. Morris LG, et al. Recurrent somatic mutation of FAT1 in multiple human cancers leads to aberrant Wnt activation. *Nat Genet* 2013;**45**(3):253–61.

274. Blair IP, et al. Positional cloning, association analysis and expression studies provide convergent evidence that the cadherin gene FAT contains a bipolar disorder susceptibility allele. *Mol Psychiatry* 2006;**11**(4):372–83.

275. Abou Jamra R, et al. Genetic variation of the FAT gene at 4q35 is associated with bipolar affective disorder. *Mol Psychiatry* 2008;**13**(3):277–84.

276. Chien WH, et al. Identification and molecular characterization of two novel chromosomal deletions associated with autism. *Clin Genet* 2010;**78**(5):449–56.

277. Rosenfeld JA, et al. Copy number variations associated with autism spectrum disorders contribute to a spectrum of neurodevelopmental disorders. *Genet Med* 2010;**12**(11):694–702.

278. Chong WW, et al. Performance of chromosomal microarray for patients with intellectual disabilities/developmental delay, autism, and multiple congenital anomalies in a Chinese cohort. *Mol Cytogenet* 2014;**7**:34.

279. Youngs EL, et al. 12-year-old boy with a 4q35.2 microdeletion and involvement of MTNR1A, FAT1, and F11 genes. *Clin Dysmorphol* 2012;**21**(2):93–6.

280. Tanoue T, et al. New insights into Fat cadherins. *J Cell Sci* 2005;**118**(Pt 11):2347–53.

281. van Maldergem L, et al. Mental retardation with blepharo-naso-facial abnormalities and hand malformations: a new syndrome? *Clin Genet* 1992;**41**(1):22–4.

282. Zampino G, et al. Cerebro-facio-articular syndrome of Van Maldergem: confirmation of a new MR/MCA syndrome. *Clin Genet* 1994;**45**(3):140–4.

283. Alders M, et al. Hennekam syndrome can be caused by FAT4 mutations and be allelic to Van Maldergem syndrome. *Hum Genet* 2014;**133**(9):1161–7.

284. Mansour S, et al. Van Maldergem syndrome: further characterisation and evidence for neuronal migration abnormalities and autosomal recessive inheritance. *Eur J Hum Genet* 2012;**20**(10):1024–31.

285. Ishikawa HO, et al. Four-jointed is a Golgi kinase that phosphorylates a subset of cadherin domains. *Science* 2008;**321**(5887):401–4.

286. Kashevarova AA, et al. Array CGH analysis of a cohort of Russian patients with intellectual disability. *Gene* 2014;**536**(1):145–50.

287. Cooper J, et al. Molecular insights into NF2/Merlin tumor suppressor function. *FEBS Lett* 2014;**588**(16):2743–52.

288. McNeill H, et al. When pathways collide: collaboration and connivance among signalling proteins in development. *Nat Rev Mol Cell Biol* 2010;**11**(6):404–13.

289. Gillberg C. Subgroups in autism: are there behavioural phenotypes typical of underlying medical conditions? *J Intellect Disabil Res* 1992;**36**(Pt 3):201–14.

290. Bruder CE, et al. Severe phenotype of neurofibromatosis type 2 in a patient with a 7.4-MB constitutional deletion on chromosome 22: possible localization of a neurofibromatosis type 2 modifier gene? *Genes Chromosomes Cancer* 1999;**25**(2):184–90.

291. Bruder CE, et al. High resolution deletion analysis of constitutional DNA from neurofibromatosis type 2 (NF2) patients using microarray-CGH. *Hum Mol Genet* 2001;**10**(3):271–82.

292. Davidson TB, et al. Microdeletion del(22)(q12.2) encompassing the facial development-associated gene, MN1 (meningioma 1) in a child with Pierre-Robin sequence (including cleft palate) and neurofibromatosis 2 (NF2): a case report and review of the literature. *BMC Med Genet* 2012;**13**:19.

293. Beck M, et al. Craniofacial abnormalities and developmental delay in two families with overlapping 22q12.1 microdeletions involving the MN1 gene. *Am J Med Genet A* 2015;**167**(5):1047–53.

294. Sudol M, et al. Characterization of the mammalian YAP (Yes-associated protein) gene and its role in defining a novel protein module, the WW domain. *J Biol Chem* 1995;**270**(24):14733–41.

295. Komuro A, et al. WW domain-containing protein YAP associates with ErbB-4 and acts as a co-transcriptional activator for the carboxyl-terminal fragment of ErbB-4 that translocates to the nucleus. *J Biol Chem* 2003;**278**(35):33334–41.

296. Plouffe SW, et al. Disease implications of the Hippo/YAP pathway. *Trends Mol Med* 2015;**21**(4):212–22.

297. Williamson KA, et al. Heterozygous loss-of-function mutations in YAP1 cause both isolated and syndromic optic fissure closure defects. *Am J Hum Genet* 2014;**94**(2):295–302.

298. Collum LM. Uveal colobomata and other anomalies in three generations of one family. *Br J Ophthalmol* 1971;**55**(7):458–61.

299. Kingston HM, et al. An autosomal dominant syndrome of uveal colobomata, cleft lip and palate, and mental retardation. *J Med Genet* 1982;**19**(6):444–6.

300. Goddard AD, et al. Cloning of the murine homolog of the leukemia-associated PML gene. *Mamm Genome* 1995;**6**(10): 732–7.

301. Lapi E, et al. PML, YAP, and p73 are components of a proapoptotic autoregulatory feedback loop. *Mol Cell* 2008;**32**(6):803–14.

302. Smith M, et al. Analysis of a 1-megabase deletion in 15q22-q23 in an autistic patient: identification of candidate genes for autism and of homologous DNA segments in 15q22-q23 and 15q11-q13. *Am J Med Genet* 2000;**96**(6):765–70.

303. Jovanovic-Privrodski JD, et al. Autism and hypoplastic corpus callosum in a case of monocentric marker chromosome 15. *Pediatr Neurol* 2009;**41**(1):65–7.

304. Humbert PO, et al. Control of tumourigenesis by the Scribble/ Dlg/Lgl polarity module. *Oncogene* 2008;**27**(55):6888–907.

305. Crespi B. Autism and cancer risk. *Autism Res* 2011;**4**(4):302–10.

306. Yates LL, et al. The PCP genes Celsr1 and Vangl2 are required for normal lung branching morphogenesis. *Hum Mol Genet* 2010; **19**(11):2251–67.

307. Tissir F, et al. Lack of cadherins Celsr2 and Celsr3 impairs ependymal ciliogenesis, leading to fatal hydrocephalus. *Nat Neurosci* 2010;**13**(6):700–7.

308. Yasunaga T, et al. Regulation of basal body and ciliary functions by Diversin. *Mech Dev* 2011;**128**(7–10):376–86.

309. Ikeda M, et al. Expression and proliferation-promoting role of Diversin in the neuronally committed precursor cells migrating in the adult mouse brain. *Stem Cells* 2010;**28**(11):2017–26.

310. Wilkinson MB, et al. A novel role of the WNT-dishevelled-GSK3beta signaling cascade in the mouse nucleus accumbens in a social defeat model of depression. *J Neurosci* 2011;**31**(25): 9084–92.

311. Wang J, et al. Dishevelled genes mediate a conserved mammalian PCP pathway to regulate convergent extension during neurulation. *Development* 2006;**133**(9):1767–78.

312. Hamblet NS, et al. Dishevelled 2 is essential for cardiac outflow tract development, somite segmentation and neural tube closure. *Development* 2002;**129**(24):5827–38.

313. Wang J, et al. Regulation of polarized extension and planar cell polarity in the cochlea by the vertebrate PCP pathway. *Nat Genet* 2005;**37**(9):980–5.

314. Etheridge SL, et al. Murine dishevelled 3 functions in redundant pathways with dishevelled 1 and 2 in normal cardiac outflow tract, cochlea, and neural tube development. *PLoS Genet* 2008; **4**(11):e1000259.

315. Ohata S, et al. Loss of *Dishevelleds* disrupts planar polarity in ependymal motile cilia and results in hydrocephalus. *Neuron* 2014;**83**(3):558–71.

316. Hua ZL, et al. Frizzled3 controls axonal development in distinct populations of cranial and spinal motor neurons. *Elife* 2013;**2**: e01482.

317. Wang L, et al. Impaired methylation modifications of FZD3 alter chromatin accessibility and are involved in congenital hydrocephalus pathogenesis. *Brain Res* 2014;**1569**:48–56.

318. Wang Y, et al. Progressive cerebellar, auditory, and esophageal dysfunction caused by targeted disruption of the frizzled-4 gene. *J Neurosci* 2001;**21**(13):4761–71.

319. Xu Q, et al. Vascular development in the retina and inner ear: control by Norrin and Frizzled-4, a high-affinity ligand-receptor pair. *Cell* 2004;**116**(6):883–95.

320. Ishikawa T, et al. Mouse Wnt receptor gene Fzd5 is essential for yolk sac and placental angiogenesis. *Development* 2001;**128**(1): 25–33.

321. Ye X, et al. The Norrin/Frizzled4 signaling pathway in retinal vascular development and disease. *Trends Mol Med* 2010;**16**(9): 417–25.

322. Majumdar A, et al. Wnt11 and Ret/Gdnf pathways cooperate in regulating ureteric branching during metanephric kidney development. *Development* 2003;**130**(14):3175–85.

323. Tao H, et al. Mouse prickle1, the homolog of a PCP gene, is essential for epiblast apical-basal polarity. *Proc Natl Acad Sci USA* 2009; **106**(34):14426–31.

324. Okuda H, et al. Mouse Prickle1 and Prickle2 are expressed in postmitotic neurons and promote neurite outgrowth. *FEBS Lett* 2007;**581**(24):4754–60.

325. Liu C, et al. Null and hypomorph Prickle1 alleles in mice phenocopy human Robinow syndrome and disrupt signaling downstream of Wnt5a. *Biol Open* 2014;**3**(9):861–70.

326. Sowers LP, et al. Defective motile cilia in Prickle2-deficient mice. *J Neurogenet* 2014;**28**(1–2):146–52.

327. Kibar Z, et al. Ltap, a mammalian homolog of Drosophila Strabismus/Van Gogh, is altered in the mouse neural tube mutant Loop-tail. *Nat Genet* 2001;**28**(3):251–5.

328. Murdoch JN, et al. Severe neural tube defects in the loop-tail mouse result from mutation of Lpp1, a novel gene involved in floor plate specification. *Hum Mol Genet* 2001;**10**(22):2593–601.

329. Greene ND, et al. Abnormalities of floor plate, notochord and somite differentiation in the loop-tail (Lp) mouse: a model of severe neural tube defects. *Mech Dev* 1998;**73**(1):59–72.

330. Torban E, et al. Independent mutations in mouse Vangl2 that cause neural tube defects in looptail mice impair interaction with members of the Dishevelled family. *J Biol Chem* 2004;**279**(50): 52703–13.

331. Shafer B, et al. Vangl2 promotes Wnt/planar cell polarity-like signaling by antagonizing Dvl1-mediated feedback inhibition in growth cone guidance. *Dev Cell* 2011;**20**(2):177–91.

332. Darken RS, et al. The planar polarity gene strabismus regulates convergent extension movements in Xenopus. *EMBO J* 2002; **21**(5):976–85.

333. Jessen JR, et al. Zebrafish trilobite identifies new roles for Strabismus in gastrulation and neuronal movements. *Nat Cell Biol* 2002;**4**(8):610–5.

334. Torban E, et al. Van Gogh-like2 (Strabismus) and its role in planar cell polarity and convergent extension in vertebrates. *Trends Genet* 2004;**20**(11):570–7.

335. Marlow F, et al. Functional interactions of genes mediating convergent extension, knypek and trilobite, during the partitioning of the eye primordium in zebrafish. *Dev Biol* 1998;**203**(2): 382–99.

336. Bingham S, et al. The Zebrafish trilobite gene is essential for tangential migration of branchiomotor neurons. *Dev Biol* 2002; **242**(2):149–60.

337. Vivancos V, et al. Wnt activity guides facial branchiomotor neuron migration, and involves the PCP pathway and JNK and ROCK kinases. *Neural Dev* 2009;**4**:7.

338. Glasco DM, et al. The mouse Wnt/PCP protein Vangl2 is necessary for migration of facial branchiomotor neurons, and functions independently of Dishevelled. *Dev Biol* 2012;**369**(2):211–22.

339. Caddy J, et al. Epidermal wound repair is regulated by the planar cell polarity signaling pathway. *Dev Cell* 2010;**19**(1):138–47.

340. Vandenberg AL, et al. Non-canonical Wnt signaling regulates cell polarity in female reproductive tract development via van gogh-like 2. *Development* 2009;**136**(9):1559–70.

341. Katoh M. WNT/PCP signaling pathway and human cancer (review). *Oncol Rep* 2005;**14**(6):1583–8.

342. Coyle RC, et al. Membrane-type 1 matrix metalloproteinase regulates cell migration during zebrafish gastrulation: evidence for an interaction with non-canonical Wnt signaling. *Exp Cell Res* 2008; **314**(10):2150–62.

343. Cantrell VA, et al. The planar cell polarity protein Van Gogh-Like 2 regulates tumor cell migration and matrix metalloproteinase-dependent invasion. *Cancer Lett* 2010;**287**(1):54–61.

344. Devenport D, et al. Planar polarization in embryonic epidermis orchestrates global asymmetric morphogenesis of hair follicles. *Nat Cell Biol* 2008;**10**(11):1257–68.

345. May-Simera HL, et al. Bbs8, together with the planar cell polarity protein Vangl2, is required to establish left-right asymmetry in zebrafish. *Dev Biol* 2010;**345**(2):215–25.

346. Borovina A, et al. Vangl2 directs the posterior tilting and asymmetric localization of motile primary cilia. *Nat Cell Biol* 2010;**12**(4):407–12.

347. Song H, et al. Planar cell polarity breaks bilateral symmetry by controlling ciliary positioning. *Nature* 2010;**466**(7304):378–82.

348. Yates LL, et al. The planar cell polarity gene Vangl2 is required for mammalian kidney-branching morphogenesis and glomerular maturation. *Hum Mol Genet* 2010;**19**(23):4663–76.

349. Li D, et al. Dishevelled-associated activator of morphogenesis 1 (Daam1) is required for heart morphogenesis. *Development* 2011;**138**(2):303–15.

350. Lopez-Escobar B, et al. The effect of maternal diabetes on the Wnt-PCP pathway during embryogenesis as reflected in the developing mouse eye. *Dis Model Mech* 2015;**8**(2):157–68.

351. Yang X, et al. SEC14 and spectrin domains 1 (Sestd1) and Dapper antagonist of catenin 1 (Dact1) scaffold proteins cooperatively regulate the Van Gogh-like 2 (Vangl2) four-pass transmembrane protein and planar cell polarity (PCP) pathway during embryonic development in mice. *J Biol Chem* 2013;**288**(28):20111–20.

352. Wen J, et al. Loss of Dact1 disrupts planar cell polarity signaling by altering dishevelled activity and leads to posterior malformation in mice. *J Biol Chem* 2010;**285**(14):11023–30.

353. Schoen CJ, et al. Diaphanous homolog 3 (Diap3) overexpression causes progressive hearing loss and inner hair cell defects in a transgenic mouse model of human deafness. *PLoS One* 2013;**8**(2):e56520.

354. Mahoney ZX, et al. Discs-large homolog 1 regulates smooth muscle orientation in the mouse ureter. *Proc Natl Acad Sci USA* 2006;**103**(52):19872–7.

355. Cuthbert PC, et al. Synapse-associated protein 102/dlgh3 couples the NMDA receptor to specific plasticity pathways and learning strategies. *J Neurosci* 2007;**27**(10):2673–82.

356. Cox BJ, et al. Phenotypic annotation of the mouse X chromosome. *Genome Res* 2010;**20**(8):1154–64.

357. Horev G, et al. Dosage-dependent phenotypes in models of 16p11.2 lesions found in autism. *Proc Natl Acad Sci USA* 2011;**108**(41):17076–81.

358. Portmann T, et al. Behavioral abnormalities and circuit defects in the basal ganglia of a mouse model of 16p11.2 deletion syndrome. *Cell Rep* 2014;**7**(4):1077–92.

359. Mazzucchelli C, et al. Knockout of ERK1 MAP kinase enhances synaptic plasticity in the striatum and facilitates striatal-mediated learning and memory. *Neuron* 2002;**34**(5):807–20.

360. Satoh Y, et al. Extracellular signal-regulated kinase 2 (ERK2) knockdown mice show deficits in long-term memory; ERK2 has a specific function in learning and memory. *J Neurosci* 2007;**27**(40):10765–76.

361. Satoh Y, et al. ERK2 contributes to the control of social behaviors in mice. *J Neurosci* 2011;**31**(33):11953–67.

362. Yin A, et al. The developmental pattern of the RAS/RAF/Erk1/2 pathway in the BTBR autism mouse model. *Int J Dev Neurosci* 2014;**39**:2–8.

363. Satoh Y, et al. Deletion of ERK1 and ERK2 in the CNS causes cortical abnormalities and neonatal lethality: Erk1 deficiency enhances the impairment of neurogenesis in Erk2-deficient mice. *J Neurosci* 2011;**31**(3):1149–55.

364. Mochizuki T, et al. Molecular cloning of a gene for inversion of embryo turning (inv) with cystic kidney. *Nephrol Dial Transplant* 2002;**17**(Suppl. 9):68–70.

365. Mochizuki T, et al. Cloning of inv, a gene that controls left/right asymmetry and kidney development. *Nature* 1998;**395**(6698):177–81.

366. McQuinn TC, et al. Cardiopulmonary malformations in the inv/inv mouse. *Anat Rec* 2001;**263**(1):62–71.

367. Phillips CL, et al. Renal cysts of inv/inv mice resemble early infantile nephronophthisis. *J Am Soc Nephrol* 2004;**15**(7):1744–55.

368. Belgardt BF, et al. Hypothalamic and pituitary c-Jun N-terminal kinase 1 signaling coordinately regulates glucose metabolism. *Proc Natl Acad Sci USA* 2010;**107**(13):6028–33.

369. Dong C, et al. Defective T cell differentiation in the absence of Jnk1. *Science* 1998;**282**(5396):2092–5.

370. Weston CR, et al. The c-Jun NH2-terminal kinase is essential for epidermal growth factor expression during epidermal morphogenesis. *Proc Natl Acad Sci USA* 2004;**101**(39):14114–9.

371. Kuan CY, et al. The Jnk1 and Jnk2 protein kinases are required for regional specific apoptosis during early brain development. *Neuron* 1999;**22**(4):667–76.

372. Sabapathy K, et al. Defective neural tube morphogenesis and altered apoptosis in the absence of both JNK1 and JNK2. *Mech Dev* 1999;**89**(1–2):115–24.

373. Hunot S, et al. JNK-mediated induction of cyclooxygenase 2 is required for neurodegeneration in a mouse model of Parkinson's disease. *Proc Natl Acad Sci USA* 2004;**101**(2):665–70.

374. Yang DD, et al. Absence of excitotoxicity-induced apoptosis in the hippocampus of mice lacking the Jnk3 gene. *Nature* 1997;**389**(6653):865–70.

375. Huang KM, et al. Xcat, a novel mouse model for Nance-Horan syndrome inhibits expression of the cytoplasmic-targeted Nhs1 isoform. *Hum Mol Genet* 2006;**15**(2):319–27.

376. Laird DJ, et al. Ror2 enhances polarity and directional migration of primordial germ cells. *PLoS Genet* 2011;**7**(12):e1002428.

377. Takeuchi S, et al. Mouse Ror2 receptor tyrosine kinase is required for the heart development and limb formation. *Genes Cells* 2000;**5**(1):71–8.

378. Raz R, et al. The mutation ROR2W749X, linked to human BDB, is a recessive mutation in the mouse, causing brachydactyly, mediating patterning of joints and modeling recessive Robinow syndrome. *Development* 2008;**135**(9):1713–23.

379. Haegel H, et al. Lack of beta-catenin affects mouse development at gastrulation. *Development* 1995;**121**(11):3529–37.

380. Tsukiyama T, et al. Mice lacking Wnt2b are viable and display a postnatal olfactory bulb phenotype. *Neurosci Lett* 2012;**512**(1):48–52.

381. Boyer A, et al. WNT4 is required for normal ovarian follicle development and female fertility. *FASEB J* 2010;**24**(8):3010–25.

382. Yamaguchi TP, et al. A Wnt5a pathway underlies outgrowth of multiple structures in the vertebrate embryo. *Development* 1999;**126**(6):1211–23.

383. Zhao C, et al. Hippocampal and visuospatial learning defects in mice with a deletion of frizzled 9, a gene in the Williams syndrome deletion interval. *Development* 2005;**132**(12):2917–27.

384. Sowers LP, et al. Disruption of the non-canonical Wnt gene PRICKLE2 leads to autism-like behaviors with evidence for hippocampal synaptic dysfunction. *Mol Psychiatry* 2013;**18**(10):1077–89.

14

Protocadherin Mutations in Neurodevelopmental Disorders

Duyen Pham[1,2,], Chuan Tan[1,*], Claire Homan[2],*
Lachlan Jolly[1,2], Jozef Gecz[1,2]

[1]School of Medicine, University of Adelaide, Adelaide, Australia;
[2]Robinson Research Institute, University of Adelaide, Adelaide, Australia

INTRODUCTION

Neurodevelopmental disorders are characterized by early impairment of growth and function of the brain, resulting in cognitive, neurological, and/or psychiatric dysfunction.[1,2] Children with neurodevelopmental disorders can experience difficulties with language, speech, motor skills, behavior, memory, learning, and/or other neurological functions.[3] These disorders have significant psychosocial consequences resulting in both economic and mental burden not only for the patients but also for their families and society as a whole. This predominantly stems from a loss of independence in self-care, social interaction, decision-making, academic achievement, work, leisure, health, and safety.[4] An estimated 70% of intellectual disability (ID) families sacrifice work opportunities to care for the affected individuals, incurring an annual cost of $15 billion in Australia alone.[4] These factors, along with the prevalence of neurodevelopmental disorders and resulting lifestyle limitations, highlight the need for continuing research in this field.

Some common forms of these disorders (on which this review will focus) include ID, epilepsy, autism spectrum disorders (ASDs), bipolar disorder (BD), and schizophrenia (SZ).[5] Intellectual disability is the most common neurodevelopmental disorder, affecting up to 3% of the global population.[4] Epilepsy and ASD, on the other hand, account for approximately 0.5%[6] and 0.62%[7] of the total global burden of disease, respectively. Similar prevalence rates are also recorded for BD (2%)[8] and SZ (0.7%).[9] These disorders are highly heterogeneous and are caused by multiple, genetic, and environmental factors. In addition, the highly overlapping nature of the clinical phenotypes makes it extremely difficult to diagnose or differentiate accurately between the different disorders.[1,10] For example, social cognitive impairment is a common feature in both ASD and SZ,

---

*These two authors contributed equally.

and psychosis is frequently observed in SZ and BD. Children with epilepsy may also have other comorbidities such as developmental delay, ASD, and SZ. Taken together, this creates an enormous challenge for diagnosing these disorders.

Recent advances in deoxyribonucleic acid (DNA) sequencing technologies including whole exome sequencing, whole genome sequencing, and genome-wide association studies (GWAS) have contributed to more accurate and reliable diagnosis for some of these disorders.[11,12] These new technologies have also led to a substantial increase in the identification of novel genes associated with neurodevelopmental disorders. These include genes with a wide range of roles in early brain development, including, for example, neurogenesis, neuronal migration, neurite growth, and synaptogenesis.[13–15] The genes themselves encode many different types of proteins and include a number of cell adhesion molecules, a focus of this review.[16] Various genes in the protocadherin (PCDH) family, specifically the delta-2-protocadherin ($\delta2$-PCDH) family, have been shown to be associated with epilepsy, ID, ASD, SZ, and BD (Table 1). Currently, information about how mutations in the PCDH gene family affect the function and/or structure of these proteins is limited. As such, how they contribute to the molecular, cell and developmental mechanisms underlying neurodevelopmental disorders remains to be resolved. In this review,

we discuss different neurodevelopmental disorders and the role of their respective associated $\delta2$-PCDHs, including new insights into potential novel mechanisms. We will primarily focus on previously published mutations in PCDH19, a member of the $\delta2$-PCDHs, and how these mutations contribute to PCDH19-Female Epilepsy (PCDH19-FE). We will also focus on the different mutations identified in PCDH19, which have resulted in several distinct neurodevelopmental phenotypes with varying levels of severity.

PROTOCADHERINS IN EPILEPSY AND ID

Epilepsy is a neurological disorder characterized by recurrent episodes of sensory disturbance, loss of consciousness, and/or convulsions, and is associated with abnormal electrical activity in the brain.[17] Intellectual disability is a neurodevelopmental disorder characterized by impaired intellect and adaptive functioning, which is defined by an intellect quotient (IQ) score below 70 and diagnosed before the age of 18 years.[18] These two disorders are independent in their classification, owing to their distinct characteristics; however, varying degrees of overlapping clinical phenotypes are observed. It is therefore unsurprising that the genetic abnormalities causing these conditions can be either

TABLE 1 Protocadherins Associated with Neurodevelopmental Disorders

Symbol	Name	Synonyms	Related Neurodevelopmental Disorders	References
PCDH-α	Protocadherin-α	Cadherin-like neuronal receptor	ASD, Bipolar, Schizophrenia (SZ)	15–17
PCDH-β	Protocadherin-β		Bipolar, SZ	18,19
PCDH-γ	Protocadherin-γ		Bipolar, SZ	18,19
PCDH7	Protocadherin-7	BH-protocadherin NF-protocadherin	Epilepsy	20
PCDH8	Protocadherin-8	Arcadlin	SZ	21
PCDH9			ASD	22,23
PCDH10	OL-protocadherin		ASD	24
PCDH11X	Protocadherin-11X	Protocadherin-X	SZ	25,26
PCDH11Y	Protocadherin 11Y	Protocadherin-Y Protocadherin-PC	ASD	25
PCDH17	Protocadherin-17	Protocadherin-68	Depression, SZ, ASD	27,28
PCDH18		Protocadherin-68-like protein (PCDH68L)	ID	29
PCDH19	Protocadherin-19		PCDH19-FE, epilepsy, ID, ASD, SZ	26,30–34

unique or shared among the disorders. Multiple mutations (genetic pleiotropy) in the same gene can lead to several distinct clinical phenotypes. A good example is mutations in the Aristaless-related homeobox gene (*ARX*).[19] In contrast, one disorder can result from mutations in multiple different genes (genetic heterogeneity). A classical demonstration of this is Dravet syndrome, in which approximately 80% of genetically solved cases have mutations in *SCN1A* and the remaining 20% of cases mostly have mutations in *SCN2A, SCN1B,* or *GABARG2*.[20]

The *δ2-PCDH* subfamily is part of the larger cadherin superfamily consisting of over 100 members.[21] δ2-Protocadherins are predominately expressed in the central nervous system, with roles in neuronal development and function, in particular, neuronal migration, specification, and synaptic plasticity.[21] Hence, genetic alterations in any one of these genes could be detrimental to normal brain development, resulting in an underlying neurodevelopmental disorder. *PCDH19* is a good example of this, because mutations in *PCDH19* result in *PCDH19*-FE (previously known as epilepsy and mental retardation limited to females (EFMR); OMIM #300088). This disorder was first identified in a large multigenerational family in which only females were affected.[22] Twenty years later, the causative mutation was mapped to the X-chromosome using linkage analysis,[23] but only recently was the responsible gene, *PCDH19*, identified.[24]

PCDH19 encodes a protein with typical features of the δ2-PCDH subfamily, with six conserved cadherin repeats in the extracellular domain, a transmembrane domain, and conserved CM1-CM2 motifs in the C-terminal region.[25] Protocadherin-19 is thought to be predominantly expressed at the cell membrane and involved in cell adhesion.[25] In contrast to the classical cadherins, which associate through strong homophilic interactions, PCDH19 forms only weak homophilic interactions, although these are likely crucial for specific cellular mechanisms. For example, PCDH17, another δ2-PCDH family member most closely related to PCDH19, has been shown to have weak homophilic interactions important for axon bundling.[26] Thus, despite facilitating weak interactions, the specificity of PCDH interactions is crucial for downstream signaling pathways.

To date, more than 100 unique germline *PCDH19* mutations in females and one somatic mutation in a male have been reported in *PCDH19*-FE. Mutations have been identified, both in small families and in singleton cases.[27,28] Most mutations are observed in the extracellular domain of the protein, and all missense mutations cluster exclusively within this region. That nonsense mutations which lead to nonsense-mediated messenger ribonucleic acid (mRNA) decay and complete loss of protein have been described in patients

with typical clinical presentation of *PCDH19*-FE suggests that all mutations are likely loss of function.[29,30] *PCDH19* is one of the most commonly mutated genes causing infantile encephalopathy.[31] *PCDH19*-FE pedigrees are characterized by heterozygous females being symptomatic whereas hemizygous males are spared. Affected females show early-onset (6- to 36-month) clusters of seizures, often triggered by febrile illness. These clusters of seizures can be brief or prolonged, occurring up to 10 times a day and lasting over several days, with most seizures resistant to current drug treatments. The phenotypic spectrum of this disorder is extremely heterogeneous, ranging from benign focal epilepsies with normal intelligence to severe generalized or multifocal epilepsy resembling Dravet syndrome.[31,32] Seizure frequency and severity tend to decrease with age; most patients are seizure-free by the time they reach adulthood. Several other comorbidities including, ID, autism, and SZ are also common in these patients.[29,31] Furthermore, although most mutations show complete penetrance, incomplete penetrance has also been observed in mothers with a severely affected daughter.[33]

Why only females are affected remains a difficult question. There appears to be no major difference between the clinical phenotypes of patients with either partial or complete loss of the PCDH19 protein. Compared with other known X-chromosome disorders,[19,34] the X-linked inheritance of this disorder is unusual, with affected females and normal carrier males. One theory behind this unusual mode of inheritance for *PCDH19*-FE is cellular interference, which is observed in craniofrontonasal syndrome, caused by mutations in ephrin-B1 (*EFNB1*).[35] Both *PCDH19* and *EFNB1* loci are subjected to random X-chromosome inactivation. We postulated that the coexistence of a mosaic population of PCDH19-positive and PCDH19-negative cells in affected females could underlie the pathogenesis of the disorder through altered cell–cell interactions and/or signaling.[24] Support for this model has come from the discovery of a male with a somatic mutation in *PCDH19*, presenting with the *PCDH19*-FE phenotype.[30] Although this proposed model of cellular interference has not yet been experimentally validated, supportive evidence in principal has been derived through studies of *Pcdh17*; expression of a wild type and a mutant *Pcdh17* in amygdala explants of *Pcdh17* knockout mouse resulted in homotypic axonal contacts (i.e., wild-type–wild-type and mutant–mutant) leading to the mutant axons having migration and growth cone defects.[26] It remains a challenge to address this mechanism for *PCDH19* mutations.

By studying the mechanism of *PCDH19*-FE, we have shown that neurosteroid metabolism may be an additional mechanism underlying the disorder.[36] We have shown that the blood levels of the neurosteroid, allopregnanolone, and the enzyme aldo-keto reductase (AKR1C2/3), involved in reducing progesterone to allopregnanolone, were decreased in *PCDH19*-FE patients compared with normal controls.[36] The role of steroid hormones in seizure susceptibility has been widely studied and is highly controversial. This is particularly well demonstrated in women with catamenial epilepsy, in whom seizure activity has been linked to fluctuating estrogen and progesterone levels during the menstrual cycle.[37] Because the seizure onset and offset age of *PCDH19*-FE patients falls within the period when steroid hormone levels are low and high, respectively, it is therefore plausible to speculate that fluctuations in steroid hormones may be associated with both the onset and offset of seizures in patients. However, the downstream mechanism by which neurosteroids are involved in *PCDH19*-FE is still being elucidated.

Other investigations have been directed toward compensatory mechanisms, which may protect boys from this disorder. Previously we and others[23] speculated that *PCDH11Y*, a Y-chromosome *PCDH* also expressed in brain, could compensate for the loss of *PCDH19*.[23,24] Although *PCDH19* and *PCDH11Y* are expressed in the brain, they have distinct expression patterns, a feature that is also common among other family members. Several studies have investigated the expression pattern of a number of different *PCDHs* *Pcdh7*, *Pcdh9*, *Pcdh10*, *Pcdh11*, *Pcdh17*, *Pcdh18*, and *Pcdh19* in mouse and rat brains.[38,39] They showed that the expression patterns of different *PCDHs* are unique, even within the same subfamily of *PCDHs* , with region specific expression observed.[40] Interestingly, *Pcdh19* and *Pcdh17* appear to have some expression overlap in specific brain regions.[38] Protocadherin 17 is evolutionary the most closely related *δ2-PCDH* to *PCDH19*.[21] These two genes appear to have arisen from the same locus by duplication; therefore, it is conceivable that if there were a compensatory mechanism in the absence of *PCDH19*, *PCDH17* is the likely molecule compensating for PCDH19. Mouse knockout studies have established that *Pcdh17* may have a role in depression, another neurodevelopmental disorder.[41] The authors demonstrated that *Pcdh17* knockout mice were more resistant to depression compared with wild-type mice, which suggests that *Pcdh17* is involved in the emotional networks. Although depression has not been seen in *PCDH19*-FE patients, obligate carrier males show some level of anxiety and rigid inflexible behavior.[32] This suggests that although evolutionary similar, *PCDH19* and *PCDH17* may have some level of overlapping functional roles but cannot fully substitute each other.

Still other molecular mechanisms are likely important for the development of *PCDH19*-FE. For example,

zebrafish pcdh19 forms a heterotypic complex with N-cadherin through the extracellular domain in a calcium-dependent manner.[42,43] This interaction between pcdh19 and N-cadherin appears to be crucial for neuronal migration during zebrafish anterior neurulation.[43] In addition to N-cadherin, both chicken and mouse Pcdh19 have been shown to interact with Nck-associated protein 1 (NAP1)[44,45] and cytoplasmic fragile X mental retardation 1 (FMR1) interacting protein 2 (CYFIP2)[44,45] through the C-terminal region. Together, these three proteins form part of the WAVE regulatory complex (WRC) that controls actin cytoskeletal dynamics within the cell (Figure 1).[45,46] The WRC has been reported to form a complex with the C-terminal region of a range of PCDHs including PCDH8, PCDH10, PCDH17, and PCDH18. Although this may suggest a generalized role for PCDHs in the regulation and formation of actin cytoskeletal networks through an association with the WAVE complex, the molecular mechanism mediating these networks has not yet been established. Based on current evidence, it is reasonable to predict that by acting through the WRC, other PCDHs could partially compensate for the loss of PCDH19.

In addition to the well-known association of *PCDH19* with both epilepsy and ID, additional members of the *δ2-PCDHs* family have been associated with these disorders. A GWAS reported *PCDH7* as a possible epilepsy-associated locus.[47] This is the first evidence indicating involvement of PCDH7 in a neuronal disorder, because there is limited study on *PCDH7* aside from its association with cancer. Interestingly, *PCDH7* is regulated by methyl CpG binding protein 2 (MECP2) in neuronal cells.[48] *MECP2* is a well-known gene; mutations in *MECP2* cause Rett syndrome, a dominant neurodevelopmental disorder that is similar to *PCDH19*-FE. Severely affected girls have developmental delay, seizures, ID, and loss of purposeful use of the hands.

A 1.53-Mb deletion at 4q28.3 was detected in a boy with severe ID by array study.[40] This genomic region contains *PCDH18*. The deletion was inherited from a healthy mother and grandmother. As a result, haploinsufficiency with reduced expressivity and incomplete penetrance may be the mechanism contributing to ID in this patient. The authors raised the possibility that *PCDH18* may have a role in ID and could be a novel ID gene.

PROTOCADHERINS IN ASD

Autism spectrum disorders are group of neurodevelopmental disorders characterized by repetitive behavior, deficits in both language and communication skills, and inability to engage in reciprocal social

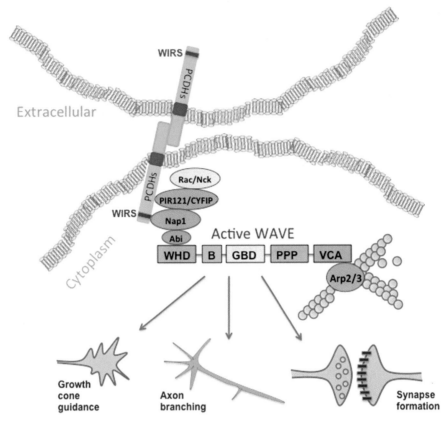

FIGURE 1 **Protocadherins associate with the WAVE regulatory complex (WRC).** Protocadherins including PCDH8, PCDH10, PCDH17, PCDH18, and PCDH19 interact with the WRC through its peptide motif known as WIRS in the C-terminal region of the protein. Association of these membrane proteins to the WRC and actin cytoskeleton could result in various downstream signaling.

interactions.[49] Similar to other neurodevelopmental disorders, the onset of ASD occurs in the first 3 years of life. According to the fifth edition of the *Diagnostic and Statistical Manual of Mental Disorder*, ASDs are made up of four separate disorders including autistic disorder, Asperger disorder, childhood disintegrative disorder, and pervasive developmental disorder, not otherwise specified (PDD-NOS).[50] The global prevalence of ASD is estimated to be 6.2 per 1000 individuals, with a four times higher ratio in males compared with females.[7] This prevalence rate of ASD has risen significantly over the past 2 decades owing to increased awareness of the disorder, broadening of the diagnostic criteria,[50] and environmental factors acting on genetically vulnerable backgrounds.[51,52] In addition to variable severity of the core deficits, ASD patients also often present with other comorbidities such as epilepsy, ID, motor control problems, attention-deficit hyperactivity disorder, anxiety, sleep disorders, and gastrointestinal problems.[53,54]

Family studies show that ASDs have a strong genetic contribution and are highly heritable. Concordance rates in monozygotic twins have been reported to be around 86–100% versus 20–40% in dizygotic twins,[55] and

siblings with ASD patients have significantly (25-fold) increased risk of presenting with ASD.[56,57] Moreover, ASD with a genetic cause from association with a known genetic or chromosomal syndrome accounts for around 10% of cases. A further 10% of cases result from de novo mutations, copy number variants (CNVs), or chromosomal rearrangements. In some cases, both genetic and environmental factors are involved.[58]

The genetic etiology of ASD is extremely heterogeneous. Whereas in epilepsy and ID single *PCHD* gene mutations of major effect have been shown to be causative, for ASD the relationship is more complex. Most of the reported links of ASD to *PCHD* genes come from the association studies. This is most likely due to the high variability in genetic background and diversity of symptoms of ASD, which makes it a multidomain disorder. Genomic and genetic studies have found a large number of genes and genomic loci that are associated with the risk and/or occurrence of ASD. Rare and de novo mutations pose a substantial risk for ASD and common polymorphisms have also been shown to increase the risk factor for ASD.[59–61] It has been previously suggested that ASD may result from a combination of both rare and common variants,[62] as seen with SZ.

There are several lines of published evidence suggesting that deregulation of *PCDH19* may contribute to the pathogenesis of ASD. The phenotypes of this disorder are a common feature observed in patients with *PCDH19*-FE, with around 60% of *PCDH19*-FE patients diagnosed with ASD.[63] It is currently unknown whether mutations in *PCDH19* directly cause ASD or the clinical phenotype of ASD is secondary, stemming from defects in developmental process triggered by early-onset seizures. Current evidence supports that hemizygous males with *PCDH19* mutations are unaffected, with no epilepsy or ID reported to date.[31,32] However, initial data suggest that carrier males can present with obsessive, rigid inflexible behavior.[32] Both phenotypic features could resemble a mild clinical phenotype of ASD, but to date no extensive examination has been conducted.

Aside from the coexisting phenotypes observed between *PCDH19*-FE and ASD, a number of *PCDH19* mutations in male patients diagnosed with ASD have been identified in targeted sequencing studies. A rare missense variant H645Q in PCDH19 (reported as H146Q using the older version of RefSeq NM_020766.1) was first identified in a male patient with ASD from direct sequencing of 111 X-linked synaptic genes in a cohort of 143 ASD patients.[64] Furthermore, another rare missense variant V590A (reported as V91Q using the older version of RefSeq NM_020766.1) was reported in the same study allegedly causing SZ. Mutations of *PCDH19* causing ASD or SZ are not unexpected because both of these disorders are common comorbidities often seen in *PCDH19*-FE patients. However, one needs to be careful when implicating such variants in these disorders, and in particular in males, without thorough experimental or statistical genetic evidence. A sequencing study using a cohort of 20 males with ASD also revealed a single missense variant in *PCDH19* in a boy diagnosed with Asperger syndrome without epilepsy and ID.[65] In silico prediction software revealed that this amino acid is highly conserved across species. Unlike all other missense changes in *PCDH19* associated with *PCDH19*-FE, all of which affect the extracellular domain of the protein involved in homophilic cell adhesion interactions, this mutation leads to an amino acid change in the C-terminal, intracellular region of the protein, which is likely involved in signal transduction. This is the first missense variant reported in the C-terminus region of the PCDH19 to be linked to a disorder. This leads us to speculate that mutations in different regions of *PCDH19* could result in different disease phenotypes; however, more experimental work is required to affirm this hypothesis.

Other PCDHs also been associated with ASD: for example, PCDH10 (also known as OL-PCDH) is another δ2-PCDH that has been implicated in ASD. Like *PCDH19*, *PCDH10* is expressed predominantly in the central nervous system. Within the brain, Pcdh10 is present in the olfactory bulb, the limbic system, and the cerebellum.[66,67] Evidence supporting *PCDH10* as a candidate gene for ASD was first reported in a study in which homozygous deletion of 321 kb on 4q28, in close proximity to *PCDH10*, was identified.[68] This deletion was more prevalent in ASD cases compared with controls, but evidence to support the involvement of PCDH10 was only speculative. However, knockout mice studies have provided significant evidence for the importance of the role of *Pcdh10* in brain development, where it is required for axon guidance through the ventral telencephalon.[69] Mice lacking *Pcdh10* show misguiding of axons in the ventral telencephalon, which suggests that *PCDH10* may be responsible for the underlying deficits in communication and behavioral function observed in patients with ASD. Thus, PCDH10 may be considered a candidate gene warranting further investigation.

Copy number variants in *PCDH9* introns have also been reported in ASD patients,[70] although to date, no mutations have been reported in the exonic regions. Again, the expression and functional studies on *PCDH9* provide evidence that this gene is important for brain development. Protocadherin-9 is a δ1-PCHD that is predominately expressed in the cortex and cranial ganglia, with expression highest during development.[39,71] Pcdh9 was also found in various brain nuclei and fibers of the vestibular and oculomotor systems in a developing mouse brain.[71] In cultured cells, Pcdh9 localized at cell—cell contact sites, in the growth cone, and along neurites.[71] Furthermore, it is expressed in specific cortical layers during development,[39,72] all of which suggests that it may be involved in the formation of correct neural circuits during development. Thus, although the genetic evidence for its involvement is only speculative and the exact mechanism of how PCDH9 is involved in ASD is still being determined, it should be considered an ASD candidate gene in future studies.

Other PCDHs, including PCHD-α (PCDHA) and PCDHA13, have also been reported to be associated with ASD.[73,74] This includes a single de novo deletion in PCDHA13 detected in a male patient with autism through exome sequencing of 343 families.[74] In a genetic association study of over 3000 patients, one single nucleotide polymorphism (SNP) (rs1119032) of PCDHA was significantly associated with autism. Protocadherin-α has a crucial role in neuronal survival, synaptic activity, and axonal convergence and is important in learning and memory.[75,76] PcdhA knockout mice showed abnormal distribution of serotonin in various brain regions,[77] a signaling pathway that is linked to behavioral abnormalities.[78] Therefore, it is plausible that genetic defects in *PCDHA* may also contribute to ASD.

Aside from genetic studies, evidence suggests that PCDH9, PCDH10, and PCDH17 participate in molecular pathway featuring the monocyte enhancer factor-2 (MEF2), which is potentially relevant to ASD. The expression of *PCDH17*, *PCDH10*, and *PCDH9* is regulated by MEF2.[48,79] Monocyte enhancer factor-2 is a transcription factor that has essential function in cell differentiation during embryonic development.[80] For example, activation of *MEF2* has been shown to lead to rapid elimination of unused synapses, a process required for normal learning.[81–83] This was demonstrated in studies showing that activation of *MEF2* drives the localization of ubiquitin ligase Mdm2 to the synaptic compartment where postsynaptic scaffolding protein PSD-95 is polyubiquitinated.[79] Monocyte enhancer factor-2 activation has also been reported to promote the association of PSD-95 with Pcdh10 via its C-terminal region, thereby facilitating proteasomal degradation leading to synapse elimination. Because all three PCDHs act downstream of MEF2, it is reasonable to predict that they may have roles in the formation of synapses, and deficits in these pathways either directly or indirectly cause cognitive dysfunction and thus also ASD.[13]

It has also been shown that the RNA-binding protein FMR1 functions downstream of MEF2.[81,84] Interestingly, FMR1 interacts with CYFIP2, a component of the WRC complex, which also interacts with PCDH10, PCDH17, and PCDH19 (as described earlier), which suggests an intricate interplay among these molecules.[45] Involvement of the WRC complex in ASD has been demonstrated, and mutations in the genes encoding components of the complex, including NAP1 (which binds PCDH19, PCDH17, and PCDH10) and CYFIP1 (another interactor of FMR1) have been reported in patients with ASD.[13] Taken together, these data portray the involvement of multiple PCDHs in pathways relevant to ASDs.

PROTOCADHERINS IN BD AND SZ

Bipolar disorder is a complex genetic disorder involving severe mood swings. Patients experience periods of elevated mood (mania) and depression. In severe cases (bipolar I), symptoms of psychosis, hallucinations, and delusions are also present.[85] Although BD is commonly diagnosed during adolescence and early adulthood, the impairment or alteration of neuronal networks leading to BD has been postulated to occur during early development.[86] Similar to ASD and SZ, BD is a multifactorial disorder with a strong genetic contribution. Monozygotic twin studies showed a concordance rate of around 60–80%.[87] In contrast to classical Mendelian disorders in which the causative gene is inherited from multiple generations, there is not yet a confirmed causative gene for BD and large families with multiple affected individuals are rare. This suggests that in addition to genetic causes, other factors including environmental and social risk factors are likely to contribute to the manifestation of BD.

Schizophrenia and BD share a high degree of similarity in disease epidemiology, and these two disorders are commonly misdiagnosed as each other. Schizophrenia is a severe emotional disorder characterized by patients who have symptoms including confusion, hallucinations, and delusions. Unlike BD patients, people with SZ generally do not function well in normal society because symptoms of this disorder result in irrational thinking processes that make it difficult for them to care for themselves. This has resulted in a scenario similar to that seen with ID: SZ causes a financial burden not only to the public health care system but in many cases to the family of patients. The similarity between BD and SZ is clearly illustrated by the fact that the two disorders have the same symptom manifestation period (adolescence to early adulthood) and similar concordance rate (about 50%) in twin, family, and adoption studies.[88] Furthermore, half of the BD patients also have hallucinations and delusions, which are the major symptoms of SZ.[89] Both positive and negative symptoms found in SZ patients resemble the manic and depressive states of BD, respectively. Atypical antipsychotic drugs such as clozapine and olanzapine, which target serotonin and dopamine signaling pathways, are currently prescribed to treat the symptoms of both BD and SZ. These medications are also prescribed to ASD patients because serotonin signaling pathways are reported to have a role in ASD (see the section on ASD). Taken together, these three psychotic disorders are likely to affect highly similar wiring networks in the brain.

The unusually high degree of overlapping clinical phenotypes between BD and SZ suggests that these two disorders may result from defects in the same or overlapping genetic networks. Linkage studies comparing BD and SZ patients with their respective control populations have found gene locus 5q31 to be a highly susceptible region.[90–92] The clustered *PCDHs* α, β, and γ are located within this region. These are cell adhesion molecules that have roles in neuronal differentiation, synaptogenesis, and neurite self-avoidance[93]; therefore, functional impairment of these proteins is thought to contribute to BD and SZ. These *PCDHs* harbor more than 50 exons, and different isoforms are translated through alternative promoter usage and cis-alternative splicing. These proteins are expressed widely in the brain and central nervous system, with specificity achieved by expressing only one or two variable exons (isoforms) within a single neuron in an allele-specific manner.[93] A study has linked a PCDHA enhancer SNP (rs31745) to BD by showing a significant increase in homozygotes for the minor allele (T) in a Czech BD population.[94] This allele is thought to be an ancestral allele, which is conserved across multiple species. Changing expression from the major (C; human-specific) to minor allele (T) could be a risk factor for BD. An enrichment, although not statistically significant, of T allele was also found in European Caucasian SZ patients from the United States. The increase in the T minor allele was shown by electrophoretic mobility shift assay to alter the binding affinity toward an unknown brain protein,[94,95] which in turn might impair the transcription of PCDHA. Copy number variants in PCDHA have also been investigated for a possible link to BD and SZ.[96] Although there is no clear association of a polymorphic CNV (a 16.7-kb deletion affecting PCDH exons A8—10) to BD and SZ, a genome-wide association study has shown an association of PCDHA with other neurodevelopmental disorders: for example, ASD.[73] This provides further support for the importance of PCDHA in the pathophysiology of psychiatric disorders.

In addition to clustered PCDH, nonclustered PCDHs have been implicated in BD and SZ. PCDH11X/Y is one of the earliest PCDHs investigated in psychiatric disorders owing to the hominoid lineage specificity of PCDH11Y.[95] Direct sequencing of PCDH11Y from 30 males with autism found two variants: F885V and K980N. However, subsequent testing of these two SNPs against a small cohort of obsessive compulsive disorder, BD, SZ, ADHD, and ASD showed no statistical differences compared with population-based controls.[95] The authors noted that these two variants were expressed differently between control populations (French versus Swiss) and the study itself may have been underpowered. A more recent study used a much larger cohort ($n = 142$ for ASD and $n = 143$ for SZ) and reported a single splice mutation (c.3034-1G > A) of PCDH11X in a single case (female) of SZ.[64] In the same study, a rare variant of nonclustered PCDH (PCDH19) mentioned earlier was also implicated in SZ (see the section on ASD).

Protocadherin 8, another δ2 PCDH, has also been associated with SZ. Analysis of an SNP (SNP001493931) showed enrichment of minor allele (R) in United Kingdom—based 520 SZ patients compared with 535 matched-control cohorts.[97] Although the same enrichment was not found in Bulgarian patient—parents trios, this study showed a high association of PCDH8 to SZ within a particular ethnic background. Based on

the aggregate evidence, it is likely that mutations in cell-adhesion molecules, especially PCDHs (clustered and nonclustered), are implicated in BD and SZ.

In addition to genetic studies, gene expression analysis has been employed to investigate mechanisms underlying SZ. A microarray study of Brodmann's area 46 from SZ patients showed significantly increased PCDH17 mRNA expression in patients who had SZ of shorter duration.[98] Apart from PCDH17, there were an additional 62 differentially expressed genes in which pathway analyses predicted involvement of cell adhesion molecules. As is the state of studies focusing on the genetic etiology of BD and SZ, the genetic evidence implicating PCDHs is speculative and will require future interrogation using much larger cohorts. The aggregate evidence to date suggests an important role of cell adhesion molecules, and in particular PCDHs in the pathophysiology of psychiatric disorders.

CONCLUSIONS

Neurodevelopmental disorders are clinically and genetically heterogeneous and share common comorbidities, which makes precise diagnosis difficult. Whereas the pathogenesis of these neurodevelopmental disorders remains largely unknown, genetic or functional defects in various PCDHs during early brain development have been shown to be responsible for some of the phenotypes of these disorders. Our understanding of the etiology and genetics of these disorders has increased significantly over the past few years, primarily a result of much improved DNA sequencing technologies and involvement of large cohorts of patients.

Large international efforts involving tens if not hundreds of thousands of patients will be necessary to resolve the genetic architecture of neurodevelopmental disorders. These are extremely heterogeneous disorders with single gene as well as complex and multifactorial genetic contributions.

We have reviewed published evidence of the involvement of PCDHs, a family of cell adhesion molecules, in multiple neurodevelopment disorders. Overall, there is still little evidence, except the case of the PCDH19 gene, that PCDH gene mutations are broadly involved in the etiology of neurodevelopmental disorders. δ2-Protocadherins belong to a family of proteins that have similar but highly specific expression patterns throughout the brain, as well as common interacting partners (at least for PCDH10, 17, 18, and 19). In addition, these proteins are involved in the similar wiring networks during development. Therefore, it is expected that genetic defects in δ2-PCDHs will lead to at least partially overlapping clinical phenotypes. It is also likely that a single mutation in any of these genes alone will not always lead to the disorder, but mutations in more than one *PCDH* or interacting molecules within the same network may contribute to the disorder. Molecular functions of many *PCDHs* and as such also their mutations are still not fully elucidated, and more detailed functional analyses are required at both the cellular and molecular level. Understanding the molecular pathways in which *PCDHs* are involved will provide new insights into the understanding of neurodevelopmental disorders.

References

1. Moreno-De-Luca A, Myers SM, Challman TD, Moreno-De-Luca D, Evans DW, Ledbetter DH. Developmental brain dysfunction: revival and expansion of old concepts based on new genetic evidence. *Lancet Neurol* 2013;**12**(4):406–14.

2. Wills CD. DSM-5 and neurodevelopmental and other disorders of childhood and adolescence. *J Am Acad Psychiatry Law* 2014;**42**(2):165–72.

3. Andrews G, Pine DS, Hobbs MJ, Anderson TM, Sunderland M. Neurodevelopmental disorders: cluster 2 of the proposed meta-structure for DSM-V and ICD-11. *Psychol Med* 2009;**39**(12):2013–23.

4. Doran CM, Einfeld SL, Madden RH, et al. How much does intellectual disability really cost? First estimates for Australia. *J Intellect Dev Disabil* 2012;**37**(1):42–9.

5. Mullin AP, Gokhale A, Moreno-De-Luca A, Sanyal S, Waddington JL, Faundez V. Neurodevelopmental disorders: mechanisms and boundary definitions from genomes, interactomes and proteomes. *Transl Psychiatry* 2013;**3**:e329.

6. Lancet T. Wanted: a global campaign against epilepsy. *Lancet* 2012;**380**(9848):1121.

7. Elsabbagh M, Divan G, Koh YJ, et al. Global prevalence of autism and other pervasive developmental disorders. *Autism Res* 2012;**5**(3):160–79.

8. SANE Australia. 2014. http://www.sane.org/information/factsheets-podcasts/199-bipolar-disorder.

9. World Health Organization (WHO). 2014. http://www.who.int/mental_health/management/schizophrenia/en/.

10. Clegg J, Gillott A, Jones J. Conceptual issues in neurodevelopmental disorders: lives out of synch. *Curr Opin Psychiatry* 2013;**26**(3):289–94.

11. Coe BP, Girirajan S, Eichler EE. The genetic variability and commonality of neurodevelopmental disease. *Am J Med Genet C Semin Med Genet* 2012;**160C**(2):118–29.

12. Sherr EH, Michelson DJ, Shevell MI, Moeschler JB, Gropman AL, Ashwal S. Neurodevelopmental disorders and genetic testing: current approaches and future advances. *Ann Neurol* 2013;**74**(2):164–70.

13. De Rubeis S, He X, Goldberg AP, et al. Synaptic, transcriptional and chromatin genes disrupted in autism. *Nature* 2014;**515**(7526):209–15.

14. Homan CC, Kumar R, Nguyen LS, et al. Mutations in USP9X are associated with X-linked intellectual disability and disrupt neuronal cell migration and growth. *Am J Hum Genet* 2014;**94**(3):470–8.

15. Kahler AK, Djurovic S, Kulle B, et al. Association analysis of schizophrenia on 18 genes involved in neuronal migration: MDGA1 as a new susceptibility gene. *Am J Med Genet B Neuropsychiatr Genet* 2008;**147B**(7):1089–100.

16. Redies C, Hertel N, Hubner CA. Cadherins and neuropsychiatric disorders. *Brain Res* 2012;**1470**:130–44.

17. Fisher RS, Acevedo C, Arzimanoglou A, et al. ILAE official report: a practical clinical definition of epilepsy. *Epilepsia* 2014;**55**(4):475–82.

18. Srour M, Shevell M. Genetics and the investigation of developmental delay/intellectual disability. *Arch Dis Child* 2014;**99**(4):386–9.

19. Shoubridge C, Fullston T, Gecz J. ARX spectrum disorders: making inroads into the molecular pathology. *Hum Mutat* 2010;**31**(8):889–900.

20. Chopra R, Isom LL. Untangling the dravet syndrome seizure network: the changing face of a rare genetic epilepsy. *Epilepsy Curr* 2014;**14**(2):86–9.

21. Kim SY, Yasuda S, Tanaka H, Yamagata K, Kim H. Non-clustered protocadherin. *Cell Adh Migr* 2011;**5**(2):97–105.

22. Juberg RC, Hellman CD. A new familial form of convulsive disorder and mental retardation limited to females. *J Pediatr* 1971;**79**(5):726–32.

23. Ryan SG, Chance PF, Zou CH, Spinner NB, Golden JA, Smietana S. Epilepsy and mental retardation limited to females: an X-linked dominant disorder with male sparing. *Nat Genet* 1997;**17**(1):92–5.

24. Dibbens LM, Tarpey PS, Hynes K, et al. X-linked protocadherin 19 mutations cause female-limited epilepsy and cognitive impairment. *Nat Genet* 2008;**40**(6):776–81.

25. Kahr I, Vandepoele K, van Roy F. Delta-protocadherins in health and disease. *Prog Mol Biol Transl Sci* 2013;**116**:169–92.

26. Hayashi S, Inoue Y, Kiyonari H, et al. Protocadherin-17 mediates collective axon extension by recruiting actin regulator complexes to interaxonal contacts. *Dev Cell* 2014;**30**(6):673–87.

27. Jamal SM, Basran RK, Newton S, Wang Z, Milunsky JM. Novel de novo PCDH19 mutations in three unrelated females with epilepsy female restricted mental retardation syndrome. *Am J Med Genet A* 2010;**152A**(10):2475–81.

28. Hynes K, Tarpey P, Dibbens LM, et al. Epilepsy and mental retardation limited to females with PCDH19 mutations can present de novo or in single generation families. *J Med Genet* 2010;**47**(3):211–6.

29. Higurashi N, Nakamura M, Sugai M, et al. PCDH19-related female-limited epilepsy: further details regarding early clinical features and therapeutic efficacy. *Epilepsy Res* 2013;**106**(1–2):191–9.

30. Depienne C, Bouteiller D, Keren B, et al. Sporadic infantile epileptic encephalopathy caused by mutations in PCDH19 resembles Dravet syndrome but mainly affects females. *PLoS Genet* 2009;**5**(2):e1000381.

31. Depienne C, LeGuern E. PCDH19-related infantile epileptic encephalopathy: an unusual X-linked inheritance disorder. *Hum Mutat* 2012;**33**(4):627–34.

32. Scheffer IE, Turner SJ, Dibbens LM, et al. Epilepsy and mental retardation limited to females: an under-recognized disorder. *Brain* 2008;**131**(Pt 4):918–27.

33. Terracciano A, Specchio N, Darra F, et al. Somatic mosaicism of PCDH19 mutation in a family with low-penetrance EFMR. *Neurogenetics* 2012;**13**(4):341–5.

34. Tylki-Szymanska A. Mucopolysaccharidosis type II, Hunter's syndrome. *Pediatr Endocrinol Rev* 2014;**12**(Suppl. 1):107–13.

35. Zafeiriou DI, Pavlidou EL, Vargiami E. Diverse clinical and genetic aspects of craniofrontonasal syndrome. *Pediatr Neurol* 2011;**44**(2):83–7.

36. Tan C, Shard C, Ranieri E, Hynes K, Pham DH, Leach D, et al. Mutations of protocadherin 19 in female epilepsy (PCDH19-FE) lead to allopregnanolone deficiency. *Hum Mol Genet* September 15, 2015;**24**(18):5250–9.

37. Verrotti A, Laus M, Coppola G, Parisi P, Mohn A, Chiarelli F. Catamenial epilepsy: hormonal aspects. *Gynecol Endocrinol* 2010;**26**(11):783–90.

38. Kim SY, Chung HS, Sun W, Kim H. Spatiotemporal expression pattern of non-clustered protocadherin family members in the developing rat brain. *Neuroscience* 2007;**147**(4):996–1021.

39. Krishna KK, Hertel N, Redies C. Cadherin expression in the somatosensory cortex: evidence for a combinatorial molecular code at the single-cell level. *Neuroscience* 2011;**175**:37–48.

40. Kasnauskiene J, Ciuladaite Z, Preiksaitiene E, et al. A single gene deletion on 4q28.3: PCDH18–a new candidate gene for intellectual disability? *Eur J Med Genet* 2012;**55**(4):274–7.

41. Hoshina N, Tanimura A, Yamasaki M, et al. Protocadherin 17 regulates presynaptic assembly in topographic corticobasal Ganglia circuits. *Neuron* 2013;**78**(5):839–54.

42. Emond MR, Biswas S, Blevins CJ, Jontes JD. A complex of Protocadherin-19 and N-cadherin mediates a novel mechanism of cell adhesion. *J Cell Biol* 2011;**195**(7):1115–21.

43. Biswas S, Emond MR, Jontes JD. Protocadherin-19 and N-cadherin interact to control cell movements during anterior neurulation. *J Cell Biol* 2010;**191**(5):1029–41.

44. Tai K, Kubota M, Shiono K, Tokutsu H, Suzuki ST. Adhesion properties and retinofugal expression of chicken protocadherin-19. *Brain Res* 2010;**1344**:13–24.

45. Chen B, Brinkmann K, Chen Z, et al. The WAVE regulatory complex links diverse receptors to the actin cytoskeleton. *Cell* 2014;**156**(1–2):195–207.

46. Nakao S, Platek A, Hirano S, Takeichi M. Contact-dependent promotion of cell migration by the OL-protocadherin-Nap1 interaction. *J Cell Biol* 2008;**182**(2):395–410.

47. ILAE. Genetic determinants of common epilepsies: a meta-analysis of genome-wide association studies. *Lancet Neurol* 2014;**13**(9):893–903.

48. Miyake K, Hirasawa T, Soutome M, et al. The protocadherins, *PCDHB1* and *PCDH7*, are regulated by MeCP2 in neuronal cells and brain tissues: implication for pathogenesis of Rett syndrome. *BMC Neurosci* 2011;**12**:81.

49. Woods AG, Wormwood KL, Wetie AG, et al. Autism spectrum disorder: an omics perspective. *Proteomics Clin Appl* 2014;**9**(1–2):159–68.

50. APA. *Diagnostic and statistical manual of mental disorders*. 5th ed. Arlington (VA): American Psychiatric Association; 2013.

51. Landrigan PJ, Lambertini L, Birnbaum LS. A research strategy to discover the environmental causes of autism and neurodevelopmental disabilities. *Environ Health Perspect* 2012;**120**(7):a258–60.

52. Shelton JF, Hertz-Picciotto I, Pessah IN. Tipping the balance of autism risk: potential mechanisms linking pesticides and autism. *Environ Health Perspect* 2012;**120**(7):944–51.

53. Abbeduto L, McDuffie A, Thurman AJ. The fragile X syndrome-autism comorbidity: what do we really know? *Front Genet* 2014;**5**:355.

54. Kohane IS, McMurry A, Weber G, et al. The co-morbidity burden of children and young adults with autism spectrum disorders. *PLoS One* 2012;**7**(4):e33224.

55. Rosenberg RE, Law JK, Yenokyan G, McGready J, Kaufmann WE, Law PA. Characteristics and concordance of autism spectrum disorders among 277 twin pairs. *Arch Pediatr Adolesc Med* 2009;**163**(10):907–14.

56. Abrahams BS, Geschwind DH. Advances in autism genetics: on the threshold of a new neurobiology. *Nat Rev Genet* 2008;**9**(5):341–55.

57. Ozonoff S, Young GS, Carter A, et al. Recurrence risk for autism spectrum disorders: a Baby Siblings Research Consortium study. *Pediatrics* 2011;**128**(3):e488–495.

58. Geschwind DH. Genetics of autism spectrum disorders. *Trends Cogn Sci* 2011;**15**(9):409–16.

59. O'Roak BJ, Deriziotis P, Lee C, et al. Exome sequencing in sporadic autism spectrum disorders identifies severe de novo mutations. *Nat Genet* 2011;**43**(6):585–9.

60. Anney R, Klei L, Pinto D, et al. Individual common variants exert weak effects on the risk for autism spectrum disorderspi. *Hum Mol Genet* 2012;**21**(21):4781–92.

61. Talkowski ME, Minikel EV, Gusella JF. Autism spectrum disorder genetics: diverse genes with diverse clinical outcomes. *Harv Rev Psychiatry* 2014;**22**(2):65–75.

62. Gaugler T, Klei L, Sanders SJ, et al. Most genetic risk for autism resides with common variation. *Nat Genet* 2014;**46**(8):881–5.

63. PCDH19 Alliance. 2014. http://www.pcdh19info.org/pcdh19-epilepsy.html.

64. Piton A, Gauthier J, Hamdan FF, et al. Systematic resequencing of X-chromosome synaptic genes in autism spectrum disorder and schizophrenia. *Mol Psychiatry* 2011;**16**(8):867–80.

65. van Harssel JJ, Weckhuysen S, van Kempen MJ, et al. Clinical and genetic aspects of PCDH19-related epilepsy syndromes and the possible role of PCDH19 mutations in males with autism spectrum disorders. *Neurogenetics* 2013;**14**(1):23–34.

66. Aoki E, Kimura R, Suzuki ST, Hirano S. Distribution of OL-protocadherin protein in correlation with specific neural compartments and local circuits in the postnatal mouse brain. *Neuroscience* 2003;**117**(3):593–614.

67. Williams EO, Sickles HM, Dooley AL, Palumbos S, Bisogni AJ, Lin DM. Delta protocadherin 10 is regulated by activity in the mouse main olfactory system. *Front Neural Circuits* 2011;**5**:9.

68. Morrow EM, Yoo SY, Flavell SW, et al. Identifying autism loci and genes by tracing recent shared ancestry. *Science* 2008;**321**(5886):218–23.

69. Uemura M, Nakao S, Suzuki ST, Takeichi M, Hirano S. OL-Protocadherin is essential for growth of striatal axons and thalamocortical projections. *Nat Neurosci* 2007;**10**(9):1151–9.

70. Marshall CR, Noor A, Vincent JB, et al. Structural variation of chromosomes in autism spectrum disorder. *Am J Hum Genet* 2008;**82**(2):477–88.

71. Asahina H, Masuba A, Hirano S, Yuri K. Distribution of protocadherin 9 protein in the developing mouse nervous system. *Neuroscience* 2012;**225**:88–104.

72. Hertel N, Redies C. Absence of layer-specific cadherin expression profiles in the neocortex of the reeler mutant mouse. *Cereb Cortex* 2011;**21**(5):1105–17.

73. Anitha A, Thanseem I, Nakamura K, et al. Protocadherin alpha (PCDHA) as a novel susceptibility gene for autism. *J Psychiatry Neurosci* 2013;**38**(3):192–8.

74. Iossifov I, Ronemus M, Levy D, et al. De novo gene disruptions in children on the autistic spectrum. *Neuron* 2012;**74**(2):285–99.

75. Hasegawa S, Hirabayashi T, Kondo T, et al. Constitutively expressed protocadherin-alpha regulates the coalescence and elimination of homotypic olfactory axons through its cytoplasmic region. *Front Mol Neurosci* 2012;**5**:97.

76. Hasegawa S, Hamada S, Kumode Y, et al. The protocadherin-alpha family is involved in axonal coalescence of olfactory sensory neurons into glomeruli of the olfactory bulb in mouse. *Mol Cell Neurosci* 2008;**38**(1):66–79.

77. Katori S, Hamada S, Noguchi Y, et al. Protocadherin-alpha family is required for serotonergic projections to appropriately innervate target brain areas. *J Neurosci* 2009;**29**(29):9137–47.

78. Kepser LJ, Homberg JR. The neurodevelopmental effects of serotonin: a behavioural perspective. *Behav Brain Res* 2014;**277**:3–13.

79. Tsai NP, Wilkerson JR, Guo W, et al. Multiple autism-linked genes mediate synapse elimination via proteasomal degradation of a synaptic scaffold PSD-95. *Cell* 2012;**151**(7):1581–94.

80. Potthoff MJ, Olson EN. MEF2: a central regulator of diverse developmental programs. *Development* 2007;**134**(23):4131–40.

81. Pfeiffer BE, Zang T, Wilkerson JR, et al. Fragile X mental retardation protein is required for synapse elimination by the activity-dependent transcription factor MEF2. *Neuron* 2010;**66**(2):191–7.

82. Dietrich JB. The MEF2 family and the brain: from molecules to memory. *Cell Tissue Res* 2013;**352**(2):179–90.

83. Rashid AJ, Cole CJ, Josselyn SA. Emerging roles for MEF2 transcription factors in memory. *Genes Brain Behav* 2014;**13**(1):118–25.

84. Zang T, Maksimova MA, Cowan CW, Bassel-Duby R, Olson EN, Huber KM. Postsynaptic FMRP bidirectionally regulates excitatory synapses as a function of developmental age and MEF2 activity. *Mol Cell Neurosci* 2013;**56**:39–49.

85. Stratford HJ, Cooper MJ, Di Simplicio M, Blackwell SE, Holmes EA. Psychological therapy for anxiety in bipolar spectrum disorders: a systematic review. *Clin Psychol Rev* 2014;**35C**:19–34.

86. Sanches M, Keshavan MS, Brambilla P, Soares JC. Neurodevelopmental basis of bipolar disorder: a critical appraisal. *Prog Neuropsychopharmacol Biol Psychiatry* 2008;**32**(7):1617–27.

87. Smoller JW, Finn CT. Family, twin, and adoption studies of bipolar disorder. *Am J Med Genet C Semin Med Genet* 2003;**123C**(1):48–58.

88. Berrettini W. Review of bipolar molecular linkage and association studies. *Curr Psychiatry Rep* 2002;**4**(2):124–9.

89. Vandeleur CL, Merikangas KR, Strippoli MP, Castelao E, Preisig M. Specificity of psychosis, mania and major depression in a contemporary family study. *Mol Psychiatry* 2014;**19**(2):209–13.

90. Schwab SG, Eckstein GN, Hallmayer J, et al. Evidence suggestive of a locus on chromosome 5q31 contributing to susceptibility for schizophrenia in German and Israeli families by multipoint affected sib-pair linkage analysis. *Mol Psychiatry* 1997;**2**(2):156–60.

91. Straub RE, MacLean CJ, Ma Y, et al. Genome-wide scans of three independent sets of 90 Irish multiplex schizophrenia families and follow-up of selected regions in all families provides evidence for multiple susceptibility genes. *Mol Psychiatry* 2002;**7**(6):542–59.

92. Hong KS, McInnes LA, Service SK, et al. Genetic mapping using haplotype and model-free linkage analysis supports previous evidence for a locus predisposing to severe bipolar disorder at 5q31-33. *Am J Med Genet B Neuropsychiatr Genet* 2004;**125B**(1):83–6.

93. Chen WV, Maniatis T. Clustered protocadherins. *Development* 2013;**140**(16):3297–302.

94. Pedrosa E, Stefanescu R, Margolis B, et al. Analysis of protocadherin alpha gene enhancer polymorphism in bipolar disorder and schizophrenia. *Schizophr Res* 2008;**102**(1–3):210–9.

95. Durand CM, Kappeler C, Betancur C, et al. Expression and genetic variability of PCDH11Y, a gene specific to Homo sapiens and candidate for susceptibility to psychiatric disorders. *Am J Med Genet B Neuropsychiatr Genet* 2006;**141B**(1):67–70.

96. Noonan JP, Li J, Nguyen L, et al. Extensive linkage disequilibrium, a common 16.7-kilobase deletion, and evidence of balancing selection in the human protocadherin alpha cluster. *Am J Hum Genet* 2003;**72**(3):621–35.

97. Bray NJ, Kirov G, Owen RJ, et al. Screening the human protocadherin 8 (PCDH8) gene in schizophrenia. *Genes Brain Behav* 2002;**1**(3):187–91.

98. Dean B, Keriakous D, Scarr E, Thomas EA. Gene expression profiling in Brodmann's area 46 from subjects with schizophrenia. *Aust NZ J Psychiatry* 2007;**41**(4):308–20.

15

Mutations of Voltage-Gated Sodium Channel Genes *SCN1A* and *SCN2A* in Epilepsy, Intellectual Disability, and Autism

Kazuhiro Yamakawa

Laboratory for Neurogenetics, RIKEN Brain Science Institute, Saitama, Japan

INTRODUCTION

Epilepsy and autism have high concordant rates in monozygotic twin studies and indicated high genetic contributions[109] (see also Chapter 22). These two diseases overlap each other at high rates (15–30%) and many patients have both diseases.[40,55] Although epilepsy itself could be an initiation or causal factor for autistic feature to some degree, a large portion of patients show only autism at first and later start to have epileptic seizures even if to a less severe grade. These observations suggest common or overlapping pathological (genetic, molecular, cellular, or circuit) bases for epilepsy and autism. Mutations of voltage-gated sodium channel genes *SCN1A* and *SCN2A* are such cases and have been well described in patients with autism and/or epilepsy. In particular, *SCN2A* has been listed among top-ranked genes that show frequent de novo loss-of-function mutations in patients with autism (see subsequent discussion). In this review, I will investigate how prevalent the *SCN1A* and *SCN2A* mutations are in patients with epilepsy and autism. I will also describe how mouse models of *SCN1A* mutations were useful to elucidate the pathological mechanisms and to define appropriate therapeutic targets.

VOLTAGE-GATED SODIUM CHANNELS AND DISEASES

Voltage-gated sodium channels are essential for the generation and propagation of action potential in electrically excitable tissues. Voltage-gated sodium channels consist of one pore-forming alpha-subunit and one or two subsidiary beta-subunits that regulate kinetics or subcellular trafficking of the channel[15] (Figure 1). Nine alpha- (Nav1.1 to Nav1.9) (Table 1) and four beta-subunits (β1–β4) have been identified in humans. Although diffusely expressed throughout the body, the main expression sites of these subunits are distinct from each other and thus their mutations correlate with different diseases phenotypes according to their expression location. For example, *SCN4A* is mainly expressed in skeletal muscle and its mutations cause skeletal muscle impairments such as myotonia and paralysis.[84,111] *SCN5A* is mainly expressed in the heart and its mutations lead to heart diseases such as long-QT syndrome.[145] *SCN9A*, *SCN10A*, and *SCN11A* are dominantly expressed in peripheral nervous system and theirs mutations have been described in patients with pain disorders.[19,31,32,69,154,155] *SCN9A* mutations have also been reported in patients with epilepsies.[119] Four alpha-subunits, *SCN1A*, *SCN2A*, *SCN3A*, and *SCN8A*, are mainly expressed in the central nervous system. *SCN3A* is mainly expressed in embryonic stages[12] and a few *SCN3A* mutations in patients with epilepsies have been reported.[51,138] Multiple *SCN8A* mutations were described in patients with cognitive impairments or early-infantile epileptic encephalopathies.[14,98,136,139] Several beta-1 gene also shows mutations in patients with epilepsies, including inherited missense mutations in generalized epilepsy with febrile seizures plus (GEFS+)[7,143] and homozygous mutation in Dravet syndrome.[95] Even with these observations, *SCN1A* and

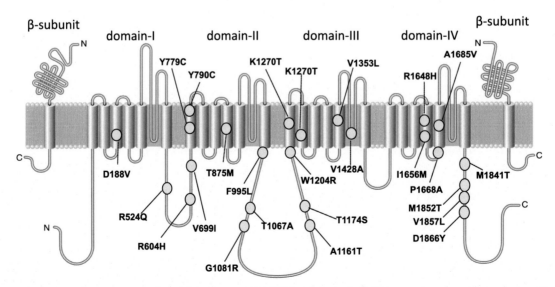

FIGURE 1 **Inherited *SCN1A* mutations found in patients with GEFS+.** Inherited *SCN1A* mutations found in patients with generalized epilepsy with febrile seizures plus (GEFS+) are described on Nav1.1 voltage-gated sodium channel.[3,30,90,122,125,142,156] Note that all are missense mutations.

TABLE 1 Voltage-Gated Sodium Channel Alpha-Subunits and Diseases

Protein (Gene)	Ch. Loci	Expression Sites	Diseases
Nav1.1 (SCN1A)	2q24.3	CNS, PNS	Epilepsy, autism, ID
Nav1.2 (SCN2A)	2q24.3	CNS, PNS	Epilepsy, autism, ID
Nav1.3 (SCN3A)	2q24.3	CNS, PNS	Epilepsy (?)
Nav1.4 (SCN4A)	17q23.3	Skeletal muscle	Myotonia, paralysis
Nav1.5 (SCN5A)	3p22.2	Heart muscle	Heart block, long-QT syndrome
Nav1.6 (SCN8A)	12q13.13	CNS, PNS	ID, ataxia, epilepsy
Nav1.7 (SCN9A)	2q24.3	PNS	Episodic pain
Nav1.8 (SCN10A)	3p22.2	PNS	Episodic pain
Nav1.9 (SCN11A)	3p22.2	PNS	Sensory loss, episodic pain

ch. loci, chromosomal loci; CNS, Central nervous system; PNS, Peripheral nervous system; ID, Intellectual disability; Note: NaX channel encoded by SCN6A/SCN7A is sodium ion concentration-gated but not voltage-gated.

SCN2A are still the two major genes whose mutations have been described in patients with epilepsy and autism. In this review, I will focus on SCN1A and SCN2A.

SCN1A AND EPILEPSY, INTELLECTUAL DISABILITY, AND AUTISM

SCN1A Mutations in Patients with Epilepsies; GEFS+, and Dravet Syndrome

Mutations in SCN1A have been reported in a wide spectrum of epilepsies including generalized epilepsy with febrile seizures plus (GEFS+)[3,30,90,122,125,142,156] (Figure 1) and Dravet syndrome[17,18,22,34,36,38,44,67,89,92,99,127,141] (Figure 2). Generalized epilepsy with febrile seizures plus is characterized by autosomal-dominant inheritance, febrile seizures that persist beyond age 6 years, and variable afebrile seizures including generalized tonic-clonic, myoclonic, and absence seizures. Dravet syndrome is a sporadic intractable epileptic encephalopathy characterized by early-onset epileptic seizures, intellectual disability, ataxia, and increased risk of sudden unexpected death in epilepsy (SUDEP). Patients with Dravet syndrome experience fever-induced tonic, clonic, and tonic-clonic seizures beginning in the first year of life; myoclonic and absence seizures occasionally follow in subsequent years.[25,26,97] Seizures are intractable and often prolonged, frequently resulting in convulsive status epilepticus. Early psychomotor development is normal but patients have acquired severe intellectual disability and ataxia by age 2 years.[25] Patients with Dravet syndrome often exhibit autism. Li and colleagues[70] studied 37 patients with Dravet syndrome and found that nine patients (24.3%) met the criteria for autism but 89.3%, 46.4%, and 39.9% of patients without autism still had speech delay, short temper, and narrow interests, respectively. The clinical features of epilepsy did not statistically differ between the patients with and without autism. Previously, the name "severe myoclonic epilepsy in infancy (SMEI)" was alternatively used for Dravet syndrome; however, it has been avoided partly because myoclonic epilepsy is not always associated.

SCN1A mutations have been found in 10–20% of patients with GEFS+ and approximately 80% of patients with Dravet syndrome. GEFS+ mutations are mostly inherited missense mutations, whereas Dravet syndrome mutations are mostly de novo. Two-thirds of those are truncation mutations such as nonsense and frameshift; the remaining one-third are missense mutations. GEFS+ and Dravet syndrome mutations are distributed along the channel structure (Figure 1). We also reported microdeletion mutations affecting SCN1A 5′ promoter region in a minor number of patients.[92] GEFS+ families with SCN1A mutations occasionally associate with autistic and psychiatric phenotypes such as Asperger syndrome and panic disorder.[104]

As mentioned, Dravet syndromes are mostly sporadic in that disease occurs only in patients but are not observed in their parents. This would be consistent with the fact that Dravet syndrome mutations are mostly de novo. However, there are a small number of familial Dravet syndrome cases in which identical SCN1A mutations were found in different members of the family who manifest Dravet syndrome or mild diseases (such as GEFS+) or were healthy.[34,67,89] Mosaicisms in those parents were reported[39,88] and it may explain the familial cases. These observations indicate that a risk of Dravet syndrome in successive children of parents who had an affected baby should be higher than that in general population, and emphasize the clinical importance of prenatal or preimplantation diagnoses.

SCN1A Mutations in Patients with Autism

SCN1A has also long been discussed as a promising candidate gene for sporadic autism. Early genome scans of autism families[56,107] reported positive log of odds scores on chromosome 2q24 in which SCN1A, SCN2A, and SCN3A are located tandem in the region spanning about 175 cM (centi-morgan). Weiss and colleagues[146] sequenced SCN1A in 117 multiplex autism families and identified an R542Q mutation that had previously been identified in a patient with juvenile myoclonic epilepsy. In recent years, studies of whole-exome sequencing on

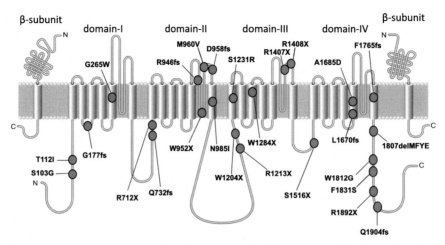

FIGURE 2   **De novo *SCN1A* mutations found in patients with Dravet syndrome.** De novo *SCN1A* mutations found in patients with typical Dravet syndrome extracted from our study[34] are described on Nav1.1 voltage-gated sodium channel. Dravet syndrome is an intractable epileptic encephalopathy associating with severe intellectual disability, ataxia, and autism. Note that 17 of 26 mutations (65%) are truncated, such as nonsense, frameshift, or deletion.

hundreds of patients with sporadic autism further showed multiple de novo loss-of-function mutations of *SCN1A*.[102,103] In the first study[102], O'Roak and colleagues sequenced the exomes of 20 individuals with sporadic ASD (autism spectrum disorder) cases and identified 21 de novo mutations including potentially causative de novo events in four probands, particularly among more severely affected individuals, in *SCN1A*, *FOXP1*, *GRIN2B*, and *LAMC3*. In the second study[103], they performed whole-exome sequencings on new 189 cases and found 248 de novo events, 225 single nucleotide variants, 17 small insertions/deletions, and six copy number variants (CNVs) including 120 severe nonsynonymous changes. De novo point mutations are overwhelmingly paternal in origin (4:1) and are positively correlated with paternal age. Of the 126 most severe or disruptive de novo mutations, 49 map to a highly interconnected β-catenin/chromatin remodeling protein network and recurrent protein-disruptive mutations were observed in netrin G1 and chromodomain helicase deoxyribonucleic acid (DNA) binding protein 8. Mutation screening of six candidate genes in 1703 ASD probands identified additional de novo protein-altering mutations in *GRIN2B*, *LAMC3*, and again *SCN1A*. These observations surely indicate that *SCN1A* mutations contribute to autism; however, *SCN2A* mutations dominate by far in autism (see subsequent discussion).

In Vitro Patch-Clamp Analyses on *SCN1A* Mutant Channels Showed Complex Results

A number of in vitro patch-clamp analyses on *SCN1A* mutations have been reported,[1,2,78,79,113,114,120,121,128] but

conclusions remain illusive. Even within GEFS+ mutations, some studies have suggested an increased activity of the channel that will probably increase neuronal excitability[78,121]; some other studies showed reduced[2,120] or complete absence of sodium current.[79] A computer simulation experiment reported increased neuronal firing with GEFS+ mutations.[123] Mantegazza and colleagues[81] described an association of *SCN1A* loss-of-function mutation with familial simple febrile seizures. *SCN1A* mutations found in patients with Dravet syndrome revealed that not only nonsense mutations but also missense mutations showed drastically attenuated sodium currents.[8,79,128] On the contrary, some Dravet syndrome missense mutations have been described to show noninactivating channel activity with abnormal kinetics similar to those of GEFS+.[113] I previously proposed that functional effects of these mutations would be loss-of-function, in which milder GEFS+ phenotypes are explained by intermediate or partial loss-of-function of mutant Nav1.1 channels, and Dravet syndrome mutation would result in complete loss-of-function or complete elimination of channel protein that should lead to a haploinsufficiency of Nav1.1 because of the nature of heterozygous mutations in patients.[152]

Nav1.1-Deficient Mouse Models Showed Epileptic Seizures, Sudden Death, and Functional Impairments of Inhibitory Neurons

To understand the actual functional consequences of *SCN1A* mutations in patients' brains, it is important to develop in vivo mouse models. Yu and colleagues[153] reported a mouse with *SCN1A* deficiency in which they deleted the last exon encoding Nav1.1 domain IV downstream of the S3 segment and cytoplasmic tail. The heterozygous mouse ($SCN1A^{+/-}$) brain expressed half the amount of normal Nav1.1 protein. The $SCN1A^{+/-}$ mouse had spontaneous seizures and sporadic deaths after postnatal day 21. Patch-clamp analyses of hippocampal cultured neurons from the mouse revealed that the sodium current density was reduced specifically in inhibitory neurons but not in excitatory neurons.[153] Subsequently, we reported a knock-in mice with an SCN1A nonsense mutation (R1407X) that actually was found in three independent Dravet syndrome patients.[94] The heterozygous mouse ($SCN1A^{RX/+}$) brain also expressed half the amount of normal Nav1.1 protein but not the truncated protein, possibly because the mutated mRNA was degraded by a nonsense-mediated mRNA decay mechanism. These observations indicated that rather than the toxicity of truncated proteins, the haploinsufficiency of Nav1.1 (becoming half the amount of normal Nav1.1 protein) is really the basis for the pathology of Dravet syndrome. Seizures and sudden death phenotypes of $SCN1A^{RX/+}$ mice were almost identical to those of $SCN1A^{+/-}$ mice.[153] Our path-clamp recordings on neurons of $SCN1A^{RX/+}$ mice visual cortex slices also revealed that electrophysiological function of inhibitory neurons was impaired whereas that of excitatory neurons remained intact.[94] Epileptic phenotypes of these mice are highly temperature-sensitive, well reproducing febrile seizures in patients.[13,93]

Nav1.1 Is Densely Expressed in Parvalbumin-Positive Inhibitory Neurons and Moderately in a Subpopulation of Excitatory Neurons

To understand pathomechanisms and further develop effective therapies for diseases, it is always important to know the exact tissue, cellular, and subcellular distributions of disease-responsible proteins. Although the epileptic and electrophysiological observations for the $SCN1A^{+/-}$ mouse[153] and $SCN1A^{RX/+}$ mouse[94] are similar to each other, as mentioned, the descriptions of Nav1.1 tissue and subcellular distributions are somehow distinct in these two studies. Yu and colleagues[153] reported that Nav1.1 expression was restricted to somata of both pyramidal and inhibitory neurons in hippocampus, which was similar to previous immunohistochemical studies describing somatodendritic distributions of Nav1.1.[41,148,149] However, our immunohistochemical study using three independent anti-Nav1.1 antibodies and using $SCN1A^{RX/RX}$ mouse as a negative control showed that in hippocampus and neocortex of wild-type mice, the Nav1.1 protein is densely expressed in parvalbumin-positive (PV+) inhibitory interneurons and at their axons and somata, but not in dendrites (Figure 3), and suggested that Nav1.1 haploinsufficiency in PV+ inhibitory neurons is a critical cause of Dravet syndrome.[94] Parvalbumin has been widely used as a specific biochemical marker for a subclass of forebrain

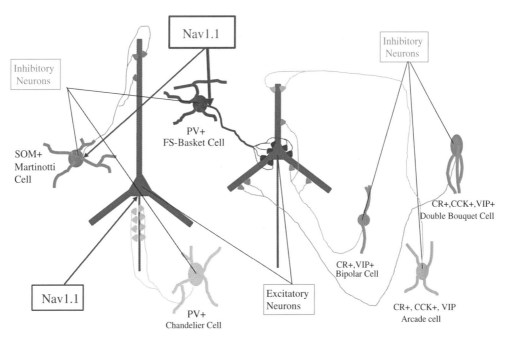

FIGURE 3 **Nav1.1 is dominantly expressed in PV+ inhibitory neurons and moderately in a subpopulation of excitatory neurons.** Nav1.1 is dominantly expressed in PV+ inhibitory neurons and moderately in Som+ inhibitory neurons. Nav1.1 is also moderately expressed in a distinct subpopulation of neocortical excitatory neurons and thalamic relay neurons, but not in hippocampal excitatory neurons. PV: parvalbumin, CR: calretinin, Som: somatostatin, CCK: cholecystokinin, VIP: vasoactive intestinal polypeptide.

GABAergic inhibitory neurons that can also be grouped electrophysiologically as fast-spiking neurons, or morphologically as basket cells and chandelier cells. Signals at the periphery of somata of neocortical or hippocampal pyramidal cells suggested Nav1.1 expression in axon terminals of PV+ basket cells. The dominant Nav1.1 expression in PV+ inhibitory neurons was further confirmed by multiple subsequent studies.[76,96,134,140] Our studies on *SCN1A*[+/−] mice and conditional knockout (KO) mice also showed that Nav1.1 is not expressed in hippocampal excitatory neurons,[94,96] which is again inconsistent with previous observations.[41,148,149,153] Several subsequent studies further reported that Nav1.1 is absent in most hippocampal excitatory neurons.[27,76,77,137] With regard to neocortical excitatory neurons, although our first study on *SCN1A*[RX/RX] mice suggested that Nav1.1 is absent,[94] and Tian and colleagues[134] reported that Nav1.1 is not expressed but instead Nav1.2 and Nav1.6 are expressed, our subsequent study on *SCN1A* conditional KO mice[96] revealed that Nav1.1 is actually expressed in a subpopulation of neocortical excitatory neurons and also thalamic relay neurons, and suggested that Nav1.1 haploinsufficiency in those cells is ameliorating for seizures and sudden death (see subsequent discussion for details).

Nav1.1 Haploinsufficiency in PV+ Inhibitory Neurons Is the Primary Cause for Epilepsy and Sudden Death in Dravet Syndrome whereas That in Excitatory Neurons Has an Ameliorating Effect

To further investigate the roles of neuron subclasses (excitatory neurons, inhibitory neurons, and their subtypes) for the pathology of Dravet syndrome, several groups studied multiple lines of *SCN1A* conditional KO mice. Cheah and colleagues[16] reported spontaneous epileptic seizures in mice with a conditional Nav1.1 deletion mediated by the distal-less homeobox (Dlx)1/2-I12b enhancer + β-globin promoter Cre driver (*Dlx1/2*-Cre), which express Cre recombinase selectively in nearly all forebrain GABAergic inhibitory neurons.[110] The phenotype of heterozygous Nav1.1 deletion with Dlx1/2-Cre (*SCN1A*[f/+];*Dlx*-Cre) mice was comparable to constitutive heterozygous *SCN1A* KO mice (*SCN1A*[+/−] and *SCN1A*[RX/+]). Subsequently, Dutton and colleagues[27] reported mice with conditional Nav1.1 elimination mediated by the protein phosphatase-1 regulatory subunit 2 (Ppp1r2) promoter-driven Cre driver (Ppp1r2-Cre), which express Cre recombinase in a subset of forebrain GABAergic neurons mainly consisting of PV interneurons, but also including reelin- and neuropeptide

Y-positive inhibitory neurons.[9] Mice with heterozygous Ppp1r2-Cre-dependent deletion of Nav1.1 (*SCN1A*[f/+];*Ppp1r2*-Cre) showed increased flurothyl- and hyperthermia-induced seizure susceptibilities, but *SCN1A*[fl/+];*Ppp1r2*-Cre mice had a normal lifespan and less spontaneous seizures compared with *SCN1A*[+/−] or *SCN1A*[RX/+] mice. We subsequently reported mice with conditional Nav1.1 elimination in global inhibitory neurons using a vesicular GABA transporter (VGAT)-Cre recombination.[96] Mice with heterozygous VGAT-Cre-dependent deletion of Nav1.1 (*SCN1A*[f/+];*VGAT*-Cre) had severe epileptic seizures and sudden death, but notably those disease phenotypes of *SCN1A*[f/+],*VGAT*-Cre mice were much more severe than that of the *SCN1A*[+/−] or *SCN1A*[RX/+] mice. As mentioned, Ppp1r2-Cre or Dlx1/2-Cre-driven elimination of Nav1.1 leads to comparable or even milder phenotypes compared with *SCN1A*[+/−] and *SCN1A*[RX/+]. These suggested that VGAT-Cre−dependent deletion can efficiently eliminate Nav1.1 in global inhibitory interneurons compared with that of Dlx1/2-Cre or Ppp1r2-Cre, and furthermore, that the remaining Nav1.1 in VGAT-negative cells has an aggravating effect(s) in the mice with VGAT-Cre−dependent elimination.

We[96] and Dutton and colleagues[27] reported similar results: Mice with conditional Nav1.1 elimination mediated by Emx1 (empty spiracles homolog 1) promoter-driven Cre driver (*Emx1*-Cre), which express Cre recombinase in neocortical and hippocampal excitatory neurons,[58] were viable and did not have epileptic seizures or any noticeable behavioral abnormalities. However, our immunohistochemical studies on *SCN1A*[f/+];*Emx1*-Cre mice showed that in wild-type mice Nav1.1 is also moderately expressed in a distinct subpopulation of excitatory neurons including medial but not lateral entorhino-hippocampal projection neurons, a subpopulation of neocortical layer V excitatory neurons, thalamocortical projection neurons, but not in hippocampal excitatory neurons[96] in addition to the dominant expression in PV+ inhibitory neurons (Figure 3). As mentioned, we showed that *SCN1A*[f/+];*VGAT*-Cre mice have more severe epileptic seizures and sudden death than those of *SCN1A*[+/−] or *SCN1A*[RX/+] mice,[96] and suggest that remaining Nav1.1 in VGAT-negative cells, which would be excitatory neurons, has an aggravating effect. Consistent with this, our study further showed that additional Emx1-Cre−dependent elimination of Nav1.1 in mice with *VGAT*-Cre−dependent Nav1.1 elimination largely improved their seizure and sudden death phenotypes.[96] These findings suggest a protective or ameliorating effect of Nav1.1 haploinsufficiency in excitatory neurons for the risk of epileptic seizures or SUDEP in Dravet syndrome (Figure 4). Although therapeutic approaches to compensate for Nav1.1 haploinsufficiency are potential

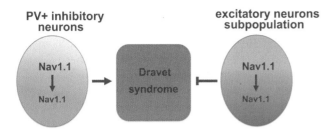

PV+ inhibitory neurons

excitatory neurons subpopulation

FIGURE 4 **Opposite roles of Nav1.1 haploinsufficiency in inhibitory interneurons and excitatory neurons for epilepsy and sudden death in Dravet syndrome.** Haploinsufficiency (becoming half the amount) of Nav1.1 in PV+ inhibitory neurons is a primary cause for epilepsy and sudden death in Dravet syndrome. In contrast, haploinsufficiency of Nav1.1 in excitatory neurons (a subpopulation of neocortical pyramidal cells, thalamic relay neurons, etc.) has the opposite and ameliorating effect in Dravet syndrome.[96]

treatments for Dravet syndrome, preferential targeting of therapeutic approaches to inhibitory rather than excitatory neurons is critically required.

We further reported that a minimal amount of PV-Cre–driven Nav1.1 deletion, using a low-efficient driver PV-IRES-Cre,[4,49,80,147] is sufficient to cause spontaneous epileptic seizures, ataxia, and sudden death in $SCN1A^{f/+}$;PV-Cre-KI mice,[96] and it further strengthened the proposal that Nav1.1 haploinsufficiency in PV+ inhibitory neurons is a primary cause for epileptic seizures and SUDEP in patients with Dravet syndrome. The milder phenotypes of mice with Nav1.1 elimination in PV+ cells ($SCN1A^{f/+}$;PV-Cre-TG) using a high-efficient PV-Cre driver,[130] compared with that of VGAT-Cre–dependent elimination,[96] could be explained by the facts that (1) it has been known that the high-efficient PV-Cre driver expresses Cre-recombinase in thalamocortical projection neurons[130] and that functional impairments of thalamocortical projection neurons have ameliorating effects for epileptic seizures,[105] and therefore the expected functional impairment of thalamocortical projection neurons caused by Nav1.1 haploinsufficiency may have an ameliorating effect for seizure phenotypes; (2) the high-efficient PV-Cre driver also expressed in a subpopulation of neocortical excitatory neurons,[130] and the resulting Nav1.1 elimination in those excitatory neurons may also have ameliorating effects; (3) the late onset of PV expression[10,20,21] may lead to incomplete elimination of Nav1.1 in PV+ cells by using PV-Cre drivers; and (4) PV-negative inhibitory interneurons may express Nav1.1, and Nav1.1 haploinsufficiency in these cells may also contribute to the aggravation of epileptic phenotypes in $SCN1A^{f/+}$;VGAT-Cre mice. Actually, Tai and colleagues[129] reported that in addition to PV+ interneurons, Nav1.1 is expressed in somatostatin-positive (Som+) inhibitory interneurons, and excitability of Som+ inhibitory

neurons is also impaired. It is interesting to study whether Nav1.1 elimination only in Som+ inhibitory interneurons in mice shows any seizure phenotypes. Anyway, these observations indicated that functional impairment of PV+ inhibitory neurons is truly the critical basis for epilepsy and SUDEP in patients with Dravet syndrome and suggests PV+ interneurons as promising therapeutic targets.

Hippocampus Is a Critical Site for the Epileptic Pathology of Dravet Syndrome

In $SCN1A^{f/f}$;PV-Cre-KI mice at postnatal day 21.5, when they began to have recurrent seizures, Nav1.1 expression in hippocampal PV+ inhibitory neurons was reduced compared with wild-type mice, whereas in neocortical PV+ inhibitory neurons remained unchanged.[96] This result indicated that modest reductions of Nav1.1 in hippocampal PV+ interneurons were sufficient to cause epileptic seizures in mouse. Liautard and colleagues[74] also reported specific signs of hyperexcitability in pre-epileptic and epileptic periods and a generation of specific epileptiform activity upon application of convulsant in the hippocampus of $SCN1A^{+/-}$ mice. Together, these results possibly suggest that hippocampus is a critical site for the epileptic pathology of Dravet syndrome and could be a primary target for therapeutic approaches.

Parasympathetic Hyperactivity Causes Ictal Bradycardia and Results in SUDEP of Dravet Syndrome

Kalume and colleagues[63] reported that sudden death in $SCN1A^{+/-}$ or $SCN1A^{-/-}$ mice occurred immediately after generalized tonic-clonic seizures and ictal bradycardia (slower heart rate) associated with the tonic phases of generalized tonic-clonic seizures. They also showed that the cardiac and sudden death phenotypes were reproduced in forebrain GABAergic neurons ($SCN1A^{f/+}$;Dlx-Cre) but not cardiac ($SCN1A^{f/+}$;Mer-Cre), conditional SCN1A KO mice. They further showed that ictal bradycardia and sudden death itself can be suppressed by a drug atropine, which is a competitive antagonist for muscarinic acetylcholine receptors and therefore counteracts against the parasympathetic nervous system. N-Methyl scopolamine, a muscarinic receptor antagonist that does not cross the blood–brain barrier, also eliminated bradycardia, which indicates that peripheral blockade of muscarinic receptors is sufficient to reduce sudden death in the mice. These observations suggested that epileptic seizures cause parasympathetic hyperactivity, which then cause ictal bradycardia and finally result in seizure-associated sudden death. It is interesting to study whether PV+ inhibitory neuron-specific elimination of Nav1.1 also sufficiently causes parasympathetic hyperactivity, and if so, which neural circuit (in brain stem) is responsible for it?

Genetic Modifiers for Dravet Syndrome

SCN1A heterozygous truncation/loss-of-function mutations or Nav1.1 haploinsufficiency are highly penetrant and always or exclusively lead to Dravet syndrome or similarly severe epileptic encephalopathies, and no truncation mutations of SCN1A have been found in healthy individuals. However, severities of disease phenotypes in patients with Dravet syndrome are variable, and therefore modifying factors such as genetic backgrounds or environmental factors are expected. It is known that in mice with Nav1.1 haploinsufficiency, genetic backgrounds also largely affect seizure severity.[94,153] The mixed C57BL6/129 (75%/25%) background resulted in 25% lethality at 1 week of age and 40% at 3 weeks, whereas the 129 dominant mixed background (C57BL6/129 = 25%/75%) did not lead to premature lethality.[94] Similarly, Rubinstein and colleagues[115] reported that SCN1A$^{+/-}$ mice in pure 129/SvJ genetic background have many fewer seizures and much less premature death than in pure C57BL/6 background, and further showed that excitability is less impaired in inhibitory neurons of Dravet syndrome mice in 129/SvJ genetic background. These observations in mice also support the notion that functional polymorphisms in genes other than SCN1A may critically modify the disease severities in patients with Dravet syndrome. Martin and colleagues[82] found that Scn8a mutant allele was able to rescue the premature lethality of SCN1A$^{+/-}$ mice and extend their lifespan. Singh and colleagues[119] found that the homozygous knock-in mouse with a missense mutation of SCN9A, which was originally identified in a large Utah family with significant linkage to chromosome 2q24 where SCN1A locates, exhibited significantly reduced thresholds to electrically induced clonic and tonic-clonic seizures, and further identifications of multiple SCN9A mutations in patients with Dravet syndrome harboring SCN1A mutations lead to their proposal of SCN9A as a modifier for Dravet syndrome. Gaily and colleagues[37] suggested heterozygous X;9 translocation and POLG variants as new genetic modifiers in patients with Dravet syndrome. Ohmori and colleagues[100,101] also proposed CACNA1A and CACNB4 as such modifiers. They first identified one Dravet syndrome patient harboring a de novo SCN1A nonsense mutation and another missense mutation (R468Q) of CACNB4, which was inherited from his father who had a history of febrile seizures, and found that the CACNB4-R468Q

mutant showed greater Cav2.1 current density.[100] Subsequently, they performed a mutational analysis of CACNA1A in 48 subjects with Dravet syndrome and found nine CACNA1A variants. Most of these are common polymorphisms; however, electrophysiological analyses revealed that many of those have gain-of-function effects and patients harboring SCN1A mutations and CACNA1A variants had absence seizures more frequently and exhibited earlier onset of seizures and more frequent prolonged seizures than those with only SCN1A mutations.[101]

Studies of Induced Pluripotent Stem Cells from Dravet Syndrome Showing Contradictory Results

Several studies of neurons derived from induced pluripotent stem (iPS) cells from Dravet syndrome patients were reported.[48,62,75] Liu and colleagues[75] reported increased sodium current in both bipolar-shaped (inhibitory) and pyramidal-shaped (excitatory) neurons differentiated from iPS cells of two Dravet syndrome patients harboring SCN1A-IVS14+3A > T splice donor site mutation or SCN1A-Y325X truncation mutation. Both types of neurons showed spontaneous bursting. Jiao and colleagues[62] also reported that excitatory neurons derived from iPS cells of a Dravet syndrome patient harboring SCN1A-F1415I mutation revealed a hyperexcitable state of enlarged and persistent sodium channel activation, and intensive evoked and spontaneous epileptic action potentials; they suggested that this intrinsic hyperexcitability of excitatory neurons in patients with Dravet syndrome is the basis for the pathology. However, if excitatory neurons with haploinsufficiency of Nav1.1 is hyperexcitable and is the basis for epileptic seizures in Dravet syndrome, as suggested by these two iPS studies,[62,75] Emx1-Cre—dependent elimination of Nav1.1 in mice should show epileptic behaviors, but actually they did not[27,96]; Nav1.1 haploinsufficiency in excitatory neurons showed an ameliorating epileptic phenotype in mice.[96] In the third iPS cell study, Higurashi and colleagues[48] reported significant impairment in action potential generation in GABAergic neurons derived from iPS cells of a Dravet syndrome patient with an SCN1A-R1645X truncation mutation. This study is the only one that is consistent with the previous results of mouse disease models.[16,27,94,96,153] It is highly important to confirm whether the hyperexcitable nature found in excitatory neurons derived from iPS cells of Dravet syndrome patients can be described in mouse models as well or is related only to the patients' iPS cells model, to design efficient therapies and avoid undesirable side-effects (see also Chapter 18).

Zebrafish Model for Dravet Syndrome and Drug Screening

Baraban and colleagues[5] described a zebrafish model for Dravet syndrome that was used for a drug screening. They selected Nav1.1 (scn1Lab) mutants in a chemical mutagenesis screening of zebrafish. The mutants had spontaneous abnormal electrographic activity, hyperactivity, convulsive behaviors that were effectively attenuated by a ketogenic diet, diazepam, valproate, potassium bromide, and stiripentol. They also identified that clemizole, a histamine blocker, is effective for seizures in zebrafish mutants. However, generally, clemizole has aggravating effects on epilepsies in patients and should be avoided. An understanding of the effectiveness of the mechanism of clemizole for seizures in the Dravet syndrome zebrafish model may lead to developments of new effective drugs without undesirable side effects.

Impairment of Inhibitory Neurons Is also the Basis for Abnormalities of Social and Cognitive Behaviors in Dravet Syndrome

As mentioned, Dravet syndrome patients have autistic features and cognitive impairment in addition to epileptic seizures. We studied cognitive and social aspects of the $SCN1A^{RX/+}$ mice using behavioral analyses such as the Barns maze and three-chamber test, and found that the mouse also has cognitive and social impairments that mimic intellectual disability and autistic features of Dravet syndrome patients.[60] Han and colleagues[43] reported similar abnormal social and cognitive behaviors in the $SCN1A^{+/-}$ mouse and showed that Dlx1/2-Cre—dependent elimination of Nav1.1 is sufficient to reproduce these sociobehavioral and cognitive

impairments. They also showed that low-dose clonazepam, an agonist for GABA-A receptor, effectively rescued these abnormalities in the mice, and suggested that they are caused by impaired GABAergic neurotransmission and not by neuronal damage from recurrent seizures. It is interesting to determine whether alterations of PV+ inhibitory neurons function also have critical and sufficient roles for those abnormalities or whether any other neuron subtype(s) are involved, and of course what may be the critical neural circuit(s) for these social and cognitive abnormalities. Further studies are awaited.

SCN2A AND EPILEPSY, INTELLECTUAL DISABILITY, AND AUTISM

SCN2A Mutations in Patients with Epilepsies

Mutations in another voltage-gated sodium channel α-subunit gene, $SCN2A$, encoding the α2-subunit have also been reported in patients with a wide spectrum of epilepsies (Table 1). We first reported an $SCN2A$ missense mutation in a patient with epilepsy.[126] The patient had atypical GEFS+ and an $SCN2A$-R188W mutation (corrected in erratum, 2001). Whole-cell patch-clamp recording of the mutant channel revealed kinetic abnormalities including slowed inactivation in the mutant protein. However, we looked for additional $SCN2A$ mutations in more than 100 GEFS+ patients but could find no further mutations (unpublished data). Since then, multiple inherited missense mutations in $SCN2A$ have been described in another milder type of epilepsy, benign familial neonatal-infantile seizures (BFNIS)[11,46,47,68,72,124] (Figure 5). Benign familial

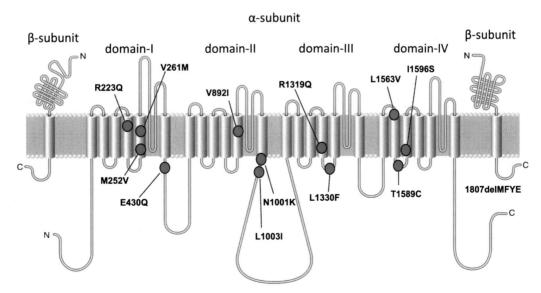

FIGURE 5 **Inherited *SCN2A* mutations found in patients with BFNIS.** Inherited *SCN2A* mutations found in patients with BFNIS are described on Nav1.2 voltage-gated sodium channel.[11,46,47,68,72,124] Note that all are missense mutations.

neonatal-infantile seizure is characterized by onset in early infancy, typically beginning with partial seizures that often become generalized. These seizures are well treated by antiepileptic drugs; generally they remit by age 1 year.[11] Subsequently, we found a de novo heterozygous nonsense mutation *SCN2A*-R102X in a female patient with sporadic intractable epilepsy, severe intellectual disability, and autism.[64] Her psychomotor development was unremarkable before onset but atonic seizures appeared at age 1 year 7 months followed by hyperkinesia and autism. Absence-like and/or partial epilepsy appeared with no seizure-inducing factors including temperature sensitivity. We further reported two additional de novo *SCN2A* missense mutations in patients with severe epilepsies: *SCN2A*-E1211K in a patient with sporadic infantile spasm (West syndrome) and *SCN2A*-I1473M in a patient with neonatal epileptic encephalopathy with suppression burst (Ohtahara syndrome).[157] Whole-cell patch recordings on these two mutant channels showed electrophysiologic properties compatible with both augmented and reduced channel activities. Wong and colleagues[150] reported an identical mutation *SCN2A*-E1211K in a Chinese patient who also had infantile spasm. Furthermore, a significant number of additional de novo *SCN2A* mutations have been reported in patients with early-onset epileptic encephalopathies (EOEEs) including Ohtahara syndrome and West syndrome[14,24,29,42,83,91,135] (Figure 6). *SCN2A* mutations account for 13% of Ohtahara syndrome mutations, which are highly prevalent next to the most prevalent *STXBP1* mutations.[91] Liao and colleagues[73] reported a de novo *SCN2A* missense mutation in a

patient with neonatal epilepsy, late-onset episodic ataxia, myoclonus, headache, and back pain. Shi and colleagues[118] described a de novo *SCN2A*-R1312T missense mutation in a patient with Dravet syndrome. Fukasawa and colleagues[35] reported a de novo *SCN2A*-L1660T missense mutation in a patient with recurrent acute encephalopathy who was born by normal delivery and developed repetitive apneic episodes at age 2 days. Although *SCN2A* mutations in patients with BFNIS and EOEEs are all missense as mentioned earlier, Carvill and colleagues[14] reported a truncation mutation *SCN2A*-I1021YfsX16 in a patient with Lennox–Gastaut syndrome, which is an additional case to our report of *SCN2A*-R102X in a patient with intractable epilepsy, severe intellectual disability, and autism.[64]

SCN2A Mutations in Patients with Autism and/or Intellectual Disability

An association of autism and *SCN2A* missense mutations was suggested by Weiss and colleagues.[146] They screened for variations in *SCN2A* coding exons and splice sites in 117 multiplex autism families and found five coding variants and one lariat branch point mutation; some showed functional changes. We subsequently reported the de novo *SCN2A*-R102X mutation in a patient with intractable epilepsy, severe intellectual disability, and autism,[64] as mentioned earlier. This is the first report of *SCN2A* de novo truncation mutation in a patient with autism. Subsequently, several whole-exome sequencing studies using

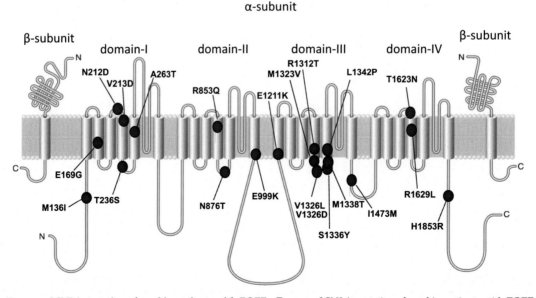

FIGURE 6   **De novo *SCN2A* mutations found in patients with EOEEs.** De novo *SCN2A* mutations found in patients with EOEEs (early onset, before age 1 year, epileptic encephalopathies), including Ohtahara syndrome and West syndrome, are described on Nav1.2 voltage-gated sodium channel.[14,24,29,42,83,91,118,135,157] Note that all are missense mutations.

hundreds or more than 1000 autism patients' genomes reported multiple de novo loss-of-function mutations of *SCN2A*, and now *SCN2A* is ranked among the top five genes for autism[23,33,57,61,112,116] (Figure 7). Sanders and colleagues[116] performed a whole-exome sequencing study on 200 patients with autism, identified 279 de novo coding mutations, and mentioned in the abstract of their report that "there is a single instance in probands, and none in siblings, in which two independent nonsense variants disrupt the same gene, *SCN2A* (sodium channel, voltage-gated, type II, α subunit), a result that is highly unlikely by chance." These two patients did not have a history of seizure. Rauch and colleagues[112] also performed whole-exome sequencing on 51 patients with sporadic intellectual disability and identified three de novo *SCN2A* mutations (two frameshift and one missense). All three patients had autoaggressive behaviors and similar facial features, but none had a history of seizures. At least two were associated with ASD. De Rubeis and colleagues[23] analyzed 3871 ASD cases (2270 ASD trios) and identified four loss-of-function and five probably damaging missense variants in *SCN2A*. Tavassoli and colleagues[132] reported de novo splice-site mutation of *SCN2A* in a patient with autism but without apparent epilepsy. However, the patient showed "frequent episodes of becoming stone faced and limp in the first year of life that may have been indicative of seizure activity," which is reminiscent of the atonic or absence-like seizures observed in the patient with de novo *SCN2A* nonsense mutation.[64]

Functional Consequences of SCN2A Mutations; Gain- or Loss-of-Function?

To date, all of the *SCN2A* mutations found in patients with BFNIS[11,46,47,68,72,124] (Figure 5) and EOEEs[14,24,29,42,83,91,118,135,157] (Figure 6) are missense mutations. In contrast, most of the *SCN2A* mutations described in patients with autism with or without later-onset (after age 1 year) epilepsy are truncation mutations[14,23,57,61,64,112,116,132] (Figure 7). What are the primary differences of functional consequences for these mutations?

Conclusions regarding in vitro electrophysiological analyses of Nav1.2 channels with *SCN2A* mutations found in patients with BFNIS remain ambiguous. Scalmani and colleagues[117] investigated the functional effects of four *SCN2A* missense mutations found in patients with BFNIS using patch-clamp recording on transfected pyramidal and bipolar neocortical neurons and found that *SCN2A*-L1330F caused a positive shift of the inactivation curve; *SCN2A*-L1563V caused a negative shift of the activation curve, with the effects consistent with neuronal hyperexcitability; and *SCN2A*-R223Q and *SCN2A*-R1319Q mainly caused positive shifts of both activation and inactivation curves, with effects that cannot be directly associated with a specific modification of excitability. They further used physiological stimuli in voltage-clamp experiments and showed that these mutations increase both subthreshold and action Na+ currents, consistent with hyperexcitability. With these results, they suggested that increased Na+ current

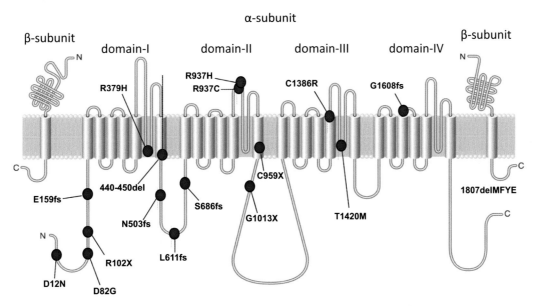

FIGURE 7 De novo *SCN2A* mutations found in patients with autism with or without later-onset epileptic encephalopathy. De novo *SCN2A* mutations found in patients with autism are described on Nav1.2 voltage-gated sodium channel.[14,23,57,61,64,112,116,132] Some patients have epileptic encephalopathy with later onset (after age 1 year), such as Lennox–Gastaut syndrome, but a significant number of patients have been reported to have no seizure history. Note that a major number of these are truncation mutations.

is the functional consequence of these mutations and is the basis for the BFNIS pathology. Misra and colleagues[86] reported the results of three *SCN2A* missense mutations found in patients with BFNIS using whole-cell patch-clamp recording of heterologously expressed human Nav1.2; *SCN2A*-R1319Q displayed mixed effects on activation and fast inactivation gating leading to a net loss of channel function, *SCN2A*-L1563V exhibited impaired fast inactivation predicting a net gain of channel function, and *SCN2A*-L1330F decreased overall channel availability during repetitive stimulation. Cells expressing these BFNIS mutants exhibited lower levels of sodium current and exhibited a significant reduction in cell surface expressions. Xu and colleagues[151] reported the computer model of a BFNIS *SCN2A* missense mutation and showed that the mutation increased the excitability of Nav1.2 neonatal splice form, which is intrinsically less excitable, compared with the adult form, to a level similar to adult one, and suggested that this adult-like increased excitability is likely to be the basis underlying BFNIS. However, Liao and colleague[72] reported that two Nav1.2 mutant channels with different BFNIS mutations showed significant gating changes leading to a gain-of-function, such as an increased persistent Na+ current, accelerated recovery from fast inactivation, or altered voltage-dependence of steady-state activation, but "those were restricted to the neonatal splice form for one mutation and more pronounced for the adult form for the other, suggesting that a differential developmental splicing does not provide a general explanation for seizure remission." Instead, they suggested that the replacing Nav1.6 expression in later developmental stages is the basis for transient nature of seizures in BFNIS.[72] Lauxman and colleagues[68] showed that the *SCN2A*-Y1589C missense mutation found in BFNIS family members revealed a depolarizing shift of steady-state inactivation, increased persistent Na+ current, a slowing of fast inactivation, and an acceleration of its recovery, thus suggesting that the mutation cause a gain-of-function of the channel.

The number of in vitro electrophysiological analyses of Nav1.2 channels harboring *SCN2A* mutations found in patients with EOEEs has remained few, and their results have remained ambiguous. We previously reported that the mutant Nav1.2 channel with *SCN2A*-E1211K mutation found in a patient with infantile spasm had altered electrophysiologic properties compatible with both augmented (hyperpolarizing shift in the voltage dependence of activation) and reduced (hyperpolarizing shift in the voltage dependence of steady-state inactivation and a slowed recovery from inactivation) channel activities and the one with *SCN2A*-I1473M found in a patient with Ohtahara syndrome revealed a hyperpolarizing shift in the voltage

dependence of activation which suggested an augmented channel function.[157] Lossin and colleagues[59] showed that the mutant Nav1.2 channel with the *SCN2A*-R1312T missense mutation found in a patient with Dravet syndrome revealed four parameters indicating a significant current decrease (reduced steady-state availability in fast and slow inactivation, slowed recovery from fast inactivation, and enhanced use dependence with repetitive stimulation), three parameters indicating a less significant current decrease (current density, onset of slow inactivation, and recovery from slow inactivation), and only one parameter indicating current enhancement (voltage dependence of activation), and suggested that the net effect of *SCN2A*-R1312T mutation is current reduction.

The number of in vitro electrophysiological analyses of Nav1.2 channels harboring *SCN2A* mutations found in patients with autism are also few. We previously performed a patch-clamp analysis on human embryonic kidney 293 cells co-expressing the Nav1.2 wild-type channel and a hypothetic truncated channel protein, which could possibly be generated in the patient with autism and late-infantile (onset at 1 year 7 months) epileptic encephalopathy harboring the heterozygous *SCN2A*-R102X mutation, and showed that the truncated mutant protein shifted the voltage dependence of inactivation of wild-type channels in the hyperpolarizing direction, and suggested gain-of-toxic function for the truncated protein.[64] However, as mentioned earlier, we showed that the heterozygous knock-in mice with the *Scn1a*-R1407X nonsense mutation actually did not express truncated protein in the brain, possibly because of elimination by nonsense-mediated mRNA decay, and instead was revealed to express half the amount of normal Nav1.1 protein.[94] This could also be the case for the patient with the *SCN2A*-R102X mutation, and the ultimate functional consequence could be loss-of-function and haploinsufficiency of Nav1.2 normal protein in the heterozygous mouse. Contrary to the *SCN2A* mutations found in patients with BFNIS and EOEEs that are all missense (Figures 5 and 6), most of the *SCN2A* mutations found in patients with autism are truncations (Figure 7). Therefore, it would be natural to assume that haploinsufficiency of Nav1.2 could be the basis for the pathology of autism in these patients.

As mentioned, mutations in patients with BFNIS and those with EOEEs are all missense, and patch-clamp recordings on both groups of mutants had complex functional consequences, either gain- or loss-of-function, and did not show distinct differences, which may explain the difference of disease severity. What is the intrinsic functional difference(s) between mutations for BFNIS and EOEEs that are critically responsible for disease severity? Because most patients with autism who harbor *SCN2A* truncation mutations do not have apparent epileptic seizures, we may not be able simply to assume moderate loss-of-function for mutations in patients with BFNIS and severe loss-of-function for those with EOEEs. Rather, we may have to assume gain-of-function for both BFNIS and EOEEs because of the presence of apparent epileptic seizures in those patients. One possible mechanism would be that Nav1.2 protein harboring such mutations may form toxic aggregates in which EOEEs mutations lead to higher toxicity and BFNIS mutations cause less. A change of degrees in binding affinities of Nav1.2 channel to its binding partners may be an alternative. Some patients with *SCN2A* truncation mutations still show later-onset epileptic phenotypes, and a distinct mechanism may have to be considered. These expectations for functional consequences for *SCN2A* mutations remain speculative and have to be confirmed by future studies such as those in knock-in mice harboring *SCN2A* missense and truncation mutations actually found in human patients.

Nav1.2 Is Dominantly Expressed in Neocortical and Hippocampal Excitatory Neurons but also in a Subpopulation of GABAergic Neurons

Nav1.2 has been known to express dominantly in excitatory neurons in neocortex and hippocampus.[53,76,134] However, a subpopulation of GABAergic neurons also expresses Nav1.2. Li and colleagues[71] reported that Nav1.2 is also expressed in neocortical somatostatin-positive (Som+) inhibitory interneurons and suggested that the functional impairments of Som+ interneurons would be involved in the pathology of epilepsy in patients with *SCN2A* mutations. This has to be confirmed by further studies such as Som+ interneuron-specific elimination of Nav1.2 in mice. We found that Nav1.2 is also dominantly expressed in GABAergic striatal projection neurons.[87] Immunohistochemical staining in mouse brain tissue showed that Nav1.2 was diffusely distributed in the striatal axons and it colocalized with a voltage-gated sodium channel beta-4 subunit. Because of possible involvements of impairments of corticostriatal circuit in the pathology of autism,[106] it is also interesting to study whether Nav1.2 haploinsufficiency in striatal projection neurons contributes to the pathology of autism in patients with *SCN2A* truncation mutations.

Mouse Models with *SCN2A* Mutations

Planenelis-Cases and colleagues[108] reported *Scn2a* KO mouse (*Scn2a*$^{-/-}$) that were morphologically and organogenically indistinguishable from their wild-type littermates but died perinatally with severe hypoxia and massive neuronal apoptosis, notably in the brainstem. They performed whole-cell recordings from hippocampal neurons of *Scn2a*$^{-/-}$ mouse in culture and showed that sodium currents were sharply attenuated. They did not notice any seizures or any other abnormalities in the *Scn2a*$^{+/-}$ mouse. This result is reminiscent of the observation that a large portion of patients with autism who have *SCN2A* truncation mutations do not have an apparent epileptic phenotype. Kearney and colleagues[66] reported that the transgenic mice expressing Nav1.2 with a gain-of-function mutation had seizures and behavioral abnormalities. Rat Nav1.2 channel protein harboring the mutation *Scn2a*-GAL879-881QQQ changes in the cytoplasmic S4-S5 linker of domain 2 of Nav1.2 expressed in *Xenopus* oocytes showed slowed inactivation and increased persistent current. The transgenic mice expressing a neuron-specific enolase promoter-driven Nav1.2 with *Scn2a*-GAL879-881QQQ mutation had seizures that began at age 2 months and were accompanied by behavioral arrest and stereotyped repetitive behaviors. This observation may support the notion that the functional effects of *SCN2A* missense mutations found in patients with epilepsies are gain-of-function.

EXPRESSION SIGHTS MAY DEFINE THE TEMPERATURE SENSITIVITIES OF EPILEPTIC SODIUM CHANNELOPATHIES

Temperature sensitivities in sodium channelopathy have long been discussed mostly through the viewpoint of the intrinsic nature or kinetics of each channel protein itself,[28,133] but the actual cause(s) of temperature sensitivity remain inconclusive. As mentioned, epileptic seizures in patients with *SCN1A* mutations such as GEFS+ and Dravet syndrome are highly temperature sensitive. In contrast, although some reports described temperature sensitivity in patients with *SCN2A* mutations,[118,126] most epilepsy cases with *SCN2A* mutations such as BFNIS[11,46,47] and Ohtahara syndrome[83,91,135] are largely temperature insensitive. Mice with Nav1.1 haploinsufficiency have temperature-dependent seizures,[13,93] whereas no temperature-dependent phenotypes were described in studies of mice with Nav1.2 haploinsufficiency[108] or gain-of-function mutation.[66] What is the basis for the deference of temperature sensitivity between epilepsies caused by *SCN1A* mutations and those caused by *SCN2A* mutations? Although Nav1.1 and Nav1.2 have a minor kinetic difference,[28,133] they are largely similar and intrinsic in nature and therefore the electrophysiological properties of sodium channel proteins themselves may not explain the difference in temperature sensitivity. Rather, it would depend on their distinct expression sites and functional consequences of mutations. Increased temperature itself may lower the sodium channel net activity.[50] Nav1.2 gain-of-function mutations in excitatory neurons may be the basis for BFNIS and EOEEs, and therefore the lowered channel activity caused by high temperature would be counteracting and not sufficient to affect the ultimate disease phenotypes. On the contrary, Nav1.1 haploinsufficiency in GABAergic neurons is the basis for Dravet syndrome, and therefore lowered channel activity caused by high temperature would initiate or aggravate the disease phenotypes. Even wild-type animals have seizures at very high temperature, especially at young ages.[52,85,131] This may also be explained by temperature-dependent inactivation of Nav1.1 in GABAergic neurons, and their recovery or the appearance of seizure resistance at older age may be explained by the increase in Nav1.6 expression at maturity.[71] The intrinsic fragility of the GABAergic system against high temperature may also contribute. Several mutations in the GABAA receptor gamma-2 subunit gene *GABRG2* were reported to be associated with febrile seizures[6,45,144] and Kang and colleagues[65] further showed that α1β2γ2 GABA-A receptors containing *GABRG2* mutations are highly temperature sensitive (trafficking is impaired at high temperature). In that study, they reported that wild-type α1β2γ2 GABA-A receptors are also slightly temperature sensitive, which suggests the intrinsic fragility of the α1β2γ2 GABA-A receptor-dependent GABAergic system at high temperature. This fragility may possibly contribute to the temperature-sensitive nature of epilepsies caused by *SCN1A* mutations. Of course, these hypotheses are still highly speculative and have to be investigated by further studies.

ENDING REMARKS

In this review, I introduced studies on epilepsies, intellectual disability, and autism caused by the voltage-gated sodium channel genes *SCN1A* and *SCN2A*.

Studies on those with *SCN1A* mutations revealed that functional impairments of PV+ inhibitory neurons (fast-spiking basket cells) caused by those mutations are the primary cause for the pathology; especially for Dravet syndrome, Nav1.1 haploinsufficiency in PV+ cells has been shown to be the critical basis for epileptic seizures and sudden death from the disease. Functional impairments of inhibitory neurons have also been shown to be critically involved in the pathology of autism in patients with Dravet syndrome. It has also been shown that Nav1.1 haploinsufficiency in excitatory neurons is contrarily ameliorating, at least for epileptic seizures and sudden death. These studies presented a critical cellular target for therapeutic approaches and show that specific targeting is required

to avoid undesirable side effects. Because of recent advances in genome-editing technologies, it is desirable to design such specific-targeting approaches. Cell implantation would be another promising approach. Hunt and colleagues[54] showed that the implantation of medial ganglionic eminence (MGE) into the hippocampus of mice that had been induced to have epileptic seizures and cognitive impairments by injection of pilocarpine markedly reduced epileptic seizures and restored spatial learning ability. Because MGE is the source of PV+ interneuron progenitors, this MGE transplantation to Dravet syndrome mouse models may be a promising approach to improving epileptic seizures and sudden death, and possibly also for cognitive impairments or even autism.

Surely *SCN1A* de novo truncation mutations also appear in studies of whole-exome sequencing on patients with sporadic autism; however, those *SCN1A* mutations do not dominate in those studies. In contrast, de novo truncation mutations of *SCN2A* are highly dominated in those exome studies, which revealed that *SCN2A* is one of the most important genes for autism. Although both *SCN1A* and *SCN2A* mutations are associated with epilepsies, intellectual disability, and autism, the studies described here suggest that the pathological mechanisms are critically distinct between these two groups, possibly not because of the differences of kinetics of Nav1.1 and Nav1.2 but because of differences in their expression sites. It is great importance to understand what the specific pathological cascade for autism is that is caused by *SCN2A* truncation mutations. Further studies are eagerly awaited.

References

1. Alekov AK, Rahman MM, Mitrovic N, Lehmann-Horn F, Lerche H. A sodium channel mutation causing epilepsy in man exhibits defects in fast inactivation and activation in vitro. *J Physiol (Lond)* 2000;**529**:533—9.
2. Alekov AK, Rahman M, Mitrovic N, Lehmann-Horn F, Lerche H. Enhanced inactivation and acceleration of activation of the sodium channel associated with epilepsy in man. *Eur J Neurosci* 2001;**13**:2171—6.
3. Annesi G, Gambardella A, Carrideo S, Incorpora G, Labate A, Pasqua AA, et al. Two novel *SCN1A* missense mutations in generalized epilepsy with febrile seizures plus. *Epilepsia* 2003;**44**:1257—8.
4. Atallah BV, Bruns W, Carandini M, Scanziani M. Parvalbumin-expressing interneurons linearly transform cortical responses to visual stimuli. *Neuron* 2012;**73**:159—70.
5. Baraban SC, Dinday MT, Hortopan GA. Drug screening in Scn1a zebrafish mutant identifies clemizole as a potential Dravet syndrome treatment. *Nat Commun* 2013;**4**:2410.
6. Baulac S, Huberfeld G, Gourfinkel-An I, Mitropoulou G, Beranger A, Prud'homme JF, et al. First genetic evidence of GABA(A) receptor dysfunction in epilepsy: a mutation in the gamma2-subunit gene. *Nat Genet* 2001;**28**:46—8.

7. Audenaert D, Claes L, Ceulemans B, Lofgren A, Van Broeckhoven C, De Jonghe P. A deletion in SCN1B is associated with febrile seizures and early-onset absence epilepsy. *Neurology* 2003;**61**:854–6.

8. Barela AJ, Waddy SP, Lickfett JG, Hunter J, Anido A, Helmers SL, et al. An epilepsy mutation in the sodium channel *SCN1A* that decreases channel excitability. *J Neurosci* 2006;**26**:2714–23.

9. Belforte JE, Zsiros V, Sklar ER, Jiang Z, Yu G, Li Y, et al. Postnatal NMDA receptor ablation in corticolimbic interneurons confers schizophrenia-like phenotypes. *Nat Neurosci* 2010;**13**:76–83.

10. Bergmann I, Nitsch R, Frotscher M. Area-specific morphological and neurochemical maturation of non-pyramidal neurons in the rat hippocampus as revealed by parvalbumin immunocytochemistry. *Anat Embryol (Berl)* 1991;**184**:403–9.

11. Berkovic SF, Heron SE, Giordano L, Marini C, Guerrini R, Kaplan RE, et al. Benign familial neonatal-infantile seizures: characterization of a new sodium channelopathy. *Ann Neurol* 2004;**55**: 550–7.

12. Brysch W, Creutzfeldt OD, Lüno K, Schlingensiepen R, Schlingensiepen KH. Regional and temporal expression of sodium channel messenger RNAs in the rat brain during development. *Exp Brain Res* 1991;**86**(3):562–7.

13. Cao D, Ohtani H, Ogiwara I, Ohtani S, Takahashi Y, Yamakawa K, et al. Efficacy of stiripentol in hyperthermia-induced seizures in a mouse model of Dravet syndrome. *Epilepsia* July 2012;**53**(7): 1140–5.

14. Carvill GL, Heavin SB, Yendle SC, McMahon JM, O'Roak BJ, Cook J, et al. Targeted resequencing in epileptic encephalopathies identifies de novo mutations in CHD2 and SYNGAP1. *Nat Genet* 2013;**45**:825–30.

15. Catterall WA. From ionic currents to molecular mechanisms: the structure and function of voltage-gated sodium channels. *Neuron* 2000;**26**:13–25.

16. Cheah CS, Yu FH, Westenbroek RE, Kalume FK, Oakley JC, Potter GB, et al. Specific deletion of NaV1.1 sodium channels in inhibitory interneurons causes seizures and premature death in a mouse model of Dravet syndrome. *Proc Natl Acad Sci USA* 2012;**109**:14646–51.

17. Claes L, Del-Favero J, Ceulemans B, Lagae L, Van Broeckhoven C, De Jonghe P. De novo mutations in the sodium-channel gene *SCN1A* cause severe myoclonic epilepsy of infancy. *Am J Hum Genet* 2001;**68**:1327–32.

18. Claes L, Ceulemans B, Audenaert D, Smets K, Lofgren A, Del-Favero J, et al. De novo *SCN1A* mutations are a major cause of severe myoclonic epilepsy of infancy. *Hum Mutat* 2003;**21**:615–21.

19. Cox JJ, Reimann F, Nicholas AK, Thornton G, Roberts E, Springell K, et al. An SCN9A channelopathy causes congenital inability to experience pain. *Nature* 2006;**444**:894–8.

20. del Río JA, de Lecea L, Ferrer I, Soriano E. The development of parvalbumin-immunoreactivity in the neocortex of the mouse. *Brain Res Dev Brain Res* 1994;**81**:247–59.

21. de Lecea L, del Río JA, Soriano E. Developmental expression of parvalbumin mRNA in the cerebral cortex and hippocampus of the rat. *Brain Res Mol Brain Res* 1995;**32**:1–13.

22. Depienne C, Trouillard O, Saint-Martin C, Gourfinkel-An I, Bouteiller D, Carpentier W, et al. Spectrum of SCN1A gene mutations associated with Dravet syndrome: analysis of 333 patients. *J Med Genet* 2009;**46**:183–91.

23. De Rubeis S, He X, Goldberg AP, Poultney CS, Samocha K, Cicek AE, et al. Synaptic, transcriptional and chromatin genes disrupted in autism. *Nature* November 13, 2014;**515**(7526):209–15.

24. Dhamija R, Wirrell E, Falcao G, Kirmani S, Wong-Kisiel LC. Novel de novo SCN2A mutation in a child with migrating focal seizures of infancy. *Pediatr Neurol* December 2013;**49**(6):486–8.

25. Dravet C. Les epilepsies graves de l'enfant. *Vie Med* 1978;**8**: 543–8.

26. Dravet C, Bureau M, Oguni H, Fukuyama Y, Cokar O. Severe myoclonic epilepsy in infancy (Dravet syndrome). In: Roger J, Bureau M, Dravet C, Genton P, Tassinari CA, Wolf P, editors. *Epileptic syndromes in infancy, childhood and adolescence*. 4th ed. (Montrouge, France): John Libbey Eurotext Ltd.; 2005. p. 89–113.

27. Dutton SB, Makinson CD, Papale LA, Shankar A, Balakrishnan B, Nakazawa K, et al. Preferential inactivation of *SCN1A* in parvalbumin interneurons increases seizure susceptibility. *Neurobiol Dis* 2013;**49**:211–20.

28. Egri C, Ruben PC. A hot topic: temperature sensitive sodium channelopathies. *Channels (Austin)* 2012 March–April;**6**(2):75–85. http://dx.doi.org/10.4161/chan.19827. Epub 2012 March 1.

29. Epi4K Consortium, Epilepsy Phenome/Genome Project, Allen AS, Berkovic SF, Cossette P, Delanty N, et al. De novo mutations in epileptic encephalopathies. *Nature* September 12, 2013; **501**(7466):217–21.

30. Escayg A, Heils A, MacDonald BT, Haug K, Sander T, Meisler MH. A novel *SCN1A* mutation associated with generalized epilepsy with febrile seizures plus—and prevalence of variants in patients with epilepsy. *Am J Hum Genet* 2001;**68**:866–73.

31. Faber CG, Lauria G, Merkies ISJ, Cheng X, Han C, Ahn HS, et al. Gain-of-function Nav1.8 mutations in painful neuropathy. *Proc Nat Acad Sci USA* 2012;**109**:19444–9.

32. Finley WH, Lindsey Jr JR, Fine JD, Dixon GA, Burbank MK. Autosomal dominant erythromelalgia. *Am J Med Genet* 1992;**42**: 310–5.

33. Fitzgerald TW, Gerety SS, Jones WD, van Kogelenberg M, King DA, McRae J, et al. Large-scale discovery of novel genetic causes of developmental disorders. *Nature* December 24, 2014. http://dx.doi.org/10.1038/nature14135 [Epub ahead of print].

34. Fujiwara T, Sugawara T, Mazaki-Miyazaki E, Takahashi Y, Fukushima K, Watanabe M, et al. Mutations of sodium channel alpha subunit type 1 (SCN1A) in intractable childhood epilepsies with frequent generalized tonic-clonic seizures. *Brain* 2003;**126**: 531–46.

35. Fukasawa T, Kubota T, Negoro T, Saitoh M, Mizuguchi M, Ihara Y, et al. A case of recurrent encephalopathy with SCN2A missense mutation. *Brain Dev* June 2015;**37**(6):631–4.

36. Fukuma G, Oguni H, Shirasaka Y, Watanabe K, Miyajima T, Yasumoto S, et al. Mutations of neuronal voltage-gated Na$^+$ channel alpha 1 subunit gene *SCN1A* in core severe myoclonic epilepsy in infancy (SMEI) and in borderline SMEI (SMEB). *Epilepsia* 2004;**45**:140–8.

37. Gaily E, Anttonen AK, Valanne L, Liukkonen E, Träskelin AL, Polvi A, et al. Dravet syndrome: new potential genetic modifiers, imaging abnormalities, and ictal findings. *Epilepsia* September 2013;**54**(9):1577–85.

38. Gennaro E, Veggiotti P, Malacarne M, Madia F, Cecconi M, Cardinali S, et al. Familial severe myoclonic epilepsy of infancy: truncation of Nav1.1 and genetic heterogeneity. *Epileptic Disord* 2003;**5**:21–5.

39. Gennaro E, Santorelli FM, Bertini E, Buti D, Gaggero R, Gobbi G, et al. Somatic and germline mosaicisms in severe myoclonic epilepsy of infancy. *Biochem Biophys Res Commun* 2006;**341**:489–93.

40. Gillberg C, Coleman M. *The biology of the autistic syndromes*. Clinics in Developmental Medicine No.153/4. 3rd ed. London: Mac Keith Press; 2000.

41. Gong B, Rhodes KJ, Bekele-Arcuri Z, Trimmer JS. Type I and type II Na$^+$ channel α-subunit polypeptides exhibit distinct spatial and temporal patterning, and association with auxiliary subunits in rat brain. *J Comp Neurol* 1999;**412**:342–52.

42. Hackenberg A, Baumer A, Sticht H, Schmitt B, Kroell-Seger J, Wille D, et al. Infantile epileptic encephalopathy, transient choreoathetotic movements, and hypersomnia due to a de novo missense mutation in the SCN2A gene. *Neuropediatrics* August 2014;**45**(4):261–4.

43. Han S, Tai C, Westenbroek RE, Yu FH, Cheah CS, Potter GB, et al. Autistic-like behaviour in *SCN1A*$^{+/-}$ mice and rescue by enhanced GABA-mediated neurotransmission. *Nature* 2012;**489**: 385–90.

44. Harkin LA, McMahon JM, Iona X, Dibbens L, Pelekanos JT, Zuberi SM, et al. The spectrum of SCN1A-related infantile epileptic encephalopathies. *Brain* 2007;**130**:843–52.

45. Harkin LA, Bowser DN, Dibbens LM, Singh R, Phillips F, Wallace RH, et al. Truncation of the GABA(A)-receptor gamma2 subunit in a family with generalized epilepsy with febrile seizures plus. *Am J Hum Genet* 2002;**70**:530–6.

46. Herlenius E, Heron SE, Grinton BE, Keay D, Scheffer IE, Mulley JC, et al. *SCN2A* mutations and benign familial neonatal-infantile seizures: the phenotypic spectrum. *Epilepsia* June 2007;**48**(6):1138–42. Epub 2007 March 26.

47. Heron SE, Crossland KM, Andermann E, Phillips HA, Hall AJ, Bleasel A, et al. Sodium-channel defects in benign familial neonatal-infantile seizures. *Lancet* 2002;**360**:851–2. Note: Erratum: Lancet 360: 1520 only, 2002.

48. Higurashi N, Uchida T, Lossin C, Misumi Y, Okada Y, Akamatsu W, et al. A human Dravet syndrome model from patient induced pluripotent stem cells. *Mol Brain* May 2, 2013;**6**:19.

49. Hippenmeyer S, Vrieseling E, Sigrist M, Portmann T, Laengle C, Ladle DR, et al. A developmental switch in the response of DRG neurons to ETS transcription factor signaling. *PLoS Biol* 2005;**3**:e159.

50. Hodgkin AL, Katz B. The effect of temperature on the electrical activity of the giant axon of the squid. *J Physiol* 1949;**109**:240–9. PMID:15394322.

51. Holland KD, Kearney JA, Glauser TA, Buck G, Keddache M, Blankston JR, et al. Mutation of sodium channel SCN3A in a patient with cryptogenic pediatric partial epilepsy. *Neurosci Lett* March 5, 2008;**433**(1):65–70.

52. Holtzman D, Obana K, Olson J. Hyperthermia- induced seizures in the rat pup: a model for febrile convulsions in children. *Science* 1981;**213**:1034–6.

53. Hu WQ, Tian CP, Li T, Yang MP, Hou H, et al. Distinct contributions of Na(v)1.6 and Na(v)1.2 in action potential initiation and backpropagation. *Nat Neurosci* 2009;**12**:996–1002.

54. Hunt RF, Girskis KM, Rubenstein JL, Alvarez-Buylla A, Baraban SC. GABA progenitors grafted into the adult epileptic brain control seizures and abnormal behavior. *Nat Neurosci* June 2013;**16**(6):692–7.

55. Inoue Y, Nishida T, Sugiyama O, Tanaka M. Psychiatric aspects of childhood epilepsy. *Jpn J Child Adolesc Psychiatr* 2005;**48**(2): 147–65.

56. International Molecular Genetic Study of Autism Consortium (IMGSAC). A full genome screen for autism with evidence for linkage to a region on chromosome 7q. *Hum Mol Genet* 1998;**7**: 571–8.

57. Iossifov I, O'Roak BJ, Sanders SJ, Ronemus M, Krumm N, Levy D, et al. The contribution of de novo coding mutations to autism spectrum disorder. *Nature* November 13, 2014;**515**(7526):216–21.

58. Iwasato T, Inan M, Kanki H, Erzurumlu RS, Itohara S, Crair MC. Cortical adenylyl cyclase 1 is required for thalamocortical synapse maturation and aspects of layer IV barrel development. *J Neurosci* 2008;**28**:5931–43.

59. Lossin C, Shi X, Rogawski MA, Hirose S. Compromised function in the Na(v)1.2 Dravet syndrome mutation R1312T. *Neurobiol Dis* September 2012;**47**(3):378–84.

60. Ito S, Ogiwara I, Yamada K, Miyamoto H, Hensch T, Osawa M, et al. Mouse with Nav1.1 haploinsufficiency, a model for Dravet syndrome, exhibits lowered sociability and learning impairment. *Neurobiol Dis* 2013;**49**:29–40 (Available online August 16, 2012).

61. Jiang YH, Yuen RK, Jin X, Wang M, Chen N, Wu X, et al. Detection of clinically relevant genetic variants in autism spectrum disorder by whole-genome sequencing. *Am J Hum Genet* August 8, 2013; **93**(2):249–63.

62. Jiao J, Yang Y, Shi Y, Chen J, Gao R, Fan Y, et al. Modeling Dravet syndrome using induced pluripotent stem cells (iPSCs) and directly converted neurons. *Hum Mol Genet* November 1, 2013; **22**(21):4241–52.

63. Kalume F, Westenbroek RE, Cheah CS, Yu FH, Oakley JC, Scheuer T, et al. Sudden unexpected death in a mouse model of Dravet syndrome. *J Clin Invest* April 1, 2013;**123**(4):1798–808.

64. Kamiya K, Kaneda M, Sugawara T, Mazaki E, Okamura N, Montal M, et al. A nonsense mutation of the sodium channel gene *SCN2A* in a patient with intractable epilepsy and mental decline. *J Neurosci* 2004;**24**:2690–8.

65. Kang JQ, Shen W, Macdonald RL. Why does fever trigger febrile seizures? GABAA receptor gamma2 subunit mutations associated with idiopathic generalized epilepsies have temperature-dependent trafficking deficiencies. *J Neurosci* 2006;**26**:2590–7.

66. Kearney JA, Plummer NW, Smith MR, Kapur J, Cummins TR, Waxman SG, et al. A gain-of-function mutation in the sodium channel gene *SCN2A* results in seizures and behavioral abnormalities. *Neuroscience* 2001;**102**(2):307–17.

67. Kimura K, Sugawara T, Mazaki-Miyazaki E, Hoshino K, Nomura Y, Tateno A, et al. A missense mutation in *SCN1A* in brothers with severe myoclonic epilepsy in infancy (SMEI) inherited from a father with febrile seizures. *Brain Dev* 2005;**27**: 424–30.

68. Lauxmann S, Boutry-Kryza N, Rivier C, Mueller S, Hedrich UB, Maljevic S, et al. An SCN2A mutation in a family with infantile seizures from Madagascar reveals an increased subthreshold Na(+) current. *Epilepsia* September 2013;**54**(9):e117–21.

69. Leipold E, Liebmann L, Korenke GC, Heinrich T, Giesselmann S, Baets J, et al. A de novo gain-of-function mutation in SCN11A causes loss of pain perception. *Nat Genet* 2013;**45**:1399–404.

70. Li BM, Liu XR, Yi YH, Deng YH, Su T, Zou X, et al. Autism in Dravet syndrome: prevalence, features, and relationship to the clinical characteristics of epilepsy and mental retardation. *Epilepsy Behav* July 2011;**21**(3):291–5.

71. Li T, Tian C, Scalmani P, Frassoni C, Mantegazza M, Wang Y, et al. Action potential initiation in neocortical inhibitory interneurons. *PLoS Biol* September 9, 2014;**12**(9):e1001944.

72. Liao Y, Deprez L, Maljevic S, Pitsch J, Claes L, Hristova D, et al. Molecular correlates of age-dependent seizures in an inherited neonatal-infantile epilepsy. *Brain* 2010;**133**:1403–14.

73. Liao Y, Anttonen AK, Liukkonen E, Gaily E, Maljevic S, Schubert S, et al. SCN2A mutation associated with neonatal epilepsy, late-onset episodic ataxia, myoclonus, and pain. *Neurology* 2010 October 19;**75**(16):1454–8.

74. Liautard C, Scalmani P, Carriero G, de Curtis M, Franceschetti S, Mantegazza M. Hippocampal hyperexcitability and specific epileptiform activity in a mouse model of Dravet syndrome. *Epilepsia* July 2013;**54**(7):1251–61.

75. Liu Y, Lopez-Santiago LF, Yuan Y, Jones JM, Zhang H, O'Malley HA, et al. Dravet syndrome patient-derived neurons suggest a novel epilepsy mechanism. *Ann Neurol* July 2013; **74**(1):128–39.

76. Lorincz A, Nusser Z. Cell-type-dependent molecular composition of the axon initial segment. *J Neurosci* 2008;**28**:14329–40.

77. Lorincz A, Nusser Z. Molecular identity of dendritic voltage-gated sodium channels. *Science* 2010;**328**:906–9.

78. Lossin C, Wang DW, Rhodes TH, Vanoye CG, George Jr AL. Molecular basis of an inherited epilepsy. *Neuron* 2002;**34**:877–84.

79. Lossin C, Rhodes TH, Desai RR, Vanoye CG, Wang D, Carniciu S, et al. Epilepsy-associated dysfunction in the voltage-gated neuronal sodium channel SCN1A. *J Neurosci* 2003;**23**:11289–95.

80. Madisen L, Zwingman TA, Sunkin SM, Oh SW, Zariwala HA, Gu H, et al. A robust and high-throughput Cre reporting and characterization system for the whole mouse brain. *Nat Neurosci* 2010;**13**:133–40.

81. Mantegazza M, Gambardella A, Rusconi R, Schiavon E, Annesi F, Cassulini RR, et al. Identification of an Nav1.1 sodium channel (SCN1A) loss-of-function mutation associated with familial simple febrile seizures. *Proc Natl Acad Sci USA* 2005;**102**:18177–82.

82. Martin MS, Tang B, Papale LA, Yu FH, Catterall WA, Escayg A. The voltage-gated sodium channel Scn8a is a genetic modifier of severe myoclonic epilepsy of infancy. *Hum Mol Genet* December 1, 2007;**16**(23):2892–9. Epub 2007 September 19.

83. Martin HC, Kim GE, Pagnamenta AT, Murakami Y, Carvill GL, Meyer E, et al. Clinical whole-genome sequencing in severe early-onset epilepsy reveals new genes and improves molecular diagnosis. *Hum Mol Genet* June 15, 2014;**23**(12):3200–11.

84. McClatchey AI, McKenna-Yasek D, Cros D, Worthen HG, Kuncl RW, DeSilva SM, et al. Novel mutations in families with unusual and variable disorders of the skeletal muscle sodium channel. *Nat Genet* 1992;**2**:148–52.

85. McCaughran Jr JA, Schechter N. Experimental febrile convulsions: long-term effects of hyperthermia- induced convulsions in the developing rat. *Epilepsia* 1982;**23**:173–83.

86. Misra SN, Kahlig KM, George Jr AL. Impaired NaV1.2 function and reduced cell surface expression in benign familial neonatal-infantile seizures. *Epilepsia* 2008;**49**:1535–45.

87. Miyazaki H, Oyama F, Inoue R, Aosaki T, Abe T, Kiyonari H, et al. Singular localization of sodium channel β4 subunit in unmyelinated fibres and its role in the striatum. *Nat Commun* November 21, 2014;**5**:5525.

88. Morimoto M, Mazaki E, Nishimura A, Chiyonobu T, Sawai Y, Murakami A, et al. *SCN1A* mutation Mosaicism in a family with severe myoclonic epilepsy in infancy. *Epilepsia* 2006;**47**:1732–6.

89. Nabbout R, Gennaro E, Dalla Bernardina B, Dulac O, Madia F, Bertini E, et al. Spectrum of SCN1A mutations in severe myoclonic epilepsy of infancy. *Neurology* 2003;**60**:1961–7.

90. Nagao Y, Mazaki-Miyazaki E, Okamura N, Takagi M, Igarashi T, Yamakawa K. A family of generalized epilepsy with febrile seizures plus type 2-a new missense mutation of *SCN1A* found in the pedigree of several patients with complex febrile seizures. *Epilepsy Res* 2005;**63**:151–6.

91. Nakamura K, Kato M, Osaka H, Yamashita S, Nakagawa E, Haginoya K, et al. Clinical spectrum of *SCN2A* mutations expanding to Ohtahara syndrome. *Neurology* September 10, 2013;**81**(11):992–8.

92. Nakayama T, Ogiwara I, Ito K, Kaneda M, Mazaki E, Osaka H, et al. Deletions of *SCN1A* 5′ genomic region with promoter activity in Dravet syndrome. *Hum Mutat* 2010;**31** [Epub ahead of print].

93. Oakley JC, Kalume F, Yu FH, Scheuer T, Catterall WA. Temperature- and age-dependent seizures in a mouse model of severe myoclonic epilepsy in infancy. *Proc Natl Acad Sci USA* 2009;**106**:3994–9.

94. Ogiwara I, Miyamoto H, Morita N, Atapour N, Mazaki E, Inoue I, et al. Nav1.1 Localizes to axons of parvalbumin-positive inhibitory interneurons: a circuit basis for epileptic seizures in mice carrying an *SCN1A* gene mutation. *J Neurosci* 2007;**27**:5903–14.

95. Ogiwara I, Nakayama T, Yamagata T, Ohtani H, Mazaki E, Tsuchiya S, et al. A homozygous mutation of voltage-gated sodium channel bI gene SCN1B in a patient with Dravet Syndrome. *Epilepsia* 2012;**53**(12):e200–203. http://dx.doi.org/10.1111/epi.12040.

96. Ogiwara I, Iwasato T, Miyamoto H, Iwata R, Yamagata T, Mazaki E, et al. Yamakawa K Nav1.1 haploinsufficiency in excitatory neurons ameliorates seizure-associated sudden death in a mouse model of Dravet syndrome. *Hum Mol Genet* 2013;**22**(23):4784–804.

97. Oguni H, Hayashi K, Osawa M, Awaya Y, Fukuyama Y, Fukuma G, et al. Severe myoclonic epilepsy in infancy: clinical analysis and relation to *SCN1A* mutations in a Japanese cohort. *Adv Neurol* 2005;**95**:103–17.

98. Ohba C, Kato M, Takahashi S, Lerman-Sagie T, Lev D, Terashima H, et al. Early onset epileptic encephalopathy caused by de novo SCN8A mutations. *Epilepsia* July 2014;**55**(7):994–1000.

99. Ohmori I, Ouchida M, Ohtsuka Y, Oka E, Shimizu K. Significant correlation of the *SCN1A* mutations and severe myoclonic epilepsy in infancy. *Biochem Biophys Res Commun* 2002;**295**:17–23.

100. Ohmori I, Ouchida M, Miki T, Mimaki N, Kiyonaka S, Nishiki T, et al. A CACNB4 mutation shows that altered Ca(v)2.1 function may be a genetic modifier of severe myoclonic epilepsy in infancy. *Neurobiol Dis* December 2008;**32**(3):349–54.

101. Ohmori I, Ouchida M, Kobayashi K, Jitsumori Y, Mori A, Michiue H, et al. CACNA1A variants may modify the epileptic phenotype of Dravet syndrome. *Neurobiol Dis* February 2013;**50**:209–17.

102. O'Roak BJ, Deriziotis P, Lee C, Vives L, Schwartz JJ, Girirajan S, et al. Exome sequencing in sporadic autism spectrum disorders identifies severe de novo mutations. *Nat Genet* June 2011;**43**(6):585–9.

103. O'Roak BJ, Vives L, Girirajan S, Karakoc E, Krumm N, Coe BP, et al. Sporadic autism exomes reveal a highly interconnected protein network of de novo mutations. *Nature* April 4, 2012;**485**(7397):246–50.

104. Osaka H, Ogiwara I, Mazaki E, Okamura N, Yamashita S, Iai M, et al. Patients with a sodium channel alpha 1 gene mutation show wide phenotypic variation. *Epilepsy Res* 2007;**75**:46–51.

105. Paz JT, Davidson TJ, Frechette ES, Delord B, Parada I, Peng K, et al. Closed-loop optogenetic control of thalamus as a new tool to interrupt seizures after cortical injury. *Nat Neurosci* 2013;**16**:64–70.

106. Peça J, Feliciano C, Ting JT, Wang W, Wells MF, Venkatraman TN, et al. Shank3 mutant mice display autistic-like behaviours and striatal dysfunction. *Nature* April 28, 2011;**472**(7344):437–42.

107. Philippe A, Martinez M, Guilloud-Bataille M, Gillberg C, Rastam M, Sponheim E, et al. Genome-wide scan for autism susceptibility genes. *Hum Mol Genet* 1999;**8**:805–12.

108. Planells-Cases R, Caprini M, Zhang J, Rockenstein EM, Rivera RR, Murre C, et al. Neuronal death and perinatal lethality in voltage-gated sodium channel alpha(II)-deficient mice. *Biophys J* 2000;**78**:2878–91.

109. Plomin R, Owen MJ, McGuffin P. The genetic basis of complex human behaviors. *Science* 1994;**264**:1733–9.

110. Potter GB, Petryniak MA, Shevchenko E, McKinsey GL, Ekker M, Rubenstein JL. Generation of Cre-transgenic mice using Dlx1/Dlx2 enhancers and their characterization in GABAergic interneurons. *Mol Cell Neurosci* 2009;**40**:167–86.

111. Ptacek LJ, George Jr AL, Griggs RC, Tawil R, Kallen RG, Barchi RL, et al. Identification of a mutation in the gene causing hyperkalemic periodic paralysis. *Cell* 1991;**67**:1021–7.

112. Rauch A, Wieczorek D, Graf E, Wieland T, Endele S, Schwarzmayr T, et al. Range of genetic mutations associated with severe non-syndromic sporadic intellectual disability: an exome sequencing study. *Lancet* 2012;**380**:1674–82.

113. Rhodes TH, Lossin C, Vanoye CG, Wang DW, George Jr AL. Noninactivating voltage-gated sodium channels in severe myoclonic epilepsy of infancy. *Proc Natl Acad Sci USA* 2004;**101**:11147–52.

114. Rhodes TH, Vanoye CG, Ohmori I, Ogiwara I, Yamakawa K, George Jr AL. Sodium channel dysfunction in intractable childhood epilepsy with generalized tonic-clonic seizures. *J Physiol* 2005;**569**(Pt 2):433–45.

115. Rubinstein M, Westenbroek RE, Yu FH, Jones CJ, Scheuer T, Catterall WA. Genetic background modulates impaired excitability of inhibitory neurons in a mouse model of Dravet syndrome. *Neurobiol Dis* January 2015;**73**:106–17.

116. Sanders SJ1, Murtha MT, Gupta AR, Murdoch JD, Raubeson MJ, Willsey AJ, et al. De novo mutations revealed by whole-exome sequencing are strongly associated with autism. *Nature* 2012;**485**: 237−41.

117. Scalmani P, Rusconi R, Armatura E, Zara F, Avanzini G, Franceschetti S, et al. Effects in neocortical neurons of mutations of the Na(v)1.2 Na$^+$ channel causing benign familial neonatal-infantile seizures. *J Neurosci* 2006;**26**:10100−9.

118. Shi X, Yasumoto S, Nakagawa E, Fukasawa T, Uchiya S, Hirose S. Missense mutation of the sodium channel gene SCN2A causes Dravet syndrome. *Brain Dev* 2009;**31**(10):758−62.

119. Singh NA, Pappas C, Dahle EJ, Claes LRF, Pruess TH, De Jonghe P, et al. A role of SCN9A in human epilepsies, as a cause of febrile seizures and as a potential modifier of Dravet syndrome. *PLoS Genet* 2009;**5**:e1000649.

120. Spampanato J, Escayg A, Meisler MH, Goldin AL. Functional effects of two voltage-gated sodium channel mutations that cause generalized epilepsy with febrile seizures plus type 2. *J Neurosci* 2001;**21**:7481−90.

121. Spampanato J, Escayg A, Meisler MH, Goldin AL. The generalized epilepsy with febrile seizures plus type 2 mutation W1204R alters voltage-dependent gating of Nav1.1 sodium channels. *Neuroscience* 2003;**116**:37−48.

122. Spampanato J, Kearney JA, de Haan G, McEwen DP, Escayg A, Aradi I, et al. A novel epilepsy mutation in the sodium channel *SCN1A* identifies a cytoplasmic domain for beta subunit interaction. *J Neurosci* 2004;**24**(44):10022−34.

123. Spampanato J, Aradi I, Soltesz I, Goldin AL. Increased neuronal firing in computer simulations of sodium channel mutations that cause generalized epilepsy with febrile seizures plus. *J Neurophysiol* 2004;**91**:2040−50.

124. Striano P, Bordo L, Lispi ML, Specchio N, Minetti C, Vigevano F, et al. A novel *SCN2A* mutation in family with benign familial infantile seizures. *Epilepsia* January 2006;**47**(1):218−20.

125. Sugawara T, Mazaki-Miyazaki E, Ito M, Nagafuji H, Fukuma G, Mitsudome A, et al. Nav1.1 mutations cause febrile seizures associated with afebrile partial seizures. *Neurology* 2001;**57**:703−5.

126. Sugawara T, Tsurubuchi Y, Agarwala KL, Ito M, Fukuma G, Mazaki-Miyazaki E, et al. A missense mutation of the Na$^+$ channel alpha II subunit gene Na(v)1.2 in a patient with febrile and afebrile seizures causes channel dysfunction. *Proc Natl Acad Sci USA* 2001 May 22;**98**(11):6384−9. Erratum in: *Proc Natl Acad Sci USA* 2001b August 28;**98**(18):10515.

127. Sugawara T, Mazaki-Miyazaki E, Fukushima K, Shimomura J, Fujiwara T, Hamano S, et al. Frequent mutations of *SCN1A* severe myoclonic epilepsy in infancy. *Neurology* 2002;**58**:1122−4.

128. Sugawara T, Tsurubuchi Y, Fujiwara T, Mazaki-Miyazaki E, Nagata K, Montal M, et al. Nav1.1 channels with mutations of severe myoclonic epilepsy in infancy display attenuated currents. *Epilepsy Res* 2003;**54**:201−7.

129. Tai C, Abe Y, Westenbroek RE, Scheuer T, Catterall WA. Impaired excitability of somatostatin- and parvalbumin-expressing cortical interneurons in a mouse model of Dravet syndrome. *Proc Natl Acad Sci USA* July 29, 2014;**111**(30):E3139−48.

130. Tanahira C, Higo S, Watanabe K, Tomioka R, Ebihara S, Kaneko T, et al. Parvalbumin neurons in the forebrain as revealed by parvalbumin-Cre transgenic mice. *Neurosci Res* 2009;**63**:213−23.

131. Tancredi V, D'Arcangelo G, Zona C, Siniscalchi A, Avoli M. Induction of epileptiform activity by temperature elevation in hippocampal slices from young rats: an in vitro model for febrile seizures? *Epilepsia* 1992;**33**:228−34.

132. Tavassoli T, Kolevzon A, Wang AT, Curchack-Lichtin J, Halpern D, Schwartz L, et al. De novo SCN2A splice site mutation in a boy with Autism spectrum disorder. *BMC Med Genet* March 20, 2014;**15**:35.

133. Thomas EA, Hawkins RJ, Richards KL, Xu R, Gazina EV, Petrou S. Heat opens axon initial segment sodium channels: a febrile seizure mechanism? *Ann Neurol* August 2009;**66**(2):219−26.

134. Tian C, Wang K, Ke W, Guo H, Shu Y. Molecular identity of axonal sodium channels in human cortical pyramidal cells. *Front Cell Neurosci* September 23, 2014;**8**:297.

135. Touma M, Joshi M, Connolly MC, Grant PE, Hansen AR, Khwaja O, et al. Whole genome sequencing identifies *SCN2A* mutation in monozygotic twins with Ohtahara syndrome and unique neuropathologic findings. *Epilepsia* May 2013;**54**(5):e81−5.

136. Trudeau MM, Dalton JC, Day JW, Ranum LPW, Meisler MH. Heterozygosity for a protein truncation mutation of sodium channel SCN8A in a patient with cerebellar atrophy, ataxia, and mental retardation. *J Med Genet* 2006;**43**:527−30.

137. Van Wart A, Trimmer JS, Matthews G. Polarized distribution of ion channels within microdomains of the axon initial segment. *J Comp Neurol* 2007;**500**:339−52.

138. Vanoye CG, Gurnett CA, Holland KD, George Jr AL, Kearney JA. Novel SCN3A variants associated with focal epilepsy in children. *Neurobiol Dis* February 2014;**62**:313−22.

139. Veeramah KR, O'Brien JE, Meisler MH, Cheng X, Dib-Hajj SD, Waxman SG, et al. De novo pathogenic SCN8A mutation identified by whole-genome sequencing of a family quartet affected by infantile epileptic encephalopathy and SUDEP. *Am J Hum Genet* 2012;**90**:502−12.

140. Verret L, Mann EO, Hang GB, Barth AM, Cobos I, Ho K, et al. Inhibitory interneuron deficit links altered network activity and cognitive dysfunction in Alzheimer model. *Cell* April 27, 2012;**149**(3):708−21.

141. Wallace RH, Hodgson BL, Grinton BE, Gardiner RM, Robinson R, Rodriguez-Casero V, et al. Sodium channel alpha1-subunit mutations in severe myoclonic epilepsy of infancy and infantile spasms. *Neurology* 2003;**61**:765−9.

142. Wallace RH, Scheffer IE, Barnett S, Richards M, Dibbens L, Desai RR, et al. Neuronal sodium-channel alpha1-subunit mutations in generalized epilepsy with febrile seizures plus. *Am J Hum Genet* 2001a;**68**:859−65.

143. Wallace RH, Wang DW, Singh R, Scheffer IE, George AL, Phillips HA, et al. Febrile seizures and generalized epilepsy associated with a mutation in the Na+-channel beta 1 subunit gene SCN1B. *Nat Genet* 1998;**19**:366−70.

144. Wallace RH, Marini C, Petrou S, Harkin LA, Bowser DN, Panchal RG, et al. Mutant GABA(A) receptor gamma2-subunit in childhood absence epilepsy and febrile seizures. *Nat Genet* 2001b;**28**:49−52.

145. Wang Q, Shen J, Splawski I, Atkinson D, Li Z, Robinson JL, et al. SCN5A mutations associated with an inherited cardiac arrhythmia, long QT syndrome. *Cell* 1995;**80**:805−11.

146. Weiss LA, Escayg A, Kearney JA, Trudeau M, MacDonald BT, Mori M, et al. Sodium channels *SCN1A, SCN2A* and SCN3A in familial autism. *Mol Psychiatry* February 2003;**8**(2):186−94.

147. Wen L, Lu YS, Zhu XH, Li XM, Woo RS, Chen YJ, et al. Neuregulin 1 regulates pyramidal neuron activity via ErbB4 in parvalbumin-positive interneurons. *Proc Natl Acad Sci USA* 2010;**107**:1211−6.

148. Westenbroek RE, Merrick DK, Catterall WA. Differential subcellular localization of the RI and RII Na$^+$ channel subtypes in central neurons. *Neuron* 1989;**3**:695−704.

149. Westenbroek RE, Noebels JL, Catterall WA. Elevated expression of type II Na$^+$ channels in hypomyelinated axons of shiverer mouse brain. *J Neurosci* 1992;**12**:2259−67.

150. Wong VC, Fung CW, Kwong AK. SCN2A mutation in a Chinese boy with infantile spasm − response to Modified Atkins Diet. *Brain Dev* November 7, 2014. pii: S0387-7604(14) 00256−00263.

151. Xu R, Thomas EA, Jenkins M, Gazina EV, Chiu C, Heron SE, et al. A childhood epilepsy mutation reveals a role for developmentally

regulated splicing of a sodium channel. *Mol Cell Neurosci* 2007;**35**: 292–301.

152. Yamakawa K. Epilepsy and sodium channel gene mutations: gain or loss of function? *Neuroreport* 2005;**16**(1).

153. Yu FH, Mantegazza M, Westenbroek RE, Robbins CA, Kalume F, Burton KA, et al. Reduced sodium current in GABAergic interneurons in a mouse model of severe myoclonic epilepsy in infancy. *Nat Neurosci* 2006;**9**:1142–9.

154. Zhang XY, Wen J, Yang W, Wang C, Gao L, Zheng LH, et al. Gain-of-function mutations in SCN11A cause familial episodic pain. *Am J Hum Genet* 2013;**93**:957–66.

155. Yang Y, Wang Y, Li S, Xu Z, Li H, Ma L, et al. Mutations in SCN9A, encoding a sodium channel alpha subunit, in patients with primary erythermalgia. *J Med Genet* March 2004;**41**(3):171–4.

156. Escayg A, MacDonald BT, Meisler MH, Baulac S, Huberfeld G, An-Gourfinkel I, et al. Mutations of SCN1A, encoding a neuronal sodium channel, in two families with GEFS+2. *Nat Genet* April 2000;**24**(4):343–5.

157. Ogiwara I, Ito K, Sawaishi Y, Osaka H, Mazaki E, Inoue I, et al. De novo mutations of voltage-gated sodium channel alphaII gene SCN2A in intractable epilepsies. *Neurology* September 29, 2009; **73**(13):1046–53.

16

Oxytocin in the Developing Brain: Relevance as Disease-Modifying Treatment in Autism Spectrum Disorders

Bice Chini[1,2], Marianna Leonzino[1,3], Valentina Gigliucci[1]

[1]National Research Council, Institute of Neuroscience, Milan, Italy; [2]Humanitas Clinical and Research Center, Rozzano, Italy; [3]Dipartimento di Biotecnologie Mediche e Medicina Traslazionale, UNIMI, Milan, Italy

Autism spectrum disorders (ASDs) are highly heterogeneous chronic neurodevelopmental conditions for which there is no medical cure. ASDs are characterized by multiple causes and courses, a vast range of symptom severity, and several associated comorbid conditions. Substantial heterogeneity exists in the age of onset, with the possibility of early inception as well as regressive phenotypes, which may have important implications for the types and evolution of the disorder. Such heterogeneity is reflected by the complex, and still largely unknown, ASD etiology. Genetic studies suggest that autism is a polygenic disorder with a high heritability index (0.90), and more than 200 gene mutations have been described in people affected by the syndrome (see part 1 of this book). Some of these genes are involved in neuronal and cortical organization, cell adhesion, neurotransmitter, and neuropeptide systems. Nurturing factors have also been implicated in protecting or favoring the emergence of the disease, further contributing to the complexity of ASD pathogenesis. Despite our limited knowledge of the etiology of autism, the redundancy of neurodevelopmental processes, their sensitivity to regulation by a variety of environmental and endogenous factors, and evidence of cortical plasticity in compensation for early developmental alterations converge to suggest that early intervention in ASD may be beneficial and can potentially alter the course of the disorder. Accordingly, early intensive behavioral interventions have consistently demonstrated improvements in learning, communication, and social skills and have now become a standard therapeutic option. There is, however, a pressing unmet medical need to identify effective and long-lasting therapeutic options capable of normalizing the social and cognitive deficits experienced by these patients. In this respect, early treatments aimed to prevent and/or compensate abnormal brain development via mechanistic targets known to promote brain plasticity and control neurodevelopmental processes would potentially modify the course of this devastating disorder. Our increased understanding of the multiplicity of molecules and effectors involved in neurodevelopment and their complex cross-interaction has highlighted several potential areas of intervention that could be exploited to this purpose.

One of these areas of intervention is represented by oxytocin (OXT), a hypothalamic neuropeptide implicated in regulating social behavior in all vertebrates, from teleost fish to humans.[1] For its master role in the regulation of social behavior, OXT has been proposed as a treatment for several neuropsychiatric disorders characterized by deficits in the social domain, including ASD.[2] Intravenous administration of OXT has been shown to improve social cognition transiently in higher functioning patients with autism and Asperger syndrome, and patients treated with intranasal OXT have exhibited similar improvements (OXT actions in normal subjects and autistic patients have been extensively reviewed elsewhere[3,4] and will not be further summarized here). Although encouraging, to date, the results of these preliminary clinical trials have been carried out in adult autistic patients—that is, when the plastic capacity of the brain is at a minimum and the social behavioral and cognitive dysfunctions are consolidated. It is conceivable, however, that treatment with OXT early in life could produce longer-lasting effects by exploiting the higher plastic capacity of the brain, possibly (and it is hoped) acting as a true disease-modifying intervention for the disorder. However, a realistic assessment of the therapeutic potential of early OXT treatment for a complex and multifactorial disease such as ASD necessarily requires a deeper understanding of the cellular and molecular effectors of OXT in the developing brain. The neurochemical, functional, and connectional substrates of OXT in the developing brain will be reviewed here with the aim of contributing to defining OXT-based therapeutic strategies of early intervention leading to a long-term and stable correction of ASD.

OXT SYNTHESIS AND OXYTOCIN RECEPTOR EXPRESSION IN THE DEVELOPING BRAIN

OXT is a peptide that binds to and activates a G protein–coupled receptor, the oxytocin receptor (OXTR), which is widely expressed in the brain. In brain regions devoid of OXTR or when applied at high concentrations, OXT can also bind to and activate the closely related vasopressin V1a and V1b receptor subtypes, which may thus contribute to mediate some central and peripheral OXT effects. Comprehensive analysis of the trajectories of OXT production and OXTR expression in the developing brain has highlighted the perinatal period as a crucial phase for maturation of the OXT system, as reviewed in Ref. 5; here, we summarize key developmental events, referring to that work for references and extensive discussion.[5] In mammals, OXT is a neuropeptide produced in parvocellular and magnocellular neurons (MCNs) located in the supraoptic and paraventricular nuclei of the hypothalamus (SON and PVN, respectively). It is synthesized as a prohormone and stored in secretory granules bound to a carrier protein, neurophysin. The prohormone undergoes a complex maturation process during the transport of the granules to the axon terminals. Immature OXT forms are detected early in embryogenesis (embryonic day [E]16.5 in rats) but the mature peptide appears only after birth. OXT-producing neurons are also still immature at birth; in rats, they become electrophysiologically mature only at the end of the second postnatal (PN) week; however, it is only starting from the fourth PN week that OXT axons mature and reach their final targets within the brain. On the contrary, OXTRs are widely expressed in the brain well before birth and undergo extensive region-specific up- and downregulation around and after birth. It has been hypothesized that in the embryonic brain and early PN days, these receptors can be activated by several mechanisms including immature OXT forms, OXT dendritically released by immature OXT-producing neurons, the highly related neuropeptide arginine-vasopressin (AVP), which is produced and released in its mature amidated form well before birth (at E16.5 in rats), and, finally, OXT produced by the mother that reaches the pup's brain via a still immature blood—brain barrier.

BEHAVIORAL EFFECTS OF OXT ADMINISTRATION AT BIRTH

Whatever the source, OXT exerts relevant, long-lasting actions on the developing brain, as revealed by the effects of single OXT administration in wild-type and genetically modified animal models.

In prairie voles, a species used in the pioneer works of C. S. Carter and T. R. Insel and collaborators to firmly establish the role of OXT and AVP in social behavior, a single administration of OXT or OXT antagonist immediately after birth was shown to affect adult partner preference and alloparental behavior in a sexually dimorphic way (reviewed in Ref. 6). More recently, long-lasting effects of OXT at birth have been demonstrated in two mice models of neurogenetic diseases, *Magel2* knockout (KO)[7,8] and *Cntnap2* KO.[9] *Magel2* is a gene located in the chromosomal 15q11-q13 region, which is subjected to genetic imprinting in normal individuals. In healthy subjects, the maternal copy of this gene is always silenced and the expressed gene is of paternal origin. The absence of expression of the paternal allele results in the Prader—Willi syndrome, a rare genetic disease characterized by a complex phenotype, which includes feeding problems at birth with failure to thrive, followed in early infancy by insatiable appetite and obesity. Mild to moderate intellectual disability, social disturbances, repetitive and ritualistic behavior, and emotional instability are also common Prader—Willi manifestations.[10] Mice deficient for *Magel2* recapitulate several features of Prader—Willi, including adult social deficits, which are completely rescued by a single OXT administration at birth.[7,8] Similarly, a single neonatal OXT administration has been reported to normalize adult social deficits in *Cntnap2* KO mice.[9] Both animal models are characterized at birth by a deficit in OXT processing and release, which supports a key neurodevelopmental role of the neuropeptide in the early PN life.

A deficit in adult OXT synthesis and/or processing is also a feature observed in several models characterized by autistic-like symptoms (Table 1). Remarkably, in several of these models, acute OXT administration in adults has been shown to rescue altered social behaviors, which suggests that the molecular target of OXT, the OXTR, and its downstream signaling pathways are in place to mediate prosocial effects. Finally, alterations

TABLE 1 Oxytocin (OXT)/Oxytocin Receptor (OXTR) Alterations in Rodent Models of Neurodevelopmental Disease

Rodent Model		References
OXT KO	↓ OXT production and/or release	118
CD38 KO	↓ OXT production and/or release	119,120
Magel2 KO	↓ OXT production and/or release	8
Maged1 KO	↓ OXT production and/or release	121
Cntnap2 KO	↓ OXT production and/or release	9
Fmr1 KO	↓ OXT production	122
5-MT treatment	↓ OXT production and/or release	83
Oxtr KO	↓ OXTR expression	38,39,123
Reelin[+/−]	↓ OXTR expression	124
Peg3 KO	↓ OXTR expression	125
Oprm1 KO	↑ OXTR expression	117
Valproate treatment	↑ OXT and OXTR expression	126
BTBR T+ tf/J	↑ OXT production and/or release	127

in OXTR expression have been linked to autistic-like phenotypes in genetically modified mice, as summarized in Table 1.

OXT AND SOCIAL/ENVIRONMENTAL INPUT

Early PN events have been shown to influence adult OXT and OXTR levels. In particular, parental care and environmental stimuli have been recognized as the most critical factors.[11] Rodents that received scarce levels of licking and grooming in the neonatal period have reduced OXTRs in the medial preoptic area and show as adults lower levels of licking and grooming toward their offspring.[12] Remarkably, these alterations can be reversed by a socially enriched periadolescent environment, which demonstrates that the plasticity of the OXT/OXTR system is maintained until the later stages of development.[13] Maternal separation,[14] late weaning, and communal rearing[15] also have a strong impact on OXTR levels later in life.

Sensory inputs have also been recognized to be among the regulators of the OXT system during development: whisker deprivation in mice at birth resulted in reduced synthesis and secretion of OXT, whereas environmental enrichment increased OXT levels and rescued the effects of sensory deprivation.[16] Direct regulation of synaptic transmission in sensory cortices in the neonatal brain has been shown to exert a direct impact on early experience-dependent cortical development (Figure 1, bottom right drawing), and as stated by the authors, "the link between sensory experience and OXT is particularly relevant to autism, where hypersensitivity or hyposensitivity to sensory inputs is prevalent."

NEUROCHEMICAL BASIS OF OXT ACTIONS IN THE DEVELOPING BRAIN

Several targets have been implicated in mediating OXT effects on the developing brain, including a direct effect on γ-aminobutyric acid (GABA)—glutamate balance, on the GABA switch, and on the appearance of early synchronized neuronal activity (Figure 1); important reciprocal interactions are established with the serotonergic, dopaminergic, catecholaminergic, and opioid systems and with neurosteroids and their receptors (Figure 2). Moreover, for OXT to target all of these different systems, the timing of the maturation of the OXT system itself and the autocontrol exerted by OXT on its own production and maturation are crucial.

OXT Effects on the Developing OXT—AVP System

During the first PN days, through activation of its receptors, OXT has a fundamental role in the maturation of its own system and on the vasopressinergic system.[17] At this time, MCNs fire only erratic action potentials and only by the end of the second PN week they acquire the capability to generate a potential-evoked calcium entry and consequent peptide release.[5] This maturation is mainly under the control of OXT itself, through a mechanism known as autocontrol. As shown in Figure 1 (bottom left drawing), locally released OXT activates OXTRs on OXT-producing MCNs, leading to calcium mobilization, membrane depolarization, and further OXT release. Moreover, acting on incoming glutamatergic afferents, OXT increases the release of glutamate, helping maturation

of the system. The concerted action of OXT and glutamate on MCNs promotes their maturation facilitating electrical activity and neurite outgrowth.[18]

The first possible target of exogenous OXT is thus the maturation of the OXT system, a hypothesis investigated by C. S. Carter and collaborators. These authors observed that a single systemic injection of OXT to vole pups 1 day after birth induced a significant increase in the number of OXT-producing neurons in females; this increase was detectable at weaning (21 days) but was no longer present in adults (60—90 days).[19,20] In female rat pups repeatedly treated with OXT during the first week of life, an increase in OXT-expressing neurons was also observed, which was maintained until adulthood.[21] Whether these differences in the outcome in adult life are due to species differences or to dose dependence remains to be established.

No effect of single OXT treatment on PN1 was observed on OXTR binding in both male and female voles once adults.[22] Moreover, this neonatal OXT treatment resulted in decreased binding of the related vasopressin V1a receptor in several brain regions of the adult female vole brain, whereas it increased V1a binding, although only in the cingulate cortex, in adult males.

These observations demonstrate that perturbations of OXT at a critical time of development can imprint the OXTergic and the AVPergic systems in such a way that production of the two hypothalamic peptides or expression of their receptors becomes permanently altered. A feature of this imprinting that stands out from these studies is its gender dependence. When looking at studies evaluating the impact of neonatally administered OXT in the rodent brain, it becomes clearly that these effects are almost exclusively exerted in females, whereas males seem more responsive to OXT antagonists.[19,20,22—24] This suggests that OXT during the perinatal period can contribute to the sexual differentiation of the brain in concert with other endogenous stimuli, such as sexual hormones.

Dimorphic Effects of OXT and the Estrogen Receptor

OXT and estrogen cooperate during development, and a reciprocal transcriptional modulation between them has been demonstrated.[25,26] For this reason, perturbations of OXT levels at birth might influence the estrogen system and its function.

In prairie voles, perinatal OXT treatment affects estrogen receptor (ER)-α persistently throughout life. In newborn females, it rapidly augments ER-α mRNA

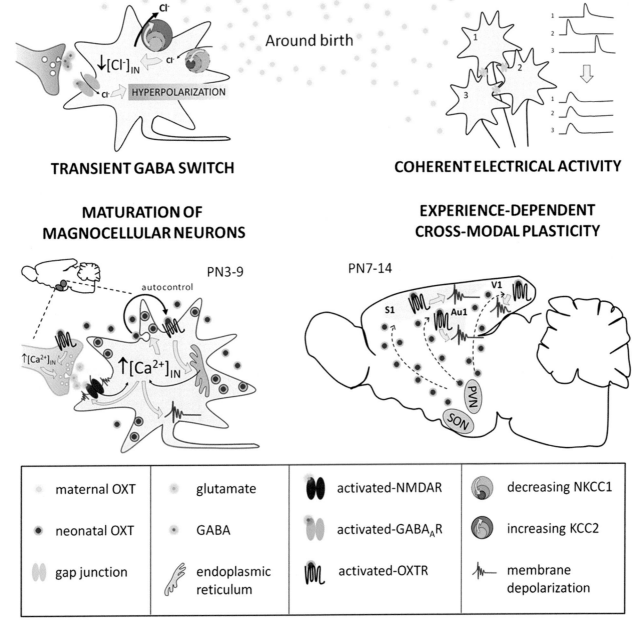

FIGURE 1 **Effects of oxytocin (OXT) on maturation of neurotransmission in rodents.** The burst of maternal OXT that reaches the fetal brain around delivery produces a decrease in intraneuronal chloride concentration by modulating the cation-chloride cotransporters NKCC1 and KCC2. As a consequence, the polarity of GABA actions switches from excitatory to inhibitory, protecting the fetal brain from anoxic insults and allowing the emergence of the first synchronized pattern of activity between small ensembles of neurons that precede the giant depolarizing potentials (GDPs) (upper drawing). Magnocellular neurons (MCNs) start to produce mature forms of OXT at PN0; during the following days, activation of OXTR expressed on MCNs themselves leads to calcium mobilization and consequently to membrane depolarization and further OXT release (autocontrol). Locally released OXT helps the maturation of incoming glutamatergic afferents by activating presynaptic OXTR and causing an increase in the release of glutamate. Because of calcium-induced membrane depolarization, NMDA receptors on MCNs become activated by glutamate and further produce calcium mobilization and electrical activity. These conditions promote the maturation of MCNs during the first 10 days of rodent life (bottom left drawing). Sensory experience positively modulates MCNs activity and local OXT release. During the second postnatal week, dendritically released OXT travels by diffusion or via cerebrospinal fluid and reaches the sensory cortices, where it increases excitatory synaptic neurotransmission, mediating an experience-dependent cross-modal plasticity (bottom right drawing). Au1, primary auditory cortex; S1, primary somatosensory cortex; V1, primary visual cortex; OXT, Oxytocin; OXTR, Oxytocin receptor.

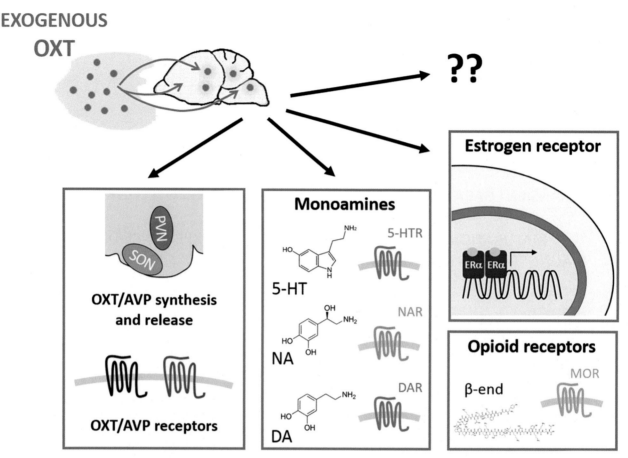

FIGURE 2   **Targets of long-term effects of exogenous OXT in the brain.** OXT administered at birth or in the first days of life affects many systems in the developing brain. The systems known to be modulated by perinatal OXT are reported in the boxes: OXT–AVP system, mono-aminergic systems, and ER. The opioid system is a highly probable target of perinatal OXT modulation because of the evidence of OXT–opioid interactions in adults. The question marks on the side represent other possible unknown targets of OXT. β-end, β-endorphin; DAR, dopamine receptor; MOR, μ-opioid receptor; NAR, noradrenaline receptor; OXT, Oxytocin.

levels in the hippocampus and hypothalamus.[27] Later in life, differential long-term effects of the treatment have been observed in regions of the brain involved in emotionality. Indeed, the number of ER-α–expressing neurons was increased in the ventromedial hypothalamus (VMH) at weaning[24] and in the VMH and central amygdala at adulthood.[21,23]

ER-α is crucial for modulation of the OXTergic system by estrogen, and the influence that perinatal OXT administration has on its expression and function suggests that OXT might regulate itself through this pathway. Testosterone also needs ER-α to fulfill its role in shaping the masculine OXTergic system.[28]

OXT's differential effects in the two sexes might be explained by the different action of estrogen and testosterone on ER-α. One speculation might be that the peak of OXT at delivery induces ER-α transcription and expression in the hypothalamus of both males and females, but this provokes diverse long-term outcomes because of the different actions of the two sexual hormones on this receptor. Further investigation to validate

this hypothesis is needed because unfortunately the study by Pournajafi-Nazarloo et al.[27] analyzed ER-α mRNA levels after OXT administration only in female pups, which leaves the question open about the immediate effects of OXT on ER-α in neonate males.

The sexual dimorphism of OXT might be relevant for autism, because males are affected with a higher prevalence than females and gender-dependent responses to OXT-based therapy can be expected.

OXT and E/I Balance

The levels of GABA- and glutamate-mediated transmission are crucial for overall balance between neuronal excitation and inhibition, which reflects the contribution of each neuronal microcircuit to its final output. Impairments in this balance (henceforth called excitation/inhibition (E/I) balance) are currently under intense investigation as pathological aspects and putative causes of several neuropsychiatric disorders, including ASD.[29,30] Diverse physiopathological findings support this idea: many autism-related genes encode for ion channels or synaptic proteins,[31] cortical hyperactivity is frequently reported in autistic children, and seizures affect about 30% of ASD patients.[32–34] This proposed neurophysiological substrate could be the consequence of a wide range of seemingly unrelated genetic abnormalities and could account for social and cognitive deficits observed in such disorder. Notably, an impaired E/I balance could produce noxious effects both during development by disturbing neural circuits formation[35,36] and in the mature brain by acutely modifying the contribution of selected brain networks involved in specific behaviors.[37] In particular, it has been shown in combinatorial optogenetic studies that even an acute state of elevated E/I balance leads to profound (but reversible) impairments in social and cognitive function.[37]

The involvement of OXT in the modulation of this balance is evident in the phenotype of $Oxtr^{-/-}$ mice: these animals display increased susceptibility to seizures and their hippocampal neurons exhibit an altered ratio between glutamatergic and GABAergic synapses. These defects accompany a strong autistic-like phenotype characterized by reduced sociability, impaired cognitive flexibility, and increased aggression.[38] The social deficits are shared by heterozygous $Oxtr^{+/-}$ mice, which points to $Oxtr$ as a haploinsufficient gene in modulating autistic-like symptoms.[39]

The neuromodulatory effect of OXT is involved in the fine-tuning of neurotransmission in many areas controlling autistic-relevant behaviors.

In the hippocampus, OXT has been described to excite GABAergic neurons and inhibit pyramidal ones.[40,41] This modulation of hippocampal neurotransmission has at least two consequences for E/I balance that are relevant to autism. On the one hand, by dampening neurotransmission, OXT may act as an endogenous anticonvulsant. Indeed, activation of OXTergic neurons and an increase in OXT mRNA levels have been observed after generalized seizures.[42,43] Moreover, treatment in zebrafish with OXT, AVP, and their nonmammalian homologues isotocin and vasotocin protected the brain from pharmacologically-induced seizures.[44] On the other hand, by selectively exciting the fast-spiking interneurons, OXT suppresses spontaneous pyramidal cell firing (noise) but also improves the fidelity and temporal precision of spike transmission (signal) through a feed-forward inhibitory mechanism. The resulting improvement in signal—noise ratio may provide a cue for salience, enhancing information processing and cognitive performance.[45] Through an analogous inhibitory pathway involving a specific subpopulation of interneurons in the medial prefrontal cortex, OXT also modulates sociosexual behavior.[46] Moreover, by modulating synaptic plasticity (in the form of long-term potentiation and depression) in

many brain regions, OXT controls several autism-relevant processes: in the olfactory bulb[47] and the medial amygdala,[48] it mediates social recognition memory; in the lateral septum, it induces the social buffering of fear and also social fear itself.[49]

OXT, the GABA Switch, and the Emergence of Synchronized Neuronal Activity

Different from what happens in the mature central nervous system where GABA is generally hyperpolarizing, at early stages of development, the activation of $GABA_A$ receptors ($GABA_ARs$) generates membrane depolarization.[50] This is because of chloride (Cl^-) efflux resulting from the high intracellular Cl^- concentration present in immature neurons. At these stages, both GABA and glutamate are released through an unconventional nonvescicular process[51] well before synapses are functional and activate their postsynaptic receptors generating depolarization and thus calcium (Ca^{2+}) influx from the voltage-gated Ca^{2+} channels.[52,53] Therefore, GABA and glutamate work in synergy in the early stages of development by depolarizing the neurons and cooperate in the removal of the Mg^{2+} blockade of NMDA receptors.[54,55] The resulting Ca^{2+} influx and electrical activity produce important trophic effects on neuronal proliferation, migration, maturation, and differentiation.[56–59] However, maturation of the two systems does not completely overlap in time; indeed, GABA-induced currents are established before glutamatergic ones in different areas (hippocampal CA1,[60] dentate gyrus,[61] and neocortex[62]). This implies that GABA is the principal excitatory neurotransmitter in the very first steps of development. The dramatic relevance of excitatory GABA makes the switch in its polarity from depolarizing (excitatory) to hyperpolarizing (inhibitory), and its proper timing fundamental for a correct development of neural circuits. This switch occurs in rodents by the end of the first PN week,[63] driven by the modulation of the expression of two neuronal cation-chloride cotransporters (CCCs), NKCC1 and KCC2. Gradual and concomitant downregulation of NKCC1, the Cl^- importer, and upregulation of KCC2, the Cl^- exporter, decrease intracellular Cl^- concentration and modify its electrochemical gradient leading to hyperpolarizing GABA activity.[64]

In the past decade, it was reported that OXT released by the mother during labor was able to induce a temporary switch in GABA polarity in the fetal rat hippocampus, possibly by modulating CCCs[65] (Figure 1, upper left drawing); through this modulation of GABA polarity, OXT was found to exert a neuroprotective role against oxygen deprivation at parturition[65] and to protect immature neurons from glucose-oxygen deprivation and reoxygenation.[66] Moreover, OXT produces an important analgesic effect in the newborn rat by increasing the GABAergic inhibition of the primary nociceptive afferents. This is the result of both an increased GABA release and a change in the GABA driving force toward more hyperpolarizing values.[67] Clinical findings suggest that a similar analgesic effect may be exerted by OXT in humans as well, because the pain threshold is reported to be higher in vaginally delivered than in cesarean newborns.[68] The dramatic relevance of OXT-induced GABA inhibition during delivery was clearly established by Ben-Ari's group.[69,70] In two different rodent models of autism in which this transient GABA switch is absent (the valproate rat and the $Fmr1^{-/-}$/fragile X mouse model), maternal pretreatment with OXT or with a selective NKCC1 inhibitor (bumetanide) was able to restore GABA inhibition in pups and to rescue behavioral deficits in the offspring. Moreover, treating mothers the day before labor with an OXTR antagonist was sufficient to induce in the offspring electrophysiological and behavioral deficits similar to those observed in autistic models.[69,70] The CCCs involved in the GABA inhibition are receiving much attention as therapeutic targets for the treatment of neuropsychiatric disorders linked to E/I imbalance, such as epilepsy and autism, and some clinical trials with bumetanide are ongoing, with promising results.[71,72] We thus hypothesize that they represent molecular targets mediating the OXT-induced amelioration of autistic symptoms.

OXT-induced GABA switch has been also linked to the appearance of the first coherent neuronal activity pattern, named synchronous plateau assemblies (SPAs) (Figure 1, upper right drawing).[73] These are spontaneous nonsynaptic gap junction—mediated calcium plateaus that synchronize small groups of neurons. SPAs appear around birth, gradually substituting the brief and sporadic calcium spikes that appear in the late embryonic development. They precede (and are shut down by) the more complex and synapse-dependent giant depolarizing potentials (GDPs), which synchronize entire neuronal networks. Crepel et al. observed that the number of cells displaying SPAs is increased by the application of $GABA_AR$ blockers only between PN2 and PN5, during the period of excitatory GABA activity, which indicates that excitatory GABA prevents SPAs. An analogous effect was also described when OXT or bumetanide was applied on E18. On the contrary, an OXTR antagonist given at PN0 reduced the appearance of these synchronous events.[73] Mechanisms controlling the generation of primitive patterns of synchronous activity and their proper evolution into synapse-driven GDPs ensure the correct formation and wiring of functional neural units; thus, their failure could reasonably be linked to the emergence of neuropsychiatric conditions. The

prominent role of OXT in these processes represents a strong neurobiological base for the involvement of this neuropeptide in such diseases.

Long-term Effects of OXT on Other Neurotransmitter Systems

In relation to the long-term neurodevelopmental effects of OXT on other neurotransmitting systems, serotonin (5-hydroxytryptamine [5-HT]), dopamine (DA), noradrenaline (NA), and opioids are particularly interesting because their function is strictly connected to the emotional domains as well as to a wide range of social/affiliative behaviors. 5-HT is linked to aggression and stress[74,75] and DA to pair bonding and reward,[76–78] NA is fundamental for social attachment and recognition,[79,80] whereas opioids mediate reward and pain modulation.[81,82] The implications of these systems in psychiatric diseases such as depression, schizophrenia, addiction, and particularly autism make them an interesting target of study when analyzing how perinatal OXT shapes the brain during development.

OXT AND SEROTONIN

Serotonin is known to be altered in autism: 30% of autistic patients have increased levels of 5-HT in the bloodstream and elevated 5-HT content in platelets (reviewed in Refs 83,84), and an increase in 5-HT fibers has been found in post-mortem brains of autistic patients.[85] Whether the 5-HTergic system is a relevant target of OXT in the developing brain is not known. To our knowledge, only one study looked at the effects of perinatal OXT administration on the 5-HTergic system, demonstrating that OXT treatment to male rat pups on the first day of life resulted in increased 5-HTergic fiber density at weaning in selected brain regions. This work provided only morphological data, with no functional and behavioral correlates, nonetheless it is interesting for its suggestion of the 5-HTergic system as an OXT target possibly relevant to the emergence of autistic symptoms.[86] In the same line are results obtained in the developmental hyperserotonemia (DHS) model of autism, in which autistic-like symptoms are induced by chronic hyperstimulation of the 5-HT receptors. In this model, a reduction in OXT-producing cells in the hypothalamus and of efferent OXTergic projections was demonstrated,[83] strongly suggesting a bidirectional influence between the developing OXT and 5-HT systems. It would be interesting to progress further along this line, to investigate whether treatment with OXT at birth can prevent long-term inhibition of the OXTergic system and detrimental effects on the

5-HT system induced by chronic 5-HT hyperstimulation in the DHS model.

In the adult brain, OXT has clearly been shown to modulate 5-HTergic transmission. The main 5-HTergic center in the brain is the raphe nucleus, where OXTR is expressed by almost half of the 5-HTergic neurons. Here the activation of OXTRs modulates 5-HT release both within the raphe nucleus itself [87,,88] and in the nucleus accumbens (NAcc).[89] Finally, in humans, a single intranasal OXT administration alters binding affinity of the brain 5-HT$_1$A receptors and seems to act directly on the coupling of the 5-HT$_1$A receptor to its intracellular G-proteins,[90] thus directly modulating the function of the 5-HTergic system.

OXT AND NORADRENALINE

Noradrenaline has a fundamental role in social recognition and its maintenance.[91] It is the key neurotransmitter for mother–infant bonding, and in ewes it is essential for the development of maternal recognition toward the newborn lamb.[92] Most important, NA is fundamental in the formation of attachment in neonates. In rats, soon after birth the locus coeruleus, the main noradrenergic nucleus in the brain, couples odor receptivity toward the caregiver with reward, ensuring higher chances of survival to the newborn. This region is highly activated during the odor sensitive-learning period in infancy (1–9 days from birth), but with age its activity gradually declines to reach the adult conformation, in which it no longer has a role in odor learning (reviewed in Refs 79,80).

To our knowledge almost nothing is known about the effects of neonatal OXT on the NAergic system. Only one study looked at chronic OXT administration in the first 2 weeks of life in rats, and found increased binding of the α_2-adrenoceptors in some brain regions in adulthood.[93] In two other studies, similar results were obtained after subchronic treatment with OXT in adults.[94,95] However, the levels and functionality of α_1-adrenoceptors, which are expressed in the PVN and SON, were not analyzed. It is known that a loop circuitry between OXT and NA exists in the SON of rats[96] and that OXT-producing MCNs in the PVN respond to NA stimulation directly via activation of α_1-adrenoceptors on the cells.[97]

These evidences suggest that a deeper study of the interactions between the OXTergic and NAergic systems during the perinatal time might reveal new factors involved in neurodevelopment and in the insurgence of ASD.

OXT AND DOPAMINE

Dopamine is fundamental to the development of social bonding because of its involvement in social reward; however, little is known about its role in neonates and pups, for which extensive literature appointed NA as a major player (see earlier section). This is surprising because it is well-established that in adults, OXT exerts relevant effects in the ventral tegmental area (VTA), the main DAergic nucleus of the brain. OXT fibers often run close to DA neurons in this region,[98] and OXTR mRNA has been detected there.[99] Tang and colleagues also demonstrated that in the mouse VTA, OXTRs are functional, at least on a subset of dopaminergic neurons.[100]

At the behavioral level, it has been found that OXT enhances the importance of social interactions, via activation of the DAergic social reward system. In rats, injection of OXT directly into the VTA increases extracellular DA in the medial prefrontal cortex and in the NAcc,[98,101] a key area for social reward and affiliation.[89,102] OXT-induced activation of the VTA is also seen in humans during anticipation of salient socially relevant stimuli (either positive or negative), likely through modulation of the DAergic system.[103] Accordingly, OXT can induce activation of the VTA in post-partum and nulliparous women, in response to sexual- and infant-related images.[104]

Moreover, an OXT–DA brain circuitry has been described, in which OXT neurons of the PVN send projections to the VTA and activate DA neurons, which in turn release DA in the NAcc. This DA can activate pathways that eventually lead to the activation of incerto-hypothalamic DA neurons that project back to the PVN to stimulate further release of OXT.[105] At the same time, OXT in the prefrontal cortex, amygdala, and hippocampus modulates the release of DA through activation of glutamatergic projections to the VTA.[106,107] This system has been widely studied in relation to penile erection, but the centrality of the NAcc and the contribution of limbic regions such as the amygdala and the hippocampus make it a potential hub for the integration of emotionality, social reward, and control of stereotyped behavior. Indeed, the NAcc seems to be the site of elaboration of several sensorial inputs relevant to social affiliation, and it is fundamental for OXT-driven social behavior.[108]

From reviewing the literature on interactions between OXT and monoamines, it is clearly seen that whereas several studies investigated the impact of aminergic manipulation on the OXT–OXTR system, few studies considered the reverse, i.e., how OXT affects the monoaminergic systems, in particular when administered at birth. The levels of monoamines were analyzed by high-performance liquid chromatography in several brain regions of 4-month-old rats that had received a single injection of OXT 1 day after birth.[109] Selective and specific effects of OXT on the metabolism of 5-HT and DA in the brain in the long term were reported; once again, gender differences were observed. Even if preliminary, these data suggest that OXT can influence the aminergic systems, and they strongly call for a detailed neurochemical and molecular analysis of the underlying mechanisms. Knowledge of developmental links between OXT and the monoaminergic systems is fundamental in light of possible treatments with OXT for children with ASD, and studies in which OXT is administered to animal models of autism based on monoaminergic dysfunctions are urgently needed.

OXT AND OPIOIDS

The desire to interact socially with conspecifics is based on reward and motivation, thus calling for an implication not only of the dopaminergic system but also of the opioid brain network. The brain opioid hypothesis of social attachment, originally formulated by Panksepp,[110] posits that reductions in opioid activity should increase the desire for social companionship, and increases in this system should reduce the need for affiliation.[111] Observations consistent with this hypothesis have been collected in a large variety of species using several distinct behavioral measures.[112] The μ-opioid system is a crucial component of the social reward processes, and in relation to mother-infant bonding it modulates the positive affective states associated with maternal stimuli.[113] Resilience to bonding could therefore likely result from a diminished capacity to experience pleasure and reward in response to maternal stimuli. Because social attachment is normally formed to conspecifics, Burkett and Young[114] suggested that the OXT system may integrate social information and attachment behavior to interact meaningfully with the reward circuitry. However, it is not yet clear how OXT and opioids mutually interact and how a defect in one system could influence the other, particularly during the first stages of social brain development. Knockout mice for the μ-opioid receptor (Oprm1$^{-/-}$ mice) have a deficit in social behavior and communication from infancy onward (i.e., a deficit in attachment behavior in infancy and reduced sociability during adolescence and in adult life).[115,116] Interestingly, these animals display increased OXTR expression in selected brain regions (medial anterior olfactory nucleus, central and medial amygdala, and NAcc), which provides evidence for an interaction between OXT and opioids in socially relevant brain areas. Moreover, a single intranasal OXT administration in adult mice shortly before the test was shown to rescue the social impairments of Oprm1$^{-/-}$ male mice, which suggests that the OXTergic system may act as a compensatory mechanism to bypass and/or restore alterations in circuits linked to impaired social behavior.[117]

CONCLUSIONS

In animal models characterized by autistic-like symptoms, OXT administration has been reported to rescue social deficits when given to young adults[8,38,39,117] and pups.[7,9,69,70] However, there is still no definitive evidence for consistent and reproducible ameliorating effects of OXT administration on social dysfunction in patients affected by psychiatric or neurodevelopmental disorders.[3,4] Such bias can be due to our incomplete knowledge of the complex effects of OXT at birth and during PN development, which hampers a successful selection of patients, dose, and time schedule for effective OXT treatment. A detailed neurochemical and molecular analysis of the developmental role of OXT in preclinical models is strongly needed to provide a solid mechanism-based therapeutic strategy focused on early and long-lasting restoration of neuronal function in ASD.

LIST OF ABBREVIATIONS

5-HT 5-Hydroxytryptamine; serotonin
ASD Autism spectrum disorder
AVP Arginine-vasopressin
DA Dopamine
E/I Excitation/inhibition
ER Estrogen receptor
GABA γ-Aminobutyric acid
KO Knockout
MCN Magnocellular neuron
NA Noradrenaline
NAcc Nucleus accumbens
OXT Oxytocin
OXTR Oxytocin receptor
PN Postnatal
PVN Paraventricular nucleus of the hypothalamus
SON Supraoptic nucleus
VTA Ventral tegmental area

Acknowledgments

Preparation of this review was supported by Telethon Foundation grant GGP12207 and CNR Research Project on Aging and Regione Lombardia (Project MbMM-convenzione no. 18099/RCC) (to BC). M. L. is the recipient of a Fondazione Confalonieri fellowship.

References

1. Donaldson ZR, Young LJ. Oxytocin, vasopressin, and the neurogenetics of sociality. *Science* November 7, 2008;**322**(5903):900–4.

2. Young LJ, Barrett CE. Neuroscience. Can oxytocin treat autism? *Science* February 20, 2015;**347**(6224):825–6.

3. Anagnostou E, Soorya L, Brian J, Dupuis A, Mankad D, Smile S, et al. Intranasal oxytocin in the treatment of autism spectrum disorders: a review of literature and early safety and efficacy data in youth. *Brain Res* September 11, 2014;**1580**:188–98.

4. Bakermans-Kranenburg MJ, van I Jzendoorn MH. Sniffing around oxytocin: review and meta-analyses of trials in healthy and clinical groups with implications for pharmacotherapy. *Transl Psychiatry* 2013;**3**:e258.

5. Grinevich V, Desarménien MG, Chini B, Tauber M, Muscatelli F. Ontogenesis of oxytocin pathways in the mammalian brain: late maturation and psychosocial disorders. *Front Neuroanatomy* 2015;**8**.

6. Carter CS, Boone EM, Pournajafi-Nazarloo H, Bales KL. Consequences of early experiences and exposure to oxytocin and vasopressin are sexually dimorphic. *Dev Neurosci* 2009;**31**(4):332–41.

7. Schaller F, Watrin F, Sturny R, Massacrier A, Szepetowski P, Muscatelli F. A single postnatal injection of oxytocin rescues the lethal feeding behaviour in mouse newborns deficient for the imprinted Magel2 gene. *Hum Mol Genet* December 15, 2010;**19**(24):4895–905.

8. Meziane H, Schaller F, Bauer S, Villard C, Matarazzo V, Riet F, et al. An early postnatal oxytocin treatment prevents social and learning deficits in adult mice deficient for Magel2, a gene involved in Prader-Willi syndrome and autism. *Biol Psychiatry* November 20, 2014;**78**.

9. Penagarikano O, Lazaro MT, Lu XH, Gordon A, Dong H, Lam HA, et al. Exogenous and evoked oxytocin restores social behavior in the Cntnap2 mouse model of autism. *Sci Transl Med* January 21, 2015;**7**(271):271ra278.

10. Rice LJ, Einfeld SL. Cognitive and behavioural aspects of Prader-Willi syndrome. *Curr Opin Psychiatry* March 2015;**28**(2):102–6.

11. Hammock EA. Developmental perspectives on oxytocin and vasopressin. *Neuropsychopharmacology* January 2015;**40**(1):24–42.

12. Champagne F, Diorio J, Sharma S, Meaney MJ. Naturally occurring variations in maternal behavior in the rat are associated with differences in estrogen-inducible central oxytocin receptors. *Proc Natl Acad Sci USA* October 23, 2001;**98**(22):12736–41.

13. Champagne FA, Meaney MJ. Transgenerational effects of social environment on variations in maternal care and behavioral response to novelty. *Behav Neurosci* December 2007;**121**(6):1353–63.

14. Lukas M, Bredewold R, Neumann ID, Veenema AH. Maternal separation interferes with developmental changes in brain vasopressin and oxytocin receptor binding in male rats. *Neuropharmacology* January 2010;**58**(1):78–87.

15. Curley JP, Davidson S, Bateson P, Champagne FA. Social enrichment during postnatal development induces transgenerational effects on emotional and reproductive behavior in mice. *Front Behav Neurosci* 2009;**3**:25.

16. Zheng JJ, Li SJ, Zhang XD, Miao WY, Zhang D, Yao H, et al. Oxytocin mediates early experience-dependent cross-modal plasticity in the sensory cortices. *Nat Neurosci* March 2014;**17**(3):391–9.

17. Brown CH, Bains JS, Ludwig M, Stern JE. Physiological regulation of magnocellular neurosecretory cell activity: integration of intrinsic, local and afferent mechanisms. *J Neuroendocrinol* August 2013;**25**(8):678–710.

18. Chevaleyre V, Moos FC, Desarmenien MG. Interplay between presynaptic and postsynaptic activities is required for dendritic plasticity and synaptogenesis in the supraoptic nucleus. *J Neurosci* January 1, 2002;**22**(1):265–73.

19. Yamamoto Y, Cushing BS, Kramer KM, Epperson PD, Hoffman GE, Carter CS. Neonatal manipulations of oxytocin alter expression of oxytocin and vasopressin immunoreactive cells in the paraventricular nucleus of the hypothalamus in a gender-specific manner. *Neuroscience* 2004;**125**(4):947–55.

20. Kramer KM, Choe C, Carter CS, Cushing BS. Developmental effects of oxytocin on neural activation and neuropeptide release in response to social stimuli. *Horm Behav* February 2006;**49**(2):206–14.

21. Perry AN, Paramadilok A, Cushing BS. Neonatal oxytocin alters subsequent estrogen receptor alpha protein expression and estrogen sensitivity in the female rat. *Behav Brain Res* December 14, 2009;**205**(1):154–61.

22. Bales KL, Plotsky PM, Young LJ, Lim MM, Grotte N, Ferrer E, et al. Neonatal oxytocin manipulations have long-lasting, sexually dimorphic effects on vasopressin receptors. *Neuroscience* January 5, 2007;**144**(1):38–45.

23. Kramer KM, Yoshida S, Papademetriou E, Cushing BS. The organizational effects of oxytocin on the central expression of estrogen receptor alpha and oxytocin in adulthood. *BMC Neurosci* 2007;**8**:71.

24. Yamamoto Y, Carter CS, Cushing BS. Neonatal manipulation of oxytocin affects expression of estrogen receptor alpha. *Neuroscience* 2006;**137**(1):157–64.

25. Richard S, Zingg HH. The human oxytocin gene promoter is regulated by estrogens. *J Biol Chem* April 15, 1990;**265**(11):6098–103.

26. Cassoni P, Catalano MG, Sapino A, Marrocco T, Fazzari A, Bussolati G, et al. Oxytocin modulates estrogen receptor alpha expression and function in MCF7 human breast cancer cells. *Int J Oncol* August 2002;**21**(2):375–8.

27. Pournajafi-Nazarloo H, Carr MS, Papademeteriou E, Schmidt JV, Cushing BS. Oxytocin selectively increases ERalpha mRNA in the neonatal hypothalamus and hippocampus of female prairie voles. *Neuropeptides* February 2007;**41**(1):39–44.

28. Israel JM, Cabelguen JM, Le Masson G, Oliet SH, Ciofi P. Neonatal testosterone suppresses a neuroendocrine pulse generator required for reproduction. *Nat Commun* 2014;**5**:3285.

29. Markram K, Markram H. The intense world theory – a unifying theory of the neurobiology of autism. *Front Hum Neurosci* 2010;**4**:224.

30. Rubenstein JL, Merzenich MM. Model of autism: increased ratio of excitation/inhibition in key neural systems. *Genes Brain Behav* October 2003;**2**(5):255–67.

31. Bourgeron T. A synaptic trek to autism. *Curr Opin Neurobiol* April 2009;**19**(2):231–4.

32. Hara H. Autism and epilepsy: a retrospective follow-up study. *Brain Dev* September 2007;**29**(8):486–90.

33. Bolton PF, Carcani-Rathwell I, Hutton J, Goode S, Howlin P, Rutter M. Epilepsy in autism: features and correlates. *Br J Psychiatry* April 2011;**198**(4):289–94.

34. Deykin EY, MacMahon B. The incidence of seizures among children with autistic symptoms. *Am J Psychiatry* October 1979;**136**(10):1310–2.

35. Ramocki MB, Zoghbi HY. Failure of neuronal homeostasis results in common neuropsychiatric phenotypes. *Nature* October 16, 2008;**455**(7215):912–8.

36. Rubenstein JL. Three hypotheses for developmental defects that may underlie some forms of autism spectrum disorder. *Curr Opin Neurol* April 2010;**23**(2):118–23.

37. Yizhar O, Fenno LE, Prigge M, Schneider F, Davidson TJ, O'Shea DJ, et al. Neocortical excitation/inhibition balance in information processing and social dysfunction. *Nature* September 8, 2011;**477**(7363):171–8.

38. Sala M, Braida D, Lentini D, Busnelli M, Bulgheroni E, Capurro V, et al. Pharmacologic rescue of impaired cognitive flexibility, social deficits, increased aggression, and seizure susceptibility in oxytocin receptor null mice: a neurobehavioral model of autism. *Biol Psychiatry* May 1, 2011;**69**(9):875–82.

39. Sala M, Braida D, Donzelli A, Martucci R, Busnelli M, Bulgheroni E, et al. Mice heterozygous for the oxytocin receptor gene (Oxtr(+/−)) show impaired social behaviour but not increased aggression or cognitive inflexibility: evidence of a selective haploinsufficiency gene effect. *J Neuroendocrinol* February 2013;**25**(2):107–18.

40. Muhlethaler M, Charpak S, Dreifuss JJ. Contrasting effects of neurohypophysial peptides on pyramidal and non-pyramidal neurones in the rat hippocampus. *Brain Res* August 6, 1984; **308**(1):97–107.

41. Zaninetti M, Raggenbass M. Oxytocin receptor agonists enhance inhibitory synaptic transmission in the rat hippocampus by activating interneurons in stratum pyramidale. *Eur J Neurosci* November 2000;**12**(11):3975–84.

42. Piekut DT, Pretel S, Applegate CD. Activation of oxytocin-containing neurons of the paraventricular nucleus (PVN) following generalized seizures. *Synapse* August 1996;**23**(4): 312–20.

43. Sun Q, Pretel S, Applegate CD, Piekut DT. Oxytocin and vasopressin mRNA expression in rat hypothalamus following kainic acid-induced seizures. *Neuroscience* March 1996;**71**(2): 543–54.

44. Braida D, Donzelli A, Martucci R, Ponzoni L, Pauletti A, Sala M. Neurohypophyseal hormones protect against pentylenetetrazole-induced seizures in zebrafish: role of oxytocin-like and V1a-like receptor. *Peptides* October 2012;**37**(2):327–33.

45. Owen SF, Tuncdemir SN, Bader PL, Tirko NN, Fishell G, Tsien RW. Oxytocin enhances hippocampal spike transmission by modulating fast-spiking interneurons. *Nature* August 22, 2013;**500**(7463):458–62.

46. Nakajima M, Gorlich A, Heintz N. Oxytocin modulates female sociosexual behavior through a specific class of prefrontal cortical interneurons. *Cell* October 9, 2014;**159**(2):295–305.

47. Fang LY, Quan RD, Kaba H. Oxytocin facilitates the induction of long-term potentiation in the accessory olfactory bulb. *Neurosci Lett* June 20, 2008;**438**(2):133–7.

48. Gur R, Tendler A, Wagner S. Long-term social recognition memory is mediated by oxytocin-dependent synaptic plasticity in the medial amygdala. *Biol Psychiatry* September 1, 2014;**76**(5):377–86.

49. Guzman YF, Tronson NC, Sato K, Mesic I, Guedea AL, Nishimori K, et al. Role of oxytocin receptors in modulation of fear by social memory. *Psychopharmacology (Berl)* May 2014; **231**(10):2097–105.

50. Ben-Ari Y, Cherubini E, Corradetti R, Gaiarsa JL. Giant synaptic potentials in immature rat CA3 hippocampal neurones. *J Physiol* September 1989;**416**:303–25.

51. Demarque M, Represa A, Becq H, Khalilov I, Ben-Ari Y, Aniksztejn L. Paracrine intercellular communication by a Ca^{2+}- and SNARE-independent release of GABA and glutamate prior to synapse formation. *Neuron* December 19, 2002;**36**(6):1051–61.

52. LoTurco JJ, Blanton MG, Kriegstein AR. Initial expression and endogenous activation of NMDA channels in early neocortical development. *J Neurosci* March 1991;**11**(3):792–9.

53. LoTurco JJ, Owens DF, Heath MJ, Davis MB, Kriegstein AR. GABA and glutamate depolarize cortical progenitor cells and inhibit DNA synthesis. *Neuron* December 1995;**15**(6):1287–98.

54. Leinekugel X, Medina I, Khalilov I, Ben-Ari Y, Khazipov R. Ca^{2+} oscillations mediated by the synergistic excitatory actions of GABA(A) and NMDA receptors in the neonatal hippocampus. *Neuron* February 1997;**18**(2):243–55.

55. Groc L, Gustafsson B, Hanse E. Spontaneous unitary synaptic activity in CA1 pyramidal neurons during early postnatal development: constant contribution of AMPA and NMDA receptors. *J Neurosci* July 1, 2002;**22**(13):5552–62.

56. Borodinsky LN, Root CM, Cronin JA, Sann SB, Gu X, Spitzer NC. Activity-dependent homeostatic specification of transmitter expression in embryonic neurons. *Nature* June 3, 2004;**429**(6991): 523–30.

57. Komuro H, Rakic P. Intracellular Ca^{2+} fluctuations modulate the rate of neuronal migration. *Neuron* August 1996;**17**(2):275–85.

58. Tang F, Kalil K. Netrin-1 induces axon branching in developing cortical neurons by frequency-dependent calcium signaling pathways. *J Neurosci* July 13, 2005;**25**(28):6702–15.

59. Zheng JQ, Wan JJ, Poo MM. Essential role of filopodia in chemotropic turning of nerve growth cone induced by a glutamate gradient. *J Neurosci* February 1, 1996;**16**(3):1140–9.

60. Tyzio R, Represa A, Jorquera I, Ben-Ari Y, Gozlan H, Aniksztejn L. The establishment of GABAergic and glutamatergic synapses on CA1 pyramidal neurons is sequential and correlates with the development of the apical dendrite. *J Neurosci* December 1, 1999;**19**(23):10372–82.

61. Ambrogini P, Orsini L, Mancini C, Ferri P, Ciaroni S, Cuppini R. Learning may reduce neurogenesis in adult rat dentate gyrus. *Neurosci Lett* April 8, 2004;**359**(1–2):13–6.

62. Dammerman RS, Flint AC, Noctor S, Kriegstein AR. An excitatory GABAergic plexus in developing neocortical layer 1. *J Neurophysiol* July 2000;**84**(1):428–34.

63. Valeeva G, Valiullina F, Khazipov R. Excitatory actions of GABA in the intact neonatal rodent hippocampus in vitro. *Front Cell Neurosci* 2013;**7**:20.

64. Rivera C, Voipio J, Payne JA, Ruusuvuori E, Lahtinen H, Lamsa K, et al. The K+/Cl- co-transporter KCC2 renders GABA hyperpolarizing during neuronal maturation. *Nature* January 21, 1999; **397**(6716):251–5.

65. Tyzio R, Cossart R, Khalilov I, Minlebaev M, Hubner CA, Represa A, et al. Maternal oxytocin triggers a transient inhibitory switch in GABA signaling in the fetal brain during delivery. *Science* December 15, 2006;**314**(5806):1788–92.

66. Ceanga M, Spataru A, Zagrean AM. Oxytocin is neuroprotective against oxygen-glucose deprivation and reoxygenation in immature hippocampal cultures. *Neurosci Lett* June 14, 2010;**477**(1): 15–8.

67. Mazzuca M, Minlebaev M, Shakirzyanova A, Tyzio R, Taccola G, Janackova S, et al. Newborn analgesia mediated by oxytocin during delivery. *Front Cell Neurosci* 2011;**5**:3.

68. Bergqvist LL, Katz-Salamon M, Hertegard S, Anand KJ, Lagercrantz H. Mode of delivery modulates physiological and behavioral responses to neonatal pain. *J Perinatol* January 2009; **29**(1):44–50.

69. Tyzio R, Nardou R, Ferrari DC, Tsintsadze T, Shahrokhi A, Eftekhari S, et al. Oxytocin-mediated GABA inhibition during delivery attenuates autism pathogenesis in rodent offspring. *Science* February 7, 2014;**343**(6171):675–9.

70. Eftekhari S, Shahrokhi A, Tsintsadze V, Nardou R, Brouchoud C, Conesa M, et al. Response to Comment on "Oxytocin-mediated GABA inhibition during delivery attenuates autism pathogenesis in rodent offspring". *Science* October 10, 2014;**346**(6206):176.

71. Lemonnier E, Degrez C, Phelep M, Tyzio R, Josse F, Grandgeorge M, et al. A randomised controlled trial of bumetanide in the treatment of autism in children. *Transl Psychiatry* 2012;**2**:e202.

72. Nardou R, Yamamoto S, Chazal G, Bhar A, Ferrand N, Dulac O, et al. Neuronal chloride accumulation and excitatory GABA underlie aggravation of neonatal epileptiform activities by phenobarbital. *Brain* April 2011;**134**(Pt 4):987–1002.

73. Crepel V, Aronov D, Jorquera I, Represa A, Ben-Ari Y, Cossart R. A parturition-associated nonsynaptic coherent activity pattern in the developing hippocampus. *Neuron* April 5, 2007;**54**(1):105−20.

74. Olivier B. Serotonin and aggression. *Ann NY Acad Sci* December 2004;**1036**:382−92.

75. Chaouloff F, Berton O, Mormede P. Serotonin and stress. *Neuropsychopharmacology* August 1999;**21**(2 Suppl):28S−32S.

76. Curtis JT, Liu Y, Aragona BJ, Wang Z. Dopamine and monogamy. *Brain Res* December 18, 2006;**1126**(1):76−90.

77. Bromberg-Martin ES, Matsumoto M, Hikosaka O. Dopamine in motivational control: rewarding, aversive, and alerting. *Neuron* December 9, 2010;**68**(5):815−34.

78. Wise RA. Roles for nigrostriatal−not just mesocorticolimbic−dopamine in reward and addiction. *Trends Neurosci* October 2009;**32**(10):517−24.

79. Moriceau S, Sullivan RM. Neurobiology of infant attachment. *Dev Psychobiol* November 2005;**47**(3):230−42.

80. Sullivan RM. Developing a sense of safety: the neurobiology of neonatal attachment. *Ann NY Acad Sci* December 2003;**1008**: 122−31.

81. Lutz PE, Kieffer BL. The multiple facets of opioid receptor function: implications for addiction. *Curr Opin Neurobiol* August 2013;**23**(4):473−9.

82. Fields HL. Understanding how opioids contribute to reward and analgesia. *Reg Anesth Pain Med* May;**32**(3):242−6.

83. Whitaker-Azmitia PM. Behavioral and cellular consequences of increasing serotonergic activity during brain development: a role in autism? *Int J Dev Neurosci* February 2005;**23**(1):75−83.

84. Lam KS, Aman MG, Arnold LE. Neurochemical correlates of autistic disorder: a review of the literature. *Res Dev Disabil* May-June 2006;**27**(3):254−89.

85. Azmitia EC, Singh JS, Whitaker-Azmitia PM. Increased serotonin axons (immunoreactive to 5-HT transporter) in postmortembrains from young autism donors. *Neuropharmacology* June 2011;**60**(7−8): 1347−54.

86. Eaton JL, Roache L, Nguyen KN, Cushing BS, Troyer E, Papademetriou E, et al. Organizational effects of oxytocin on serotonin innervation. *Dev Psychobiol* January 2012;**54**(1):92−7.

87. Yoshida M, Takayanagi Y, Inoue K, Kimura T, Young LJ, Onaka T, et al. Evidence that oxytocin exerts anxiolytic effects via oxytocin receptor expressed in serotonergic neurons in mice. *J Neurosci* February 18, 2009;**29**(7):2259−71.

88. Spaethling JM, Piel D, Dueck H, Buckley PT, Morris JF, Fisher SA, et al. Serotonergic neuron regulation informed by in vivo single-cell transcriptomics. *FASEB J* February 2014;**28**(2):771−80.

89. Dolen G, Darvishzadeh A, Huang KW, Malenka RC. Social reward requires coordinated activity of nucleus accumbens oxytocin and serotonin. *Nature* September 12, 2013;**501**(7466):179−84.

90. Mottolese R, Redoute J, Costes N, Le Bars D, Sirigu A. Switching brain serotonin with oxytocin. *Proc Natl Acad Sci USA* June 10, 2014;**111**(23):8637−42.

91. Shahrokh DK, Zhang TY, Diorio J, Gratton A, Meaney MJ. Oxytocin-dopamine interactions mediate variations in maternal behavior in the rat. *Endocrinology* May 2010;**151**(5):2276−86.

92. Pissonnier D, Thiery JC, Fabre-Nys C, Poindron P, Keverne EB. The importance of olfactory bulb noradrenalin for maternal recognition in sheep. *Physiol Behav* September 1985;**35**(3):361−3.

93. Diaz-Cabiale Z, Olausson H, Sohlstrom A, Agnati LF, Narvaez JA, Uvnas-Moberg K, et al. Long-term modulation by postnatal oxytocin of the alpha 2-adrenoceptor agonist binding sites in central autonomic regions and the role of prenatal stress. *J Neuroendocrinol* March 2004;**16**(3):183−90.

94. Petersson M, Diaz-Cabiale Z, Angel Narvaez J, Fuxe K, Uvnas-Moberg K. Oxytocin increases the density of high affinity alpha(2)-adrenoceptors within the hypothalamus, the amygdala and the nucleus of the solitary tract in ovariectomized rats. *Brain Res* July 12, 2005;**1049**(2):234−9.

95. Diaz-Cabiale Z, Petersson M, Narvaez JA, Uvnas-Moberg K, Fuxe K. Systemic oxytocin treatment modulates alpha 2-adrenoceptors in telencephalic and diencephalic regions of the rat. *Brain Res* December 29, 2000;**887**(2):421−5.

96. Onaka T, Ikeda K, Yamashita T, Honda K. Facilitative role of endogenous oxytocin in noradrenaline release in the rat supraoptic nucleus. *Eur J Neurosci* December 2003;**18**(11):3018−26.

97. Daftary SS, Boudaba C, Szabo K, Tasker JG. Noradrenergic excitation of magnocellular neurons in the rat hypothalamic paraventricular nucleus via intranuclear glutamatergic circuits. *J Neurosci* December 15, 1998;**18**(24):10619−28.

98. Melis MR, Melis T, Cocco C, Succu S, Sanna F, Pillolla G, et al. Oxytocin injected into the ventral tegmental area induces penile erection and increases extracellular dopamine in the nucleus accumbens and paraventricular nucleus of the hypothalamus of male rats. *Eur J Neurosci* August 2007;**26**(4):1026−35.

99. Vaccari C, Lolait SJ, Ostrowski NL. Comparative distribution of vasopressin V1b and oxytocin receptor messenger ribonucleic acids in brain. *Endocrinology* December 1998;**139**(12):5015−33.

100. Tang Y, Chen Z, Tao H, Li C, Zhang X, Tang A, et al. Oxytocin activation of neurons in ventral tegmental area and interfascicular nucleus of mouse midbrain. *Neuropharmacology* February 2014; **77**:277−84.

101. Sanna F, Argiolas A, Melis MR. Oxytocin-induced yawning: sites of action in the brain and interaction with mesolimbic/mesocortical and incertohypothalamic dopaminergic neurons in male rats. *Horm Behav* September 2012;**62**(4):505−14.

102. Depue RA, Morrone-Strupinsky JV. A neurobehavioral model of affiliative bonding: implications for conceptualizing a human trait of affiliation. *Behav Brain Sci* June 2005;**28**(3):313−50. discussion 350−395.

103. Groppe SE, Gossen A, Rademacher L, Hahn A, Westphal L, Grunder G, et al. Oxytocin influences processing of socially relevant cues in the ventral tegmental area of the human brain. *Biol Psychiatry* August 1, 2013;**74**(3):172−9.

104. Gregory R, Cheng H, Rupp HA, Sengelaub DR, Heiman JR. Oxytocin increases VTA activation to infant and sexual stimuli in nulliparous and postpartum women. *Horm Behav* January 3, 2015;**69C**:82−8.

105. Melis MR, Argiolas A. Central control of penile erection: a re-visitation of the role of oxytocin and its interaction with dopamine and glutamic acid in male rats. *Neurosci Biobehav Rev* January 2011;**35**(3):939−55.

106. Succu S, Sanna F, Argiolas A, Melis MR. Oxytocin injected into the hippocampal ventral subiculum induces penile erection in male rats by increasing glutamatergic neurotransmission in the ventral tegmental area. *Neuropharmacology* July-August 2011;**61**(1−2):181−8.

107. Young KA, Liu Y, Gobrogge KL, Wang H, Wang Z. Oxytocin reverses amphetamine-induced deficits in social bonding: evidence for an interaction with nucleus accumbens dopamine. *J Neurosci* June 18, 2014;**34**(25):8499−506.

108. Keverne EB, Curley JP. Vasopressin, oxytocin and social behaviour. *Curr Opin Neurobiol* December 2004;**14**(6):777−83.

109. Hashemi F, Tekes K, Laufer R, Szegi P, Tothfalusi L, Csaba G. Effect of a single neonatal oxytocin treatment (hormonal imprinting) on the biogenic amine level of the adult rat brain: could oxytocin-induced labor cause pervasive developmental diseases? *Reprod Sci* October 2013;**20**(10):1255−63.

110. Panksepp J, Herman B, Conner R, Bishop P, Scott JP. The biology of social attachments: opiates alleviate separation distress. *Biol Psychiatry* October 1978;**13**(5):607−18.

111. Stein DJ, van Honk J, Ipser J, Solms M, Panksepp J. Opioids: from physical pain to the pain of social isolation. *CNS Spectr* September 2007;**12**(9):669−70. 672-664.

112. Nelson EE, Panksepp J. Brain substrates of infant-mother attachment: contributions of opioids, oxytocin, and norepinephrine. *Neurosci Biobehav Rev* May 1998;**22**(3):437−52.

II. FUNCTION OF MUTATED GENES IN INTELLECTUAL DISABILITY (ID) AND AUTISM

113. Panksepp J, Nelson E, Siviy S. Brain opioids and mother-infant social motivation. *Acta Paediatr Suppl* June 1994;**397**:40−6.

114. Burkett JP, Young LJ. The behavioral, anatomical and pharmacological parallels between social attachment, love and addiction. *Psychopharmacology (Berl)* November 2012;**224**(1):1−26.

115. Moles A, Kieffer BL, D'Amato FR. Deficit in attachment behavior in mice lacking the mu-opioid receptor gene. *Science* June 25, 2004;**304**(5679):1983−6.

116. Becker JA, Clesse D, Spiegelhalter C, Schwab Y, Le Merrer J, Kieffer BL. Autistic-like syndrome in mu opioid receptor null mice is relieved by facilitated mGluR4 activity. *Neuropsychopharmacology* August 2014;**39**(9):2049−60.

117. Gigliucci V, Leonzino M, Busnelli M, Luchetti A, Palladino VS, D'Amato FR, et al. Region specific up-regulation of oxytocin receptors in the opioid oprm1 (-/-) mouse model of autism. *Front Pediatr* 2014;**2**:91.

118. Ferguson JN, Young LJ, Hearn EF, Matzuk MM, Insel TR, Winslow JT. Social amnesia in mice lacking the oxytocin gene. *Nat Genet* 2000;**25**:284−8.

119. Higashida H, Yokoyama S, Munesue T, Kikuchi M, Minabe Y, Lopatina O. CD38 gene knockout juvenile mice: a model of oxytocin signal defects in autism. *Biol Pharm Bull* 2011;**34**: 1369−72.

120. Jin D, Liu HX, Hirai H, Torashima T, Nagai T, et al. CD38 is critical for social behaviour by regulating oxytocin secretion. *Nature* 2007; **446**:41−5.

121. Dombret C, Nguyen T, Schakman O, Michaud JL, Hardin-Pouzet H, et al. Loss of Maged1 results in obesity, deficits of social interactions, impaired sexual behavior and severe alteration of mature oxytocin production in the hypothalamus. *Hum Mol Genet* 2012;**21**:4703−17.

122. Francis SM, Sagar A, Levin-Decanini T, Liu W, Carter CS, Jacob S. Oxytocin and vasopressin systems in genetic syndromes and neurodevelopmental disorders. *Brain Res* 2014;**1580**:199−218.

123. Takayanagi Y, Yoshida M, Bielsky IF, Ross HE, Kawamata M, et al. Pervasive social deficits, but normal parturition, in oxytocin receptor-deficient mice. *Proc Natl Acad Sci USA* 2005;**102**: 16096−101.

124. Liu W, Pappas GD, Carter CS. Oxytocin receptors in brain cortical regions are reduced in haploinsufficient (+/−) reeler mice. *Neurol Res* 2005;**27**:339−45.

125. Champagne FA, Curley JP, Swaney WT, Hasen NS, Keverne EB. Paternal influence on female behavior: the role of Peg3 in exploration, olfaction, and neuroendocrine regulation of maternal behavior of female mice. *Behav Neurosci* 2009;**123**:469−80.

126. Stefanik P, Olexova L, Krskova L. Increased sociability and gene expression of oxytocin and its receptor in the brains of rats affected prenatally by valproic acid. *Pharmacol Biochem Behav* 2015;**131C**:42−50.

127. Silverman JL, Yang M, Turner SM, Katz AM, Bell DB, et al. Low stress reactivity and neuroendocrine factors in the BTBR T+tf/J mouse model of autism. *Neuroscience* 2010;**171**:1197−208.

EXPERIMENTAL MODELS, CLINICAL AND PHARMACOLOGICAL ASPECTS OF MAJOR ASDS, AND INTELLECTUAL DISABILITY SYNDROMES

Mouse Behavior and Models for Autism Spectrum Disorders

Laura Ricceri, Caterina Michetti, Maria Luisa Scattoni

Department of Cell Biology and Neuroscience, Istituto Superiore di Sanità, Rome, Italy

OUTLINE

Neuronal and Synaptic Dysfunction in Autism Spectrum Disorder and Intellectual Disability
http://dx.doi.org/10.1016/B978-0-12-800109-7.00017-0

INTRODUCTION

Animal models provide essential translational tools for studying mechanisms underlying human genetic disorders and for developing treatment strategies.[1] In principle, an effective mouse model should incorporate face validity (i.e., strong analogies to the endophenotypes of the human syndrome), construct validity (i.e., the same biological dysfunction that causes the human disease, such as a gene mutation or anatomical abnormality), and predictive validity (i.e., an analogous response to treatments that prevent or reverse symptoms in human disease). However, no animal model will ever fully recapitulate a uniquely human disorder such as autism spectrum disorders (ASDs). Moreover, because the etiopathogenesis of autism remain unknown, and to date no treatments consistently improve the core symptoms, it is currently not possible to incorporate definitive construct and predictive validity into an animal model of autism.

In the absence of consistent biological markers, the diagnosis of ASDs is currently based on well-defined behavioral symptoms, and animal models therefore focus on behavioral phenotypes with face validity to the diagnostic symptoms of autism. Validation of ASD rodent models is based on a parallel identification of one or more of the distinctive clinical features of autism through a set of behavioral tasks measuring social interaction and communication deficits and repetitive behaviors.[2–7]

Several data strongly support the role of genetic factors in autism etiology.[8–15] For this reason, preclinical research has generated transgenic and knockout mice, and more recently also rats, with mutations in genes identified in ASD children, with the main aim of: (1) understanding the role of those genes in ASD etiology, (2) discovering the biological mechanisms underlying autistic behaviors detected in these mutant lines, and (3) evaluating potential treatments.

Mice and rats may be helpful to model neurodevelopmental disorders in which unusual social behaviors are major components. In fact, they are both social species with a wide repertoire of social behaviors that range from parenting and communal nesting their pups, to juvenile play, and to sexual and aggressive behaviors.

The American Psychiatric Association published the fifth edition of the *Diagnostic and Statistical Manual of Mental Disorders* (DSM-5), which introduced some changes in diagnostic criteria.[16] Two of the previous diagnostic criteria, qualitative impairments in reciprocal social interactions and in communication, have been merged into "Persistent deficits in social communication and social interaction across contexts."[16] This change became necessary to acknowledge that deficits in communication are intimately related to social deficits. Such an issue has led neuroscientists to develop and apply (or reapply) in preclinical settings behavioral methods to simultaneously record and evaluate these two key aspects of the mouse social repertoire: social motivation and bioacoustic communication.

The following paragraphs present the state of the art of behavioral phenotyping tasks to assess autism core symptoms in autism animal models.

Behavioral phenotyping can be addressed by using standardized (and thus comparable) methodology targeting ASD core symptoms. In many cases, however, other behavioral tests have been performed as well, providing additional information about other aspects of the phenotype (e.g., other comorbidity traits such us learning and memory, including flexibility, anxiety, response to novelty, etc.).

BEHAVIORAL PARADIGMS USED IN MOUSE MODELS OF ASDs

Modeling the First ASD Core Symptom: Persistent Deficits in Social Communication and Social Interaction across Contexts

Social Interaction Tests

Social interaction tests allow a fine-grained evaluation of social responses that the subject mouse exhibits when directly facing a co-specific (i.e., a freely moving stimulus mouse). Importantly, these tests also allow a concomitant measurement of mouse ultrasonic vocalizations (USVs), to assess social and vocal repertoires simultaneously, in line with the recent revision of DSM-5 concerning the ASD core symptoms classification.

During social interaction tests, mice investigate each other primarily by sniffing their anogenital region, their head, or the rest of their body, by crawling over and under each other, and reciprocal following. This test can be performed in same-sex pairs (male—male or female—female) or in male—female pairs. Moreover, both in the male—female and female—female social interaction tests, emission of USVs (ranging from 40 to 80 kHz) is a consistent and robust phenomenon and is considered an index of social interest and motivation.[17–19] These vocalizations have been positively correlated with social investigation such as anogenital sniffing.[17,20–22] Digital spectrographic analysis currently allows to collect further information upon genetic factors shaping the ultrasonic vocalization response and upon USV qualitative features (waveforms of the calls) (Figure 1). Ultrasonic vocalizations can be classified into up to 10 categories defined according to internal frequency changes, duration, and spectrographic shape.[22–26]

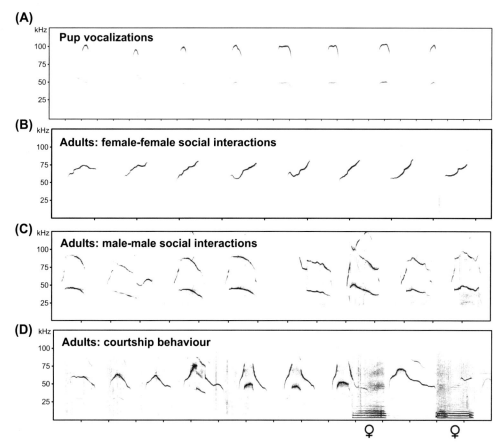

FIGURE 1   Sequences of calls emitted by mice at different ages during varied social contexts. (A) Pup separation calls collected from an 8-day-old mouse of the C57BL/6J strain after removal from the nest and placement in a 23 °C soundproof chamber. (B) Calls emitted by a resident female in response to the presence of an intruder female. Both mice were of the C57BL/6J strain. (C) Calls emitted during male—male interactions were collected after an intruder male of the C57BL/6J strain was inserted into the cage of a resident male mouse of the C57BL/6J strain in his home cage environment after 3 days of social isolation. (D) Calls emitted by a C57BL/6J male when a female of the same strain was inserted into the cage; some audible (< 20-kHz) female calls are also indicated. On the x-axis time (ms); on the y-axis frequency (kHz).

To assess USV rates in female[27] and juvenile[28] mice, an anesthetized female was used as social stimulus. This procedure can be useful to elicit vocalization in juveniles, ruling out the possibility that two animals vocalize during social interaction, but it needs detailed characterization (a developmental profile, the role of the sex of the anesthetized partner). Importantly, it would be necessary to assess the possibility of a simultaneous collection of social investigation responses, which would render this test a new informative behavioral assay for juvenile mice, also suitable for studying developmental trajectories of social behavior extremely relevant to neurodevelopmental disorders such as ASDs.

Male–Female Social Interaction

Because children with autism have a sex ratio of 4:1 (male to female), behavioral phenotyping of animal models has primarily focused on male mice; the male—female interaction has been therefore the most popular interaction test to detect communication deficits in ASD mouse models at adulthood.[22,29–39] Indeed, males vocalize during encounters with a female (whereas the female does not vocalize), and such vocalizations are usually associated with anogenital sniffing responses.[22,40,41] Moreover, as illustrated in Table 1, in most ASD mouse models considered, sniffing levels and vocalization rate alterations (compared with wild types) go in the same direction.

Despite the wide use of male—female tests in behavioral phenotyping of ASD mouse models, some methodological considerations need to be raised to control for undesirable sources of variability.

Because the session length has not been standardized and varies from 3[34,35,37] to 5[22,29–32,38,39] and up to 10 min,[33] it is thus useful to present these data as the mean value per minute throughout the session, to allow meaningful direct comparisons among different experiments, mouse lines, and laboratories.

TABLE 1   Schematic Data from Tests Addressing Autistic Core Symptomatology in ASD Mouse Models

ASD Mouse Models	Social Behaviors											Repetitive Behaviors				References
	Social Interactions							Social Approach		Social Recognition		Motor Stereotypies		Inflexibility		
	M–F		F–F		M–M											
	Sniff	USVs	Sniff	USVs	Sniff	USVs	A	Soc	Nov	Fam	Unfam	Self Grooming	Marble Burying	T/Y Maze	Water Maze	
Avpr1aR −/−							−			−	−					99
													↓			295
Avpr1bR +/−	−		−													46
Avpr1bR −/−	−		−	↓												46
								↑	↑							55
						↓(RI)										296
						↑(RI)				↑	↑					298
Cadm1 −/−		↓						↑		↑	↑	↑				74
Cntnap2 −/−		−			−			↓	↓			↑	↑	↑	↑	61
Dlg4 −/−			−		↓			↓	↓			↑	↑	↑		31
En2 +/−	−							−				−				30
En2 −/−	↓							↑				−				30
Fmr1						↓(RI)										279
		↓			−		−	−	−	−	−					182
					↓			↑	↑	↑	↑					73
					−											255
																256
					↓			↑	↑							254
					−								−			135
	−				−											36
Fmr1−/−mGlu1R+/−													−			135
Fmr1−/−mGluR5+/−													−			135
Gabrb3 −/−								↑	↑							304
Glut3 +/−								↑	−	−(OF)	−(Juv)	−		↑		145
Nlg1 −/−								−(OF)	−(OF)			↑			↑	218
Nlgn2 +/−								−	−	−			−			159

Continued

Model		Reference
Nlgn2 −/−		159
Nlgn3 −/−		35
Nlgn3 KI		144
Nlgn3 (R451C) KI		63
Nlgn4 −/−		33
Nrxn1α −/−		27
		205
NMDA−Nr1-Neo −/−		32
Oxt −/−		72
		288
Oxtr +/−		56
Oxtr −/−		56
		57
Pten −/−		123
		66
SertAla56		162
Shank1 +/−		169
Shank1 −/−		169
Shank2 +/−		37
Shank2 −/−		38
		37
		23
Shank3 +/−		29
Shank3 −/−		39
		39
Shank3B −/−		54
Shank3 e4-9		42
Syn1 −/−		64
Syn2 −/−		64
Syn3 −/−		64
Tsc1 +/−		58

III. EXPERIMENTAL MODELS, CLINICAL AND PHARMACOLOGICAL ASPECTS OF MAJOR ASDS

TABLE 1　Schematic Data from Tests Addressing Autistic Core Symptomatology in ASD Mouse Models—cont'd

ASD Mouse Models	Social Behaviors											Repetitive Behaviors				References
	Social Interactions							Social Approach		Social Recognition		Motor Stereotypies		Inflexibility		
	M–F		F–F		M–M							Self Grooming	Marble Burying	T/Y Maze	Water Maze	
	Sniff	USVs	Sniff	USVs	Sniff	USVs	A	Soc	Nov	Fam	Unfam					
Tsc1 −/−								→	→			↑		↓(W)		58
		↓(2F)														248
TS2-neo								−		−	−		↑		→	142
Tsc2cc/+								−	−					↓(W)		246
Tsc2Kc/+								−	→					↓(W)		246
Tsc2f/−													−		−	237
Tsc2f/− Cre													↑M; −F		−	237
Uba6NKO								→						→		60
Ube3a 1x						−		→				−				273
Ube3a 2x						→		→				↓				273
5htt +/−					−(RI)		↓(RI)									314
5htt −/−					−(RI)		↓(RI)									314
MIA (BTBR)								→					↑			322
MIA (C57)						→		→				↑	↑			322
VPA (CD1)			↓(E12.5)					↓(Ind)				↑	↑			34
								−	→							318
BTBR	→	→			↓	→		→				↓		−		22
														→	→	65
												↓		↑		144
												↑	↑			326
			↑	↑												59
			→											→		143
						→										325

Blue panel (evaluation of social behaviors): male–female interactions (M–F); female–female interactions (F–F); male–male interactions (M–M); social approach test and social recognition test. Red panel (evaluation of repetitive behaviors): self grooming; marble burying; inflexibility behaviors in reversal phase of T-maze, Y-maze (T/Y maze) or water maze. –, no change; ↑, increased response; ↓, decreased response; –, no change; 2F, modified paradigm with two female stimuli; A, number of attacks; E12.5, day of treatment; F, female mouse; Ind, index of sociability (not absolute sniffing value); Juv, data collected in juvenile mice; M, male; Nov, novelty phase; OF, modified protocol on open field arena; RI, Resident-Intruder paradigm; Sniff, sniffing levels; Soc, sociability phase; Unfam, unfamiliar mouse; USVs, number of Ultrasonic Vocalizations; W, water modified protocol.

Male previous experience with females is also a key factor modulating male vocalization rates[34,37] and needs to be carefully considered, because repeated prior exposures to females maximize probabilities of male vocalizations, whereas inexperienced males may not vocalize at all.

Another crucial aspect is the sexual receptivity of the female partner; in most studies the estrus status of the female is appropriately evaluated.[22,29–39]

The genotype (or strain) of the female partner can also affect male behavioral responsiveness: The most common choice is a wild-type female[29–32,37–39]; alternatively, a female of the same genotype of the tested mice,[22,33,35,36] more rarely a different mouse strain, has been used.[42]

Female–Female Social Interaction

During encounters with same-sex co-specifics, female mice emit a large number of USVs at rates comparable to those of the male–female interaction.[43] When the female–female encounter occurs within a resident–intruder experimental paradigm, the resident female investigates the partner and emits a great number of ultrasonic calls whereas the intruder female does not, as demonstrated by alternatively anesthetizing members of the pair.[17,40,44,45] Similar to the male–female one, high levels of social investigation are associated with high vocalization rates in female–female interactions. This paradigm has been applied to ASD models and has generally found a reduction in both vocalizations and social investigation compared with controls.[22,37,42,46] Interestingly, in inbred mouse lines[47] as well as in ASD mouse models,[22,37] qualitative differences between vocal repertoires (detected by spectrographic analysis) in male–female and female–female encounters are much more limited than expected.

Male–Male Social Interaction

During male–male interactions between either juveniles or adult subjects of low-aggressive strains, social interactions include investigation responses and USV emissions more similar to ones displayed in male–female and female–female encounters.[22,34,37,42,48]

However, it is noteworthy that mouse males emit USVs and exhibit social investigation responses exclusively during nonaggressive encounters.

Resident–intruder tests directly target a different social domain, namely the aggressive one, which can still be relevant in the behavioral phenotyping of ASD mouse models.[27] However, these resident–intruder paradigms are characterized by a different pattern of social responses including offensive and defensive postures[49] never displayed during male–female and female–female encounters described in the previous discussion. As for vocalizations, only audible ones have been detected within this context, primarily in association with defensive postures, and therefore are considered stress-associated vocalizations.[18,44]

Social-Approach Test

Within the field of behavioral phenotyping in ASD mouse models, many researchers are interested in assessing mouse preference for a social context versus a nonsocial one as well as the ability to recognize an unfamiliar co-specific from a familiar one (social recognition). The social approach task allows an evaluation of both of these different aspects of the social domain by means of two distinct test phases conducted on the same apparatus (Figure 2).[50–52]

For several reasons this test has become extremely popular in behavioral phenotyping of ASD mouse models over the past 10 years: (1) It should not be deeply biased by individual variations in behavior of social stimuli (stranger mice) because they are confined in small wire cages; (2) it is less time-consuming than other comparable tests[53]; and (3) an automated version of social approach has been developed (Jacqueline Crawley's lab at the National Institutes of Mental Health) that detect the frequency and duration of each movement of the mouse test facilitating the work of the investigator.[51] However, more than preference for social or nonsocial chamber, time spent sniffing the co-specific (not detectable by automated systems) remains the most reliable index of sociability. An opportunity not yet exploited is that the social approach test can be performed on mice at different ages, which offers the possibility of following developmental trajectories.

As for limitations of this test, with the three-chamber apparatus it is possible to measure only the social approach initiated by the subject mouse, because the stimulus mouse is contained under a wire cup. Whereas the wire cup permits olfactory, auditory, and visual contact and avoids sexual and aggressive behaviors, it unfortunately prevents a fine-grain evaluation of the repertoire of social behaviors and, importantly, of reciprocity. For this reason, it is often useful to associate the social approach task to social interaction tests.[31,33,35,37,54]

In the social approach task, the sociability test phase allows the researcher to investigate preferences for social stimuli in ASD mouse models. Usually, mice prefer to spend time with a stranger rather than in contact with an object,[50,51] whereas ASD mouse models tested in this apparatus often spend equal interaction time with either the mouse or the object, thus showing an absence of preference for social stimuli that may be considered analogous to the deficits in social interactions observed in many cases of autism.[27,33,54–58] Of note, some ASD mouse models have performed only this first phase of the test, which is probably considered more informative for translational purposes.[30,32,59–62]

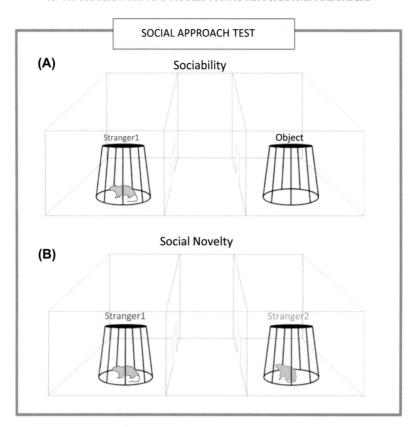

FIGURE 2   The social approach apparatus, consisting of a polycarbonate box with two partitions that divide the box into three chambers. The partitions have openings that allow the animal to move freely from one chamber to another and to choose between either an object or a mouse (sociability phase) or between a familiar mouse or an unfamiliar one (social novelty phase); time spent in each chamber, number of transitions between chambers, and time spent sniffing each wire cup are recorded. (A) Sociability phase: The test mouse is first placed in the middle chamber to explore it. After this initial habituation period, an unfamiliar adult control male mouse (stranger 1) is placed inside a small wire cup in the right or left chamber. An identical empty wire cup is placed in the opposite chamber and represents the object. (B) Social novelty phase: The social novelty test phase begins immediately after the sociability phase. The familiar mouse (stranger 1) remains under its wire cup on one side of the apparatus. On the opposite side, a new unfamiliar mouse (stranger 2) is placed in the wire cup that was empty in the previous phase.[3]

A second fundamental aspect of social competences, the ability to recognize an unfamiliar co-specific from a familiar one, can be measured in the second phase of the social approach test. Typically, control mice display a preference for stranger 2, whereas ASD mouse models often do not show a preference for the unfamiliar mouse and spent equal time in interacting with either the familiar or the unfamiliar mouse.[35,37,63–65]

This second part of the social approach test actually addresses a behavioral domain, the social recognition competences, that were previously also addressed by other tests specifically tailored to measure these aspects.[64,66]

Social Recognition Test

An intact social memory is a fundamental prerequisite to form the basis of interaction among individuals.[67] A relevant aspect of social memory is represented by social recognition, which is the ability of an animal to distinguish co-specifics and is critical for the survival of an animal; without such essential skill, animals would not discriminate between mate and intruder and would

not distinguish different degrees within a social hierarchy.[68–70] To assess social recognition, researchers primarily use the habituation-dishabituation paradigm. The test begins with a habituation phase: A test mouse is exposed to the same stimulus mouse for repeated trials and social investigation levels are expected to decrease progressively (some protocols end up with nine repeated trials[71]). Immediately after the habituation, a dishabituation trial follows in which the stimulus mouse is a novel co-specific (unfamiliar) that is supposed to elicit high levels of social investigation. This test has been performed in a limited number of ASD mouse models, with impairments evident in both habituation and response to novelty phases.[72–74]

Olfactory Tasks Relevant to Mouse Social Behaviors

Mice mainly use olfactory cues to discriminate individuals.[1,75–84] Odor cues influence a wide range of social activities in mice, including kin recognition, bond information, mate recognition and selection, sexual maturation, inbreeding avoidance, and juvenile dispersal.[1,79,80,85−88] The ability to differentiate familiar and unfamiliar individuals has advantages in many social contexts, enabling animals to form and maintain affiliative relationship while avoiding potential conspecific threats.[77,78,89−91] Two anatomical distinct pathways regulate the mouse olfactory system.[77,78,90,92−94] The first olfactory system consists of the main olfactory epithelium, which connects to the main olfactory bulbs. The second one, represented by the accessory olfactory system, consists of the vomeronasal organ whose sensory neurons send signals to the accessory olfactory bulb. Recent advances have shown complementary roles of the main and accessory systems (such as the medial amygdala, which is important for social behaviors).[1,93,95]

Olfactory Habituation−Dishabituation Test

This test measures the ability to detect and differentiate different odors. Almond and vanilla extracts (1:1000 dilutions) can be used as nonsocial odors, and soiled cage bedding or fresh urine can be used as social odors.[1,95−102] Habituation, a progressive decrease in olfactory investigation (sniffing) following repeated exposure to the same odor stimulus, indicates that the subject can recognize that identical odors are the same. Dishabituation, a reinstatement of sniffing when a novel odor is presented, reflects that the subject can differentiate a new odor from a now-familiar odor. The peak of the habituation−dishabituation curves reflects the animal's interest in the each odor.[1,103−105]

Buried Food Test

This test measures the latency to uncover a piece of odorous food such as cookies, cereals, chocolate chips, or food pellets, which is hidden underneath a layer of bedding.[1] The assumption is that food-restricted mice that fail to use odor cues to locate the food within a 15-min period are likely to have deficits in olfactory abilities. Most mice with normal olfaction can find the hidden food piece within a few minutes.[105]

Scent Marking Behavior Test

Besides USVs, mice also communicate by means of olfactory signals.[106−108] Mice deposit urinary pheromones that act as territorial scent marks[109,110] and show high interest for urinary scents left by co-specifics.[105,110−114] The deposition of urinary pheromone traces in strategic locations may serve communicative functions because, by means of pheromones, mice can discriminate among strains, sexes, and individuals.[115] A number of studies identified scent marks as a key signal through which male mice announce their identity as a negative advertisement to exclude other adult males from their territory and prevent potential competition[109,115,116]; male scent marks may also function as a positive advertisement directed toward females.[112,117−119] Male mice actively scent mark to adult females and female urinary cues,[113,114,120,121] more than to adult or juvenile males and more than to juvenile females.[111]

Because of the high relevance of scent marking behavior for mouse social behavior, in the past few years scent marking behavior has been measured in mouse models of autism.[34,39,113,114,121−123] Results of these studies suggest that scent marking may serve as an ethologically valid approach for assessing communication deficits. A reduction in male scent marking behavior was observed in the BTBR mouse model of autism[124] after exposure to female urinary cues, compared with males from the C57BL/6J strain. Because no strain differences in scent marking behavior were detected under nonsocial baseline conditions, the reduced scent marking behavior in BTBR mice in the social context likely reflects a specific deficit in the social domain.[113] Reduced scent marking behavior along with changed USV emission was also found in a genetic model of autism, the *Shank1* knockout mouse,[114] whereas in *Shank3* knockout mice no deficits in scent marking behavior and USV emission were detected, in line with a weaker autism-like phenotype.[39]

As a whole, parallel assessment of acoustic and olfactory communication usually led to consistent results. Interestingly, the same measures were associated in male C57BL/6J mice, but only when these males had previous female experience, and not in inexperienced ones.[121]

Modeling the Second ASD Core Symptom: Restricted, Repetitive Patterns of Behavior, Interests, or Activities

Repetitive Behavior

In ASD, the second diagnostic core symptom consists of restricted, repetitive patterns of behavior, interests, or activities, manifested by repetitive motor movements stereotypies (i.e., repetitive sequences of motor behavior, topographically and morphologically invariant, often rhythmical), inflexible adherence to routines, or ritualized patterns or excessively circumscribed or perseverative interest. Part of these behaviors can be measured in ASD mouse models, although it should not be forgotten that laboratory conditions per se may favor the onset of stereotypies in caged animals primarily because of low environmental complexity.[125]

Repetitive behaviors have been usefully subdivided in two classes: one (also called lower-order) including repetition of movements and stereotypies, and another (higher-order) concerning insistence on sameness, lack of behavioral flexibility, thus also having a distinct cognitive component. Both classes of repetitive behaviors can be measured in rodents.[126]

Motor Stereotypies

Mice may exhibit several spontaneous motor stereotypies such as high levels of vertical jumping, back flipping, circling, and digging, but excessive self-grooming has been by far the most common stereotyped response studied in ASD mouse models, probably because it is common in the mouse species and is certainly easy to measure.[126-133]

Another test largely used in the context of animal models of repetitive behavior is marble burying, which measures repetitive behavior related to digging not correlated with anxiety traits and primarily stimulated by novelty.[134,135]

Interestingly, motor repetitive behaviors (measured in terms of grooming and marble burying) are sensitive targets (often more sensitive than social responses) in preclinical studies testing different pharmacological strategies in ASD mouse models (mGLUR5 antagonist in BTBR mice[6] and acetylcholine esterase inhibitors in BTBR mice[136]).

Restricted Interests

Restricted interests have been modeled in mice analyzing the motivation to explore novel objects and spatial pattern of nose poking into holes in the wall or floor.[137] Perseverative exploration of only a limited set of the available objects or holes, rather than exploring all available ones, has been considered analogous to restricted interests in human subjects with ASD.[131] To date, however, these tests have rarely been used among ASD mouse models; yet, they could be useful in phenotyping repetitive behavior in mouse lines that do not present excessive grooming as motor stereotypy.[138]

Behavioral Inflexibility

Children with ASD prefer to follow fixed routines and are resistant to change.[139-141] In mice, it is possible to model this insistence on sameness and assess their flexibility in switching from an established habit to a new one through reversal learning tasks, within dry or water T-mazes or the common Morris water maze. After establishing a spatial habit (e.g., reinforcing entries into the left arm of a T-maze or locating the hidden escape platform in one quadrant of a Morris water maze), the experimental setup is changed and the mouse is required to abandon the previously acquired habit and shift to a new location. Autism spectrum disorder mouse models that display repetitive behaviors perform well during the acquisition phase but are slower in acquiring new information during the reversal phase.[32,42,56,57,60,61,65,142-145]

Behavioral Phenotyping in ASD Mouse Pups

Because ASDs are neurodevelopmental disorders with early-onset symptoms, neuroscientists highlight the importance of conducting behavioral phenotyping during the early developmental period.[146,147]

Ultrasonic vocalizations emitted by mouse pups in response to separation from the lactating mother and littermates are considered a reliable index of social motivation[148-150] and thus may represent a suitable tool for identifying early communication deficits in autism mouse models.[7] Importantly, pup isolated-induced vocalizations are considered the sign of an aversive affective state, eliciting maternal exploratory and retrieval behaviors.[151-153] Usually pups vocalize for a brief period after separation from the nest, and rapidly habituate. During early postnatal days, the emission of USVs follows a clear strain-dependent ontogenetic profile, with a typical peak between the fifth and eighth day after birth and a progressive decrease around the second postnatal week.[154-156] Unusual calling patterns, frequently reduced vocalization rates, sometimes associated with a restricted vocal repertoire,[157] are detected in several genetic mouse models of neurodevelopmental disorders,[19] including autism.[25,29,37-39,158,159] When evaluating the development of vocal response, it is crucial to check for potential confounders such as alterations of body temperature, body weight, and general somatic growth; all of these physical parameters can deeply influence both quantitative and qualitative neonatal vocalizations.[24,29,39,48,158,160-162] Moreover, evidence has been collected concerning the presence of early motor abnormalities in ASD neonates and children,[163-165] as well as in infants at risk for ASD.[166] Because motor dysfunctions can anticipate the onset of the other symptoms in ASD, preclinical studies in ASD and Rett mouse models have addressed this issue, and fine-grain characterizations of spontaneous motor behavior throughout the first 2 postnatal weeks have been performed.[158,160] These studies indicated that subtle delays are detectable in acquiring specific motor patterns in both *Reeler* mutant and *MeCP2-308* pups, which clearly point to the altered development of motor coordination capacities. Interestingly, these latter studies represent a useful strategy in terms of the reduction of number of animals to be used, because the analysis of spontaneous motor behavior can occur during the experimental session dedicated to USV recording.[167]

Other evaluations of early motor development in ASD models have been based on scoring a battery of reflexes during postnatal life, an experimental strategy initially developed for behavioral teratology experiments.[25,29,159,168,169]

As a whole, it appears that in pups, USVs and fine-grained motor characterization allow an autistic-like phenotype to be identified at an early stage during development, during which social deficits and other associated behavioral measurements are often difficult to detect.

Behavioral Tests Targeting Other ASD Symptoms

In association with ASD core symptoms, autistic patients commonly exhibit a variety of comorbid traits including seizures, anxiety disorders, altered sensory processing, sleep disturbances, and gastrointestinal problems.[170–174] Although treatments addressing these symptoms can significantly improve quality of life for patients and their families, relative underlying biological mechanisms are still barely known within the ASD context. If comorbid traits associated with ASD are integral to the disorder, we expect that many of these traits will be also present in ASD mouse models.[175] Besides the large body of evidence concerning core behavioral traits in ASD mouse models,[7,175] it is also possible to perform behavioral tests targeting associated symptoms.[121,127] Importantly, the presence of comorbid traits such as the occurrence of low-intensity seizures (inducing immobility) or altered anxiety levels could interfere with spontaneous social responses, thus confounding the interpretation of these results.[121]

An evaluation of comorbid traits (selected on the basis of information already available on the phenotype or on the basis of the role played by gene alteration on central nervous system function) is therefore recommended when performing a fine-grain behavioral characterization of the ASD mouse model.

Anxiety

Studies have estimated that 40% of ASD cases are associated with at least one comorbid anxiety disorder.[173,175,176] Standardized mouse assays used to measure anxiety-related behaviors are primarily based on approach–avoidance conflicts: Mice are nocturnal and prefer dark or enclosed environments.[121,127] Currently, the most popular anxiety-related tests include the elevated plus-maze and light–dark test.[177,178] The first test consists of two open and two enclosed arms, whereas the second is a two-compartment apparatus in which one chamber is dark and enclosed and the other is open and bright.[179] An unusually high preference for the closed arm and for the dark compartment is considered as excessive anxiety-like trait. Interestingly, several ASD mouse models such as the *Nlgn2*, *5htt*, *Fmr1*, *Avpr1b*, *Shank2*, and *Shank3* and other lines of mice with mutations that may be relevant to autism have increased anxiety profiles in addition to at least one of the core symptoms.[37,38,54,180–183] In contrast, BTBR mice show conflicting/inconsistent results to anxiety responses, depending on several experimental conditions (apparatus, lighting conditions, and previous handling procedures) (see references 62 and 130 for a discussion of such inconsistencies).

Epilepsy

Several forms of epilepsy are observed in the ASD population (with a range between 8% and 25%[184–186]); the common is in ASD patients with intellectual disabilities.[174] Interestingly, 60% of the ASD population not diagnosed with epilepsy has abnormal epileptiform activity on electroencephalograph (EEG).[172,184,187,188] Similarly, children diagnosed with epilepsy often exhibit ASD-like behaviors.[189] The presence of the seizures can be also evaluated in mice by means of tonic-clonic rating scales and EEG recordings. Tonic-clonic rating scales measure the duration and severity of seizures. Seizures can be spontaneous or drug induced; in both cases, when the seizure starts, activities such as walking, exploring, sniffing, and grooming are interrupted and mice progressively exhibit severe seizure-related behaviors ranging from immobility to motionless body/tail rigidity, and to convulsions.[190]

Different from tonic-clonic rating scales based on behavioral observations, EEG recordings evaluate neuronal activity and identify seizures as a spike-wave pattern.[180,191,192] Seizure susceptibility and high levels of seizures have been reported in several ASD mouse models such as *Shank3B*, *Cntnap2*, *Pten*, and *Gabrb3* knockout mice.[54,61,192–194] Conversely, selected epileptic mouse lines such as *Synapsin I* and *Synapsin II* knockout mice also have ASD-like traits.[64]

AUTISM SPECTRUM DISORDER MUTANT MOUSE MODELS

Autism basic research evaluates the role of ASD etiology for each of many candidate genes for autism susceptibility,[195] generating mouse models with targeted mutations in genes homologous or orthologous to the human candidate gene. Table 1 includes a selection of genetic, nongenetic, and idiopathic ASD mouse models. In particular, genetic models include gene deletion/mutations coding for proteins involved in: (1) cell-adhesion molecules and synapse scaffolding (e.g., neurexins, the neuroligin family, contactins, neuronal cell adhesion molecules, and the Shank family); (2) intracellular signaling cascades related to extracellular events (phosphatase and tensin homolog, tuberosclerotic complex, fragile X mental retardation protein, E3 ubiquitin-protein ligase, and engrailed 2); (3) neuropeptides and their receptors (oxytocin, oxytocin receptor, and vasopressin receptor 1a and 1b); and (4) neurotransmitter metabolism and neurotransmitter receptors (Synapsin family, gamma aminobutyric acid receptor subunit 3b, neuronal glucose transporter isoform 3, monoamine oxidase a, and serotonin transporter). Nongenetic models consist of two gestational pharmacological treatments and include offspring of valproic acid and poly(I:C) mothers (maternal immune activation model).

Cell-Adhesion Molecules and Synapse Scaffolding

Neurexins

Neurexins (NRXN1 to NRXN3) are neuronal presynaptic cell-adhesion molecules and binding partners of the postsynaptic neuroligins in a Ca^{2+}-dependent manner.[196,197] Moreover, NRXNs are expressed postsynaptically, where they block the synaptogenic activity of neuroligins by modulating the strength of neuroligin–neurexin interactions.[196,198] The distribution of NRXNs in excitatory or inhibitory synapses as well the interaction with neuroligins are regulated by alternative splicing.[199] There are three *Nrxn* genes (1–3) encoding for long (a) and short (b) isoforms, which differ in their extracellular domains.[196,200] Abnormalities in a-NRXNs but not b-NRXNs have been found associated with ASD.[200,201] Whereas Neuroligins (NLGNs) induce presynaptic differentiation in contacting axons (a response mediated by neurexin),[202,203] NRXNs induce postsynaptic differentiation in glutamatergic synapses through interactions with NLGN1, NLGN3, and NLGN4 and in GABAergic synapses through interactions with NLGN2.[204] In addition, NRXNs regulate postsynaptic N-methyl-D-aspartate (NMDA) receptor function through a cell-autonomous postsynaptic mechanism.[205]

Single-deletion α-NRXN1 altered excitatory transmission in the hippocampus[206]: behavioral studies showed decreased sensory gating (prepulse inhibition), impaired nest building activity, and improved motor learning ability but no obvious social defects in these knockout mice.[200,206] Double and triple α-*Nrxn* knockout mice showed synaptic transmission defects with no obvious impairment in axon guidance or synapse formation[196,207,208]; Ca^{2+}-triggered neurotransmitter release was severely depressed in these animals owing to altered functional coupling of Ca^{2+} channels to the presynaptic membrane, an effect specifically rescued by α-NRXN1 but not by β-NRXNs.[209]

Neuroligins

Neuroligins (NLGNs) are postsynaptic proteins that, together with their presynaptic and intracellular binding partners, the neurexins and PSD-95, are involved in synaptic maturation and transmission.[210–212] Genetic association to ASD has been found for three of five known isoforms of NLGNs: copy number variations in the *Nlgn1* gene and rare mutations in the *Nlgn3-4* genes[197,213] (see also Chapter 11).

In rodents, only four NLGNs exist (NLGN1–4), showing different synaptic localization: NLGN1 is localized exclusively in the excitatory synapses, NLGN2 and 4 in the inhibitory synapses and NLGN3 in the inhibitory and excitatory synapses.[214–217] The effects of the targeted deletion of all NLGNs have been extensively studied in mice. With the exception of *Nlgn2* knockout mice, all *Nlgn* mutant mice show some ASD-like traits.[217] *Nlgn1* knockout mice show impaired spatial memory in the Morris water maze and increased repetitive stereotyped grooming.[218] These mice also exhibit reduced NMDA/α-amino-3-hydroxy-5-methyl-4-isoxazolepropionic acid ratios in corticostriatal synapses and impaired hippocampal long-term depression.[200,218] Administration of the NMDA receptor partial co-agonist (and anti-inflammatory agent) D-cycloserine was able to rescue the excessive grooming behavior in adult *Nlgn1* knockout mice but not their cognitive deficits.[218,219]

Several studies performed on *Nlgn3* and *Nlgn4* mutant mice support the functional significance of NLGNs in synaptic function and social behavior.[217] Male mice bearing the R451C mutation found in the human *Nlgn3* gene (*Nlgn3R451C* knock-in mice) emitted fewer ultrasonic vocalizations at postnatal day 8 and slower righting reflex latencies compared with wild-type pups on postnatal days 2, 4, and 6.[168] At adulthood, *Nlgn3R451C* knock-in mice showed an increased excitatory transmission followed by a deficit in social novelty.[63] Mice with a targeted deletion of *Nlgn3* (*Nlgn3* knockout mice) showed a partial loss of parvalbumin-positive basket cells in the cerebral cortex.[220] At behavioral level, *Nlgn3* knockout mice displayed decreased social novelty in the three-chamber social approach test and decreased ultrasonic vocalizations when exposed to a female mouse in estrous but no deficits in social interaction.[35,200] Finally, *Nlgn3* knockout mice exhibited olfactory deficits in the buried food test, which may account for the deficits in the olfactory systems. Interestingly, some ASD patients also exhibit olfactory deficits.[200,221,222]

Nlgn4 knockout mice appeared to be deficient in all experimental settings selected to test their social competences, ranging from social interaction to social approach and social memory in the three-chamber apparatus.[27,33] In addition, both male and female *Nlgn4* knockout mice showed decreased ultrasonic vocalization when in interaction with a stimulus mouse.[27,33] Interestingly, they did not display repetitive behaviors or impairments in some of the other autism symptoms such as sensory sensitivity, sensorimotor gating, locomotion, exploratory activity, anxiety, or learning and memory.[33,219] These observations are consistent with those seen in patients with the*Nlgn4* mutation, who also do not show these comorbid features.[219]

Altogether, these studies performed on different *Nlgn* mutant lines suggest that *Nlgn* variations could have a role in ASD etiology.[200] In vitro studies clarified the role of NLGNs in synapse formation: studies with triple *Nlgn1-Nlgn2-Nlgn3* knockout mice showed that elimination of neuroligins does not affect synapse numbers in the brain but alters the recruitment of postsynaptic receptors to glutamatergic, γ-aminobutyric acid (GABA) ergic, and glycinergic synapses.[196,223,224] These findings indicate that NLGNs are essential for proper synapse maturation and function but not for the initial formation of synaptic contacts.[196,197]

Contactin-Associated Protein-Like 2

A well-validated ASD susceptibility gene is contactin-associated protein-like 2 (*Cntnap2*), a member of the contactin family, involved in neuron—glial interactions and crucial in brain development[225] (see also Chapter 12). It is intriguing that *Cntnap2* expression is elevated in circuits in the human cortex that are important for language development. In fact, *Cntnap2* polymorphisms have been associated with language disorders. A single nucleotide polymorphism (SNP) (rs2710102) in the *Cntnap2* has been shown to affect language development in the general population[226] and age at first word in children with ASD.[225] In addition, the expression of can be regulated by *Foxp2*, a gene whose mutations can cause language and speech disorders.[227] Behavioral studies performed on *Cntnap2* mutants showed deficits in knockout mice during the sociability phase of the social approach test as well as repetitive and inflexibility behaviors in the T- and Morris water mazes.[61]

Shank

Shank family proteins (SHANK1−3) are multidomain scaffold proteins forming postsynaptic density complexes (PSD)[217] (see also Chapter 10). SHANK proteins interact with many synaptic proteins including NLGNs, glutamate receptor complexes, and the cytoskeleton, acting as a master scaffold in the PSD.[200,228] Several studies found a correlation between ASD and single mutations in *Shank3*.[229−231] The *Shank* family seems to have a role in synaptic strength and dendritic spine maturation, as demonstrated by studies performed in *Shank1* and *Shank3* knockout mice. Interestingly, overexpression of *Shank1* in vitro resulted in dendritic spine enlargement,[232] and expression of *Shank3* was sufficient to induce dendritic spine formation in spiny neurons.[233] Moreover, knockdown of *Shank3* had a small spine size in hippocampal neurons in vitro.[200,233]

At the behavioral level, *Shank1* null mutant mice displayed motor impairments, increased anxiety-like behaviors, reduced vocalizations in the scent marking test, and impaired fear conditioning memory.[114,169] In contrast, these mutants also had enhanced radial arm maze spatial learning and memory.[234]

In *Shank2* mice, mild alterations were found in ultrasonic vocalization in both pups and adults, impaired social interaction in the three-chamber task, increased locomotor activity, and anxiety-like behaviors.[23,37,38]

Several *Shank3* mutant mouse lines have been generated,[29,39,42,54,235] leading to either a truncated SHANK3 protein or to possible disruption of full-length ribonucleic acid (RNA) or protein isoforms. Extensive behavioral analyses have been carried out in these lines. Reduced social interaction and reduced USVs, reduced behavioral flexibility, and increased stereotypic responses were repeatedly observed. In contrast, results concerning learning and memory performances are less consistent, with deficits observed only in one line with exons 4−9^J (Δex4−9$^{J-/-}$ mice)[42] and exon 21.[235]

Intracellular Signaling Cascades Related to Extracellular Events

Phosphatase and Tensin Homologue Deleted on Chromosome 10

The tumor suppressor Phosphatase and Tensin homologue on chromosome 10 (*Pten*) is a negative regulator of the phosphatidylinositol 3-kinase signaling pathway, which mediates several processes in various tissues.[90,217] Genetic studies showed that some ASD patients have variations in the *Pten* gene.[236] *Pten* variations have also been identified in some ASD patients with macroencephaly.[237]

Conditional deletion of *Pten* in a selected population of mature neurons in the cortex and hippocampus resulted in low levels of social approach when paired with a stimulus mouse in a neutral cage or in the three-chamber social approach test, and high levels of activity in the open field.[66,200,238] In addition, these mice had progressive macroencephaly. This feature resembles the increased head circumference seen in autistic children.[239] In addition to the macroencephaly and behavioral abnormalities observed in the *Pten* mice, there are also changes in neuronal morphology, including loss of polarity and neuronal hypertrophy.[66,238] Interestingly, mammalian target of rapamycin complex 1 (mTORC1) is a downstream target of PTEN[240] and a study has shown that rapamycin, a specific inhibitor of mTORC1, can rescue many of the behavioral abnormalities seen in *Pten* mice.[192] These studies suggest that downstream targets of PTEN may be useful therapeutic targets for treating ASD, particularly in cases associated with macroencephaly.[200]

Tuberous Sclerosis

Tuberous sclerosis complex (TSC) is a dominant tumor suppressor disorder caused by mutations in either *Tsc1* or *Tsc2*. Tuberous sclerosis complex causes substantial neuropathology, often leading to ASDs in up to 60% of patients.[241] Hamartin and tuberin, the protein products of TSC1 and TSC2, inhibit mammalian target of rapamycin (mTOR).[242] Interestingly, mTOR signaling is deregulated in a mouse model of fragile X.[243] Loss of TSC1/2 function leads to activation of the mTOR cascade and results in increased cell proliferation.[244,245] Different *Tsc* mutant lines have been studied and all displayed behavioral inflexibility in the T/Y maze.[58,142,246] Heterozygous and knockout for *Tsc1* also showed impairments in the social approach test and high levels of self grooming.[58] In addition to the behavioral changes, synaptic abnormalities were observed in the hippocampus of *Tsc2* heterozygous and in mice with a conditional homozygous deletion of *Tsc1* in astrocytes.[247,248] Furthermore, *Tsc1* conditional knockout mice showed abnormal dendritic spine morphology and density, enhanced cortical excitability, and seizures.[249,250] Brief administration of the mTOR inhibitor rapamycin rescues synaptic plasticity and behavioral deficits in the *Tsc* models.[251]

Fragile Mental Retardation 1 Locus

Fragile X syndrome (FXS) is the most frequent inherited cause of mental retardation and an identified cause of autism.[217,252] The Fragile Mental Retardation 1 locus (*Fmr1*) resides in the X chromosome. Fragile X syndrome results from the expansion of triplet repeats in the untranslated region of the *Fmr1* gene, preventing synthesis of the *Fmr1* gene product (FMRP). The *Fmr1* gene product is an RNA-binding protein that modulates mRNA trafficking, dendritic maturation, and synaptic plasticity[253] (see also Chapter 8). The phenotype of *Fmr1* knockout mice has been extensively studied.[36,73,134,182,254–256] Behavioral tests performed on *Fmr1* mice to evaluate their social competences produced conflicting results. Some groups identified deficits in social approach and social anxiety using the three-chamber social approach test,[73,254] whereas others found equal or increased social approach.[182,200,254,255] To date, it is not clear why there are contradictory results. Differences in experimental design, controls, and animal age could be potential reasons.[200,257]

The altered behaviors were accompanied by a series of anatomical and synaptic plasticity deficits primarily affecting neurotransmission at the level of GABAA and group I metabotropic glutamate (mGluR1/5) receptors. Several studies showed a severe reduction in the expression of GABAA receptor subunit mRNAs and proteins in adult *Fmr1* knockout mice,[258,259] along with an abnormal GABAergic transmission[260,261] and deficits of parvalbumin expressing cortical GABAergic interneurons.[262] A "metabotropic glutamate receptor theory" of FXS pathogenesis has also been proposed, based on a series of findings indicating that in the absence of FMRP, the FMRP-dependent consequences of mGluR5 activation are exaggerated.[263] In support of this hypothesis, a 50% reduction in *mGluR5* on the *FMR1* null background in transgenic mice normalizes dendrite morphology, seizure susceptibility, and inhibitory avoidance extinction.[264] Also, the mGluR5 antagonist, MPEP, can rescue PPI in *FMR1* null mice.[265] In addition, inhibition of p21-activated kinase, a downstream target of FMRP, rescues some phenotypes of *Fmr1* null mice. Fragile X syndrome, as several ASD-related disorders, exhibits an imbalance between excitation and inhibition in brain circuitry.[200,219]

Ubiquitin-Protein Ligase E3A

Angelman syndrome is a neurodevelopmental disorder characterized by mental retardation, the absence of language development, EEG abnormalities, and epilepsy.[217] The genetic defects underlying Angelman syndrome are heterogeneous, including large maternal deletions of chromosome 15q11-q13, disomies of chromosome 15, and mutations in the E6-AP ubiquitin ligase gene (*Ube3A*), located on chromosome 15.[217,266,267] Also duplication of the 15q11-13 chromosomal region is associated with ASD and is most commonly maternally derived, although evidence for paternally derived duplications is accumulating.[108,200,268–270] Interestingly, decreased *Ube3A* expression has been observed in a small number of cases of ASD and Rett syndrome.[200,271]

In mice, *Ube3A* is required for experience-dependent maturation of the neocortex,[102] and a deficiency of the maternal allele of *Ube3A* results in impaired motor function, inducible seizures, learning deficits, abnormal hippocampal EEG, and severely impaired LTP.[272] Increased gene dosage of *Ube3A* results in decreased glutamate synaptic transmission in mice and ASD-like traits represented by a high rate of self grooming and deficits in social interaction and the social approach test.[273] These studies suggest that *Ube3A* gene dosage may contribute to the autism traits of individuals with maternal 15q11-13 duplication.[217,273]

Engrailed 2

Engrailed 2 (*En2*) is a transcription factor important in neurodevelopment and is critical in the formation of specific serotonergic and noradrenergic nuclei in the mid and hindbrain.[200,274] *En2* is also important for the survival of specific subpopulations of dopaminergic neurons.[275] Genetic studies showed that SNPs of *En2* are associated with ASD.[276,277]

En2 knockout mice displayed cerebellar hypoplasia and a reduced number of Purkinje cells.[217,278] *En2* knockout mice had social deficits as juveniles (reduced social play) and as adults (decreased aggression when paired in a neutral environment[279] and decreased social behaviors during social interaction and social approach tests[30]). Moreover, *En2* knockout mice are hyperactive with impaired motor coordination as observed in the open field test.[279] *En2* knockout mice also showed an increased susceptibility to experimentally induced seizures that is accompanied by altered GABAergic connectivity in the hippocampus, which suggests that *En2* knockout mice might be used as model to study the role of GABAergic system dysfunction in the genesis of autism and epilepsy.[217,280]

Neuropeptides and Their Receptors

Oxytocin

Oxytocin (OXT) stimulates uterine contraction during labor and milk ejection during nursing and is involved in the central mediation of attachment behavior.[281] Oxytocin effects are mediated by the OXT receptor (OXTr). In the brain, OXTrs are found in several regions including the hypothalamus, hippocampus, and limbic and autonomic areas.[282,283] Reduced OXT plasma levels are observed in autistic children, and OXTr mRNA is decreased in postmortem samples of temporal cortex from ASD patients.[283] Genetic variations in *Oxtr* have been associated with autism.[284–287] Mice with targeted deletion of *Oxt* or *Oxtr* genes have been generated and their behavior analyzed to evaluate the presence of ASD-like traits.[56,57,62,72,288] Adult *Oxtr* knockout mice displayed more aggressive behavior than wild-type mice during male–male interaction and reduced anxiety behaviors.[56,57] In addition, both *Oxt* and *Oxtr* knockout males emitted fewer USVs as neonates, which suggests decreased anxiety during maternal separation but is also consistent with the lack of communication in ASD.[289,290] *Oxt* knockout mice failed to recognize familiar co-specifics after repeated social encounters, despite intact olfactory and nonsocial memory functions.[291] Also *Oxtr* knockout mice showed severe impairments in social recognition, as observed in the social novelty test.[56,57,289] Functional alterations in the oxytocinergic system may contribute not only to social deficits in autism but also to repetitive behaviors,[247,292] as shown by the high levels of repetitive behaviors in *Oxtr* null mice[123] (see also Chapter 16).

Vasopressin

Normal vasopressin (*Avp*) function is implicated in typical male social behaviors in animals, including aggression, scent marking, courtship, and pair-bonding.[293] Two AVP receptors are expressed in the central nervous system: A1aR localized throughout the brain, and AVP1bR, most highly expressed in the amygdala.[294] *Avp1aR* knockout mice showed profound deficits in male–male social interaction, and, similar to *Oxt* mice, they showed decreased anxiety in the elevated-plus maze and the light–dark emergence test.[103,295] *Avp1bR* knockout mice showed reduced social aggression, reduced social motivation, and impaired social memory.[296–298] Moreover, *Avp1bR* knockout mice

exhibited decreased USVs in social environments as both pups and adults.[46] Overall, *Avp* and *Oxt* models show great promise for understanding mechanisms involved in social interactions and recognition, behaviors that are severely affected in ASD.

Neurotransmitter Metabolism and Neurotransmitter Receptors

GABA

GABAergic signaling has an important role in brain development,[299] and altered GABAergic signaling has been found in some patients with ASD.[300] In addition, polymorphisms in *Gabrb3* have been associated with autism by a linkage and association study.[301] *Gabrb3* knockout mice have a high mortality rate and cerebellar hypoplasia together with poor motor skills, tremors, seizures, and learning and memory deficits in contextual fear conditioning and passive avoidance.[193,302,303] *Gabrb3* knockout mice also have ASD-like traits such as reduced sociability in the social approach test[304] and some forms of stereotyped behaviors such as running in tight circles.[303] Altogether, these observations support the face validity of the *Gabrb3* mutant line.

Serotonin

Serotonin (5-HT) signaling is involved in many neurodevelopmental processes ranging from neurogenesis to synaptogenesis including cell migration, cell survival, and plasticity.[122] Platelet hyperserotonemia is one of the most consistent findings in patients with ASD.[305] In addition, genetic studies in ASD patients identified mutations in genes involved in serotonin signaling.[306] Finally, treatment with selective serotonin re-uptake inhibitors, in particular fluoxetine, mildly improves social behavior and decreases aggression and stereotyped behavior in children with autism.[307,308]

Mice with targeted disruption of the serotonin transporter such as (5-HTT) were generated to investigate the role of serotonin signaling. The *5-htt* null mice showed alterations in cortical thickness and cell density.[309,310] Interestingly, patients with variations in the *5-htt* gene have decreased gray matter volumes.[311] In addition, these mice have altered hypothalamic–pituitary–adrenal axis signaling.[312] At a behavioral level, *5-htt* null mice had hyperactivity, reduction of aggressive behavior, and greater anxiety in the elevated-plus maze and in the open field.[313–315]

Nongenetic Mouse Models (Pharmacologically Induced)

Valproic acid (VPA), an anticonvulsant and mood stabilizer drug, is one of the most studied chemical agents linked to autism, because maternal use of VPA during pregnancy is associated with a significantly increased risk of ASD and other developmental disabilities.[316] When VPA is administered during pregnancy in rats or mice,[317,318] it causes behavioral deficits to a varying extent, including motor symptoms, social deficits, and cognitive impairment at the adult stage. The mechanisms by which VPA causes such neurobehavioral changes are not yet fully known, but among VPA biological effects, the inhibition of histone deacetylase (HDAC) might have an important epigenetic role. Indeed, HDAC inhibition in the offspring after mild doses of gestational VPA resulted in significant increases in histone H3 and H4 acetylation and histone H3 lysine 4 trimethylation; these changes throughout development, together with likely parallel changes in deoxyribonucleic acid methylation, might lead to long-term behavioral alterations in both the social communication and repetitive behavior domains.[319]

As for VPA, the maternal immune activation (MIA) paradigm has been developed on the basis of several epidemiological studies showing that maternal viral and bacterial infections during gestation are associated with an increased risk of several neurodevelopmental disorders including ASD in the offspring.[320,321] In laboratory mice, the MIA paradigm usually consists of transient activation of the immune system of the dam (during the second half of gestation) by means of viral mimic, synthetic double-stranded RNA (polyinosinic–polycytidylic acid), which stimulates an inflammatory response (via Toll-like receptor 3) in the absence of specific pathogens. Such prenatal perturbation induces behavioral alterations in social and repetitive behavior comparable to those shown by genetic ASD mouse models.[34] Interestingly, these behavioral alterations—together with immune dysregulations—appear to be exacerbated in two different genetic models of vulnerability to ASD: namely, BTBR mice[322] and mice hypomorphic for α7 nicotinic receptors.[323]

One statistical caveat is necessary for these nongenetic models: Both VPA and MIA studies to date have had poor experimental designs that did not account for the statistical requirements of an adequate number of subjects that are not littermates (in the case of prenatal treatments in multiple litters). This requirement is obvious for developmental neurotoxicologists but not as obvious in the field of mouse models of neurodevelopmental disorders. Indeed, these features are not considered (or even mentioned) in many studies, and certainly this statistical flaw may render many of the neurobehavioral results weak, as wisely pointed out for VPA studies by Lazic and Essioux.[324] The same biases and limitations are often found in MIA studies, a mouse model for which there is great interest and growing use in the field of the mouse model of autism.

Model of Idiopathic Autism: BTBR Mouse Strain

BTBR T + tf/J (BTBR) is an inbred mouse strain that displays several behavioral traits relevant to autism, including impairments in social and communication domains as shown by reduced social interest/motivation, alterations in emission of USVs,[22,25,325] and poor behavioral flexibility and high levels of repetitive behaviors.[124,326] The inherited genetic changes that lead to autistic-like behaviors in these mice are incompletely known and are still under active investigation. Unlike transgenic knockout mouse models, whose altered phenotype may be causally related to diminished or absent expression of single major genes, the impaired sociability of BTBR mice may reflect subtle epistatic interactions within a network of related genes, many of which may be normal polymorphisms.[59,130]

FUTURE DIRECTIONS

More Than One Test Is Recommended and Global Tests in ASD Mouse Models Are Mandatory

As in autistic patients, there is often huge variability in the severity of the diverse symptom-related deficits among individual mice, even when they carry the same autism-related mutation. El-Kordi et al.[27] thus proposed the use of a global score rather than a selection of singe readouts, also in preclinical research. Using the validated Nlgn4 null mutant mouse model,[33] they constructed an autism severity score for both sexes. In males, it includes seven behavioral categories covering all three core symptoms: namely, qualitative impairments in social interaction (social approach behavior, nest building, and aggression), communication deficits (USVs emitted during male—female interactions), and restricted, repetitive, and stereotyped patterns of behavior (marble burying and circling behavior). In females, similar behavioral categories were included. When applying the autism severity score, individual male mice were assigned to the correct genotype in almost 100% of cases, whereas accuracy was slightly lower (80%) in females (likely because of their weaker phenotype). The high level of accuracy obtained clearly confirms that a composite score is a more reliable starting point for treatment studies than use of a single behavioral test. Although it is unlikely that a single treatment for autism will be found, owing to the diversity of symptoms, the autism severity score as well as other global scores to evaluate the entire phenotype could certainly be of great advantage in preclinical ASD research.

Not Only Mouse Models: Potential Beneficial Effects of Development Rat ASD Models for ASD Preclinical Research

Another important development in the field of animal models of autism is certainly the generation of rat knockout models. The rat was the first mammalian species domesticated with the aim of conducting scientific research and it has become the most widely used animal model in behavioral neuroscience.[327] For the mammalian geneticist, however, the mouse soon became the model of choice, and with the generation of the first knockout mice, mouse models have often been used by the behavioral neuroscience community. A few years ago, however, the first targeted knockout rat models were developed using zinc-finger nuclease methodology. Among the first releases were a number of autism models, including *Fmr1*, *Nlgn3*, *Nrxn1*, *mGluR5*, and *MeCP2* knockout rats (http://www.sageresearchmodels.com).

The development of knockout rats promises several advantages. Rats are highly social animals with a richer social behavioral repertoire[328] and a richer acoustic communication system than the mouse species, including aversive alarm calls and appetitive ones.[329,330] The richness of the rat's social and communication repertoire allows study social-cognitive processes to be studied that are not readily accessible in the mouse, such as cooperative behavior[331] and social acoustic memory using playback of USVs.[332] Such a rich social behavior repertoire of rats might also render genetic rat models of autism a more sensitive tool to evaluate the efficacy of potential drug treatments for autism.

Need for Gene—Environment Interaction Studies

It has become progressively clear that the etiology of ASD (and its increase in prevalence) includes environmental factors.[333-335] Despite the availability of genetic mouse models of ASD in past years, to date a limited number of studies have evaluated gene—environment interactions in the development of neurobehavioral phenotype features in these mouse lines. The paucity of data is probably due to feasibility constraints in setting neurotoxicological experiments with developmental exposures in mouse lines that do not breed easily. Indeed, the few studies available have been carried out with inbred BTBR mice (that show outstanding reproductive/breeding performances among the mouse ASD lines).

As for developmental exposure to environmental contaminants in ASD,[336] the effect of organophosphates has been tested only in *Reeler* mice[337,338] and more recently in BTBR mice.[339] Epidemiological studies[339-341] suggest hypotheses of synergistic effects between environmental contaminants and selected genetic vulnerabilities that certainly need to be carefully investigated in ASD rodent models.

Acknowledgments

Supported by the Italian Ministry of Health Grant (GR3), Young Researcher 2008, "Noninvasive tools for early detection of Autism Spectrum Disorders."

References

1. Yang M, Scattoni ML, Chadman KK, Silverman JL, Crawley JN. Behavioral evaluation of genetic mouse models of autism. In: David G, Amaral GD, Geschwind DH, editors. *Autism spectrum disorders*. Oxford University Press; 2011.
2. Bishop SL, Lahvis GP. The autism diagnosis in translation: shared affect in children and mouse models of ASD. *Autism Res* October 2011;**4**(5):317—35.
3. Crawley JN. Designing mouse behavioral tasks relevant to autistic-like behaviors. *Ment Retard Dev Disabil Res Rev* 2004; **10**(4):248—58.
4. Hunsaker MR. Comprehensive neurocognitive endophenotyping strategies for mouse models of genetic disorders. *Prog Neurobiol* February 2012;**96**(2):220—41.
5. Lahvis G, Black L. Social interactions in the clinic and the cage: toward a more valid mouse model of autism. In: Raber J, editor. *Animal models of behavioral analysis neuromethods*, vol. 50; 2011. p. 153—92.
6. Silverman JL, Yang M, Lord C, Crawley JN. Behavioural phenotyping assays for mouse models of autism. *Nat Rev Neurosci* July 2010;**11**(7):490—502.
7. Wohr M, Scattoni ML. Behavioural methods used in rodent models of autism spectrum disorders: current standards and new developments. *Behav Brain Res* August 15, 2013;**251**:5—17.
8. Anderson GM. Genetics of childhood disorders: XLV. Autism, part 4: serotonin in autism. *J Am Acad Child Adolesc Psychiatry* December 2002;**41**(12):1513—6.
9. Constantino JN, Zhang Y, Frazier T, Abbacchi AM, Law P. Sibling recurrence and the genetic epidemiology of autism. *Am J Psychiatry* November 2010;**167**(11):1349—56.
10. Folstein S, Rutter M. Genetic influences and infantile autism. *Nature* February 24, 1977;**265**(5596):726—8.
11. Kleijer KT, Schmeisser MJ, Krueger DD, et al. Neurobiology of autism gene products: towards pathogenesis and drug targets. *Psychopharmacol Berl* March 2014;**231**(6):1037—62.
12. Lauritsen MB, Pedersen CB, Mortensen PB. Effects of familial risk factors and place of birth on the risk of autism: a nationwide register-based study. *J Child Psychol Psychiatry* September 2005; **46**(9):963—71.
13. Ozonoff S, Young GS, Carter A, et al. Recurrence risk for autism spectrum disorders: a Baby Siblings Research Consortium study. *Pediatrics* September 2011;**128**(3):e488—495.
14. Persico AM, Napolioni V. Autism genetics. *Behav Brain Res* August 15, 2013;**251**:95—112.
15. Rosti RO, Sadek AA, Vaux KK, Gleeson JG. The genetic landscape of autism spectrum disorders. *Dev Med Child Neurol* January 2014; **56**(1):12—8.
16. American Psychiatric Association Washington DC. *Diagnostic and statistical manual of mental disorders DSM-5*. 5th ed. Washington, DC: American Psychiatric Publishing; 2013.

17. Moles A, Costantini F, Garbugino L, Zanettini C, D'Amato FR. Ultrasonic vocalizations emitted during dyadic interactions in female mice: a possible index of sociability? *Behav Brain Res* September 4, 2007;**182**(2):223–30.

18. Nyby JG. Auditory communication among adults. In: Willott JF, editor. *Handbook of mouse auditory research: from behavior to molecular biology.* New York: CRC; 2001. p. 3–18.

19. Scattoni ML, Crawley J, Ricceri L. Ultrasonic vocalizations: a tool for behavioural phenotyping of mouse models of neurodevelopmental disorders. *Neurosci Biobehav Rev* April 2009;**33**(4):508–15.

20. Nyby J. Ultrasonic vocalizations during sex behavior of male house mice (*Mus musculus*): a description. *Behav Neural Biol* September 1983;**39**(1):128–34.

21. Sales GD. Ultrasound and aggressive behaviour in rats and other small mammals. *Anim Behav* February 1972;**20**(1):88–100.

22. Scattoni ML, Ricceri L, Crawley JN. Unusual repertoire of vocalizations in adult BTBR T+tf/J mice during three types of social encounters. *Genes Brain Behav* February 2011;**10**(1):44–56.

23. Ey E, Torquet N, Le Sourd AM, et al. The Autism ProSAP1/Shank2 mouse model displays quantitative and structural abnormalities in ultrasonic vocalisations. *Behav Brain Res* November 1, 2013;**256**:677–89.

24. Roy S, Watkins N, Heck D. Comprehensive analysis of ultrasonic vocalizations in a mouse model of fragile x syndrome reveals limited, call type specific deficits. *PLoS One* 2012;**7**(9):e44816.

25. Scattoni ML, Gandhy SU, Ricceri L, Crawley JN. Unusual repertoire of vocalizations in the BTBR T+tf/J mouse model of autism. *PLoS One* 2008;**3**(8):e3067.

26. Tyzio R, Nardou R, Ferrari DC, et al. Oxytocin-mediated GABA inhibition during delivery attenuates autism pathogenesis in rodent offspring. *Science* February 7, 2014;**343**(6171):675–9.

27. El-Kordi A, Winkler D, Hammerschmidt K, et al. Development of an autism severity score for mice using Nlgn4 null mutants as a construct-valid model of heritable monogenic autism. *Behav Brain Res* August 15, 2013;**251**:41–9.

28. Ju A, Hammerschmidt K, Tantra M, Krueger D, Brose N, Ehrenreich H. Juvenile manifestation of ultrasound communication deficits in the neuroligin-4 null mutant mouse model of autism. *Behav Brain Res* August 15, 2014;**270**:159–64.

29. Bozdagi O, Sakurai T, Papapetrou D, et al. Haploinsufficiency of the autism-associated Shank3 gene leads to deficits in synaptic function, social interaction, and social communication. *Mol Autism* 2010;**1**(1):15.

30. Brielmaier J, Matteson PG, Silverman JL, et al. Autism-relevant social abnormalities and cognitive deficits in engrailed-2 knockout mice. *PLoS One* 2012;**7**(7):e40914.

31. Feyder M, Karlsson RM, Mathur P, et al. Association of mouse Dlg4 (PSD-95) gene deletion and human DLG4 gene variation with phenotypes relevant to autism spectrum disorders and Williams' syndrome. *Am J Psychiatry* December 2010;**167**(12):1508–17.

32. Gandal MJ, Sisti J, Klook K, et al. GABAB-mediated rescue of altered excitatory-inhibitory balance, gamma synchrony and behavioral deficits following constitutive NMDAR-hypofunction. *Transl Psychiatry* 2012;**2**:e142.

33. Jamain S, Radyushkin K, Hammerschmidt K, et al. Reduced social interaction and ultrasonic communication in a mouse model of monogenic heritable autism. *Proc Natl Acad Sci U.S.A.* February 5, 2008;**105**(5):1710–5.

34. Malkova NV, Yu CZ, Hsiao EY, Moore MJ, Patterson PH. Maternal immune activation yields offspring displaying mouse versions of the three core symptoms of autism. *Brain Behav Immun* May 2012;**26**(4):607–16.

35. Radyushkin K, Hammerschmidt K, Boretius S, et al. Neuroligin-3-deficient mice: model of a monogenic heritable form of autism with an olfactory deficit. *Genes Brain Behav* June 2009;**8**(4):416–25.

36. Rotschafer SE, Trujillo MS, Dansie LE, Ethell IM, Razak KA. Minocycline treatment reverses ultrasonic vocalization production deficit in a mouse model of Fragile X Syndrome. *Brain Res* February 23, 2012;**1439**:7–14.

37. Schmeisser MJ, Ey E, Wegener S, et al. Autistic-like behaviours and hyperactivity in mice lacking ProSAP1/Shank2. *Nature* June 14, 2012;**486**(7402):256–60.

38. Won H, Lee HR, Gee HY, et al. Autistic-like social behaviour in Shank2-mutant mice improved by restoring NMDA receptor function. *Nature* June 14, 2012;**486**(7402):261–5.

39. Yang M, Bozdagi O, Scattoni ML, et al. Reduced excitatory neurotransmission and mild autism-relevant phenotypes in adolescent Shank3 null mutant mice. *J Neurosci* May 9, 2012;**32**(19):6525–41.

40. Maggio JC, Maggio JH, Whitney G. Experience-based vocalization of male mice to female chemosignals. *Physiol Behav* September 1983;**31**(3):269–72.

41. Whitney G, Nyby J. Cues that elicit ultrasounds from adult male mice. *Am Zool* 1979;**19**(2):457–63.

42. Wang X, McCoy PA, Rodriguiz RM, et al. Synaptic dysfunction and abnormal behaviors in mice lacking major isoforms of Shank3. *Hum Mol Genet* August 1, 2011;**20**(15):3093–108.

43. Maggio JC, Whitney G. Ultrasonic vocalizing by adult female mice (*Mus musculus*). *J Comp Psychol* December 1985;**99**(4):420–36.

44. Gourbal BE, Barthelemy M, Petit G, Gabrion C. Spectrographic analysis of the ultrasonic vocalisations of adult male and female BALB/c mice. *Naturwissenschaften* August 2004;**91**(8):381–5.

45. Moles A, D'Amato FR. Ultrasonic vocalization by female mice in the presence of a conspecific carrying food cues. *Anim Behav* November 2000;**60**(5):689–94.

46. Scattoni ML, McFarlane HG, Zhodzishsky V, et al. Reduced ultrasonic vocalizations in vasopressin 1b knockout mice. *Behav Brain Res* March 5, 2008;**187**(2):371–8.

47. Hammerschmidt K, Radyushkin K, Ehrenreich H, Fischer J. The structure and usage of female and male mouse ultrasonic vocalizations reveal only minor differences. *PLoS One* 2012;**7**(7):e41133.

48. Hamilton SM, Spencer CM, Harrison WR, et al. Multiple autism-like behaviors in a novel transgenic mouse model. *Behav Brain Res* March 17, 2011;**218**(1):29–41.

49. Grant E, Mackintosh JH. A comparison of the social postures of some common laboratory rodents. *Behaviour* 1963;**21**(3/4):246–59.

50. Moy SS, Nadler JJ, Perez A, et al. Sociability and preference for social novelty in five inbred strains: an approach to assess autistic-like behavior in mice. *Genes Brain Behav* October 2004;**3**(5):287–302.

51. Nadler JJ, Moy SS, Dold G, et al. Automated apparatus for quantitation of social approach behaviors in mice. *Genes Brain Behav* October 2004;**3**(5):303–14.

52. Yang M, Silverman JL, Crawley JN. Automated three-chambered social approach task for mice. *Curr Protoc Neurosci* July 2011. Chapter 8:Unit 8.26.

53. Pearson BL, Bettis JK, Meyza KZ, Yamamoto LY, Blanchard DC, Blanchard RJ. Absence of social conditioned place preference in BTBR T+tf/J mice: relevance for social motivation testing in rodent models of autism. *Behav Brain Res* July 15, 2012;**233**(1):99–104.

54. Peca J, Feliciano C, Ting JT, et al. Shank3 mutant mice display autistic-like behaviours and striatal dysfunction. *Nature* 2011;**472**:437–42.

55. DeVito LM, Konigsberg R, Lykken C, Sauvage M, Young WS 3rd, Eichenbaum H. Vasopressin 1b receptor knock-out impairs memory for temporal order. *J Neurosci* March 4, 2009;**29**(9):2676–83.

56. Sala M, Braida D, Donzelli A, et al. Mice heterozygous for the oxytocin receptor gene (Oxtr(+/−)) show impaired social behaviour but not increased aggression or cognitive inflexibility: evidence of a selective haploinsufficiency gene effect. *J Neuroendocrinol* February 2013;**25**(2):107–18.

57. Sala M, Braida D, Lentini D, et al. Pharmacologic rescue of impaired cognitive flexibility, social deficits, increased aggression, and seizure susceptibility in oxytocin receptor null mice: a neurobehavioral model of autism. *Biol Psychiatry* May 1, 2011;**69**(9): 875–82.

58. Tsai PT, Hull C, Chu Y, et al. Autistic-like behaviour and cerebellar dysfunction in Purkinje cell Tsc1 mutant mice. *Nature* August 30, 2012;**488**(7413):647–51.

59. Jones-Davis DM, Yang M, Rider E, et al. Quantitative trait loci for interhemispheric commissure development and social behaviors in the BTBR T(+) tf/J mouse model of autism. *PLoS One* 2013; **8**(4):e61829.

60. Lee PC, Dodart JC, Aron L, et al. Altered social behavior and neuronal development in mice lacking the Uba6-Use1 ubiquitin transfer system. *Mol Cell* April 25, 2013;**50**(2):172–84.

61. Penagarikano O, Abrahams BS, Herman EI, et al. Absence of CNTNAP2 leads to epilepsy, neuronal migration abnormalities, and core autism-related deficits. *Cell* September 30, 2011;**147**(1): 235–46.

62. Pobbe RL, Defensor EB, Pearson BL, Bolivar VJ, Blanchard DC, Blanchard RJ. General and social anxiety in the BTBR T+ tf/J mouse strain. *Behav Brain Res* January 1, 2011;**216**(1):446–51.

63. Etherton M, Foldy C, Sharma M, et al. Autism-linked neuroligin-3 R451C mutation differentially alters hippocampal and cortical synaptic function. *Proc Natl Acad Sci USA* August 16, 2011; **108**(33):13764–9.

64. Greco B, Manago F, Tucci V, Kao HT, Valtorta F, Benfenati F. Autism-related behavioral abnormalities in synapsin knockout mice. *Behav Brain Res* August 15, 2013;**251**:65–74.

65. Moy SS, Nadler JJ, Young NB, et al. Mouse behavioral tasks relevant to autism: phenotypes of 10 inbred strains. *Behav Brain Res* January 10, 2007;**176**(1):4–20.

66. Kwon CH, Luikart BW, Powell CM, et al. Pten regulates neuronal arborization and social interaction in mice. *Neuron* May 4, 2006; **50**(3):377–88.

67. van der Kooij MA, Sandi C. Social memories in rodents: methods, mechanisms and modulation by stress. *Neurosci Biobehav Rev* August 2012;**36**(7):1763–72.

68. Carter C, Keverne E. The neurobiology of social affiliation and pair bonding. *Hormones Brain Behav* 2002;**1**:299–337.

69. Choleris E, Clipperton-Allen AE, Phan A, Kavaliers M. Neuroendocrinology of social information processing in rats and mice. *Front Neuroendocrinol* October 2009;**30**(4):442–59.

70. Choleris E, Kavaliers M, Pfaff DW. Functional genomics of social recognition. *J Neuroendocrinol* April 2004;**16**(4):383–9.

71. Wolstenholme JT, Goldsby JA, Rissman EF. Transgenerational effects of prenatal bisphenol A on social recognition. *Horm Behav* November 2013;**64**(5):833–9.

72. Ferguson JN, Young LJ, Hearn EF, Matzuk MM, Insel TR, Winslow JT. Social amnesia in mice lacking the oxytocin gene. *Nat Genet* July 2000;**25**(3):284–8.

73. Mineur YS, Huynh LX, Crusio WE. Social behavior deficits in the Fmr1 mutant mouse. *Behav Brain Res* March 15, 2006;**168**(1):172–5.

74. Takayanagi Y, Fujita E, Yu Z, et al. Impairment of social and emotional behaviors in Cadm1-knockout mice. *Biochem Biophys Res Commun* June 4, 2010;**396**(3):703–8.

75. Arakawa H, Arakawa K, Blanchard DC, Blanchard RJ. A new test paradigm for social recognition evidenced by urinary scent marking behavior in C57BL/6J mice. *Behav Brain Res* June 26, 2008;**190**(1):97–104.

76. Bredy TW, Barad M. Social modulation of associative fear learning by pheromone communication. *Learn Mem* January 2009;**16**(1):12–8.

77. Brennan PA, Kendrick KM. Mammalian social odours: attraction and individual recognition. *Philos Trans R Soc Lond B Biol Sci* December 29, 2006;**361**(1476):2061–78.

78. Brennan PA, Keverne EB. Something in the air? New insights into mammalian pheromones. *Curr Biol* January 20, 2004;**14**(2):R81–9.

79. Brown R. Mammalian social odors: a critical review. *Adv Study Behav* 1979;**10**:10–162.

80. Doty RL. Odor-guided behavior in mammals. *Experientia* March 15, 1986;**42**(3):257–71.

81. Kavaliers M, Choleris E, Pfaff DW. Genes, odours and the recognition of parasitized individuals by rodents. *Trends Parasitol* September 2005;**21**(9):423–9.

82. Keverne EB. Importance of olfactory and vomeronasal systems for male sexual function. *Physiol Behav* November 15, 2004;**83**(2):177–87.

83. Restrepo D, Arellano J, Oliva AM, Schaefer ML, Lin W. Emerging views on the distinct but related roles of the main and accessory olfactory systems in responsiveness to chemosensory signals in mice. *Horm Behav* September 2004;**46**(3):247–56.

84. Schellinck HM, Smyth C, Brown R, Wilkinson M. Odor-induced sexual maturation and expression of c-fos in the olfactory system of juvenile female mice. *Brain Res Dev Brain Res* July 16, 1993;**74**(1): 138–41.

85. Brennan PA, Zufall F. Pheromonal communication in vertebrates. *Nature* November 16, 2006;**444**(7117):308–15.

86. Hurst JL, Payne CE, Nevison CM, et al. Individual recognition in mice mediated by major urinary proteins. *Nature* December 6, 2001;**414**(6864):631–4.

87. Hurst JL, Thom MD, Nevison CM, Humphries RE, Beynon RJ. MHC odours are not required or sufficient for recognition of individual scent owners. *Proc Biol Sci* April 7, 2005;**272**(1564):715–24.

88. Sanchez-Andrade G, Kendrick KM. The main olfactory system and social learning in mammals. *Behav Brain Res* June 25, 2009; **200**(2):323–35.

89. Dulac C, Wagner S. Genetic analysis of brain circuits underlying pheromone signaling. *Annu Rev Genet* 2006;**40**:449–67.

90. Luo HR, Hattori H, Hossain MA, et al. Akt as a mediator of cell death. *Proc Natl Acad Sci USA* September 30, 2003;**100**(20): 11712–7.

91. Spehr M, Spehr J, Ukhanov K, Kelliher KR, Leinders-Zufall T, Zufall F. Parallel processing of social signals by the mammalian main and accessory olfactory systems. *Cell Mol Life Sci* July 2006;**63**(13):1476–84.

92. Buck LB. The molecular architecture of odor and pheromone sensing in mammals. *Cell* March 17, 2000;**100**(6):611–8.

93. Kang N, Baum MJ, Cherry JA. A direct main olfactory bulb projection to the 'vomeronasal' amygdala in female mice selectively responds to volatile pheromones from males. *Eur J Neurosci* February 2009;**29**(3):624–34.

94. Martel KL, Baum MJ. A centrifugal pathway to the mouse accessory olfactory bulb from the medial amygdala conveys gender-specific volatile pheromonal signals. *Eur J Neurosci* January 2009;**29**(2):368–76.

95. Trinh K, Storm DR. Vomeronasal organ detects odorants in absence of signaling through main olfactory epithelium. *Nat Neurosci* May 2003;**6**(5):519–25.

96. Alberts JR, Galef Jr BG. Acute anosmia in the rat: a behavioral test of a peripherally-induced olfactory deficit. *Physiol Behav* May 1971;**6**(5):619–21.

97. Del Punta K, Leinders-Zufall T, Rodriguez I, et al. Deficient pheromone responses in mice lacking a cluster of vomeronasal receptor genes. *Nature* September 5, 2002;**419**(6902):70–4.

98. Klein SL, Kriegsfeld LJ, Hairston JE, Rau V, Nelson RJ, Yarowsky PJ. Characterization of sensorimotor performance, reproductive and aggressive behaviors in segmental trisomic 16 (Ts65Dn) mice. *Physiol Behav* October 1996;**60**(4):1159–64.

99. Wersinger SR, Caldwell HK, Martinez L, Gold P, Hu SB, Young 3rd WS. Vasopressin 1a receptor knockout mice have a subtle olfactory deficit but normal aggression. *Genes Brain Behav* August 2007;**6**(6):540–51.

100. Woodley SK, Baum MJ. Effects of sex hormones and gender on attraction thresholds for volatile anal scent gland odors in ferrets. *Horm Behav* August 2003;**44**(2):110−8.

101. Yamada K, Wada E, Wada K. Female gastrin-releasing peptide receptor (GRP-R)-deficient mice exhibit altered social preference for male conspecifics: implications for GRP/GRP-R modulation of GABAergic function. *Brain Res* March 16, 2001;**894**(2):281−7.

102. Yashiro K, Riday TT, Condon KH, et al. Ube3a is required for experience-dependent maturation of the neocortex. *Nat Neurosci* June 2009;**12**(6):777−83.

103. Bielsky IF, Hu SB, Szegda KL, Westphal H, Young LJ. Profound impairment in social recognition and reduction in anxiety-like behavior in vasopressin V1a receptor knockout mice. *Neuropsychopharmacology* March 2004;**29**(3):483−93.

104. Wersinger SR, Rissman EF. Oestrogen receptor alpha is essential for female-directed chemo-investigatory behaviour but is not required for the pheromone-induced luteinizing hormone surge in male mice. *J Neuroendocrinol* February 2000;**12**(2):103−10.

105. Yang M, Crawley JN. Simple behavioral assessment of mouse olfaction. *Curr Protoc Neurosci* July 2009. Chapter 8:Unit 8.24.

106. Keverne EB. Mammalian pheromones: from genes to behaviour. *Curr Biol* December 10, 2002;**12**(23):R807−9.

107. Keverne EB. Pheromones, vomeronasal function, and gender-specific behavior. *Cell* March 22, 2002;**108**(6):735−8.

108. Roberts SE, Dennis NR, Browne CE, et al. Characterisation of interstitial duplications and triplications of chromosome 15q11-q13. *Hum Genet* March 2002;**110**(3):227−34.

109. Desjardins C, Maruniak JA, Bronson FH. Social rank in house mice: differentiation revealed by ultraviolet visualization of urinary marking patterns. *Science* November 20, 1973;**182**(4115):939−41.

110. Hurst J. Urine marking in populations of wild house mice Mus domesticus Rutty. III. Communication between the sexes. *Anim Behav* 1990;**40**:233−43.

111. Arakawa H, Arakawa K, Blanchard DC, Blanchard RJ. Scent marking behavior in male C57BL/6J mice: sexual and developmental determination. *Behav Brain Res* August 22, 2007;**182**(1):73−9.

112. Jones RB, Nowell NW. A comparison of the aversive and female attractant properties of urine from dominant and subordinate male mice. *Anim Learn Behav* May 1974;**2**(2):141−4.

113. Wohr M, Roullet FI, Crawley JN. Reduced scent marking and ultrasonic vocalizations in the BTBR T+tf/J mouse model of autism. *Genes Brain Behav* February 2011;**10**(1):35−43.

114. Wohr M, Roullet FI, Hung AY, Sheng M, Crawley JN. Communication impairments in mice lacking Shank1: reduced levels of ultrasonic vocalizations and scent marking behavior. *PLoS One* 2011;**6**(6):e20631.

115. Bowers JM, Alexander BK. Mice: individual recognition by olfactory cues. *Science* December 1, 1967;**158**(3805):1208−10.

116. Hurst J. Urine marking in populations of wild house mice *Mus domesticus rutty* I. Communication between males. *Anim Behav* 1990;**40**:209−22.

117. Caroom D, Bronson FH. Responsiveness of female mice to preputial attractant: effects of sexual experience and ovarian hormones. *Physiol Behav* November 1971;**7**(5):659−62.

118. Hurst J. Urine marking in populations of wild house mice *Mus domesticus rutty* II. Communication between females. *Anim Behav* 1990;**40**:223−32.

119. Rich TJ, Hurst JL. The competing countermarks hypothesis: reliable assessment of competitive ability by potential mates. *Anim Behav* November 1999;**58**(5):1027−37.

120. Davies VJ, Bellamy D. The olfactory response of mice to urine and effects of gonadectomy. *J Endocrinol* October 1972;**55**(1):11−20.

121. Roullet FI, Crawley JN. Mouse models of autism: testing hypotheses about molecular mechanisms. *Curr Top Behav Neurosci* 2011;**7**:187−212.

122. Azmitia EC. Modern views on an ancient chemical: serotonin effects on cell proliferation, maturation, and apoptosis. *Brain Res Bull* November 15, 2001;**56**(5):413−24.

123. Pobbe RL, Pearson BL, Defensor EB, et al. Oxytocin receptor knockout mice display deficits in the expression of autism-related behaviors. *Horm Behav* March 2012;**61**(3):436−44.

124. Meyza KZ, Defensor EB, Jensen AL, et al. The BTBR T+ tf/J mouse model for autism spectrum disorders-in search of biomarkers. *Behav Brain Res* August 15, 2013;**251**:25−34.

125. Garner JP, Mason GJ. Evidence for a relationship between cage stereotypies and behavioural disinhibition in laboratory rodents. *Behav Brain Res* October 17, 2002;**136**(1):83−92.

126. Lewis MH, Tanimura Y, Lee LW, Bodfish JW. Animal models of restricted repetitive behavior in autism. *Behav Brain Res* January 10, 2007;**176**(1):66−74.

127. Crawley JN. Mouse behavioral assays relevant to the symptoms of autism. *Brain Pathol* October 2007;**17**(4):448−59.

128. Creese I, Iversen SD. The pharmacological and anatomical substrates of the amphetamine response in the rat. *Brain Res* January 17, 1975;**83**(3):419−36.

129. Korff S, Harvey BH. Animal models of obsessive-compulsive disorder: rationale to understanding psychobiology and pharmacology. *Psychiatr Clin North Am* June 2006;**29**(2):371−90.

130. McFarlane HG, Kusek GK, Yang M, Phoenix JL, Bolivar VJ, Crawley JN. Autism-like behavioral phenotypes in BTBR T+tf/J mice. *Genes Brain Behav* March 2008;**7**(2):152−63.

131. Moy SS, Nadler JJ, Poe MD, et al. Development of a mouse test for repetitive, restricted behaviors: relevance to autism. *Behav Brain Res* March 17, 2008;**188**(1):178−94.

132. Pogorelov VM, Rodriguiz RM, Insco ML, Caron MG, Wetsel WC. Novelty seeking and stereotypic activation of behavior in mice with disruption of the Dat1 gene. *Neuropsychopharmacology* October 2005;**30**(10):1818−31.

133. Turner CA, Presti MF, Newman HA, Bugenhagen P, Crnic L, Lewis MH. Spontaneous stereotypy in an animal model of down syndrome: Ts65Dn mice. *Behav Genet* July 2001;**31**(4):393−400.

134. Thomas A, Burant A, Bui N, Graham D, Yuva-Paylor LA, Paylor R. Marble burying reflects a repetitive and perseverative behavior more than novelty-induced anxiety. *Psychopharmacol Berl* June 2009;**204**(2):361−73.

135. Thomas AM, Bui N, Graham D, Perkins JR, Yuva-Paylor LA, Paylor R. Genetic reduction of group 1 metabotropic glutamate receptors alters select behaviors in a mouse model for fragile X syndrome. *Behav Brain Res* October 1, 2011;**223**(2):310−21.

136. Karvat G, Kimchi T. Acetylcholine elevation relieves cognitive rigidity and social deficiency in a mouse model of autism. *Neuropsychopharmacology* March 2013;**39**(4):831−40.

137. Elsabbagh M, Gliga T, Pickles A, Hudry K, Charman T, Johnson MH. The development of face orienting mechanisms in infants at-risk for autism. *Behav Brain Res* August 15, 2013;**251**:147−54.

138. Moy SS, Riddick NV, Nikolova VD, et al. Repetitive behavior profile and supersensitivity to amphetamine in the C58/J mouse model of autism. *Behav Brain Res* February 1, 2014;**259**:200−14.

139. Chen YH, Rodgers J, McConachie H. Restricted and repetitive behaviours, sensory processing and cognitive style in children with autism spectrum disorders. *J Autism Dev Disord* April 2009;**39**(4):635−42.

140. Frith U, Morton J, Leslie AM. The cognitive basis of a biological disorder: autism. *Trends Neurosci* October 1991;**14**(10):433−8.

141. Goldman S, Wang C, Salgado MW, Greene PE, Kim M, Rapin I. Motor stereotypies in children with autism and other developmental disorders. *Dev Med Child Neurol* January 2009;**51**(1):30−8.

142. Bader PL, Faizi M, Kim LH, et al. Mouse model of Timothy syndrome recapitulates triad of autistic traits. *Proc Natl Acad Sci USA* September 13, 2011;**108**(37):15432−7.

143. Guariglia SR, Chadman KK. Water T-maze: a useful assay for determination of repetitive behaviors in mice. *J Neurosci Methods* October 30, 2013;**220**(1):24–9.

144. Karvat G, Kimchi T. Systematic autistic-like behavioral phenotyping of 4 mouse strains using a novel wheel-running assay. *Behav Brain Res* August 1, 2012;**233**(2):405–14.

145. Zhao Y, Fung C, Shin D, et al. Neuronal glucose transporter isoform 3 deficient mice demonstrate features of autism spectrum disorders. *Mol Psychiatry* March 2010;**15**(3):286–99.

146. Bale TL, Baram TZ, Brown AS, et al. Early life programming and neurodevelopmental disorders. *Biol Psychiatry* August 15, 2010;**68**(4):314–9.

147. Branchi I, Ricceri L. Transgenic and knock-out mouse pups: the growing need for behavioral analysis. *Genes Brain Behav* August 2002;**1**(3):135–41.

148. Branchi I, D'Andrea I, Cirulli F, Lipp HP, Alleva E. Shaping brain development: mouse communal nesting blunts adult neuroendocrine and behavioral response to social stress and modifies chronic antidepressant treatment outcome. *Psychoneuroendocrinology* June 2010;**35**(5):743–51.

149. Ehret G. Infant rodent ultrasounds – a gate to the understanding of sound communication. *Behav Genet* January 2005;**35**(1):19–29.

150. Sewell GD. Ultrasonic communication in rodents. *Nature* December 1970;**227**:410.

151. Knutson B, Burgdorf J, Panksepp J. Ultrasonic vocalizations as indices of affective states in rats. *Psychol Bull* November 2002;**128**(6):961–77.

152. Panksepp J. Can anthropomorphic analyses of separation cries in other animals inform us about the emotional nature of social loss in humans? Comment on Blumberg and Sokoloff (2001). *Psychol Rev* April 2003;**110**(2):376–88. discussion 389–396.

153. Zippelius HM, Schleidt WM. Ultraschall-laute bej jungen mausen (Ultrasonic vocalization in infant mice). *Naturwissenschaften* 1956;**43**:502–3.

154. Elwood RW, Keeling F. Temporal organization of ultrasonic vocalizations in infant mice. *Dev Psychobiol* May 1982;**15**(3):221–7.

155. Hahn ME, Karkowski L, Weinreb L, Henry A, Schanz N, Hahn EM. Genetic and developmental influences on infant mouse ultrasonic calling. II. Developmental patterns in the calls of mice 2–12 days of age. *Behav Genet* July 1998;**28**(4):315–25.

156. Roubertoux PL, Martin B, Le Roy I, et al. Vocalizations in newborn mice: genetic analysis. *Behav Genet* July 1996;**26**(4):427–37.

157. Michetti CR, Ricceri L, Scattoni ML. Modeling social communication deficits in mouse models of autism. *Autism* 2012;**S1**:007.

158. Romano E, Michetti C, Caruso A, Laviola G, Scattoni ML. Characterization of neonatal vocal and motor repertoire of reelin mutant mice. *PLoS One* 2013;**8**(5):e64407.

159. Wohr M, Silverman JL, Scattoni ML, et al. Developmental delays and reduced pup ultrasonic vocalizations but normal sociability in mice lacking the postsynaptic cell adhesion protein neuroligin2. *Behav Brain Res* July 20, 2012;**251**.

160. De Filippis B, Ricceri L, Laviola G. Early postnatal behavioral changes in the Mecp2-308 truncation mouse model of Rett syndrome. *Genes Brain Behav* March 1, 2010;**9**(2):213–23.

161. Shair HN, Brunelli SA, Masmela JR, Boone E, Hofer MA. Social, thermal, and temporal influences on isolation-induced and maternally potentiated ultrasonic vocalizations of rat pups. *Dev Psychobiol* March 2003;**42**(2):206–22.

162. Veenstra-VanderWeele J, Muller CL, Iwamoto H, et al. Autism gene variant causes hyperserotonemia, serotonin receptor hypersensitivity, social impairment and repetitive behavior. *Proc Natl Acad Sci USA* April 3, 2012;**109**(14):5469–74.

163. Iverson JM, Braddock BA. Gesture and motor skill in relation to language in children with language impairment. *J Speech Lang Hear Res* February 2013;**54**(1):72–86.

164. LeBarton ES, Iverson JM. Fine motor skill predicts expressive language in infant siblings of children with autism. *Dev Sci* November 2013;**16**(6):815–27.

165. Phagava H, Muratori F, Einspieler C, et al. General movements in infants with autism spectrum disorders. *Georgian Med News* March 2008;**156**:100–5.

166. Leonard HC, Bedford R, Charman T, Elsabbagh M, Johnson MH, Hill EL. Motor development in children at risk of autism: a follow-up study of infant siblings. *Autism* April 2013;**18**(3):281–91.

167. Branchi I, Santucci D, Puopolo M, Alleva E. Neonatal behaviors associated with ultrasonic vocalizations in mice (*mus musculus*): a slow-motion analysis. *Dev Psychobiol* January 2004;**44**(1):37–44.

168. Chadman KK, Gong S, Scattoni ML, et al. Minimal aberrant behavioral phenotypes of neuroligin-3 R451C knockin mice. *Autism Res* June 2008;**1**(3):147–58.

169. Silverman JL, Turner SM, Barkan CL, et al. Sociability and motor functions in Shank1 mutant mice. *Brain Res* March 22, 2011;**1380**:120–37.

170. Fassio A, Raimondi A, Lignani G, Benfenati F, Baldelli P. Synapsins: from synapse to network hyperexcitability and epilepsy. *Semin Cell Dev Biol* June 2011;**22**(4):408–15.

171. Gilby KL, O'Brien TJ. Epilepsy, autism, and neurodevelopment: kindling a shared vulnerability? *Epilepsy Behav* March 2013;**26**(3):370–4.

172. Kim HL, Donnelly JH, Tournay AE, Book TM, Filipek P. Absence of seizures despite high prevalence of epileptiform EEG abnormalities in children with autism monitored in a tertiary care center. *Epilepsia* February 2006;**47**(2):394–8.

173. van Steensel FJ, Bogels SM, Perrin S. Anxiety disorders in children and adolescents with autistic spectrum disorders: a meta-analysis. *Clin Child Fam Psychol Rev* September 2011;**14**(3):302–17.

174. Woolfenden S, Sarkozy V, Ridley G, Coory M, Williams K. A systematic review of two outcomes in autism spectrum disorder – epilepsy and mortality. *Dev Med Child Neurol* April 2012;**54**(4):306–12.

175. Argyropoulos A, Gilby KL, Hill-Yardin EL. Studying autism in rodent models: reconciling endophenotypes with comorbidities. *Front Hum Neurosci* 2013;**7**:417.

176. Gillott A, Furniss F, Walter A. Anxiety in high-functioning children with autism. *Autism* September 2001;**5**(3):277–86.

177. Crawley JN. Translational animal models of autism and neurodevelopmental disorders. *Dialogues Clin Neurosci* September 2012;**14**(3):293–305.

178. Finn DA, Rutledge-Gorman MT, Crabbe JC. Genetic animal models of anxiety. *Neurogenetics* April 2003;**4**(3):109–35.

179. Crawley JN. Exploratory behavior models of anxiety in mice. *Neurosci Biobehav Rev* Spring 1985;**9**(1):37–44.

180. Blundell J, Tabuchi K, Bolliger MF, et al. Increased anxiety-like behavior in mice lacking the inhibitory synapse cell adhesion molecule neuroligin 2. *Genes Brain Behav* February 2009;**8**(1):114–26.

181. Holmes A, Lit Q, Murphy DL, Gold E, Crawley JN. Abnormal anxiety-related behavior in serotonin transporter null mutant mice: the influence of genetic background. *Genes Brain Behav* December 2003;**2**(6):365–80.

182. Spencer CM, Alekseyenko O, Serysheva E, Yuva-Paylor LA, Paylor R. Altered anxiety-related and social behaviors in the Fmr1 knockout mouse model of fragile X syndrome. *Genes Brain Behav* October 2005;**4**(7):420–30.

183. Wersinger SR, Ginns EI, O'Carroll AM, Lolait SJ, Young 3rd WS. Vasopressin V1b receptor knockout reduces aggressive behavior in male mice. *Mol Psychiatry* 2002;**7**(9):975–84.

184. Hara H. Autism and epilepsy: a retrospective follow-up study. *Brain Dev* September 2007;**29**(8):486–90.

185. Jeste SS. The neurology of autism spectrum disorders. *Curr Opin Neurol* April 2011;**24**(2):132−9.

186. Sansa G, Carlson C, Doyle W, et al. Medically refractory epilepsy in autism. *Epilepsia* June 2011;**52**(6):1071−5.

187. Chez MG, Chang M, Krasne V, Coughlan C, Kominsky M, Schwartz A. Frequency of epileptiform EEG abnormalities in a sequential screening of autistic patients with no known clinical epilepsy from 1996 to 2005. *Epilepsy Behav* February 2006;**8**(1):267−71.

188. Ekinci O, Arman A, Isık U, Bez Y, Berkem M. EEG abnormalities and epilepsy in autistic spectrum disorders: clinical and familial correlates. *Epilepsy Behav* 2010;**17**(2):178−82.

189. Kanner AM. Advances in epilepsy: new perspectives on new-onset epilepsy, comorbidities, and pharmacotherapy. *F1000 Med Rep* 2010;**2**:51.

190. Morrison RS, Wenzel HJ, Kinoshita Y, Robbins CA, Donehower LA, Schwartzkroin PA. Loss of the p53 tumor suppressor gene protects neurons from kainate-induced cell death. *J Neurosci* February 15, 1996;**16**(4):1337−45.

191. Chemelli RM, Willie JT, Sinton CM, et al. Narcolepsy in orexin knockout mice: molecular genetics of sleep regulation. *Cell* August 20, 1999;**98**(4):437−51.

192. Zhou J, Blundell J, Ogawa S, et al. Pharmacological inhibition of mTORC1 suppresses anatomical, cellular, and behavioral abnormalities in neural-specific Pten knock-out mice. *J Neurosci* February 11, 2009;**29**(6):1773−83.

193. DeLorey TM, Handforth A, Anagnostaras SG, et al. Mice lacking the beta3 subunit of the GABAA receptor have the epilepsy phenotype and many of the behavioral characteristics of Angelman syndrome. *J Neurosci* October 15, 1998;**18**(20):8505−14.

194. Han K, Holder Jr JL, Schaaf CP, et al. SHANK3 overexpression causes manic-like behaviour with unique pharmacogenetic properties. *Nature* November 7, 2013;**503**(7474):72−7.

195. Abrahams BS, Geschwind DH. Advances in autism genetics: on the threshold of a new neurobiology. *Nat Rev Genet* May 2008;**9**(5):341−55.

196. Betancur C, Sakurai T, Buxbaum JD. The emerging role of synaptic cell-adhesion pathways in the pathogenesis of autism spectrum disorders. *Trends Neurosci* July 2009;**32**(7):402−12.

197. Sudhof TC. Neuroligins and neurexins link synaptic function to cognitive disease. *Nature* October 16, 2008;**455**(7215):903−11.

198. Taniguchi H, Gollan L, Scholl FG, et al. Silencing of neuroligin function by postsynaptic neurexins. *J Neurosci* March 14, 2007;**27**(11):2815−24.

199. Craig AM, Kang Y. Neurexin-neuroligin signaling in synapse development. *Curr Opin Neurobiol* February 2007;**17**(1):43−52.

200. Robertson HR, Feng G. Annual research review: transgenic mouse models of childhood-onset psychiatric disorders. *J Child Psychol Psychiatry* April 2011;**52**(4):442−75.

201. Yan J, Noltner K, Feng J, et al. Neurexin 1alpha structural variants associated with autism. *Neurosci Lett* June 27, 2008;**438**(3):368−70.

202. Dean C, Scholl FG, Choih J, et al. Neurexin mediates the assembly of presynaptic terminals. *Nat Neurosci* July 2003;**6**(7):708−16.

203. Scheiffele P, Fan J, Choih J, Fetter R, Serafini T. Neuroligin expressed in nonneuronal cells triggers presynaptic development in contacting axons. *Cell* June 9, 2000;**101**(6):657−69.

204. Graf ER, Zhang X, Jin SX, Linhoff MW, Craig AM. Neurexins induce differentiation of GABA and glutamate postsynaptic specializations via neuroligins. *Cell* December 29, 2004;**119**(7):1013−26.

205. Kattenstroth G, Tantalaki E, Sudhof TC, Gottmann K, Missler M. Postsynaptic N-methyl-D-aspartate receptor function requires alpha-neurexins. *Proc Natl Acad Sci USA* February 24, 2004;**101**(8):2607−12.

206. Etherton MR, Blaiss CA, Powell CM, Sudhof TC. Mouse neurexin-1alpha deletion causes correlated electrophysiological and behavioral changes consistent with cognitive impairments. *Proc Natl Acad Sci USA* October 20, 2009;**106**(42):17998−8003.

207. Dudanova I, Tabuchi K, Rohlmann A, Sudhof TC, Missler M. Deletion of alpha-neurexins does not cause a major impairment of axonal pathfinding or synapse formation. *J Comp Neurol* May 10, 2007;**502**(2):261−74.

208. Missler M, Zhang W, Rohlmann A, et al. Alpha-neurexins couple Ca^{2+} channels to synaptic vesicle exocytosis. *Nature* June 26, 2003;**423**(6943):939−48.

209. Zhang W, Rohlmann A, Sargsyan V, et al. Extracellular domains of alpha-neurexins participate in regulating synaptic transmission by selectively affecting N- and P/Q-type Ca^{2+} channels. *J Neurosci* April 27, 2005;**25**(17):4330−42.

210. Tsetsenis T, Boucard AA, Arac D, Brunger AT, Sudhof TC. Direct visualization of trans-synaptic neurexin-neuroligin interactions during synapse formation. *J Neurosci* November 5, 2014;**34**(45):15083−96.

211. Irie M, Hata Y, Takeuchi M, et al. Binding of neuroligins to PSD-95. *Science* September 5, 1997;**277**(5331):1511−5.

212. Song JY, Ichtchenko K, Sudhof TC, Brose N. Neuroligin 1 is a postsynaptic cell-adhesion molecule of excitatory synapses. *Proc Natl Acad Sci USA* February 2, 1999;**96**(3):1100−5.

213. Jamain S, Quach H, Betancur C, et al. Mutations of the X-linked genes encoding neuroligins NLGN3 and NLGN4 are associated with autism. *Nat Genet* May 2003;**34**(1):27−9.

214. Budreck EC, Scheiffele P. Neuroligin-3 is a neuronal adhesion protein at GABAergic and glutamatergic synapses. *Eur J Neurosci* October 2007;**26**(7):1738−48.

215. Hoon M, Soykan T, Falkenburger B, et al. Neuroligin-4 is localized to glycinergic postsynapses and regulates inhibition in the retina. *Proc Natl Acad Sci USA* February 15, 2011;**108**(7):3053−8.

216. Levinson JN, Li R, Kang R, Moukhles H, El-Husseini A, Bamji SX. Postsynaptic scaffolding molecules modulate the localization of neuroligins. *Neuroscience* February 3, 2010;**165**(3):782−93.

217. Provenzano G, Zunino G, Genovesi S, Sgado P, Bozzi Y. Mutant mouse models of autism spectrum disorders. *Dis Markers* 2012;**33**(5):225−39.

218. Blundell J, Blaiss CA, Etherton MR, et al. Neuroligin-1 deletion results in impaired spatial memory and increased repetitive behavior. *J Neurosci* February 10, 2010;**30**(6):2115−29.

219. Patterson PH. Modeling autistic features in animals. *Pediatr Res* May 2011;**69**(5 Pt 2):34R−40R.

220. Gogolla N, Leblanc JJ, Quast KB, Sudhof TC, Fagiolini M, Hensch TK. Common circuit defect of excitatory-inhibitory balance in mouse models of autism. *J Neurodev Disord* June 2009;**1**(2):172−81.

221. Bennetto L, Kuschner ES, Hyman SL. Olfaction and taste processing in autism. *Biol Psychiatry* November 1, 2007;**62**(9):1015−21.

222. Suzuki Y, Critchley HD, Rowe A, Howlin P, Murphy DG. Impaired olfactory identification in Asperger's syndrome. *J Neuropsychiatry Clin Neurosci* Winter 2003;**15**(1):105−7.

223. Chih B, Engelman H, Scheiffele P. Control of excitatory and inhibitory synapse formation by neuroligins. *Science* February 25, 2005;**307**(5713):1324−8.

224. Varoqueaux F, Aramuni G, Rawson RL, et al. Neuroligins determine synapse maturation and function. *Neuron* September 21, 2006;**51**(6):741−54.

225. Alarcon M, Abrahams BS, Stone JL, et al. Linkage, association, and gene-expression analyses identify CNTNAP2 as an autism-susceptibility gene. *Am J Hum Genet* January 2008;**82**(1):150−9.

226. Whitehouse AJ, Bishop DV, Ang QW, Pennell CE, Fisher SE. CNTNAP2 variants affect early language development in the general population. *Genes Brain Behav* June 2011;**10**(4):451−6.

227. Vernes SC, Newbury DF, Abrahams BS, et al. A functional genetic link between distinct developmental language disorders. *N Engl J Med* November 27, 2008;**359**(22):2337−45.

228. Gerrow K, El-Husseini A. Cell adhesion molecules at the synapse. *Front Biosci* 2006;**11**:2400−19.

229. Durand CM, Betancur C, Boeckers TM, et al. Mutations in the gene encoding the synaptic scaffolding protein SHANK3 are associated with autism spectrum disorders. *Nat Genet* January 2007;**39**(1):25–7.

230. Gauthier J, Spiegelman D, Piton A, et al. Novel de novo SHANK3 mutation in autistic patients. *Am J Med Genet B Neuropsychiatr Genet* April 5, 2009;**150B**(3):421–4.

231. Moessner R, Marshall CR, Sutcliffe JS, et al. Contribution of SHANK3 mutations to autism spectrum disorder. *Am J Hum Genet* December 2007;**81**(6):1289–97.

232. Sala C, Piech V, Wilson NR, Passafaro M, Liu G, Sheng M. Regulation of dendritic spine morphology and synaptic function by Shank and Homer. *Neuron* July 19, 2001;**31**(1):115–30.

233. Roussignol G, Ango F, Romorini S, et al. Shank expression is sufficient to induce functional dendritic spine synapses in aspiny neurons. *J Neurosci* April 6, 2005;**25**(14):3560–70.

234. Hung AY, Futai K, Sala C, et al. Smaller dendritic spines, weaker synaptic transmission, but enhanced spatial learning in mice lacking Shank1. *J Neurosci* February 13, 2008;**28**(7):1697–708.

235. Kouser M, Speed HE, Dewey CM, et al. Loss of predominant Shank3 isoforms results in hippocampus-dependent impairments in behavior and synaptic transmission. *J Neurosci* November 20, 2013;**33**(47):18448–68.

236. Buxbaum JD, Cai G, Chaste P, et al. Mutation screening of the PTEN gene in patients with autism spectrum disorders and macrocephaly. *Am J Med Genet B Neuropsychiatr Genet* June 5, 2007;**144B**(4):484–91.

237. Butler MG, Dasouki MJ, Zhou XP, et al. Subset of individuals with autism spectrum disorders and extreme macrocephaly associated with germline PTEN tumour suppressor gene mutations. *J Med Genet* April 2005;**42**(4):318–21.

238. Ogawa S, Kwon CH, Zhou J, Koovakkattu D, Parada LF, Sinton CM. A seizure-prone phenotype is associated with altered free-running rhythm in Pten mutant mice. *Brain Res* September 7, 2007;**1168**:112–23.

239. Hazlett HC, Poe M, Gerig G, et al. Magnetic resonance imaging and head circumference study of brain size in autism: birth through age 2 years. *Arch Gen Psychiatry* December 2005;**62**(12):1366–76.

240. Stiles BL. Phosphatase and tensin homologue deleted on chromosome 10: extending its PTENtacles. *Int J Biochem Cell Biol* April 2009;**41**(4):757–61.

241. Reith RM, McKenna J, Wu H, et al. Loss of Tsc2 in Purkinje cells is associated with autistic-like behavior in a mouse model of tuberous sclerosis complex. *Neurobiol Dis* March 2013;**51**:93–103.

242. Yates JR. Tuberous sclerosis. *Eur J Hum Genet* October 2006;**14**(10):1065–73.

243. Sharma A, Hoeffer CA, Takayasu Y, et al. Dysregulation of mTOR signaling in fragile X syndrome. *J Neurosci* January 13, 2010;**30**(2):694–702.

244. Holmes GL, Stafstrom CE. Tuberous sclerosis complex and epilepsy: recent developments and future challenges. *Epilepsia* April 2007;**48**(4):617–30.

245. Jozwiak J. Hamartin and tuberin: working together for tumour suppression. *Int J Cancer* January 1, 2006;**118**(1):1–5.

246. Yuan E, Tsai PT, Greene-Colozzi E, Sahin M, Kwiatkowski DJ, Malinowska IA. Graded loss of tuberin in an allelic series of brain models of TSC correlates with survival, and biochemical, histological and behavioral features. *Hum Mol Genet* October 1, 2012;**21**(19):4286–300.

247. Ehninger D, Han S, Shilyansky C, et al. Reversal of learning deficits in a Tsc2$^{+/-}$ mouse model of tuberous sclerosis. *Nat Med* August 2008;**14**(8):843–8.

248. Goorden SM, van Woerden GM, van der Weerd L, Cheadle JP, Elgersma Y. Cognitive deficits in Tsc1$^{+/-}$ mice in the absence of cerebral lesions and seizures. *Ann Neurol* December 2007;**62**(6):648–55.

249. Meikle L, Talos DM, Onda H, et al. A mouse model of tuberous sclerosis: neuronal loss of Tsc1 causes dysplastic and ectopic neurons, reduced myelination, seizure activity, and limited survival. *J Neurosci* May 23, 2007;**27**(21):5546–58.

250. Tavazoie SF, Alvarez VA, Ridenour DA, Kwiatkowski DJ, Sabatini BL. Regulation of neuronal morphology and function by the tumor suppressors Tsc1 and Tsc2. *Nat Neurosci* December 2005;**8**(12):1727–34.

251. Ehninger D, Silva AJ. Rapamycin for treating Tuberous sclerosis and Autism spectrum disorders. *Trends Mol Med* February 2010;**17**(2):78–87.

252. Dolen G, Bear MF. Fragile x syndrome and autism: from disease model to therapeutic targets. *J Neurodev Disord* June 2009;**1**(2):133–40.

253. Zalfa F, Giorgi M, Primerano B, et al. The fragile X syndrome protein FMRP associates with BC1 RNA and regulates the translation of specific mRNAs at synapses. *Cell* February 7, 2003;**112**(3):317–27.

254. Liu ZH, Smith CB. Dissociation of social and nonsocial anxiety in a mouse model of fragile X syndrome. *Neurosci Lett* April 17, 2009;**454**(1):62–6.

255. McNaughton CH, Moon J, Strawderman MS, Maclean KN, Evans J, Strupp BJ. Evidence for social anxiety and impaired social cognition in a mouse model of fragile X syndrome. *Behav Neurosci* April 2008;**122**(2):293–300.

256. Spencer CM, Graham DF, Yuva-Paylor LA, Nelson DL, Paylor R. Social behavior in Fmr1 knockout mice carrying a human FMR1 transgene. *Behav Neurosci* June 2008;**122**(3):710–5.

257. Brodkin ES. Social behavior phenotypes in fragile X syndrome, autism, and the Fmr1 knockout mouse: theoretical comment on McNaughton et al. (2008). *Behav Neurosci* April 2008;**122**(2):483–9.

258. Adusei DC, Pacey LK, Chen D, Hampson DR. Early developmental alterations in GABAergic protein expression in fragile X knockout mice. *Neuropharmacology* September 2010;**59**(3):167–71.

259. D'Hulst C, Heulens I, Brouwer JR, et al. Expression of the GABAergic system in animal models for fragile X syndrome and fragile X associated tremor/ataxia syndrome (FXTAS). *Brain Res* February 9, 2009;**1253**:176–83.

260. Centonze D, Rossi S, Mercaldo V, et al. Abnormal striatal GABA transmission in the mouse model for the fragile X syndrome. *Biol Psychiatry* May 15, 2008;**63**(10):963–73.

261. Curia G, Papouin T, Seguela P, Avoli M. Downregulation of tonic GABAergic inhibition in a mouse model of fragile X syndrome. *Cereb Cortex* July 2009;**19**(7):1515–20.

262. Selby L, Zhang C, Sun QQ. Major defects in neocortical GABAergic inhibitory circuits in mice lacking the fragile X mental retardation protein. *Neurosci Lett* February 2, 2007;**412**(3):227–32.

263. Bear MF, Huber KM, Warren ST. The mGluR theory of fragile X mental retardation. *Trends Neurosci* July 2004;**27**(7):370–7.

264. Dolen G, Osterweil E, Rao BS, et al. Correction of fragile X syndrome in mice. *Neuron* December 20, 2007;**56**(6):955–62.

265. de Vrij FM, Levenga J, van der Linde HC, et al. Rescue of behavioral phenotype and neuronal protrusion morphology in Fmr1 KO mice. *Neurobiol Dis* July 2008;**31**(1):127–32.

266. Kishino T, Lalande M, Wagstaff J. UBE3A/E6-AP mutations cause Angelman syndrome. *Nat Genet* January 1997;**15**(1):70–3.

267. Veltman MW, Craig EE, Bolton PF. Autism spectrum disorders in Prader-Willi and Angelman syndromes: a systematic review. *Psychiatr Genet* December 2005;**15**(4):243–54.

268. Bolton PF, Veltman MW, Weisblatt E, et al. Chromosome 15q11-13 abnormalities and other medical conditions in individuals with autism spectrum disorders. *Psychiatr Genet* September 2004;**14**(3):131–7.

269. Dykens EM, Sutcliffe JS, Levitt P. Autism and 15q11-q13 disorders: behavioral, genetic, and pathophysiological issues. *Ment Retard Dev Disabil Res Rev* 2004;**10**(4):284–91.

270. Schroer RJ, Phelan MC, Michaelis RC, et al. Autism and maternally derived aberrations of chromosome 15q. *Am J Med Genet* April 1, 1998;**76**(4):327–36.

271. Samaco RC, Hogart A, LaSalle JM. Epigenetic overlap in autism-spectrum neurodevelopmental disorders: MECP2 deficiency causes reduced expression of UBE3A and GABRB3. *Hum Mol Genet* February 15, 2005;**14**(4):483–92.

272. Miura K, Kishino T, Li E, et al. Neurobehavioral and electroencephalographic abnormalities in Ube3a maternal-deficient mice. *Neurobiol Dis* March 2002;**9**(2):149–59.

273. Smith SE, Zhou YD, Zhang G, Jin Z, Stoppel DC, Anderson MP. Increased gene dosage of Ube3a results in autism traits and decreased glutamate synaptic transmission in mice. *Sci Transl Med* October 5, 2011;**3**(103):103ra197.

274. Simon HH, Thuret S, Alberi L. Midbrain dopaminergic neurons: control of their cell fate by the engrailed transcription factors. *Cell Tissue Res* October 2004;**318**(1):53–61.

275. Sgado P, Alberi L, Gherbassi D, et al. Slow progressive degeneration of nigral dopaminergic neurons in postnatal Engrailed mutant mice. *Proc Natl Acad Sci USA* October 10, 2006;**103**(41):15242–7.

276. Benayed R, Gharani N, Rossman I, et al. Support for the homeobox transcription factor gene ENGRAILED 2 as an autism spectrum disorder susceptibility locus. *Am J Hum Genet* November 2005;**77**(5):851–68.

277. Wang L, Jia M, Yue W, et al. Association of the ENGRAILED 2 (EN2) gene with autism in Chinese Han population. *Am J Med Genet B Neuropsychiatr Genet* June 5, 2008;**147B**(4):434–8.

278. Joyner AL, Herrup K, Auerbach BA, Davis CA, Rossant J. Subtle cerebellar phenotype in mice homozygous for a targeted deletion of the En-2 homeobox. *Science* March 8, 1991;**251**(4998):1239–43.

279. Cheh MA, Millonig JH, Roselli LM, et al. En2 knockout mice display neurobehavioral and neurochemical alterations relevant to autism spectrum disorder. *Brain Res* October 20, 2006;**1116**(1):166–76.

280. Tripathi PP, Sgado P, Scali M, et al. Increased susceptibility to kainic acid-induced seizures in Engrailed-2 knockout mice. *Neuroscience* March 17, 2009;**159**(2):842–9.

281. Insel TR. A neurobiological basis of social attachment. *Am J Psychiatry* June 1997;**154**(6):726–35.

282. Gimpl G, Fahrenholz F. The oxytocin receptor system: structure, function, and regulation. *Physiol Rev* April 2001;**81**(2):629–83.

283. Insel TR, Young LJ. Neuropeptides and the evolution of social behavior. *Curr Opin Neurobiol* December 2000;**10**(6):784–9.

284. Campbell DB, Datta D, Jones ST, et al. Association of oxytocin receptor (OXTR) gene variants with multiple phenotype domains of autism spectrum disorder. *J Neurodev Disord* June 2011;**3**(2):101–12.

285. Ebstein RP, Israel S, Lerer E, et al. Arginine vasopressin and oxytocin modulate human social behavior. *Ann NY Acad Sci* June 2009;**1167**:87–102.

286. Jacob S, Brune CW, Carter CS, Leventhal BL, Lord C, Cook Jr EH. Association of the oxytocin receptor gene (OXTR) in Caucasian children and adolescents with autism. *Neurosci Lett* April 24, 2007;**417**(1):6–9.

287. Wu S, Jia M, Ruan Y, et al. Positive association of the oxytocin receptor gene (OXTR) with autism in the Chinese Han population. *Biol Psychiatry* July 1, 2005;**58**(1):74–7.

288. Lazzari VM, Becker RO, de Azevedo MS, et al. Oxytocin modulates social interaction but is not essential for sexual behavior in male mice. *Behav Brain Res* May 1, 2013;**244**:130–6.

289. Takayanagi Y, Yoshida M, Bielsky IF, et al. Pervasive social deficits, but normal parturition, in oxytocin receptor-deficient mice. *Proc Natl Acad Sci USA* November 1, 2005;**102**(44):16096–101.

290. Winslow JT, Hearn EF, Ferguson J, Young LJ, Matzuk MM, Insel TR. Infant vocalization, adult aggression, and fear behavior of an oxytocin null mutant mouse. *Horm Behav* March 2000;**37**(2):145–55.

291. Winslow JT, Insel TR. The social deficits of the oxytocin knockout mouse. *Neuropeptides* Apr-Jun 2002;**36**(2–3):221–9.

292. Eliason MJ. Neurofibromatosis: implications for learning and behavior. *J Dev Behav Pediatr* June 1986;**7**(3):175–9.

293. Carter CS, Grippo AJ, Pournajafi-Nazarloo H, Ruscio MG, Porges SW. Oxytocin, vasopressin and sociality. *Prog Brain Res* 2008;**170**:331–6.

294. de Vries GJ, Miller MA. Anatomy and function of extrahypothalamic vasopressin systems in the brain. *Prog Brain Res* 1998;**119**:3–20.

295. Egashira N, Tanoue A, Matsuda T, et al. Impaired social interaction and reduced anxiety-related behavior in vasopressin V1a receptor knockout mice. *Behav Brain Res* March 12, 2007;**178**(1):123–7.

296. Caldwell HK, Wersinger SR, Young 3rd WS. The role of the vasopressin 1b receptor in aggression and other social behaviours. *Prog Brain Res* 2008;**170**:65–72.

297. Caldwell HK, Young 3rd WS. Persistence of reduced aggression in vasopressin 1b receptor knockout mice on a more "wild" background. *Physiol Behav* April 20, 2009;**97**(1):131–4.

298. Stevenson EL, Caldwell HK. The vasopressin 1b receptor and the neural regulation of social behavior. *Horm Behav* March 2012;**61**(3):277–82.

299. Manent JB, Represa A. Neurotransmitters and brain maturation: early paracrine actions of GABA and glutamate modulate neuronal migration. *Neuroscientist* June 2007;**13**(3):268–79.

300. Blatt GJ. GABAergic cerebellar system in autism: a neuropathological and developmental perspective. *Int Rev Neurobiol* 2005;**71**:167–78.

301. Buxbaum JD, Silverman JM, Smith CJ, et al. Association between a GABRB3 polymorphism and autism. *Mol Psychiatry* 2002;**7**(3):311–6.

302. Culiat CT, Stubbs LJ, Montgomery CS, Russell LB, Rinchik EM. Phenotypic consequences of deletion of the gamma 3, alpha 5, or beta 3 subunit of the type A gamma-aminobutyric acid receptor in mice. *Proc Natl Acad Sci USA* March 29, 1994;**91**(7):2815–8.

303. Homanics GE, DeLorey TM, Firestone LL, et al. Mice devoid of gamma-aminobutyrate type A receptor beta3 subunit have epilepsy, cleft palate, and hypersensitive behavior. *Proc Natl Acad Sci USA* April 15, 1997;**94**(8):4143–8.

304. DeLorey TM, Sahbaie P, Hashemi E, Homanics GE, Clark JD. Gabrb3 gene deficient mice exhibit impaired social and exploratory behaviors, deficits in non-selective attention and hypoplasia of cerebellar vermal lobules: a potential model of autism spectrum disorder. *Behav Brain Res* March 5, 2008;**187**(2):207–20.

305. Hranilovic D, Novak R, Babic M, Novokmet M, Bujas-Petkovic Z, Jernej B. Hyperserotonemia in autism: the potential role of 5HT-related gene variants. *Coll Antropol* January 2008;**32**(Suppl. 1):75–80.

306. Huang CH, Santangelo SL. Autism and serotonin transporter gene polymorphisms: a systematic review and meta-analysis. *Am J Med Genet B Neuropsychiatr Genet* September 5, 2008;**147B**(6):903–13.

307. King BH, Hollander E, Sikich L, et al. Lack of efficacy of citalopram in children with autism spectrum disorders and high levels of repetitive behavior: citalopram ineffective in children with autism. *Arch Gen Psychiatry* June 2009;**66**(6):583–90.

308. West L, Brunssen SH, Waldrop J. Review of the evidence for treatment of children with autism with selective serotonin reuptake inhibitors. *J Spec Pediatr Nurs* July 2009;**14**(3):183–91.

309. Altamura C, Dell'Acqua ML, Moessner R, Murphy DL, Lesch KP, Persico AM. Altered neocortical cell density and layer thickness in serotonin transporter knockout mice: a quantitation study. *Cereb Cortex* June 2007;**17**(6):1394–401.

310. Bengel D, Murphy DL, Andrews AM, et al. Altered brain serotonin homeostasis and locomotor insensitivity to 3, 4-methylenedioxymethamphetamine ("Ecstasy") in serotonin transporter-deficient mice. *Mol Pharmacol* April 1998;**53**(4):649–55.

311. Canli T, Omura K, Haas BW, Fallgatter A, Constable RT, Lesch KP. Beyond affect: a role for genetic variation of the serotonin transporter in neural activation during a cognitive attention task. *Proc Natl Acad Sci USA* August 23, 2005;**102**(34):12224—9.

312. Jiang X, Wang J, Luo T, Li Q. Impaired hypothalamic-pituitary-adrenal axis and its feedback regulation in serotonin transporter knockout mice. *Psychoneuroendocrinology* April 2009;**34**(3):317—31.

313. Carroll JC, Boyce-Rustay JM, Millstein R, et al. Effects of mild early life stress on abnormal emotion-related behaviors in 5-HTT knockout mice. *Behav Genet* January 2007;**37**(1):214—22.

314. Holmes A, Murphy DL, Crawley JN. Reduced aggression in mice lacking the serotonin transporter. *Psychopharmacol Berl* May 2002;**161**(2):160—7.

315. Kalueff AV, Fox MA, Gallagher PS, Murphy DL. Hypolocomotion, anxiety and serotonin syndrome-like behavior contribute to the complex phenotype of serotonin transporter knockout mice. *Genes Brain Behav* June 2007;**6**(4):389—400.

316. Christensen J, Gronborg TK, Sorensen MJ, et al. Prenatal valproate exposure and risk of autism spectrum disorders and childhood autism. *Jama* April 24, 2013;**309**(16):1696—703.

317. Roullet FI, Lai JK, Foster JA. In utero exposure to valproic acid and autism—a current review of clinical and animal studies. *Neurotoxicol Teratol* March—April 2013;**36**:47—56.

318. Kataoka S, Takuma K, Hara Y, Maeda Y, Ago Y, Matsuda T. Autism-like behaviours with transient histone hyperacetylation in mice treated prenatally with valproic acid. *Int J Neuropsychopharmacol* February 2013;**16**(1):91—103.

319. Moldrich RX, Leanage G, She D, et al. Inhibition of histone deacetylase in utero causes sociability deficits in postnatal mice. *Behav Brain Res* November 15, 2013;**257**:253—64.

320. Brown AS, Derkits EJ. Prenatal infection and schizophrenia: a review of epidemiologic and translational studies. *Am J Psychiatry* March 2010;**167**(3):261—80.

321. Kinney DK, Munir KM, Crowley DJ, Miller AM. Prenatal stress and risk for autism. *Neurosci Biobehav Rev* October 2008;**32**(8):1519—32.

322. Schwartzer JJ, Careaga M, Onore CE, Rushakoff JA, Berman RF, Ashwood P. Maternal immune activation and strain specific interactions in the development of autism-like behaviors in mice. *Transl Psychiatry* 2013;**3**:e240.

323. Wu WLaP PH. The interaction between α7nachr and maternal infection in regulating schizophrenia- and autism-like behaviors. In: *Paper presented at: neuroscience 2013*; 2013. San Diego.

324. Lazic SE, Essioux L. Improving basic and translational science by accounting for litter-to-litter variation in animal models. *BMC Neurosci* 2013;**14**:37.

325. Scattoni ML, Martire A, Cartocci G, Ferrante A, Ricceri L. Reduced social interaction, behavioural flexibility and BDNF signalling in the BTBR T+ tf/J strain, a mouse model of autism. *Behav Brain Res* August 15, 2013;**251**:35—40.

326. Amodeo DA, Jones JH, Sweeney JA, Ragozzino ME. Differences in BTBR T+ tf/J and C57BL/6J mice on probabilistic reversal learning and stereotyped behaviors. *Behav Brain Res* February 1, 2012;**227**(1):64—72.

327. Lindsey JB. HJ historical foundations. In: Suckow MA, Weisbroth SH, Franklin CL, editors. *The laboratory rat.*, vol. 2. New York: NY: Academic Press; 2006. p. 1—152.

328. Siviy SM, Panksepp J. In search of the neurobiological substrates for social playfulness in mammalian brains. *Neurosci Biobehav Rev* October 2011;**35**(9):1821—30.

329. Brudzynski SM. Communication of adult rats by ultrasonic vocalization: biological, sociobiological, and neuroscience approaches. *Ilar J* 2009;**50**(1):43—50.

330. Wöhr M, Schwarting RKW. Activation of limbic system structures by replay of ultrasonic vocalization in rats. In: Brudzynski S, editor. *Handbook of behavioral neuroscience*, vol. 19; 2010.

331. Rutte C, Taborsky M. The influence of social experience on cooperative behaviour of rats (Rattus norvegicus): direct vs generalised reciprocity. *Behav Ecol Sociobiol* 2008;**62**(4):499—505.

332. Wohr M, Schwarting RK. Testing social acoustic memory in rats: effects of stimulus configuration and long-term memory on the induction of social approach behavior by appetitive 50-kHz ultrasonic vocalizations. *Neurobiol Learn Mem* September 2012;**98**(2):154—64.

333. Gesundheit B, Rosenzweig JP, Naor D, et al. Immunological and autoimmune considerations of Autism Spectrum Disorders. *J Autoimmun* August 2013;**44**:1—7.

334. Schwartzer JJ, Koenig CM, Berman RF. Using mouse models of autism spectrum disorders to study the neurotoxicology of gene-environment interactions. *Neurotoxicol Teratol* Mar-Apr 2013;**36**:17—35.

335. Shelton JF, Hertz-Picciotto I, Pessah IN. Tipping the balance of autism risk: potential mechanisms linking pesticides and autism. *Environ Health Perspect* July 2012;**120**(7):944—51.

336. Landrigan PJ, Lambertini L, Birnbaum LS. A research strategy to discover the environmental causes of autism and neurodevelopmental disabilities. *Environ Health Perspect* July 2012;**120**(7):a258—260.

337. Laviola G, Adriani W, Gaudino C, Marino R, Keller F. Paradoxical effects of prenatal acetylcholinesterase blockade on neurobehavioral development and drug-induced stereotypies in reeler mutant mice. *Psychopharmacol Berl* August 2006;**187**(3):331—44.

338. Mullen BR, Khialeeva E, Hoffman DB, Ghiani CA, Carpenter EM. Decreased reelin expression and organophosphate pesticide exposure alters mouse behaviour and brain morphology. *ASN Neuro* 2012;**5**(1):e00106.

339. De Felice A, Scattoni ML, Ricceri L, Calamandrei G. Prenatal exposure to a common organophosphate insecticide delays motor development in a mouse model of idiopathic autism. *PLoS One* 2015;**10**(3):e0121663.

340. Keil AP, Daniels JL, Hertz-Picciotto I. Autism spectrum disorder, flea and tick medication, and adjustments for exposure misclassification: the CHARGE (CHildhood Autism Risks from Genetics and Environment) case-control study. *Environ Health* 2014;**13**(1):3.

341. Shelton JF, Geraghty EM, Tancredi DJ, et al. Neurodevelopmental disorders and prenatal residential proximity to agricultural pesticides: the CHARGE study. *Environ Health Perspect* October 2014;**122**(10):1103—9.

18

The iPSC Technology to Study Neurodevelopmental Disorders

Alysson Renato Muotri[1,2]

[1]Department of Pediatrics, University of California San Diego, School of Medicine, Rady Children's Hospital San Diego, San Diego, CA, USA; [2]Department of Cellular & Molecular Medicine, Stem Cell Program, University of California San Diego, La Jolla, CA, USA

INTRODUCTION

People with from autism spectrum disorder (ASD) are mainly characterized by struggles in social communication and the presence of focused repetitive behaviors, appearing within the first years of life. The prevalence rate of ASD has dramatically risen over the years owing to reasons that include the improvement and availability of the diagnosis or a real increase in the rate of affected newborns.[1,2]

There is no cure for ASD. Treatment requires strong network collaboration among multiple professionals, and the cornerstone of treatment lies in individualized educational interventions, including early and intensive behavioral strategies.[3,4] As these children mature into autistic adults, most do not live independently.[5] Thus, the need for early diagnosis and better treatment of ASD is a concern that is increasing not only among scientists and physicians, but also from an economic perspective.[6] However, the human nature of ASD, with an intrinsic heterogeneity and large spectrum of clinical symptoms among patients, is a major challenge to study the disease mechanisms underlying ASD.

The lack of usable neuronal samples from postmortem brains and the inability to isolate populations of neurons from living subjects have blocked progress toward ASD research. The ASD field lacks an appropriate human experimental model and would benefit greatly from unlimited supplies of neurons so that experiments can be performed in controlled situations. This new model could nicely complement efforts from previous approaches such as postmortem brain tissues and mouse models.

Genetic reprogramming of adult somatic cells to a pluripotent state (induced pluripotent stem cells [iPSCs]) has been accomplished using human cells.[7,8] The breakthrough that led to the Nobel Prize in medicine in 2012 to Dr. Shinya Yamanaka uses a relative simple approach: a set of transcription factors to reprogram the genetic network and epigenetic landscape of a somatic cell toward a pluripotent stage. The new technique gained attention for the potential of generating disease-specific pluripotent stem cells with unprecedented simplicity. Human iPSCs are seen as attractive models for understanding complex disorders with heritable and sporadic conditions, allowing an individual's development to be played back in the lab.[9]

Disorders of monogenic origin were first reprogrammed to iPSC[10–12] and the demonstration of disease-specific pathogenesis in complex disease such as ASD is a current challenge in the field.[13] Extending the iPSC modeling technology beyond monogenic ASD to the study of nonsyndromic forms of autism is a new trend to uncover molecular and cellular pathways that may overlap among different forms of autism. Despite excitement, several pitfalls in the technology need to be optimized so the full potential of iPSC can be better explored.

CURRENT LIMITATIONS AND PITFALLS OF THE iPSC DISEASE MODELING TECHNOLOGY

It is crucial to understanding the pitfalls of the iPSC approach to make correct interpretations and extrapolations to the human brain and disease progress. Cells in culture miss important signaling pathways and interaction with other cells. Moreover, current culture conditions are not optimized but were empirically achieved based on mouse embryology. Thus, it is likely that important human-specific signaling information is misplaced in the current culture system.

Another challenge is the derivation of relevant neuronal subtypes. To date, there are only a few protocols to induce pluripotent stem cells into specific subtypes of neurons. Even for these cases, the differentiation protocols usually result in a heterogeneous population of cell types. Thus, relevant neuronal subtypes need to be sorted out or visualized using specific reporter genes. Moreover, having the relevant neuronal type in culture does not guarantee that disease neurons will behave differently from controls. Non–cell autonomous effects, three-dimensional scaffolding, or maturation timing may also contribute to neuronal phenotypes.

Another important limitation and recurrent concern among users is the use of appropriate controls. Based on previous mouse models, the ideal control seems to be one that differs from the patient only by the genetic defect(s). Genome editing allows for rigorous study designs that could substantially alleviate concerns about potential off-target effects or other confounding by clonal sequence variation.[14] Thus, iPSC can be manipulated to carry genetic mutations in control cell lines or used to add reporters, biosensors, and tagged proteins, to easily assay biological end points in a specific cell

line.[15,16] Another strategy to generate isogenic control lines is to take advantage of X-inactivation in female cell lines. Because of the fast X inactivation process during reprogramming, it is possible to generate iPSC cell clones carrying the mutant or the wild-type version of an X-linked affected gene. This strategy was used to model Rett syndrome (RTT), which affects female patients with mutations in the X-linked *MeCP2* gene.[10,17] However, it is important to consider that even isogenic clones in culture will accumulate mutations in their genome over time, and thus there will never be an ideal control line. Variability among cell lines and even between iPSC clones from the same individual can influence some cellular and molecular readout, which is a serious concern. Better stem cell protocols and the use of large cohort of individuals can help to reduce experimental variations. Consortium initiatives could also be useful to create banks of well-characterized controls that could be used to research the controls closest to ASD cases.[18]

A final challenge for the iPSC model is the validation of phenotypes observed in human neurons and to show that it can recapitulate the disease in a dish. Comparison with postmortem brain tissues is perhaps the most obvious step toward validation and it depends on the tissue condition and availability of such a material. Moreover, the lack of consistency would not mean that the phenotype is invalid, but it may not reflect alterations conserved during neurodevelopment. Validation in animals is an attractive alternative in theory (although limited by species variations) and may reveal important conserved neural pathways/circuits between different species. Again, a negative correlation with the animal model does not necessarily imply the observations are not relevant for the human disease. In the case of sporadic ASDs, in which animal models offer limited information about the human brain, validation can be especially problematic.

Undoubtedly, the iPSC technology still requires a series of optimization steps. Nonetheless, even with all of these caveats, the study of ASD-derived brain cell types is already generating new biological data.

MODELING ASDs USING iPSCs

Disorders such as fragile X, RTT, and Timothy syndrome are caused by specific genetic alterations that also present neurodevelopmental and speech delays, resulting in an autistic phenotype. Although these syndromic forms are not clinically grouped under ASD, these disorders have provided useful insights into sporadic or idiopathic (nonsyndromic) forms of autism.

The use of monogenetic forms of ASD was wisely chosen as proof-of-principle that neurons derived from these patients can recapitulate important aspects of the disease in vitro. These models can bring new insights to other forms of ASDs. Moreover, by capturing the genetic heterogeneity of ASDs in a pluripotent state, the iPSC model has the potential to determine whether patients carrying distinct mutations in disparate genes share common cellular and molecular neuronal phenotypes.

We demonstrated the utility of iPSCs to investigate the functional consequences of mutations in the gene encoding the methyl-CpG-binding protein-2 (MeCP2) in neurons from patients with RTT, a syndromic form of ASD[10] (see also Chapters 7 and 19). Neurons derived from RTT-iPSCs carrying four different MeCP2 mutations had several alterations compared with five healthy unaffected individuals, such as decreased soma size, altered dendritic spine density, and reduced excitatory synapses. Importantly, these phenotypes were validated using wild-type MeCP2 cDNA and specific small hairpin ribonucleic acids (shRNAs) against MeCP2 in gain-and-loss of function experiments. Some of these cellular defects were sequentially validated by independent groups, revealing the robustness and reproducibility of the system.[17,19,20] We were able to rescue the defects in the number of glutamatergic synapses using two candidate drugs, insulin growth factor 1 (IGF-1) and gentamicin. Insulin growth factor 1 is considered to be a candidate for pharmacological treatment of RTT and potentially other central nervous system disorders in ongoing clinical trials.[21] These observations bring valued information for RTT and, potentially, other ASD patients, because they suggest that presymptomatic defects may represent novel biomarkers to be exploited as diagnostic tools.

Since this first report, several other scientific articles were published showing that iPSCs can be used to model other syndromic types of autism, such as Timothy syndrome[12] and Phelan—McDermid syndrome[11] using similar strategies.

Based on the examples of syndromic ASD, it is possible to conclude that functional studies using iPSC-derived neuronal cultures of idiopathic or nonsyndromic ASD patients can be an important addition to an exploration of the contribution of rare variants to ASD etiology. The notion that rare mutations may point to key etiological pathways and mechanisms has been repeatedly demonstrated for a wide range of common human disorders.[22,23] A rapidly increasing number of ASD risk regions have been identified and considerable effort has been made to understand the biological substrates influenced by these various mutations.[24—28] There is strong evidence for a high degree of locus heterogeneity and a contribution by rare and de novo variants.[29,30] However, the demonstration of a causal role for these low-frequency variants is challenging, particularly

by mutations that defy Mendelian expectations and carry intermediate risks.[31—33]

Our group focused on reprogramming human dental pulp stem cells from ASD children using the deciduous tooth as a source of somatic cells, the Tooth-Fairy Project,[34] that uses social networking to connect with ASD families. The bank has now over 3500 ASD families listed and more than 300 samples successfully established. The goal is to cross-reference genotypes and cellular phenotypes with detailed clinical information. The bank will be useful to model differences in ASDs patients with distinct clinical features using reprogramming strategies. Moreover, we believe that iPSC together with genomic analyses will help stratify ASDs and reveal some of the molecular pathways that several autistic behaviors.

We have also made progress on modeling nonsyndromic autism. We have characterized the breakpoints of a de novo balanced translocation t(3; 11)(p21; q22) that disrupts the TRPC6 gene. TRPC6 encodes for the canonical transient receptor potential 6 channel, a voltage-independent, Ca^{2+}-permeable cation channel involved in dendritic spine and excitatory synapse formation.[35,36] The biological impact of the genetic alteration in the index case and its functional relationship to ASD etiology were carefully evaluated through several analyses using cortical neurons derived from iPSCs. We showed that TRPC6 haploinsufficiency leads to altered neuronal morphology and function.[37] The observed neuronal phenotypes could then be rescued by TRPC6 complementary deoxyribonucleic acid (cDNA) and by treatment with hyperforin, a TRPC6-specific agonist, which suggests that ASD individuals with alterations in this pathway might benefit from these drugs. We also demonstrate that MeCP2 levels affect TRPC6 expression, revealing common pathways among ASDs (Figure 1). Genetic sequencing of TRPC6 in ASD individuals and controls revealed significantly more nonsynonymous mutations in the ASD population.[37] Taken together, our findings suggest that TRPC6 is a novel predisposing gene for ASD, likely acting in a multiple-hit model. This was the first study to use iPSC-derived human neurons to model nonsyndromic ASD and to illustrate the potential of modeling genetically complex sporadic diseases using such cells.

A DRUG SCREENING PLATFORM USING HUMAN ASD NEURONS

The lack of pharmacological treatments for ASD core symptoms may reflect the missing relevant human model. Autism spectrum disorder preclinical assays are mostly based on transformed cell lines and animal models that cannot fully recapitulate neural cellular

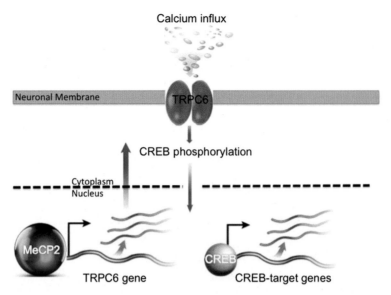

FIGURE 1   Revealing shared molecular pathways using ASD iPSC-derived neurons. A recently discovered ASD predisposition gene (TRPC6) was shown to contribute to the formation of glutamatergic synapses in human neurons by activating downstream cAMP response element-binding protein target genes. Interestingly, TRPC6 expression is activated by MeCP2, a gene implicated in RTT and nonsyndromic autism. This new overlap metabolic pathway was systematically investigated using ASD iPSCs (see text for more details).

function, with obvious interspecies differences and pharmacokinetic properties.[38,39] Drug screening platforms require robust cellular or molecular phenotypes. Late readouts such as neuronal electrophysiological activity may not be ideal and are perhaps too late for a future treatment anyway. Cellular morphology such as soma size can be measured using high-content imaging software. Biochemical and gene expression readouts are also valuable alternatives for large primary screenings.

Whereas most research has focused on neurons, the transition to a high-throughput drug screening platform has intrinsic challenges; it is notoriously difficult to produce a homogeneous population of subtypes, and human neurons are not well adapted to the high-throughput format. Therefore, the use of other well-characterized cell types that are easily adapted to high-throughput formats may bring significant advantage for drug-screening initiatives. Most research has focused on new therapeutics that would target neurons and enhance the number of functional synapses in ASD. However, research has shown that glia cells may represent exciting novel therapeutic targets that could be explored in this setting. Several studies have established that astrocytes secrete signaling molecules that stimulate the formation, pruning, and function of synapses throughout the brain.[40,41] Astrocyte dysfunctions are known to be associated with many mouse models of neurological diseases, but their specific contribution to the human disease pathology has yet to be determined. It is likely that some glia cells such as astrocytes and microglia also contribute to the disease. By mixing different cell types in co-culture experiments, it will be possible to isolate the non–cell

autonomous contribution to specific neurodevelopmental disorders. Unfortunately, there are no short and robust protocols to generate astrocytes from the human pluripotent stage. New protocols for the generation of astrocytes will allow researchers to identify the contribution of this cell type to ASD.

Several chemical libraries could be used in ASD-derived cells. It makes sense to use small molecules that cross the blood–brain barrier and have good penetration in the brain. Drug repositioning is another fantastic opportunity. Although this strategy may face some intellectual property challenges, repurposed drugs can bypass much of the early cost and time needed to bring a drug to market.

AUTISM SPECTRUM DISORDER MINI-BRAINS AND TISSUE ENGINEERING

Tissue engineering combines concepts and techniques from engineering and biology to the problem of cultivating human tissues and organs in the laboratory. This involves creating a scaffold of specific materials, seeding it with human stem cells provided with specific nutrients, and a physical environment that will populate the structure.[42] Despite success with simple tissues, the reconstruction of complex organs such as the brain is a major challenge. Interestingly, it is known that human pluripotent stem cells growing in three-dimensional cultures can self-organize into blobs that resemble a

9-week-old developing fetus human brain, forming cerebral organoids that are one step ahead from two-dimensional cultures.[43,44] Obviously, these structures are not miniatures of the human brain per se because several parts are not present in these structures. Nonetheless, the strategy offers a panoramic picture of brain development and how the process can go wrong in specific disease contexts.

Similarly, generation of human neuronal microcircuits in the dish is already a reality.[45] Multielectrode arrays (MEA) could be incorporated to record electrical impulses or stimulate the circuitry and investigate the connectivity of functional human networks.[46] By having the different cells functioning together, these circuits will replicate the dynamic interactions that take place in the brain. The use of MEA to record from these neuronal assembles can be directly correlated to electroencephalogram recordings from patients. Obviously, the "brain on a chip" does not look precisely like the natural human brain. However, breaking the brain into microcircuits has both financial and convenient advantages. A microscale version of the brain is easy to interrogate, supporting multiple variables at the same time. The system has the potential to eliminate dependence on animal models and speed drug development, helping to identify ineffective or unsafe drugs several steps earlier in the development process. In the future, doctors may no longer have to estimate blindly which of several drugs and dosages would work best for their patients—they could simply test them all and select the one with greatest efficacy and the fewest side effects.

CONCLUSIONS AND FUTURE PERSPECTIVE

The iPSC strategy is now an additional and complementary approach to model ASDs. Although this technology is still in its early stage, it potentially demonstrates the ability to recapitulate relevant neuronal defects of those diseases. This new human model has the capacity to fill gaps generated from systems biology, computer simulations, human brain imaging, and animal work, generating downstream hypotheses that could be tested in lab-controlled environment. Future work should take advantage of better-characterized ASD cohorts, with well-defined clinical endophenotypes, pharmacological history, and genetic predisposition. By generating human induced pluripotent stem cells neurons from these ASD cohorts, scientists can test whether the clinical outcome is predictive of the magnitude of cellular phenotype, whether specific mutations correlate to gene expression differences, or whether a clinical pharmacological response is predictable by human neuronal drug response. Such a strategy may also generate diagnostic tools and make clinical predictions. For this to become a reality in autism, reproducible and robust ASD phenotypes need to be validated by collaborative consortiums, involving several independent laboratories, perhaps sharing patient cohorts.

References

1. Hertz-Picciotto I, Delwiche L. The rise in autism and the role of age at diagnosis. *Epidemiology* 2009;**20**(1):84–90.
2. King M, Bearman P. Diagnostic change and the increased prevalence of autism. *Int J Epidemiol* 2009;**38**(5):1224–34.
3. Myers SM, Johnson CP, American Academy of Pediatrics Council on Children with Disabilities. Management of children with autism spectrum disorders. *Pediatrics* 2007;**120**(5):1162–82.
4. Warren Z, McPheeters ML, Sathe N, Foss-Feig JH, Glasser A, Veenstra-Vanderweele J. A systematic review of early intensive intervention for autism spectrum disorders. *Pediatrics* 2011;**127**(5): e1303–1311.
5. Bruder MB, Kerins G, Mazzarella C, Sims J, Stein N. Brief report: the medical care of adults with autism spectrum disorders: identifying the needs. *J Autism Dev Disord* 2012;**42**(11):2498–504.
6. Kogan MD, Strickland BB, Blumberg SJ, Singh GK, Perrin JM, van Dyck PC. A national profile of the health care experiences and family impact of autism spectrum disorder among children in the United States, 2005–2006. *Pediatrics* 2008;**122**(6):e1149–1158.
7. Takahashi K, Yamanaka S. Induction of pluripotent stem cells from mouse embryonic and adult fibroblast cultures by defined factors. *Cell* 2006;**126**(4):663–76.
8. Yu J, Vodyanik MA, Smuga-Otto K, Antosiewicz-Bourget J, Frane JL, Tian S, et al. Induced pluripotent stem cell lines derived from human somatic cells. *Science* 2007;**318**(5858):1917–20.
9. Freitas BC, Trujillo CA, Carromeu C, Yusupova M, Herai RH, Muotri AR. Stem cells and modeling of autism spectrum disorders. *Exp Neurol* 2012;**260**:33–43.
10. Marchetto MC, Carromeu C, Acab A, Yu D, Yeo GW, Mu Y, et al. A model for neural development and treatment of Rett syndrome using human induced pluripotent stem cells. *Cell* 2010;**143**(4): 527–39.
11. Shcheglovitov A, Shcheglovitova O, Yazawa M, Portmann T, Shu R, Sebastiano V, et al. SHANK3 and IGF1 restore synaptic deficits in neurons from 22q13 deletion syndrome patients. *Nature* 2013; **503**(7475):267–71.
12. Pasca SP, Portmann T, Voineagu I, Yazawa M, Shcheglovitov A, Pasca AM, et al. Using iPSC-derived neurons to uncover cellular phenotypes associated with Timothy syndrome. *Nat Med* 2011; **17**(12):1657–62.
13. Beltrao-Braga PC, Pignatari GC, Russo FB, Fernandes IR, Muotri AR. In-a-dish: induced pluripotent stem cells as a novel model for human diseases. *Cytometry A* 2013;**83**(1):11–7.
14. Cai M, Yang Y. Targeted genome editing tools for disease modeling and gene therapy. *Curr Gene Ther* 2014;**14**(1):2–9.
15. Soldner F, Laganiere J, Cheng AW, Hockemeyer D, Gao Q, Alagappan R, et al. Generation of isogenic pluripotent stem cells differing exclusively at two early onset Parkinson point mutations. *Cell* 2011;**146**(2):318–31.
16. Liu GH, Suzuki K, Qu J, Sancho-Martinez I, Yi F, Li M, et al. Targeted gene correction of laminopathy-associated LMNA mutations in patient-specific iPSCs. *Cell Stem Cell* 2011;**8**(6): 688–94.

17. Cheung AY, Horvath LM, Grafodatskaya D, Pasceri P, Weksberg R, Hotta A, et al. Isolation of MECP2-null Rett Syndrome patient hiPS cells and isogenic controls through X-chromosome inactivation. *Hum Mol Genet* 2011;**20**(11):2103–15.

18. Rao M. iPSC crowdsourcing: a model for obtaining large panels of stem cell lines for screening. *Cell Stem Cell* 2013;**13**(4):389–91.

19. Ananiev G, Williams EC, Li H, Chang Q. Isogenic pairs of wild type and mutant induced pluripotent stem cell (iPSC) lines from Rett syndrome patients as in vitro disease model. *PLoS One* 2011; **6**(9):e25255.

20. Kim KY, Hysolli E, Park IH. Neuronal maturation defect in induced pluripotent stem cells from patients with Rett syndrome. *Proc Natl Acad Sci USA* 2011;**108**(34):14169–74.

21. Tropea D, Giacometti E, Wilson NR, Beard C, McCurry C, Fu DD, et al. Partial reversal of Rett Syndrome-like symptoms in MeCP2 mutant mice. *Proc Natl Acad Sci USA* 2009;**106**(6):2029–34.

22. Scheuner D, Eckman C, Jensen M, Song X, Citron M, Suzuki N, et al. Secreted amyloid beta-protein similar to that in the senile plaques of Alzheimer's disease is increased in vivo by the presenilin 1 and 2 and APP mutations linked to familial Alzheimer's disease. *Nat Med* 1996;**2**(8):864–70.

23. Ji W, Foo JN, O'Roak BJ, Zhao H, Larson MG, Simon DB, et al. Rare independent mutations in renal salt handling genes contribute to blood pressure variation. *Nat Genet* 2008;**40**(5):592–9.

24. Bozdagi O, Sakurai T, Papapetrou D, Wang X, Dickstein DL, Takahashi N, et al. Haploinsufficiency of the autism-associated Shank3 gene leads to deficits in synaptic function, social interaction, and social communication. *Mol Autism* 2010;**1**(1):15.

25. Gutierrez RC, Hung J, Zhang Y, Kertesz AC, Espina FJ, Colicos MA. Altered synchrony and connectivity in neuronal networks expressing an autism-related mutation of neuroligin 3. *Neuroscience* 2009;**162**(1):208–21.

26. Sanders SJ, Ercan-Sencicek AG, Hus V, Luo R, Murtha MT, Moreno-De-Luca D, et al. Multiple recurrent de novo CNVs, including duplications of the 7q11.23 Williams syndrome region, are strongly associated with autism. *Neuron* 2011;**70**(5):863–85.

27. Levy D, Ronemus M, Yamrom B, Lee YH, Leotta A, Kendall J, et al. Rare de novo and transmitted copy-number variation in autistic spectrum disorders. *Neuron* 2011;**70**(5):886–97.

28. Gilman SR, Iossifov I, Levy D, Ronemus M, Wigler M, Vitkup D. Rare de novo variants associated with autism implicate a large functional network of genes involved in formation and function of synapses. *Neuron* 2011;**70**(5):898–907.

29. El-Fishawy P, State MW. The genetics of autism: key issues, recent findings, and clinical implications. *Psychiatr Clin North Am* 2010; **33**(1):83–105.

30. Geschwind DH. Genetics of autism spectrum disorders. *Trends Cogn Sci* 2011;**15**(9):409–16.

31. Weiss LA, Shen Y, Korn JM, Arking DE, Miller DT, Fossdal R, et al. Association between microdeletion and microduplication at 16p11.2 and autism. *N Engl J Med* 2008;**358**(7):667–75.

32. Bucan M, Abrahams BS, Wang K, Glessner JT, Herman EI, Sonnenblick LI, et al. Genome-wide analyses of exonic copy number variants in a family-based study point to novel autism susceptibility genes. *PLoS Genet* 2009;**5**(6):e1000536.

33. State MW, Levitt P. The conundrums of understanding genetic risks for autism spectrum disorders. *Nat Neurosci* 2011;**14**(12):1499–506.

34. Beltrao-Braga PI, Pignatari GC, Maiorka PC, Oliveira NA, Lizier NF, Wenceslau CV, et al. Feeder-free derivation of induced pluripotent stem cells from human immature dental pulp stem cells. *Cell Transplant* 2011;**20**(11–12):1707–19.

35. Tai Y, Feng S, Ge R, Du W, Zhang X, He Z, et al. TRPC6 channels promote dendritic growth via the CaMKIV-CREB pathway. *J Cell Sci* 2008;**121**(Pt 14):2301–7.

36. Zhou J, Du W, Zhou K, Tai Y, Yao H, Jia Y, et al. Critical role of TRPC6 channels in the formation of excitatory synapses. *Nat Neurosci* 2008;**11**(7):741–3.

37. Griesi-Oliveira K, Acab A, Gupta AR, Sunaga DY, Chailangkarn T, Nicol X, et al. Modeling non-syndromic autism and the impact of TRPC6 disruption in human neurons. *Mol Psychiatry* 2014;**11**: 1350–65.

38. Greek R, Rice MJ. Animal models and conserved processes. *Theor Biol Med Model* 2012;**9**:40.

39. van der Worp HB, Howells DW, Sena ES, Porritt MJ, Rewell S, O'Collins V, et al. Can animal models of disease reliably inform human studies? *PLoS Med* 2010;**7**(3):e1000245.

40. Diniz LP, Almeida JC, Tortelli V, Vargas Lopes C, Setti-Perdigao P, Stipursky J, et al. Astrocyte-induced synaptogenesis is mediated by transforming growth factor beta signaling through modulation of D-serine levels in cerebral cortex neurons. *J Biol Chem* 2012; **287**(49):41432–45.

41. Chung WS, Clarke LE, Wang GX, Stafford BK, Sher A, Chakraborty C, et al. Astrocytes mediate synapse elimination through MEGF10 and MERTK pathways. *Nature* 2013;**504**(7480):394–400.

42. Huh D, Matthews BD, Mammoto A, Montoya-Zavala M, Hsin HY, Ingber DE. Reconstituting organ-level lung functions on a chip. *Science* 2010;**328**(5986):1662–8.

43. Lancaster MA, Knoblich JA. Organogenesis in a dish: modeling development and disease using organoid technologies. *Science* 2014;**345**(6194):1247125.

44. Shi Y, Kirwan P, Smith J, Robinson HP, Livesey FJ. Human cerebral cortex development from pluripotent stem cells to functional excitatory synapses. *Nat Neurosci* 2012;**15**(3):477–86. S471.

45. Shi Y, Kirwan P, Livesey FJ. Directed differentiation of human pluripotent stem cells to cerebral cortex neurons and neural networks. *Nat Protoc* 2012;**7**(10):1836–46.

46. Wainger BJ, Kiskinis E, Mellin C, Wiskow O, Han SS, Sandoe J, et al. Intrinsic membrane hyperexcitability of amyotrophic lateral sclerosis patient-derived motor neurons. *Cell Rep* 2014;**7**(1):1–11.

Rett Syndrome: Clinical Aspects

Daniel C. Tarquinio[1], Alan K. Percy[2]

[1]Emory University, Children's Healthcare of Atlanta, Alanta, GA, USA; [2]University of Alabama at Birmingham, Birmingham, AL, USA

INTRODUCTION

Rett syndrome (RTT) is a rare disorder affecting almost exclusively girls, characterized by apparently normal early development followed by a period of psychomotor regression and the emergence of stereotypic hand movements. Although diagnostic criteria have been updated many times since the original descriptions, the core features of the disorder remain loss of purposeful hand skills and spoken language,

Neuronal and Synaptic Dysfunction in Autism Spectrum Disorder and Intellectual Disability
http://dx.doi.org/10.1016/B978-0-12-800109-7.00019-4

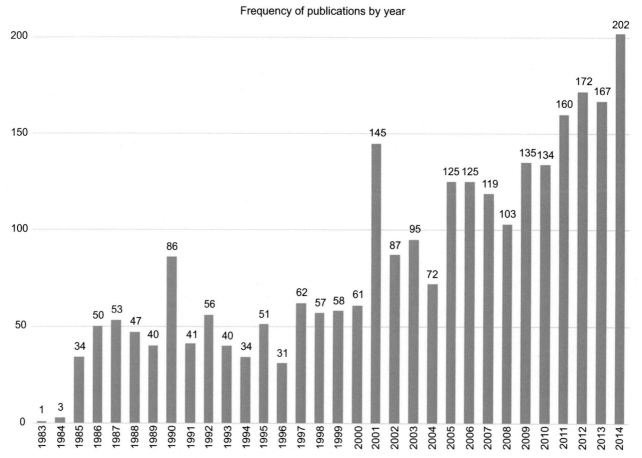

FIGURE 1   Frequency of publications cited in the US National Library of Medicine since Bengt Hagberg's publication naming the disorder. Search captured terms "Rett's syndrome" or "Rett syndrome" or "Rett's disorder" or "Rett disorder."

abnormal or absent walking, and repetitive hand movements. Many additional features can be present, and the overall disease burden of this protean disorder is often defined by the presence or absence of these additional comorbidities. In addition, because some of these afflictions, such as epilepsy, are common, and others such as cardiac conduction abnormality are less common, anticipation and appropriate treatment of these features are critical in clinical management.

Over 50 years have passed since two pediatricians, Austrian Andreas Rett in 1954 and Swedish Bengt Hagberg in 1960, first recognized this pattern in girls. Because Rett's publications in German did not circulate widely,[1,2] decades elapsed before a description of the disorder reached a larger audience. When Hagberg published a seminal paper in 1983 in a widely distributed American journal, he granted the eponym to Rett, and the disorder gained international recognition.[3] These two remarkable physicians captured most of what we now understand about the clinical aspects of the disorder in their original descriptions, although owing to aberrant assay results, Rett initially associated the disorder with hyperammonemia, which is no longer believed

to be the case. Since then, researchers have published over 2500 articles in peer-reviewed journals (Figure 1), elucidating many clinical, neurobiological, and genetic aspects of RTT, including identification of methyl CpG binding protein 2 gene (MECP2) mutations in most (see also Chapter 7).

EPIDEMIOLOGY

Rett syndrome is the leading cause of profound cognitive impairment in females. The incidence of RTT appears to be relatively stable worldwide. Since Hagberg's original prevalence estimate of 0.65 per 10,000 females in Sweden,[4] estimates of prevalence in other populations have varied from 0.22 per 10,000 in one prefecture of Japan[5] to 2.23 per 10,000 in Norway.[6] All of these studies were conducted before association with MECP2 mutations, and variability may be due to differences in ages of sampling and inclusion criteria. The largest study in the post-MECP2 era found a cumulative incidence of 1.09 per 10,000 by age 12 years in

Australia.[7] A small proportion of those with nonsyndromic autism spectrum disorder (ASD) actually have RTT; therefore, the current estimates of incidence may be low.[8] In recent years, studies have focused on the prevalence of various comorbidities and on survival within RTT, and these statistics are described below in respective sections.

Most cases of RTT are sporadic, a characteristic that RTT shares with most other X-linked dominant diseases, and most result from spontaneous mutations in the paternal germ line. However, a minority are inherited through one of two mechanisms: germ line mosaicism or transmission from an asymptomatic carrier mother with X-chromosome inactivation skewed toward silencing of the mutated X-chromosome.[9] The incidence of such familial cases is estimated at 0.5%[10]; nonetheless, some authors have recommended prenatal testing of all pregnancies in a family of a child with RTT.[11]

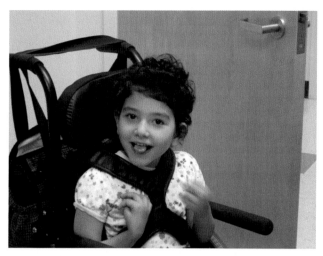

FIGURE 2 A 5-year-old girl with classic Rett syndrome after regression. Although she has severe gross and fine motor disability (nonambulatory, with truncal tone requiring substantial support, and frequent hand stereotypies), she is happy and socially engaging. *Photo used with permission.*

CLINICAL FEATURES

The pattern of development in RTT is unique and somewhat predictable. Normal early development is replaced at 6–18 months by developmental plateau, followed by developmental regression and development of a dyspraxic, wide-based gait in those who acquire ambulation, and accompanied by the emergence of growth failure and prominent hand stereotypies. Thereafter, throughout childhood and adolescence a series of associated characteristics and comorbidities may occur, some of which are more common than others. This section will elucidate the details of this series of events.

Hagberg proposed a clinical staging system with four stages of development, and although this system is rarely used to guide clinical management, a brief description of this framework helps to understand the historical course of the disorder.[12] Stage I, early-onset stagnation, begins insidiously and involves unusual eye contact, change in personality, and decreased interest in play. Stage II, the rapid destructive stage, begins between 1 and 3 years of age, and the combination of disconnection from the environment and stereotypies often leads to a diagnosis of ASD at this stage. Stage III, the pseudostationary stage, follows the period of regression, can last many years, and is variable with respect to functional decline or improvement. Although hand use and verbal language generally remain poor, these can improve. Nonverbal interaction and socialization improve in most, and those previously diagnosed as autistic generally become socially interactive and engaging (Figure 2).[13] The fourth, most poorly defined stage, late motor degeneration, can begin in childhood or adulthood and is

characterized by prominent gross motor dysfunction and the inability to walk. Because supportive care has improved dramatically since Hagberg proposed this system, many women with RTT continue to walk throughout adulthood, never entering stage IV (Figure 3). Therefore, this system can be misleading to both clinicians and families who expect a downward spiral of events that often never occurs.

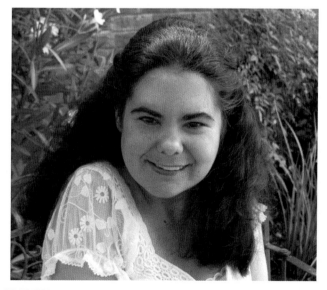

FIGURE 3 A 34-year-old woman with classic Rett syndrome, who continues to walk. Although the historical staging of the disorder implied that women eventually experience late motor degeneration and lose the ability to walk, many continue to walk into the fourth, fifth, and even sixth decades. As in the first figure, this woman continues to be happy and socially interactive. *Photo used with permission.*

Development

Development in RTT is apparently normal for the first 6–18 months of life when a period of regression occurs.[14] The modifier "apparently" is used because several studies have documented subtle abnormalities of early development using videos.[15–18] Although the 2002 diagnostic criteria required "essentially normal" early development to make the diagnosis,[19] the most recent criteria were altered to exclude "grossly abnormal" early development.[20]

Developmental abnormalities often begin with decreased velocity and then plateau of acquisition of skills, which can be subtle. The physician must conduct a detailed developmental history to elicit these findings in most parents, many of whom fail to mention regression without being prompted. The largest study of development to include direct assessment by clinicians experienced in RTT management used data on 542 females who met criteria for classic RTT and 96 females who met criteria for atypical RTT (defined in the section on diagnostic criteria) from the National Institute of Child Health and Human Development–sponsored Rare Disease Natural History Study (NHS).[14] This study found that nearly all participants acquired fundamental gross motor (e.g., rolling and sitting with support), fine motor (e.g., reaching and holding a bottle), and language (fixing/following, social smile, and babbling) skills. However, in classic RTT, fewer acquired more advanced skills; only 53% acquired the ability to walk, 74% acquired a refined pincer grasp, and 77% acquired single words. Moreover, although most acquired sitting, reaching, and the ability to fix and follow, most were delayed in onset. Social smile was acquired on time in about 75%. The NHS study also uncovered an important distinction in the atypical RTT group between higher-functioning and lower-functioning atypical individuals. These data suggest that atypical RTT patients fail to meet the criteria for classic RTT either because their development was too normal and they did not regress in one or more domains or it was too abnormal and they never acquired skills that could be lost. In the atypical mild group, 78% acquired walking, 90% acquired a pincer grasp, and 94% acquired single words, whereas in the atypical severe group only 7% acquired walking, 42% acquired a pincer grasp, and 36% acquired single words. Notably, in classic RTT, attaining motor milestones and higher-level expressive language milestones was predictive of lower severity later in life, based on the Motor Behavioral Assessment (MBA), a global measure of severity.

The pattern of developmental regression varies widely, from rapid loss of skills, in which parents describe that "someone pulled the plug" and the child lost all domains of development overnight, to an insidious process lasting for months to years.[21] Onset is most commonly between 12 and 18 months, but can occur before 6 months or after 3 years of age.[22] The NHS found that in classic RTT, fine motor regression was more common than gross motor regression, and for those who gained higher expressive language (e.g., single words, phrases, pointing, gesturing), most lost these abilities. However, receptive language was relatively well preserved, with one-third or fewer losing abilities to recognize "no" or to follow commands. Compared with classic RTT, the atypical mild group generally lost fewer abilities during regression, and the atypical severe group lost more abilities.[14]

Maintenance of skills is variable and often depends on the baseline level of function attained. One Australian 4-year longitudinal study documented maintenance or improvement in gross motor function in 40% over time and a slight decrease in function in 60%.[23] Individuals with classic RTT maintain function in many domains throughout adulthood: 40–50% continue to walk independently, 10–20% continue to use a pincer grasp, 25–45% can feed themselves, and 10–20% continue to use verbalizations (consonant–vowel combinations or words) with meaning, and 50–60% continue to make effective nonverbal choices (unpublished findings from NHS). Although skills that are lost often are never regained, both anecdotal reports and peer-reviewed research support the concept that with intensive therapy, lost skills can be regained. This is the case both for skills lost during the initial regression period, and those lost later in life during so-called "late motor degeneration." In one particularly illustrative case, a woman who lost the ability to walk at age 21 years and spent 15 years in a wheelchair regained the ability to walk with only minimal assistance at age 36 years.[24]

Stereotypical Movements

Hand movements in RTT are peculiar to this disorder. Although many other disorders, including ASD, express stereotypical hand movements, the stereotypies in RTT are frequent or continuous, occur almost exclusively in the midline, are markedly rhythmic, and are often multiple (e.g., clapping, wringing, and mouthing in the same individual). Compared with ASD, RTT stereotypies are significantly more frequent, more often unilateral, larger amplitude, more rhythmic, less likely to incorporate the use of an object, and more often in the midline.[25] Despite these unifying factors, stereotypies can vary widely among RTT patients, and at least 15 categories of stereotypies have been described.[26]

Stereotypies and other behaviors (breathing dysregulation, described below) are often exacerbated by stress and cease during sleep.[27] One study has considered interpreting stereotypies directly as a marker of stress by quantifying behavioral responses.[28] However, stereotypies naturally change over the lifespan of an individual with RTT, and the complex repertoire of movements evolves with addition and subtraction of certain movements over time.[26,29]

Many strategies have been employed to limit stereotypical hand movements. The movements are perceived to inhibit normal hand function and regression in hand use often occurs concurrently with emergence of stereotypies.[29] Individuals with some preserved hand function often demonstrate the remarkable ability to suppress stereotypies briefly, execute a purposeful hand movement, and immediately resume the stereotypies. Braces can be effective, although one study demonstrated that elbow orthoses were more effective than hand splints when the goals were both to suppress repetitive movement and enhance hand use in playing with toys.[30] Anecdotal reports describe the successful use of gloves, socks placed over the hands, and bracelets or necklaces to distract the patient and inhibit stereotypies.

Behaviors

In the presymptomatic phase during early infancy, children are often described as "too good," with little crying or irritability compared with siblings. The initial behavioral abnormalities seen in RTT develop during regression, and include irritability and disconnection from the environment. Social withdrawal and inconsolable crying often occur together during the period of regression, and can give the impression of ASD.[21] The crying spells, decreased eye contact, and poor nonverbal communication are usually transient, lasting for weeks to months, and after age 5 years only a small proportion of girls meet the diagnostic criteria for ASD in addition to RTT; this differentiation was recognized several years before RTT was introduced into the pervasive developmental disorder category of the Diagnostic and Statistical Manual *of Mental Disorders*, Fourth edition.[31] Older girls are socially engaging, although they tend to approach male adults preferentially and can often communicate their desires nonverbally. However, a host of other behaviors can emerge, some of which are problematic; these are described below.

Breathing Dysregulation

During wakefulness, most patients with RTT exhibit abnormal breathing patterns.[3,32] These may appear at any time after the regression period but they typically become evident during late childhood. They consist of episodes of disorganized breathing that can include breathing unusually fast, unusually deep, or not at all. Periods of apnea can last seconds to over a minute and

consist of either ceasing respiratory effort in inspiration or expiration, or clear breath-holding against a closed glottis, followed by forced exhalation. During hyperventilation, severe hypocapnia occurs and during breath-holding, oxygen saturations can drop well below 50%, accompanied clinically by cyanosis.[33,34] Although breathing dysregulation is generally understood to be the result of autonomic dysfunction, this phenomenon ceases almost entirely during sleep.[33]

Three distinct breathing patterns have been identified: forceful breathing, with high-amplitude breaths; feeble breathing, with weak respiration overall; and apneustic breathing, with long periods of breath-holding.[35] Forceful breathers can have tonic seizure-like movements, accompanied by spikes in heart rate and blood pressure. This behavior has been treated successfully with either administration of a paper bag (as was traditionally done to treat anxiety attacks) or a mixture of 5% CO_2 and 95% O_2 administered by a face mask.[36] Feeble breathers can develop low oxygen levels, with pO_2 as low as 26 mm Hg.[37] This has been managed with oxygen administered via continuous positive airway pressure. Apneustic breathers are generally refractory to treatment; however, one girl was treated successfully with buspirone[38] and another with a mixed forceful/apneustic pattern was successfully treated with concomitant buspirone and fluoxetine.[39]

Studies have uncovered subtle breathing dysregulation present during both sleep and wakefulness that does not clearly warrant treatment.[40,41] These studies support the theory that breathing dysregulation results from an underlying autonomic dysregulation with superimposed behavioral features. In addition, abnormal upper airway muscle function, similar to that found in Parkinson disease, may have a role.[33] No routine surveillance of breathing during sleep is recommended. However, if snoring or apnea is present, a polysomnogram should be performed (see subsequent discussion).

Anxiety

Spells of breathing dysregulation, staring, or tremulousness are often attributed to anxiety. Serotonergic medications are often prescribed, but no systematic research has demonstrated their efficacy in managing these "Rett spells." Animal evidence suggests increased cortisol release in girls with RTT.[42] However, no targeted treatments based on this finding have been assessed.

Abusive or Disruptive Behaviors

Spitting: Although no systematic review describes this behavior, forceful spitting can be problematic and can lead to removal from school environments and to social ostracism by peers. In our experience, behavioral therapy is ineffective, as are treatments for concomitant sialorrhea. Application of a mask over the mouth has been effective temporarily.

Bruxism: Another problematic behavior, teeth grinding is often loud and distracting. However, damage to the teeth is generally minimal. We do not advocate the use of mouth guards because these could be dislodged and cause injury. Occasionally, chewable necklaces or bracelets can be used to distract from this behavior.

Screaming: As described above, this is often a problem during the regression period and is rare thereafter. However, episodes of screaming can occur throughout childhood and adulthood, and this behavior is often difficult to differentiate from pain caused by a medical concern.

Epilepsy

Epilepsy is a common but not universal comorbidity in RTT. After 2–3 years of age, electroencephalogram (EEG) slowing, spikes, and polyspikes are a nearly universal finding on EEGs in children with RTT.[43] Yet, according to NHS data, at a given age, the prevalence of caregiver-reported seizures varies, from 33% at age 3–5 years to 86% at age 15–20 years.[44] However, although the overall prevalence of spells reported by parents in RTT is 60%, only 48% had epileptic seizures based on physician assessment. Rett syndome experts typically do not prescribe antiseizure medications for patients without clear epileptic seizures, despite an abnormal EEG. Because of the wide variety of behaviors seen in RTT, "spells" of uncertain significance should be investigated with long-term video EEG or ambulatory EEG before starting medications. An examination of 82 long-term video EEG studies, lasting from 8 to 120 h, found that although parents of 42% of the 55 individuals with a history of seizures identified events typical of their child's seizure, EEG showed no epileptiform correlate.[45] Although all patients had abnormal EEGs, only 16% had electroclinical seizures, including both focal and generalized, during recording. The nonepileptic spells seen in this study consisted of staring, laughing, pupillary dilatation, breathing dysregulation, and a variety of motor activities.

Electroencephalograms during sleep are generally abnormal after regression and can consist of slowing and rare epileptiform discharges, or even of a continuous spike-and-slow-wave pattern reminiscent of an epileptic encephalopathy. However, unlike epileptic encephalopathy, no evidence supports treatment of these features to normalize the EEG, because this has not historically resulted in cognitive improvement.

No specific medications have been demonstrated to have superior efficacy in RTT. However, the side-effect profiles should be considered carefully, and medications that can cause behavioral issues (e.g., levetiracetam), anorexia (e.g., topiramate), QT interval prolongation (e.g., felbamate), or marked sedation (e.g., benzodiazepines) should be used with caution. Medication choice should be based on consideration of semiology, EEG characteristics, and risk–benefit with respect to adverse effects.

Growth Failure

Decrease in height, weight, and front-occipital head circumference (FOC) are pervasive in RTT. Deceleration of FOC is one of the earliest consistent features of the disorder, and the average FOC in RTT decreases relative to the normative population as early as age 1.5 months.[46] Although microcephaly is present in most by age 2 years, about 20% of adults maintain an FOC in the normal range. Therefore, microcephaly is no longer one of the required criteria for diagnosis. Weight is significantly lower than the normative population by 13 months, and height is significantly lower by 17 months. Nonetheless, in adulthood 30% have normal or above-normal weight and 15% have normal height. Although average body mass index (BMI) is similar to the normative population, the distribution of BMI is wider, with 36% falling below the normative second percentile and 19% falling above the 98th percentile at some point during development.

Nutritional assessment and evaluation of chewing and swallowing should be performed routinely. Often girls with RTT require assistance with physical positioning during eating, special utensils, and modification of food consistency. A consensus statement recommended targeting the BMI of girls with RTT above the 25th percentile on normative charts, roughly equivalent to the 50th percentile on the RTT charts, suggesting that malnutrition occurs in most.[47] Recommendations of this consensus include discussion of when to consider gastrostomy tube placement, the benefits of which include avoidance of aspiration during feeding, improved nutrition, shorter meal times, decreased energy expenditure, decreased family burden, and, if fundoplication is performed, improvement in gastroesophageal reflux disease (GERD).

Atrophic, small distal extremities, particularly feet,[48] are present and can become cold and purple when severe. This phenomenon varies among individuals and is thought to be result from autonomic dysregulation, specifically sympathetic dominance. Individuals who have had an incidental sympathectomy (as part of scoliosis surgery) show that relief from sympathetic drive causes the foot to grow and resume normal vascular perfusion. Although sympathectomy is not considered a treatment approach, when this condition is severe the authors have referred patients to vascular specialists for medical management.

Sleep

Sleep is abnormal in RTT, with decreased rapid-eye-movement sleep.[33] Children often have difficulty falling asleep and staying asleep throughout the night, but generally wake appearing rested. Melatonin is often sufficient to induce sleep, although this will not sustain sleep if nighttime waking is a problem. If melatonin is unsuccessful, trazodone is also safe and has been used extensively. Periods of waking often go unnoticed, because children are happy and play by themselves. They can be found at 1–3 am, sitting up and laughing to themselves in bed for 1–2 h and then resuming sleep. In general, no treatment is warranted for this behavior. However, if sleep maintenance is a problem, chloral hydrate has been used in RTT successfully for this purpose.[49]

Obstructive sleep apnea occurs, although it is unclear whether this is more frequent than in the general population. However, in some cases the obstruction is severe and, particularly in medically fragile girls, can result in death. Therefore, polysomnography is recommended in all children with a history of respiratory issues during sleep.[50] Often, hypertrophy of tonsils and adenoid cause obstructive sleep apnea and are amenable to surgical correction.

Gastrointestinal

Oromotor Dysfunction

Chewing and swallowing difficulties occur to some degree in almost all girls and women with RTT. Based on family report, 81% of 983 girls and women with RTT have difficulty with feeding.[51] A videofluoroscopy study of 13 girls and women found oropharyngeal dysfunction in all and gastroesophageal dysmotility in 69%.[52] These abnormalities included poor oral transit, pooling of thin liquids in the pharynx in 50%, and laryngeal penetration or aspiration of thin liquids in over 60%. Generalized hypertonia or hypotonia were associated with aspiration of thin liquids. Because dysfunction is often not evident on bedside swallow evaluation, videofluoroscopy swallow studies help caretakers identify safety issues and adjust consistency of food.

Drooling

The severity of drooling problems in RTT ranges widely. Often this is easily managed with a towel or bib. However, many girls saturate these quickly, and caretakers can have difficulty preventing rashes and infections related to excessive moisture on the skin. Four medical options and one surgical option exist to address this problem. Glycopyrrolate and scopolamine transdermal patches have similar efficacy and side-effect profiles, although the latter offers ease of administration.

Atropine, available as an ophthalmic solution, can be administered directly to the salivary glands by placing a single drop in each cheek every 8 h as needed. This local administration technique avoids systemic side effects and allows the medication to be used as needed. Botulinum toxin can be injected directly into the salivary glands, and effects last for several months. However, the procedure for administration is the most invasive of the medical options. Finally, salivary gland excision or duct ligation is reserved for the most severe cases.

Gastroesophageal Reflux Disease

Families report symptoms of GERD in 39%.[51] In the videofluoroscopy study discussed, gastric dysmotility was present in 46% and reflux to the level of the aortic arch was present in 23%.[52] Because upper gastrointestinal studies may miss GERD in 50% of cases, esophageal pH probe is preferred as a more sensitive test, although this can be technically difficult. Treatment can be approached using acid blockade as in any child with GERD, but difficult cases should be referred to gastroenterology.

Constipation

Constipation, often resulting in pseudo-obstruction and hospitalization, is present in 80% of the RTT population, and treatment of this has resulted in one of the greatest improvements in quality of life in the RTT population.[51] Most patients require daily laxatives to maintain normal bowel movements, and without this treatment they may retain stool for several days, resulting in extreme discomfort. Although suppositories, enemas, and even manual disimpaction are still common practice, we discourage these approaches in favor of polyethylene glycol and/or magnesium hydroxide. Dietary modification and fiber supplementation are helpful, and lactulose can also be used. Mineral oil can be added as a temporary supplement; however, chronic use results in deficiencies of fat-soluble vitamins.

Abdominal Bloating

Although less common, air-swallowing with hyperventilation often leads to painful bloating. Simethicone can be helpful, and if a gastrostomy tube is present, venting can alleviate this.

Biliary Tract Disorders

Biliary tract disorders are present in over 3% of the RTT population: cholelithiasis in 2% and biliary dyskinesia in a further 1%.[51] In one study, almost half of those identified with biliary tract disorders were aged under 20 years, two-thirds had gallstones, and nearly 90% required cholecystectomy.[53] Therefore, biliary tract disorders should be considered when unexplained general discomfort is present. Although ultrasound is considered the initial diagnostic test of choice, a nuclear medicine scan (e.g., hepatobiliary iminodiacetic acid scan) is often required to rule out dyskinesia.

Motor Abnormalities

In addition to stereotypies, the etiology of which remain unclear, a number of movement disorders affect patients with RTT throughout their lifespan. These include some phenomena discussed earlier, such as bruxism, neurogenic scoliosis (discussed subsequently), as well as dystonia, and, rarely, myoclonus, athetosis, and oculogyric crises. Movement disorders in RTT display an age-related pattern: Hyperkinetic disorders occurring at younger ages are replaced by bradykinetic disorders in the third to fifth decades of life.[54,55] Parkinsonian features and rigidity are prominent in many older women and can be debilitating. Levodopa has been beneficial in some, but tetrabenazine has had mixed results and can exacerbate abnormal movements.

Orthopedic Issues and Bone Health

Scoliosis and Kyphosis

Overall, scoliosis is present in 85% after age 16 years and can be severe. Surgery was performed in 13% of the United States (US) population studied in the NHS, resulting in an overall improvement in quality of life.[56] Screening should be performed at least annually, and more frequently before the onset of puberty when scoliosis can progress more rapidly. Guidelines exist for management of scoliosis in RTT and include recommendations for referral for bracing or surgical management.[57] Kyphosis is less prevalent, and although this can be severe in some, bracing and surgery are rarely performed.

Bone Health

Girls and women with RTT are at high risk for fracture, estimated at 40% by age 15 years.[58] Vitamin D deficiency is prevalent in RTT, occurring in 20% of participants in one study, and the use of supplements or vitamin D–containing formulas is associated with higher levels.[59] Notably, antiseizure medications are not associated with low vitamin D level or bone mineral density in RTT.[59,60] Bone mineral density is in the osteoporotic range in half of those tested, independent of age, and is associated with lack of ambulation and higher disease severity, a finding also present in the murine model of a large *MECP2* deletion.[60]

Supplementation with both calcium and vitamin D is recommended. Standing, either with assistance or in a standing frame, and ambulation, if possible, should be encouraged to promote bone health. Weight-bearing exercise is preferable for bone health as opposed to weight-neutral (e.g., aquatherapy). Only one case of use of bisphosphonate has been reported, and no systematic study has examined the risk–benefit ratio in RTT.[61]

Cardiac

Prolonged QT syndrome, although rare, is more common than in the general population. Screening with a 12-lead electrocardiogram (EKG) should be performed annually. If the corrected QT interval is greater than 450 ms, the patient should be referred to cardiology. In addition, families should be informed that a long list of medications can further lengthen QTc and should be avoided. Rather than provide this list, we recommend they alert their providers to the risk of QTc prolongation when new medications are proposed. Regarding treatment, although the mainstay of treatment in the general population with prolonged QT interval is beta blockade, propranolol does not appear to prevent lethal arrhythmia in a mouse model of RTT, whereas the sodium channel blocking agent phenytoin does.[62] To date, phenytoin has not been tested clinically to treat QT prolongation.

Metabolic and Endocrine

Puberty

Precocious puberty has been documented in RTT, based on both endocrinological evidence in a single case[63] and on physician examination in a large cohort.[64] Clinically, in a study of 802 participants, 25% of girls reached thelarche early and 28% reached adrenarche early.[64] In the single case with laboratory data, these features were consistent with true precocious puberty.[63] In the cohort, menarche occurred over a wide range, with precocious onset of menses in 13% and delayed onset in 19% of the population. Higher BMI was associated with early adrenarche and thelarche but was not associated with menarche. In addition, those with milder mutation types (see discussion on *MECP2* mutations) experienced earlier menarche, and those with less severe clinical phenotype experienced earlier menarche and thelarche.

Dyslipidemia

Abnormal cholesterol metabolism has been suggested by one suppressor screen study conducted using a mouse model, and another study on cultured human fibroblasts.[65,66] Clinically, the authors have noted both elevated LDL and triglycerides (not discussed in these reports) in several girls and women with RTT; however, these abnormalities have been easily addressed with dietary modification, and none has required treatment with statin drugs. No study has compared the prevalence of dyslipidemia in RTT with the general population using age- and diet-matched controls.

Longevity

Longevity in RTT is better than one would expect based on other disorders of profound cognitive impairment, in which only 27% survive at age 35. In RTT, survival at age 35 is 60–70%, and median survival is age greater than 50 years.[67–69] Therefore, parents should expect children to live into adulthood, and in many cases to outlive them, and should plan accordingly. The obsolete notion that RTT is a neurodegenerative disorder has been dispelled by numerous anatomical and neurobiological studies that have led to the current perspective that RTT is a neurodevelopmental condition.[70] Many medical concerns, such as malnutrition and severe scoliosis, could contribute to early death, but with modern management, the contribution of these factors to mortality is largely historical. The most common causes of death include epilepsy and respiratory problems.[69] Sudden cardiac death owing to cardiac conduction abnormality may account for a small proportion of sudden death.[71] However, life expectancy is long with good medical management and anticipation of these known causes of early death.

SYMPTOMATIC MANAGEMENT

Therapies

Therapy is critical in RTT not only for improvement of function but also for prevention of loss of attained skills, and should include physical, occupational, and speech and language therapy in all cases. Because of their expressive language and speech deficits, we encourage individual speech and language therapy as opposed to group therapy. Andreas Rett reportedly urged parents to keep children walking; in fact, the ability to ambulate is more closely associated with overall disease severity than any other functional skill or symptom.[72] Longitudinal evidence suggests that patients with RTT can lose function after a short vacation from therapy and may take some time to regain lost skills.[73] Unfortunately, therapy services are often discontinued owing to the inability to demonstrate improvement, when in fact, maintaining function should be the public health goal set for this population. Many types of expenditure, including wheelchairs and other equipment, orthopedic surgery, and medically trained caretakers, could be minimized or potentially avoided if therapy were initiated early and maintained throughout life. Older women who have received excellent services can

often walk, feed themselves with minimal assistance, maintain continence, and enjoy a social role in a group home. Alternately, those in whom therapy is discontinued often lose the ability to walk, use their hands, and communicate meaningfully as they age.

Motivation appears critical in improving function, and experimentation is necessary. One girl achieved her best improvements in mobility when pushing a toy shopping cart.[74] Although no strong evidence supports a particular therapeutic regimen, the rehabilitation program at the Israeli Rett Syndrome Center offers a comprehensive approach supported by numerous successful cases.[73,75–77] In addition, music therapy can be used to augment other therapeutic approaches.[78,79] Behavioral therapy can be used to improve adaptive function, although this is labor-intensive and has been unsuccessful in some cases.[80,81]

Communication is often aided through augmentative and alternative communication devices, which can be as simple as cards or pictures at which the patient looks or gestures, or as complex as eye-gaze hardware and software. Eye-tracking has been studied in RTT with promising results; girls are able to recognize and fix on novel and salient features during testing, which suggests that eye-tracking is a valid window to communication in the disorder.[82,83] Many parents describe that children with RTT can make consistent choices and express desires when a system of communication is reinforced.[84] Caretakers generally have positive impressions of additional therapies such as aquatherapy and hippotherapy. In our experience, hippotherapy is helpful, especially to those with low truncal tone, and swimming is both enjoyable and beneficial, especially in a heated pool.

In girls with constant hand stereotypies, for whom hand use is minimal, bracing or barriers to inhibit movement can be used. Unless the movements are self-injurious, which is rare, or are causing skin breakdown, we do not recommend such barriers throughout the day. These barriers often limit whatever functional hand use remains. The one exception is that a barrier on one hand can facilitate use of the other hand; this strategy can be useful during occupational therapy and can be tested by restraining one hand during therapy. Often, girls who are profoundly dominant with one hand (commonly the left hand)[85] will use the alternate hand during therapy if the dominant hand is restrained.

Medical Surveillance and Anticipatory Guidance

Patients are typically seen in a neurology clinic for routine visits every 6 months during early childhood, and annually thereafter. Topics discussed are covered in more detail in respective sections, but are reviewed here for completeness. A multidisciplinary approach is beneficial and can include the routine involvement of a nutritionist, gastroenterologist, orthopedic surgeon, physiotherapist, and other personnel.[24]

- Diagnosis is reviewed if not firmly established based on clinical features. Once diagnosis is suspected, genetic testing is sent (see subsequent discussion). If *MECP2* testing reveals one of the more common mutations, genotype–phenotype counseling is offered. If *MECP2* testing is not revealing, other testing is considered as clinical features evolve.
- Annual EKGs are obtained to evaluate for prolonged corrected QT interval.
- Growth parameters are obtained at each visit and BMI is calculated. Nutrition consultation is recommended in most cases because of either growth failure or obesity.
- Spine examination is performed to evaluate for scoliosis, and consultation is recommended with an orthopedic surgeon when present, although surgery is not generally pursued until the Cobb angle is greater than 40°.
- Vitamin D level is tested annually; routine supplementation is recommended and additional supplementation provided if the 25-OH vitamin D level is low. If fractures have occurred, bone density is tested using dual-emission X-ray absorptiometry. In cases of low bone density, a referral to endocrinology should be made.
- Gastrointestinal issues are discussed, with attention to constipation and bowel regimen, GERD, and unexplained abdominal discomfort.
- Cholesterol is screened during childhood, and referral to an endocrinologist or cardiologist in conjunction with a nutritionist should be made if lipid panel is abnormal.
- Pubertal concerns are addressed, and if signs of precocious puberty are present, consultation with an endocrinologist can be helpful.
- Breathing dysfunction is discussed, and particularly when cyanosis or recurrent infections (rare) are present, a referral to pulmonology is made. If nighttime breathing abnormalities are present, a sleep study is ordered.
- Mobility issues are discussed in detail, with attention to equipment (wheelchair, ankle foot orthoses, etc.) and therapeutic regimen. Strategies to improve standing and walking are discussed, and efforts are made to maximize therapy sessions depending on specific needs. Medications for spasticity can be prescribed to improve function, and specific joint problems (e.g., hip dislocation) can be addressed by an orthopedic consultant.
- Stereotypies and hand use are reviewed. Skin is examined for any evidence of breakdown. If stereotypies are severe, occupational therapists can offer suggestions, and bracing or other barriers can be used intermittently.
- Communication techniques are reviewed, and suggestions are made for expanding the repertoire of communicative tools. Because girls with RTT often communicate best with eye gaze, evaluation through an alternative and augmentative communication program can result in improved communication through low-technology (e.g., picture cards) or high-technology (e.g., eye-gaze computers) means. Often, anxiety and aggression are manifestations of frustration resulting from difficulty with communication.
- Behavioral problems are discussed, and medical or therapeutic strategies for management are offered.
- Seizure burden is discussed, including seizure semiology, diagnostic testing needed, changes to medication regimen, and safety issues.
- Particularly in older girls and women, bradykinesia, dyskinesia and rigidity are assessed, and referral to a movement disorder specialist is made if these are problematic.
- Although not discussed at every visit, concerns about longevity and prognosis are elicited and answered. Many parents fear the worst and are reassured by the life expectancy and outcome in women with RTT.

DIAGNOSTIC CRITERIA

Consensus criteria were initially developed in 1985 and have undergone periodic revisions as molecular diagnosis has improved and supportive features of the disorder have been clarified.[19,20,86–88] The most recent criteria allow for two possible RTT diagnoses: classic, also known as typical RTT, and variant or atypical RTT.

Classic RTT

The four core features for diagnosis of classic RTT have remained since Hagberg's 1985 criteria: loss of communication and fine motor hand skills, apraxia or absence of gait, and hand stereotypies; however, Hagberg initially emphasized screening children with loss of hand use.[4] The penultimate criteria for classic RTT, from 2002, contained eight necessary criteria, eight supportive criteria, and five exclusion criteria. However, only four of the eight necessary criteria are now considered cardinal characteristics of the disorder, and the other four were relegated to the preamble and exclusion criteria in 2010. In their summation of the 2002 consensus criteria, the authors emphasized the need for consistency in diagnosis to achieve "accurate conduct of phenotype-genotype studies."[19] In the ensuing decade, much confusion has arisen, and the diagnosis has often been blurred to include boys with *MECP2* duplications and girls with mild intellectual disability and *MECP2* mutations.

To diagnose classic RTT based on the current criteria, an individual must undergo a period of regression followed by stabilization and meet the four main criteria and neither of the exclusion criteria (grossly abnormal development before age 6 months or traumatic, neurometabolic, or infectious brain injury). Possible RTT may be diagnosed in those with a *MECP2* mutation who may not have manifested regression owing to age, but this diagnosis should be questioned if the child achieves age 5 years without regression.

In a comparison of the 2002 and 2010 criteria using the natural history study, all participants with classic RTT expressed the four main criteria. However, supportive criteria were present variably, in as few as 23% (small hands) and as many as 91% (bruxism).[89] Presence of the supportive criteria has been eliminated from the criteria for classic RTT diagnosis, because these were never explicitly required for such a diagnosis. Moreover, the presence of these less specific features has led to confusion in diagnosis as well as the labeling of many as Rett-like, or even having RTT, when in fact they do not meet diagnostic criteria. The remainder of the confusion surrounding diagnosis stems from the fact that Rett syndrome is not synonymous with *MECP2* mutations, and *MECP2* mutations occur in individuals without RTT.[19] Thus, *MECP2*-related phenotypes involve both males and females and extend well beyond classic RTT. Head circumference deceleration was present in 82% of the natural history cohort, which supports the 2002 criteria that specified that this phenomenon occurs in the majority but is not required for diagnosis.

Atypical RTT

Atypical RTT is problematic as a diagnostic category because of the breadth of the phenotypes included. As individuals with RTT or characteristics of the disorder were discovered after Hagberg's 1983 report, unusual cases were identified. First, Hanefeld identified a girl with infantile spasms, later classified as the early-onset seizure or Hanefeld variant.[90] This variant was later associated with *CDKL5*, although many with mutations in this gene never undergo regression, and so never meet the clinical criteria for RTT.[91] Rolando reported one case of RTT with markedly abnormal early development, and although this individual exhibited many other characteristics of the disorder, no fundamental skills were acquired, so the concept of regression cannot

be applied.[31] This congenital Rolando variant was later associated with mutations in *FOXG1*.[92] Hagberg and Rasmussen identified a girl with preservation of hand use and some language,[93] a *forme fruste* of the disorder that was later elucidated when Zappella identified three girls who spoke in fully articulated phrases, yet expressed all the other core characteristics of the classic disorder.[94] Zappella formulated criteria with statistical support for a separate diagnostic category of girls with milder symptoms and preserved speech, the Zappella variant.[95]

According to the current criteria, atypical RTT can be diagnosed when individuals experience regression, exhibit two of the four main criteria discussed earlier, have none of the exclusion criteria, and display five of a list of 11 supportive criteria. Supportive criteria include: breathing disturbances while awake; bruxism (awake); impaired sleep; abnormal muscle tone; peripheral vasomotor disturbances; scoliosis or kyphosis; growth retardation; small, cold hands and feet; inappropriate laughing or screaming spells; diminished pain response; and intense eye-pointing gaze. Criteria for the three historical variant forms discussed above are presented in the most recent diagnostic criteria, however, many individuals with features of each (mild *MECP2* mutations, *CDKL5* mutations, and *FOXG1* mutations) do not meet the diagnostic criteria for atypical RTT because of a lack of regression and/or absence of stereotypies.[96] These *MECP2*-related individuals should be categorized separately; in the case of *MECP2*, labeling based on the genetic defect and predominant features is appropriate, for example, as in individuals with a *MECP2* mutation and intellectual disability, but without clinical RTT.[97] Many such individuals have small deletions in the 3′ region of the gene, and it is in their best interests, both for research purposes and clinical management, to be treated apart from classic or atypical RTT. In cases of *CDKL5* and *FOXG1*, these are likely separate clinical entities in which a minority meet the clinical criteria for RTT, and as the phenotypes of each are clarified, distinct clinical diagnostic criteria will be developed.[96]

In the natural history study, 14% of those met criteria for atypical RTT and 76% had a mutation in *MECP2*. Essentially, atypical RTT represents both the upper and lower ends of typical RTT, those who never lost hand use or language skills, and those who never attained abilities to lose (see the discussion on development).[14,72] These patterns are associated with known groupings among the common mutations (discussed subsequently) in *MECP2*, with milder mutations in classic RTT presenting with an even more mild phenotype in atypical RTT, and severe mutations in classic RTT with a more debilitating phenotype in atypical RTT.[72]

MECP2 MUTATIONS

Classic RTT is caused by mutations in *MECP2*, located at Xq28, in at least 95% of cases.[98] Most (> 99%) are the result of spontaneous mutations in the paternal germ line rather than inherited from carrier mothers. Over 200 mutations in *MECP2* have been identified as causative; of these, four missense mutations, four nonsense mutations, and several 3′ truncations and deletions of entire exons account for up to 80% of cases.[13]

Although genotype–phenotype studies have helped to explain some of the phenotypic heterogeneity in RTT, severity among mutations overlaps substantially. Only the extreme mild (R133C, R294X, R306C, and 3′ truncations) and severe (large deletions and R168X) mutations are significantly different on average when compared systematically in large groups.[99] Nonetheless, severely disabled individuals with a mild R133C mutation and higher-functioning individuals with a severe R168X mutation exist.

Variability of phenotype in X-linked dominant disease can depend on lionization, the process of (usually) random silencing of one of the X-chromosomes in each cell early in embryonic development. Cases of very mild disease and asymptomatic carriers have been documented with markedly skewed X-chromosome inactivation (XCI). In addition, monozygotic twins with different phenotypes can be attributed to skewed XCI in the milder twin.[100] Although testing can be done easily on blood or buccal tissue, peripheral silencing of the mutant gene is only presumed to represent XCI in the brain.[101,102] Nonetheless, XCI does not account for all of the phenotypic variability present in RTT[103] and may be misleading.[104] An additional variable, one that is impossible to test clinically, is the clonal expansion of the mutant X-chromosome. Perhaps the best example of this is the Calico cat, whose discrete patches are different on every cat and are the result of variable distribution of the maternal and paternal X-chromosomes, in this case during dermatogenesis. Because of variable clonal expansion during neurogenesis, the distribution of mutant *MECP2* will be different in various brain regions, even in twins with RTT, regardless of their XCI skewing, and this pattern of expansion cannot be tested in vivo.[105]

The spectrum of *MECP2* mutations extends far beyond RTT, including the following: asymptomatic carrier females described previously; females with mild learning disability; profoundly disabled females who never achieve developmental milestones beyond fixing and following or reaching, and never express stereotypical behaviors; males with intellectual disability, particularly those with the A140V mutation; and males with infantile encephalopathy. Duplication of *MECP2* is now recognized as a relatively common cause of moderate to severe intellectual disability in males, and presents with absent speech, spasticity, shuffling gait, and proclivity to respiratory infections, but further detail is beyond the scope of this chapter.

Mutation of *MECP2* in a male is typically lethal in utero, with four exceptions. The first, mutation A140V mentioned previously, is associated with PPM-X syndrome. The "psychosis, pyramidal signs, and macro-orchidism" syndrome also includes parkinsonian features (resting tremor) and manic depression.[106,107] This has been found in a female with the same mutation.[108] The second, infantile encephalopathy, carries a poor prognosis. In this case, babies with mutations that would typically cause lethality in utero are born alive, and most survive fewer than 2 years. In one review of 11 boys, one patient survived until 36 months, with respiratory insufficiency, rigidity, axial hypotonia, and movement disorder, and another has been ventilator dependent and is aged 11 years at the time of this writing.[109] In the third case, a male can experience spontaneous mutation early in embryogenesis, resulting in somatic mosaicism, although reported cases do not have classic RTT by the current definition, but rather a severe variant form.[110,111] The final scenario involves the extremely rare co-occurrence of a *MECP2* mutation and Klinefelter syndrome (XXY), in which case the individual has one normally functioning X chromosome as do females with RTT.[112]

GENETIC TESTING STRATEGIES

Testing for an *MECP2* mutation should be performed in the following individuals:

- all who meet criteria for classic or atypical RTT
- females with features of RTT who have:
  - unexplained developmental delay
  - low muscle tone
  - head circumference deceleration
  - molecularly unconfirmed Angelman syndrome (negative methylation/mutation studies)
- males with X-linked intellectual disability and normal fragile X testing
- unexplained neonatal or infantile encephalopathy

Testing should be performed stepwise, beginning with sequencing for exons 1–4, followed by deletion/duplication analysis if sequencing is normal. Because exon one mutations are rare, some laboratories sequence exons 2–4 before exon 1, but all should be done to evaluate an individual who meets the above criteria. If a mutation is found, testing of all first-degree female relatives should be offered regardless of their phenotype, and first-degree male relatives who have neurologic or neurodevelopmental abnormalities (X-linked male intellectual disability).

Some authors advocate testing children who have characteristics of the disorder, but have not expressed the full phenotype.[7] However, the presence of a mutation in *MECP2* is not synonymous with RTT, and no reliable prognosis can be given to the parents of a young infant with mild developmental delay and an *MECP2* mutation who is otherwise asymptomatic. Therefore, others advocate restricting testing to the categories mentioned.

Widespread prenatal testing is currently impractical. Although the incidence of RTT, similar to that of phenylketonuria, supports testing, no proven presymptomatic treatment approach exists to justify the expense of such a program.[113] However, it is appropriate to offer both prenatal testing of families who have already had a child with RTT, and preimplantation genetic testing (if the disease-causing mutation is known).[11]

NEUROBIOLOGY AND PATHOPHYSIOLOGY

Early autopsy studies in RTT patients revealed global abnormalities. Brain weight in RTT is reduced in all age groups to 60—88% of expected weight.[114] The frontal cortex and deep nuclei have reduced volume, and melanin pigmentation is decreased in the substantia nigra. Although the overall appearance of the brain is normal in RTT, it is smaller and characterized by diffuse abnormalities. The neuropil is denser with smaller, more tightly packed neurons, short, primitive dendrites, and reduced arborizations,[115] all features suggesting an immature pattern or a developmental arrest of synaptic connections.[116] Pathological studies found no support for the clinical motor deterioration observed, and no evidence of active degeneration.[117] Normal neuronal migration, involvement of multiple neurotransmitter (NT) systems, and immature dendrites also suggest developmental arrest late in the third trimester or early in infancy, rather than a progressive disorder.[118]

After the association with mutations in the MeCP2 gene was discovered, experimental models of RTT with deficient or absent protein revealed that both immature synapses and deficient synaptic reorganization begin after early development. Current evidence suggests that synaptic reorganization is disrupted, in part, because of abnormal calcium-dependent activation in response to synaptic stimulation as well as loss of MeCP2's epigenetic function. Long-term potentiation (LTP), which is normal in presymptomatic Mecp2-deficient mice, becomes abnormal in symptomatic mice, which supports the concept that a synaptopathy accounts for most clinical phenomena in RTT, including regression.[119] Decreased Mecp2 levels are associated with reductions in the key postsynaptic protein PSD-95, as well as abnormal excitatory and inhibitory signaling.[120]

The abnormal excitatory-inhibitory balance in Mecp2 deficiency seems to reflect changes in multiple NT systems.[121] For instance, abnormal GABA release may explain prevalent seizures,[122] whereas abnormal excitatory NT release may be associated with motor and cardiorespiratory manifestations.[123] Mice with abnormal MeCP2 in only GABA-releasing neurons express the phenotype of repetitive behaviors, which suggests that stereotypies may also be associated with abnormal GABAergic function. The brain stem in RTT exhibits inappropriate serotonin transporter binding in the dorsal motor nucleus of the vagus compared with age-matched controls, which could explain poor autonomic control over gastrointestinal and cardiac functions.[124] Abnormal synaptic connections in the hippocampus are associated with abnormal socialization and motor apraxia.[125] Dysfunction in the hypothalamic—pituitary—adrenal axis and enhanced corticotropin-releasing hormone expression may contribute to anxiety.[42] Low brain-derived neurotrophic factor (BDNF) levels in the nucleus tractus solitarius are associated with abnormal neuronal gating, a phenomenon thought to be associated with the cardiorespiratory abnormalities in RTT.[126]

MeCP2 has many epigenetic roles, including both repression and induction of gene transcription, and regulation of chromatin organization. Although MeCP2 is expressed in all tissues, central nervous system expression predominates. Faulty or absent MeCP2 results in immature neurons through several mechanisms: abnormal gene repression, increased transcriptional noise, overtranscription of certain genes, and downstream effects on other processes.[127] The level of affinity of MeCP2 for methylated DNA is associated with the phenotypic severity in the case of missense mutations. For example, an R106W mutation (associated with a severely affected phenotype) results in 100-fold reduced affinity, whereas T158M (associated with a less severe phenotype) causes a moderate reduction in binding.[128] Affinity of R133C (the least affected phenotype) displays similar DNA binding to that of the wild-type protein.[129]

MECP2 dosing is tightly regulated to control neuronal morphologic characteristics and dendritic spine density. In cultured rat embryonic hippocampal neurons, knockdown of normal MECP2 produces shorter dendrites with normal axon length, whereas mutant MECP2 results in shorter axons and dendrites.[130] Conversely, overexpression (approximately twofold) of MECP2 yields longer axons and dendrites.

Regulation of BDNF by MeCP2 and subsequent neurosecretory signaling is particularly critical.[131] Both knockdown and overexpression (approximately twofold) of MECP2 produce higher BDNF levels; overexpression of BDNF partially corrects the adverse effect of mutant MECP2. However, in Mecp2 knockout (KO) mice, a model that recapitulates features of RTT, BDNF levels are paradoxically low,[132] possibly owing to global reductions in synaptic activity or to overtranscription of neuronal transcriptional repressors that subsequently downregulate BDNF. Also, in postnatal rat hippocampal slice cultures, knockdown of MECP2 reduces spine density, whereas overexpression results in spine density similar to that of controls.[133]

Although much remains to be learned about the roles of Mecp2, an encouraging experiment asked the question, Could mature individuals with defective Mecp2 benefit from presence of the normal protein? Researchers silenced Mecp2 in mice with a genetic switch and activated the gene after the RTT phenotype was evident, resulting in restoration of function. This proof-of-principle experiment showed that neurological defects, including those in synaptic plasticity, can be reversed in the mouse model by the presence of a normal Mecp2 gene.[134] Restoration of function is more pronounced when Mecp2 is activated earlier in postnatal life, but still occurs in adult mice.[135] (More details on the function of Mecp2 are described in Chapter 7.)

TARGETED THERAPEUTICS

The concept that the synaptopathy in RTT could possibly be reversed is encouraging, yet neurobiologically targeted treatment for RTT is in its infancy. Over the past 10 years, numerous mechanisms for treatment have been proposed, and several preclinical trials have shown promising results. One summary of preclinical investigations into targeted treatments identified 11 strategies, many of which have yet to be explored fully.[136] To date, no clinical trials have yielded dramatic, sustained improvements in function; however, the equivocal or failed trials in the past are instructive, and are summarized below.

Several challenges exist in designing a targeted treatment for RTT. Because MeCP2 is expressed variably in different cells in the brain and at different times in development, restoration of MeCP2 production may result in four scenarios: complete restoration of function, no restoration of function, decline in function resulting from overproduction of MeCP2, or restoration of function in certain cells but not those in which MeCP2 was critical at a certain period of development.[137] Moreover, targeted treatments that restore function to processes regulated by MeCP2, without replacing MeCP2 itself,

may only improve certain symptoms. Because MeCP2 production is prominent in early postnatal life, treatment may need to begin during the early stages of regression or even before regression to be effective, which raises the issue of neonatal screening discussed earlier. The fact that loss of previously normal MECP2 function in adult mice leads to a severe phenotype supports the notion that treatment would need to be administered throughout a patient's life.[138]

Preclinical Studies

Genetic Manipulation

The most attractive strategy from a mechanistic standpoint is insertion or activation of a normally functioning MECP2 gene or MeCP2 protein. Patients with RTT typically have random XCI, resulting in approximately 50% of cells expressing normal MeCP2 and 50% expressing either no protein or a mutated version. In the abnormal cells, a normal MECP2 gene is present that was methylated early in embryonic life to inactivate its transcription. Reactivation of this normal gene is a strategy that could potentially cure the disease; however, barriers to successful implementation are profound. Reactivation of an inactive X chromosome is possible in theory but has never been accomplished. Moreover, if the entire silenced X chromosome is reactivated, the dose of MeCP2 would approach normal levels in those cells; however, the dose of all other genes on the X chromosome would likely reach pathological levels. Therefore, a strategy for selective activation of silenced MECP2 must also be developed.

Gene Replacement

A working copy of the MECP2 gene could be transfected to specific cell types using a viral vector and raise production of the normal protein in those cells. As in the reactivation strategy mentioned earlier, overexpression in normal cells is a concern. Strategies to overcome this include engineering feedback inhibition of gene expression into the treatment, or silencing the normal endogenous gene in the hope that all normal neurons would only begin expressing the transfected gene (transgene) at a uniform dose. However, if more than one viral particle transfects a neuron, the dose of MeCP2 will be unpredictable. In addition, barriers such as in vivo transfection of sufficient cells are technically challenging. Many researchers have attempted transfection with a variety of vectors, with limited success and inconsistent functional improvement.[139]

Additional genetic strategies include improving the binding function of mutated MeCP2,[140] using molecular chaperones to help mutated MeCP2 protein folding,[141] and increasing the number of methyl groups present on DNA for MeCP2 to bind to using methyl donors.[142] A process known as posttranscriptional regulation, which suppresses premature stop codons, converting them to random missense mutations, has been employed with varying success in vivo in other disorders,[143] and has been associated with increased levels of BDNF in RTT.[144] However, because genetic manipulation is the most challenging strategy to implement, targeting processes regulated by MeCP2 (downstream) is a less complete but more realistic strategy.

Neurotransmitters

Many girls with RTT have low levels of cerebrospinal fluid (CSF) dopamine metabolites (19%) and serotonin metabolites (23%), especially those with severe mutations.[145] Mouse models with prominent behavioral disruption and parkinsonian features exhibit low dopamine, serotonin, and norepinephrine (NE) levels, along with low levels of the enzymes responsible for production of these NTs (e.g., tyrosine hydroxylase [TH]). Respiratory abnormalities in MECP2-deficient mice are associated with abnormalities in the medulla, and further brain stem and forebrain dysfunction can be associated with hyperexcitability in the locus ceruleus. Both regions exhibit a paucity of TH-expressing neurons and low levels of NE.[146] However, these low levels may be inherently result from abnormal Mecp2, or may be due to an aberrant response to chronic hypoxia.[147] In vitro administration of NE results in improvement in the rhythm of the respiratory network. Two follow-up studies demonstrated that MECP2-deficient mice treated with desipramine, which specifically inhibits NE reuptake, had improved respiratory rhythm and a longer lifespan. Moreover, one study showed that desipramine treatment increases the number of TH-expressing neurons in the medulla to normal,[148] and the other study found that despite an improved respiratory pattern, desipramine selectively decreases NE levels in the medulla.[149]

Based on direct assessment in postmortem tissue and case reports of improvement in respiratory function when girls with RTT were treated with serotonin agonists, serotonin receptors in the brain stem were implicated in cardiorespiratory dysregulation. To examine this hypothesis, researchers attempted to induce Mecp2 expression by injecting male Wistar rats with fluoxetine, cocaine, a dopamine reuptake inhibitor, a norepinephrine reuptake inhibitor, or saline. The fluoxetine and cocaine groups showed increased expression of Mecp2 as well as another methyl CpG binding domain protein, MBD1, which suggests that extracellular serotonin concentration is a regulator of MeCP2 expression.[150]

Choline acetyltransferase (an enzyme involved in acetylcholine production) levels are low in the forebrain of girls with RTT.[151] Similarly, a knock-in mouse model demonstrated reduced choline levels in the striatum and increased levels in the hippocampus.[152] Researchers administered supplemental choline to these mice from birth to postnatal day 25 and found restoration of central choline levels and increased BDNF and nerve growth factor expression. Although no major behavioral changes were observed, mice treated with choline maintained normal locomotion well beyond the period of choline supplementation, whereas control mice exhibited abnormal locomotor activity. Other studies have reported improvement in motor and behavioral function with choline treatment. Rett syndrome is almost never diagnosed in the perinatal period, and the impact of choline supplementation later in life has not been examined in a preclinical model.

Postmortem studies of patients with RTT have demonstrated age-related abnormalities in the glutamatergic system and N-methyl-D-aspartate (NMDA) receptors, characterized by an early increase and late decrease in NMDA receptor levels, which have been reproduced in Mecp2 KO mice.[153] One possible mechanism is MeCP2's regulation of NMDA subunit NR1 splicing.[154] Genetic deletion of the NMDA receptor subunit NR2A prevented the progressive visual loss exhibited by Mecp2-deficient mice.[155] From a therapeutic standpoint, administration of the NMDA antagonist ketamine increased expression of the activity-dependent Fos protein in hypoactive regions such as the piriform and motor cortex of KO mice, as well as improved sensorimotor gating (a common index of cognitive function in neuropsychiatric disorders).[123] The authors interpreted these findings as indicative of a network abnormality in the default mode network, also found in ASD, which can be partially rescued by administration of an NMDA antagonist. Although their functional test was an index of forebrain circuitry, which was hypoactive, they also found synaptic hyperexcitability, a sign of immaturity, in brain stem reflex cardiorespiratory circuitry of KO mice. These authors are currently pursuing the initiation of a clinical trial of ketamine to improve cardiorespiratory function in humans. A study that administered memantine, another NMDA antagonist, transiently corrected LTP abnormalities in KO mice.[119]

Cortical GABAergic neurons express 50% more MeCP2 than other neurons, and GABAergic cell-specific KO mice recapitulate the respiratory, compulsive, motor, and social symptoms in RTT.[156] A cell- and region-specific KO model demonstrated that loss of MeCP2 in only forebrain GABAergic cells was sufficient to produce compulsive, motor, and social symptoms. Transcription of the genes responsible for intracellular GABA synthesis (GAD1/GAD2) is decreased, which suggests that the same mechanism resulting in decreased BDNF production in MeCP2 deficient cells is responsible. Although this KO model did not display seizures, this finding raises the possibility that GABA transaminase inhibitors, such as vigabatrin, could target one of the mechanisms thought to generate epilepsy in RTT.

The GABA agonist midazolam transiently reversed the breathing dysfunction in KO mice.[156] Both GABA reuptake blockers and serotonin 1a agonists partially correct breathing dysfunction in a female KO model; however, both compounds in conjunction restore respiratory function to that seen in wild-type mice.

Growth Factors

A number of neurotrophic factors are critical to both development and maintenance of nerve function.[157] Several studies targeting BDNF have demonstrated both histological and functional improvements. Using a transgene in a mouse model of RTT, BDNF overexpression resulted in an extended lifespan and improved locomotion.[126] Phosphorylation of MeCP2 releases the transcriptional repression of BDNF, leading to expansions in dendritic arborizations and synaptic maturation.[158] Exogenous administration of BDNF successfully rescued the cardiorespiratory abnormalities present in KO mice; however, BDNF does not cross the blood–brain barrier (BBB). Administration of ampakines, compounds that facilitate activation of AMPA glutamate receptors and cross the BBB, increased BDNF levels in an RTT mouse model and improved respiratory dysfunction.[126] Glatiramer acetate, an immunomodulator used in multiple sclerosis (MS) increases BDNF levels in humans and has been shown to increase BDNF expression to wild-type levels in KO mice; functional outcomes have not yet been assessed.[159] Fingolimod, a sphingosine-1-phosphate receptor modulator also used to treat MS, increased BDNF levels and improved lifespan, motor function, and the size of the striatum in KO mice.[160] Brain-derived neurotrophic factor mimetics have also shown promise in reversing the phenotype of Mecp2 KO mice.

A link between Huntington disease (HD) and RTT suggested a therapeutic target to increase BDNF levels. Huntingtin and Huntingtin-associated protein are involved in axonal transport of BDNF, and decreased levels of BDNF in a model of HD are rescued by cysteamine treatment.[161] In a KO model of RTT, the velocity of BDNF vesicle axonal trafficking was decreased, and treatment with cysteamine improved not only vesicular velocity and BDNF levels but also lifespan and motor deficits.[162] An examination of other targeted treatments being tested in HD may be indicated (e.g., calcineurin).

Further downstream, tyrosine-related kinase B (TrkB), a target of BDNF, is critical for brain stem and hippocampal function and memory consolidation through LTP.[163] Targeting this receptor with TrkB agonists improved respiratory function in heterozygous female MECP2 mutant mice.[164]

Insulin-like growth factor binding protein 3 (IGFBP3), a regulator of insulin-like growth factor 1 (IGF-1), is modulated by MeCP2.[165] MeCP2 binds directly to the promoter of IGFBP3, and in the Mecp2 KO mouse IGFBP3 levels are elevated. Moreover, IGFBP3 levels are elevated in postmortem human brain tissue in RTT. The roles of hormones such as IGF-1 in RTT are not completely understood. However, IGF-1 phosphorylates Huntingtin, resulting in increased BDNF release,[166] and the IGF-1 receptor activates intracellular pathways also regulated by the TrkB receptor.[167]

Treatment with an active peptide fragment of IGF-1 partially restored both functional and histological aspects of the disease in mice. Lifespan was extended by 50%, and locomotion, breathing abnormalities, and heart rate variability improved. Moreover, treatment increased brain weight, dendritic spine density, synaptic amplitude, and PSD-95 (a marker of postsynaptic density) levels, and matured occipital cortex plasticity to wild-type levels.[168]

Other Preclinical Approaches

Although classically conceived as a neuronal disorder, both in vitro and in vivo models of RTT have demonstrated that mutant Mecp2 in astrocytes (supportive or glial cells) affects dendritic morphology and other phenotypical features. In vitro, dendrites of both mutant and wild type neurons were abnormal when neurons were co-cultured with mutant astrocytes.[169] Dendritic and synaptic abnormalities attributable to astrocytes are thought to result from excessive secretion of glutamate; however, cultured KO astrocytes have an elevated glutamate clearance rate associated with impaired downregulation of excitatory amino acid transporters and excessive glutamate synthetase production.[170] Dendritic abnormalities were reversed in Mecp2-deficient mice when Mecp2 function was selectively restored in astrocytes, and levels of the excitatory glutamate transporter VGLUT1 were increased. Moreover, these mice exhibited improved lifespan, locomotion, anxiety, and respiratory abnormalities, which further supports astrocytes as a therapeutic target.[171] In a mouse model of RTT with atrophic and decreased numbers of astrocytes, targeting G-protein function with cytotoxic necrotizing factor 1 improved both astrocyte number and morphology. Behavior also improved in these animals, as did levels of the cytokine interleukin-6 (associated with synaptic plasticity dysfunction when elevated) and astrocytic and neuronal metabolites.[172] Bone marrow transplant in Mecp2 KO mice populated the brain with microglia with normal Mecp2 function.[173] Although this study corroborated previous in vitro evidence of microglial dysfunction in Mecp2 deficiency, the reported treatment required cranial irradiation to be effective, which limits its clinical application in patients with RTT.

TABLE 1   Clinical Trials in Rett syndrome, Including Uncontrolled Trials but Excluding Case Reports

Intervention (n)	Year	Design	Outcome Measures (Improved, *Worsened*)
Ketogenic diet (7)	1986	Open label, uncontrolled	Objective: **% seizure control, EEG features,** labs Subjective: Stereotypies, ambulation, bruxism, breathing dysregulation, social interaction
Tyrosine and tryptophan (11)	1990	Double-blind, placebo controlled, crossover	Objective: Homovanillic acid and 5-5-hydroxyindoleacetic acid in CSF and plasma Subjective: EEG visual inspection, psychologist interview of parents
Bromocriptine (10)	1990	Double-blind, placebo controlled, partial crossover	**Portage guide for early education: gross/fine motor development, cognition, socialization**
Naltrexone (25)	1994	Double-blind, placebo controlled, crossover	*Clinical stage, Bayley, Peabody, Gesell, Vineland*, MBA, EEG, **polygraphy (breathing dysregulation)**, CSF
L-Carnitine (35)	1999	Double-blind, placebo controlled, crossover	**MBA (behavioral/social, orofacial/respiratory subscales) hand apraxia scale, Patient Well-being Index**
L-Carnitine (21)	2001	Open label	RS: SSI **(communication, energy level, bruxism)**, hand apraxia scale, **sleep efficiency**, *alertness*, Short Form—36
Topiramate (8)	2004	Retrospective	**Seizure frequency, breathing dysrhythmia**
Folate/betaine (73)	2009	Double-blind, placebo controlled	MBA, growth, **overall improvement by parental report in age <5 years**
Creatine (18)	2011	Double-blind, placebo controlled, crossover	MBA, labs
IGF-1 (9[12])	2012	Phase I, open label	**Apnea Index**, CSS, MBA, RSBQ **(fear/anxiety)**, ADAMS **(social avoidance)**, **EEG alpha asymmetry**
IGF-1 (6)	2012	Open label	CGI, EEG, *seizure frequency*
IGF-1 (30)	*Incomplete end of 2014*	Double-blind crossover	Kerr, EEG, RSBQ, ADAMS, ABC, CGI, VAS, Vineland
NNZ-2566 (60)	2014	Unbalanced double-blind	EEG spikes, Behavior, autonomic function, CSS, **MBA, CGI**, visual analog scale, Vineland
Desipramine (36)	*Incomplete end of 2014*	Double-blind	Respiration
Copaxone (20)	*Incomplete end of 2014*	Open label	EEG, gait, autonomic, visual attention, behavior, QOL
Dextromethorphan (60)	*Incomplete end of 2014*	Double-blind	Mullen, Vineland, screen for social interaction

RS: SSI, Rett Syndrome Symptom Score Index; CSS, Clinical Severity Score; RSBQ, Rett Syndrome Behavioral Questionnaire; ADAMS, Anxiety Depression and Mood Scale; CGI, Clinical Global Impression.

Moreover, when performed too late in development, treatment resulted in little improvement. Subsequent studies in different laboratories failed to reproduce these beneficial effects.

Finally, in Mecp2 KO mice, the nuclear gene for ubiquinol-cytochrome c reductase core protein 1, which produces a component of mitochondrial complex III, is overexpressed because of a lack of repression by Mecp2. Functionally, this results in an increased rate and decreased efficiency of mitochondrial respiration, and correction of this imbalance is another potential avenue for treatment.[174]

Clinical Trials

Before identification of *MECP2* mutations as causative of RTT, no specific animal models were available. Nonetheless, based on evidence from pathological specimens and imaging, clinical trials were conducted using tyrosine, tryptophan, bromocriptine, L-carnitine, the ketogenic diet, and the opiate agonist naltrexone.[175] Numerous others have been conducted since association with *MECP2*, with the largest proportion since 2010 (Table 1).

Soon after Hagberg's original RTT report and not long after the ketogenic diet was proposed as a treatment for epilepsy, an uncontrolled trial of the ketogenic diet was conducted in RTT.[176] Five of seven girls tolerated the diet and experienced reduction in seizures but only slight improvements in behavior and motor function.

Early dopamine metabolite discoveries prompted treatment with tyrosine and tryptophan, which increased CSF monoamine metabolite levels but did not improve clinical outcomes over 10 weeks.[177] A double-blind, placebo-controlled trial of bromocriptine (a dopamine agonist) resulted in subtle motor, communication, and cognitive improvements in some participants.[178]

Based on the observation of increased β-endorphin levels in girls with RTT, naltrexone was administered in a randomized crossover trial to 25 girls with RTT.[179] The trial was complicated by an inadequate washout period; analysis of the first phase revealed improvement in respiratory parameters (potentially owing to sedation) but no other behavioral or motor findings.

A randomized crossover trial examined L-carnitine supplementation in 35 girls with RTT and found modest improvements in the Patient Well-Being Index as well as physician (but not parent) ratings of behavioral and orofacial/respiratory features.[180] A follow-up 6-month, open-label study of 21 girls demonstrated small but discernable improvements in sleep efficiency, energy level, and communication skills.[181] Side effects included a fishy odor and diarrhea necessitating dose adjustment in 9% of subjects.

A retrospective review of eight individuals who received topiramate for seizure control (monotherapy in two and adjunctive in six) showed improvement in seizure and/or respiratory dysfunction in seven.[182] Both outcome measures were based on parental report of severity (percent change). No follow-up clinical trial has been conducted.

In an effort to improve MeCP2 binding by increasing the number of methyl groups present in DNA, 68 participants with RTT were randomized in a double-blind, randomized, controlled trial (RCT) to receive placebo or folate (a cofactor necessary for methyl donor pools), and betaine (a methyl group donor) for 12 months.[142] No objective improvements were noted; however, subjective improvement was reported in children aged less than 5 years based on a parent questionnaire. Possible explanations for type II error included lack of controlling for genotype, and the authors cautioned that future studies should account for current knowledge about disease severity based on *MECP2* genotype.

To target serotoninergic abnormalities, six patients were treated with fluoxetine in an open-label trial at Necker Enfants Malades University Hospital. None had a beneficial response at the end of the study, and three stopped the medication owing to behavioral disturbances, sleep disorder, and/or anorexia. The study was ended prematurely by the French safety monitoring group.

A randomized crossover trial of creatine supplementation enrolled 21 girls with RTT and was completed in 2009.[183] Global DNA methylation, metabolic markers of methylation, and motor and behavioral data were collected. Global DNA methylation increased significantly; however, neither metabolic markers nor functional variables changed with supplementation.

Two phase I trials of recombinant full-length IGF-1 in girls with classic RTT were completed in 2012 and demonstrated safety and tolerability. In one, nine participants (aged 2–11 years) received the drug in escalating doses over a 4-week period with good CSF penetration and without adverse events.[184] In another, six patients (aged 4–11 years) received daily injections for 6 months without adverse events.[185] A phase II crossover RCT began in March 2013 at Boston Children's Hospital and is collecting neurological, behavioral, neurophysiological, and autonomic outcome data.

A phase IIa randomized placebo-controlled trial of NNZ-2566 (a tripeptide normally cleaved from IGF-1 in brain tissue) in RTT was completed in November 2014, as announced in a press release.[186] Fifty-three women aged 16 years and older completed the study, which collected neurological, behavioral, and neurophysiological outcome data. Benchmark improvements were achieved for the higher intervention dose compared with placebo for several outcome measures, including a modified version of the MBA discussed earlier.

Based on these animal studies using desipramine to improve norepinephrine levels, a phase II clinical trial is currently being conducted at six centers in France. However, the most recent update in clinicaltrials.gov in the summer of 2014 listed this trial as "ongoing, but not recruiting participants."

An open-label trial of glatiramer acetate (discussed previously) recruiting participants at Montefiore Medical Center and is primarily assessing effects of the drug on gait speed, with respiratory function as a secondary outcome measure. Another is recruiting in Italy and is evaluating epileptiform activity as a primary outcome measure.

An open-label study of the NMDA antagonist dextromethorphan has recruited 35 participants at the Hugo W. Moser Research Institute, and a double blind RCT began in 2012. Researchers are collecting neuropsychological and behavioral data on children with RTT aged 2–10 years during a 3-month treatment period.

CONCLUSIONS

In the generations since Andreas Rett first described the pattern of regression and stereotypies that now bears his name, enormous strides have been taken toward improving the quality of life for girls and women with

RTT and their families. Successful treatments for RTT may emerge within the next several years. These treatments will be based on the neurobiology of the disorder, but will most likely target specific aspects of the disorder and will not represent a panacea. It is hoped that these treatments will target symptoms of great distress to patients and families. However, many interventions currently available have had a dramatic impact on quality of life. If begun early in life and sustained throughout, therapy can maintain and even improve function. Life expectancy and improving quality of life in the third, fourth, and fifth decades are far beyond what Rett and Hagberg hoped for in their practices. If the practice of applying the highest standards of care currently available is applied, the next generation of women with RTT will likely extend the current life expectancy and improve the average level of functional ability in the disorder. Moreover, when targeted treatments become available, the prevention of contractures and other permanent disability will allow these treatments to have a greater effect. The continuing growth of RTT specialty clinics across the US will help to support this improvement in overall quality of care for girls and women with RTT.

References

1. Rett A. [On a unusual brain atrophy syndrome in hyperammonemia in childhood]. *Wien Med Wochenschr* September 10, 1966; **116**(37):723–6.
2. Rett A. [Hyperammonaemia and cerebral atrophy in childhood]. *Folia Hered Pathol* July 1969;**18**(3):115–23.
3. Hagberg B, Aicardi J, Dias K, Ramos O. A progressive syndrome of autism, dementia, ataxia, and loss of purposeful hand use in girls: Rett's syndrome: report of 35 cases. *Ann Neurol* October 1983;**14**(4):471–9.
4. Hagberg B. Rett syndrome: Swedish approach to analysis of prevalence and cause. *Brain Dev* 1985;**7**(3):276–80.
5. Terai K, Munesue T, Hiratani M, Jiang ZY, Jibiki I, Yamaguchi N. The prevalence of Rett syndrome in Fukui prefecture. *Brain Dev* March–April 1995;**17**(2):153–4.
6. Skjeldal OH, von Tetzchner S, Aspelund F, Herder GA, Lofterld B. Rett syndrome: geographic variation in prevalence in Norway. *Brain Dev* June 1997;**19**(4):258–61.
7. Laurvick CL, de Klerk N, Bower C, Christodoulou J, Ravine D, Ellaway C, et al. Rett syndrome in Australia: a review of the epidemiology. *J Pediatr* March 2006;**148**(3):347–52.
8. Young DJ, Bebbington A, Anderson A, Ravine D, Ellaway C, Kulkarni A, et al. The diagnosis of autism in a female: could it be Rett syndrome? *Eur J Pediatr* June 2008;**167**(6):661–9.
9. Venancio M, Santos M, Pereira SA, Maciel P, Saraiva JM. An explanation for another familial case of Rett syndrome: maternal germline mosaicism. *Eur J Hum Genet* August 2007;**15**(8):902–4.
10. Herman GE, Butter E, Enrile B, Pastore M, Prior TW, Sommer A. Increasing knowledge of PTEN germline mutations: two additional patients with autism and macrocephaly. *Am J Med Genet A* March 15, 2007;**143**(6):589–93.
11. Mari F, Caselli R, Russo S, Cogliati F, Ariani F, Longo I, et al. Germline mosaicism in Rett syndrome identified by prenatal diagnosis. *Clin Genet* March 2005;**67**(3):258–60.
12. Hagberg B, Witt-Engerström I, Opitz JM, Reynolds JF. Rett Syndrome: a suggested staging system for describing impairment profile with increasing age towards adolescence. *Am J Med Genet* 1986;**25**(S1):47–59.
13. Percy AK. Rett syndrome: exploring the autism link. *Arch Neurol* August 2011;**68**(8):985–9.
14. Neul JL, Lane JB, Lee HS, Geerts S, Barrish JO, Annese F, et al. Developmental delay in Rett syndrome: data from the natural history study. *J Neurodev Disord* 2014;**6**(1):20.
15. Einspieler C, Kerr AM, Prechtl HF. Is the early development of girls with Rett disorder really normal? *Pediatr Res* May 2005; **57**(5 Pt 1):696–700.
16. Marschik PB, Kaufmann WE, Sigafoos J, Wolin T, Zhang D, Bartl-Pokorny KD, et al. Changing the perspective on early development of Rett syndrome. *Res Dev Disabil* April 2013; **34**(4):1236–9.
17. Marschik PB, Einspieler C. Methodological note: video analysis of the early development of Rett syndrome—one method for many disciplines. *Dev Neurorehabil* 2011;**14**(6):355–7.
18. Einspieler C, Kerr AM, Prechtl HF. Abnormal general movements in girls with Rett disorder: the first four months of life. *Brain Dev* November 2005;**27**(Suppl. 1):S8–13.
19. Hagberg B, Hanefeld F, Percy A, Skjeldal O. An update on clinically applicable diagnostic criteria in Rett syndrome. Comments to Rett Syndrome Clinical Criteria Consensus Panel Satellite to European Paediatric Neurology Society Meeting, Baden Baden, Germany, 11 September 2001. *Eur J Paediatr Neurol* 2002;**6**(5): 293–7.
20. Neul JL, Kaufmann WE, Glaze DG, Christodoulou J, Clarke AJ, Bahi-Buisson N, et al. Rett syndrome: revised diagnostic criteria and nomenclature. *Ann Neurol* December 2010;**68**(6):944–50.
21. Lee J, Leonard H, Piek J, Downs J. Early development and regression in Rett syndrome. *Clin Genet* January 25, 2013;**84**(6):572–6.
22. Charman T, Cass H, Owen L, Wigram T, Slonims V, Weeks L, et al. Regression in individuals with Rett syndrome. *Brain Dev* August 2002;**24**(5):281–3.
23. Foley KR, Downs J, Bebbington A, Jacoby P, Girdler S, Kaufmann WE, et al. Change in gross motor abilities of girls and women with rett syndrome over a 3- to 4-year period. *J child Neurol* October 2011;**26**(10):1237–45.
24. Larsson G, Engerstrom IW. Gross motor ability in Rett syndrome—the power of expectation, motivation and planning. *Brain Dev* December 2001;**23**(Suppl. 1):S77–81.
25. Goldman S, Temudo T. Hand stereotypies distinguish Rett syndrome from autism disorder. *Mov Disord* July 2012;**27**(8):1060–2.
26. Carter P, Downs J, Bebbington A, Williams S, Jacoby P, Kaufmann WE, et al. Stereotypical hand movements in 144 subjects with Rett syndrome from the population-based Australian database. *Mov Disord* February 15, 2010;**25**(3):282–8.
27. Percy AK. *Rett syndrome needs your attention*. Clinton (MD): IRSA; 2007.
28. Quest KM, Byiers BJ, Payen A, Symons FJ. Rett syndrome: a preliminary analysis of stereotypy, stress, and negative affect. *Res Dev Disabil* May 2014;**35**(5):1191–7.
29. Temudo T, Oliveira P, Santos M, Dias K, Vieira J, Moreira A, et al. Stereotypies in Rett syndrome: analysis of 83 patients with and without detected MECP2 mutations. *Neurology* April 10, 2007; **68**(15):1183–7.
30. Sharpe PA. Comparative effects of bilateral hand splints and an elbow orthosis on stereotypic hand movements and toy play in two children with Rett syndrome. *Am J Occup Ther* February 1992;**46**(2):134–40.
31. Rolando S. Rett syndrome: report of eight cases. *Brain Dev* 1985; **7**(3):290–6.
32. Rett A. *Cerebral atrophy associated with hyperammonaemia*, vol. 29. New York: North-Holland Publishing Co.; 1977.

33. Glaze DG, Frost Jr JD, Zoghbi HY, Percy AK. Rett's syndrome: characterization of respiratory patterns and sleep. *Ann Neurol* April 1987;**21**(4):377–82.

34. Southall DP, Kerr AM, Tirosh E, Amos P, Lang MH, Stephenson JB. Hyperventilation in the awake state: potentially treatable component of Rett syndrome. *Arch Dis Child* September 1988;**63**(9):1039–48.

35. Julu PO, Witt Engerstrom I. Assessment of the maturity-related brainstem functions reveals the heterogeneous phenotypes and facilitates clinical management of Rett syndrome. *Brain Dev* November 2005;**27**(Suppl. 1):S43–53.

36. Smeets EE, Julu PO, van Waardenburg D, Engerstrom IW, Hansen S, Apartopoulos F, et al. Management of a severe forceful breather with Rett syndrome using carbogen. *Brain Dev* November 2006;**28**(10):625–32.

37. Julu PO, Witt Engerstrom I, Hansen S, Apartopoulos F, Engerstrom B. Treating hypoxia in a feeble breather with Rett syndrome. *Brain Dev* March 2013;**35**(3):270–3.

38. Andaku DK, Mercadante MT, Schwartzman JS. Buspirone in Rett syndrome respiratory dysfunction. *Brain Dev* September 2005;**27**(6):437–8.

39. Gokben S, Ardic UA, Serdaroglu G. Use of buspirone and fluoxetine for breathing problems in Rett syndrome. *Pediatr Neurol* March 2012;**46**(3):192–4.

40. Weese-Mayer DE, Lieske SP, Boothby CM, Kenny AS, Bennett HL, Silvestri JM, et al. Autonomic nervous system dysregulation: breathing and heart rate perturbation during wakefulness in young girls with Rett syndrome. *Pediatr Res* October 2006;**60**(4):443–9.

41. Weese-Mayer DE, Lieske SP, Boothby CM, Kenny AS, Bennett HL, Ramirez JM. Autonomic dysregulation in young girls with Rett syndrome during nighttime in-home recordings. *Pediatr Pulmonol* November 2008;**43**(11):1045–60.

42. McGill BE, Bundle SF, Yaylaoglu MB, Carson JP, Thaller C, Zoghbi HY. Enhanced anxiety and stress-induced corticosterone release are associated with increased Crh expression in a mouse model of Rett syndrome. *Proc Natl Acad Sci USA* November 28, 2006;**103**(48):18267–72.

43. Glaze DG. Neurophysiology of Rett syndrome. *J Child Neurol* September 2005;**20**(9):740–6.

44. Glaze DG, Percy AK, Skinner S, Motil KJ, Neul JL, Barrish JO, et al. Epilepsy and the natural history of Rett syndrome. *Neurology* March 16, 2010;**74**(11):909–12.

45. Glaze DG, Schultz RJ, Frost JD. Rett syndrome: characterization of seizures versus non-seizures. *Electroencephalogr Clin Neurophysiol* January 1998;**106**(1):79–83.

46. Tarquinio DC, Motil KJ, Hou W, Lee HS, Glaze DG, Skinner SA, et al. Growth failure and outcome in Rett syndrome: specific growth references. *Neurology* October 16, 2012;**79**(16):1653–61.

47. Leonard H, Ravikumara M, Baikie G, Naseem N, Ellaway C, Percy A, et al. Assessment and management of nutrition and growth in Rett syndrome. *J Pediatr Gastroenterol Nutr* October 2013;**57**(4):451–60.

48. Schultz R, Glaze D, Motil K, Hebert D, Percy A. Hand and foot growth failure in Rett syndrome. *J Child Neurol* February 1998;**13**(2):71–4.

49. Chapleau CA, Lane J, Pozzo-Miller L, Percy AK. Evaluation of current pharmacological treatment options in the management of Rett syndrome: from the present to future therapeutic alternatives. *Curr Clin Pharmacol* November 2013;**8**(4):358–69.

50. Hagebeuk EE, Bijlmer RP, Koelman JH, Poll-The BT. Respiratory disturbances in rett syndrome: don't forget to evaluate upper airway obstruction. *J Child Neurol* July 2012;**27**(7):888–92.

51. Motil KJ, Caeg E, Barrish JO, Geerts S, Lane JB, Percy AK, et al. Gastrointestinal and nutritional problems occur frequently throughout life in girls and women with Rett syndrome. *J Pediatr Gastroenterol Nutr* September 2012;**55**(3):292–8.

52. Motil KJ, Schultz RJ, Browning K, Trautwein L, Glaze DG. Oropharyngeal dysfunction and gastroesophageal dysmotility are present in girls and women with Rett syndrome. *J Pediatr Gastroenterol Nutr* July 1999;**29**(1):31–7.

53. Percy AK, Lane JB. Rett syndrome: model of neurodevelopmental disorders. *J Child Neurol* September 2005;**20**(9):718–21.

54. FitzGerald PM, Jankovic J, Glaze DG, Schultz R, Percy AK. Extrapyramidal involvement in Rett's syndrome. *Neurology* February 1990;**40**(2):293–5.

55. FitzGerald PM, Jankovic J, Percy AK. Rett syndrome and associated movement disorders. *Mov Disord* 1990;**5**(3):195–202.

56. Percy AK, Lee HS, Neul JL, Lane JB, Skinner SA, Geerts SP, et al. Profiling scoliosis in Rett syndrome. *Pediatr Res* April 2010;**67**(4):435–9.

57. Downs J, Bergman A, Carter P, Anderson A, Palmer GM, Roye D, et al. Guidelines for management of scoliosis in Rett syndrome patients based on expert consensus and clinical evidence. *Spine* August 1, 2009;**34**(17):E607–17.

58. Leonard H, Thomson MR, Glasson EJ, Fyfe S, Leonard S, Bower C, et al. A population-based approach to the investigation of osteopenia in Rett syndrome. *Dev Med Child Neurol* May 1999;**41**(5):323–8.

59. Motil KJ, Barrish JO, Lane J, Geerts SP, Annese F, McNair L, et al. Vitamin D deficiency is prevalent in girls and women with Rett syndrome. *J Pediatr Gastroenterol Nutr* November 2011;**53**(5):569–74.

60. Shapiro JR, Bibat G, Hiremath G, Blue ME, Hundalani S, Yablonski T, et al. Bone mass in Rett syndrome: association with clinical parameters and MECP2 mutations. *Pediatr Res* November 2010;**68**(5):446–51.

61. Lotan M, Reves-Siesel R, Eliav-Shalev RS, Merrick J. Osteoporosis in Rett syndrome: a case study presenting a novel management intervention for severe osteoporosis. *Osteoporos Int* December 2013;**24**(12):3059–63.

62. McCauley MD, Wang T, Mike E, Herrera J, Beavers DL, Huang TW, et al. Pathogenesis of lethal cardiac arrhythmias in Mecp2 mutant mice: implication for therapy in Rett syndrome. *Sci Transl Med* December 14, 2011;**3**(113):113ra125.

63. Bas VN, Cetinkaya S, Agladioglu SY, Aksoy A, Gulpinar B, Aycan Z. Report of the first case of precocious puberty in Rett syndrome. *J Pediatr Endocrinol Metab* April 2, 2013;**26**:1–3.

64. Killian JT, Lane JB, Cutter GR, Skinner SA, Kaufmann WE, Tarquinio DC, et al. Pubertal development in Rett syndrome deviates from typical females. *Pediatr Neurol* December 2014;**51**(6):769–75.

65. Segatto M, Trapani L, Di Tunno I, Sticozzi C, Valacchi G, Hayek J, et al. Cholesterol metabolism is altered in rett syndrome: a study on plasma and primary cultured fibroblasts derived from patients. *PLoS One* 2014;**9**(8):e104834.

66. Buchovecky CM, Turley SD, Brown HM, Kyle SM, McDonald JG, Liu B, et al. A suppressor screen in Mecp2 mutant mice implicates cholesterol metabolism in Rett syndrome. *Nat Genet* July 28, 2013;**45**(9):1013–20.

67. Kirby RS, Lane JB, Childers J, Skinner SA, Annese F, Barrish JO, et al. Longevity in Rett syndrome: analysis of the North American Database. *J Pediatr* January 2010;**156**(1):135–8. e1.

68. Percy AK. Rett syndrome. Current status and new vistas. *Neurol Clin* November 2002;**20**(4):1125–41.

69. Anderson A, Wong K, Jacoby P, Downs J, Leonard H. Twenty years of surveillance in Rett syndrome: what does this tell us? *Orphanet J Rare Dis* 2014;**9**:87.

70. Christopher AC, Jane L, Lucas P-M, Alan KP. *Rett syndrome: a model of genetic neurodevelopmental disorders.* 2013.

71. Ellaway CJ, Sholler G, Leonard H, Christodoulou J. Prolonged QT interval in Rett syndrome. *Arch Dis Child* May 1999;**80**(5):470–2.

72. Cuddapah VA, Pillai RB, Shekar KV, Lane JB, Motil KJ, Skinner SA, et al. Methyl-CpG-binding protein 2 (MECP2) mutation type is associated with disease severity in Rett syndrome. *J Med Genet* March 2014;**51**(3):152–8.

73. Lotan M, Schenker R, Wine J, Downs J. The conductive environment enhances gross motor function of girls with Rett syndrome. A pilot study. *Dev Neurorehabil* 2012;**15**(1):19–25.

74. Schaefer-Campion C, Johnson NL. Fostering Ambulation for a Preschool Child with Rett Syndrome: A Case Report. *Phys Occup Ther Pediatr* March 20, 2014.

75. Lotan M, Manor-Binyamini I, Elefant C, Wine J, Saraf E, Yoshei Y. The Israeli Rett Syndrome Center. Evaluation and transdisciplinary play-based assessment. *Sci World J* 2006;**6**:1302–13.

76. Lotan M. Assistive technology and supplementary treatment for individuals with Rett syndrome. *Sci World J* 2007;**7**:903–48.

77. Lotan M. Alternative therapeutic intervention for individuals with Rett syndrome. *Sci World J* 2007;**7**:698–714.

78. Wigram T, Lawrence M. Music therapy as a tool for assessing hand use and communicativeness in children with Rett Syndrome. *Brain Dev* November 2005;**27**(Suppl. 1):S95–6.

79. Yasuhara A, Sugiyama Y. Music therapy for children with Rett syndrome. *Brain Dev* December 2001;**23**(Suppl. 1):S82–4.

80. Bat-Haee MA. Behavioral training of a young women with Rett syndrome. *Percept Mot Skills* February 1994;**78**(1):314.

81. Smith T, Klevstrand M, Lovaas OI. Behavioral treatment of Rett's disorder: ineffectiveness in three cases. *Am J Ment Retard* November 1995;**100**(3):317–22.

82. Rose SA, Djukic A, Jankowski JJ, Feldman JF, Fishman I, Valicenti-McDermott M. Rett syndrome: an eye-tracking study of attention and recognition memory. *Dev Med Child Neurol* April 2013;**55**(4):364–71.

83. Djukic A, Valicenti McDermott M, Mavrommatis K, Martins CL. Rett syndrome: basic features of visual processing—a pilot study of eye-tracking. *Pediatr Neurol* July 2012;**47**(1):25–9.

84. Urbanowicz A, Leonard H, Girdler S, Ciccone N, Downs J. Parental perspectives on the communication abilities of their daughters with Rett syndrome. *Dev Neurorehabil* February 24, 2014.

85. Umansky R, Watson JS, Colvin L, Fyfe S, Leonard S, de Klerk N, et al. Hand preference, extent of laterality, and functional hand use in Rett syndrome. *J Child Neurol* July 2003;**18**(7):481–7.

86. Hagberg B. Clinical delineation of Rett syndrome variants. *Neuropediatrics* April 1995;**26**(2):62.

87. Diagnostic criteria for Rett syndrome. The rett syndrome diagnostic criteria work group. *Ann Neurol* April 1988;**23**(4):425–8.

88. Hagberg B, Goutieres F, Hanefeld F, Rett A, Wilson J. Rett syndrome: criteria for inclusion and exclusion. *Brain Dev* 1985;**7**(3):372–3.

89. Percy AK, Neul JL, Glaze DG, Motil KJ, Skinner SA, Khwaja O, et al. Rett syndrome diagnostic criteria: lessons from the Natural History Study. *Ann Neurol* December 2010;**68**(6):951–5.

90. Hanefeld F. The clinical pattern of the Rett syndrome. *Brain Dev* 1985;**7**(3):320–5.

91. Scala E, Ariani F, Mari F, Caselli R, Pescucci C, Longo I, et al. CDKL5/STK9 is mutated in Rett syndrome variant with infantile spasms. *J Med Genet* February 2005;**42**(2):103–7.

92. Ariani F, Hayek G, Rondinella D, Artuso R, Mencarelli MA, Spanhol-Rosseto A, et al. FOXG1 is responsible for the congenital variant of Rett syndrome. *Am J Hum Genet* July 2008;**83**(1):89–93.

93. Hagberg B, Rasmussen P, Opitz JM, Reynolds JF. "Forme fruste" of rett syndrome – a case report. *Am J Med Genet* 1986;**25**(S1):175–81.

94. Zappella M. The Rett girls with preserved speech. *Brain Dev* March 1992;**14**(2):98–101.

95. Renieri A, Mari F, Mencarelli MA, Scala E, Ariani F, Longo I, et al. Diagnostic criteria for the Zappella variant of Rett syndrome (the preserved speech variant). *Brain Dev* March 2009;**31**(3):208–16.

96. Fehr S, Wilson M, Downs J, Williams S, Murgia A, Sartori S, et al. The CDKL5 disorder is an independent clinical entity associated with early-onset encephalopathy. *Eur J Hum Genet* March 2013;**21**(3):266–73.

97. Christodoulou J, Ho G. MECP2-Related disorders. In: Pagon RA, Adam MP, Ardinger HH, et al., editors. *GeneReviews®*; 1993. Seattle (WA).

98. Amir RE, Van den Veyver IB, Wan M, Tran CQ, Francke U, Zoghbi HY. Rett syndrome is caused by mutations in X-linked MECP2, encoding methyl-CpG-binding protein 2. *Nat Genet* October 1999;**23**(2):185–8.

99. Neul JL, Fang P, Barrish J, Lane J, Caeg EB, Smith EO, et al. Specific mutations in methyl-CpG-binding protein 2 confer different severity in Rett syndrome. *Neurology* April 15, 2008;**70**(16):1313–21.

100. Ishii T, Makita Y, Ogawa A, Amamiya S, Yamamoto M, Miyamoto A, et al. The role of different X-inactivation pattern on the variable clinical phenotype with Rett syndrome. *Brain Dev* December 2001;**23**(Suppl. 1):S161–4.

101. Huppke P, Maier EM, Warnke A, Brendel C, Laccone F, Gartner J. Very mild cases of Rett syndrome with skewed X inactivation. *J Med Genet* October 2006;**43**(10):814–6.

102. Hardwick SA, Reuter K, Williamson SL, Vasudevan V, Donald J, Slater K, et al. Delineation of large deletions of the MECP2 gene in Rett syndrome patients, including a familial case with a male proband. *Eur J Hum Genet* December 2007;**15**(12):1218–29.

103. Xinhua B, Shengling J, Fuying S, Hong P, Meirong L, Wu XR. X chromosome inactivation in Rett syndrome and its correlations with MECP2 mutations and phenotype. *J Child Neurol* January 2008;**23**(1):22–5.

104. Takahashi S, Ohinata J, Makita Y, Suzuki N, Araki A, Sasaki A, et al. Skewed X chromosome inactivation failed to explain the normal phenotype of a carrier female with MECP2 mutation resulting in Rett syndrome. *Clin Genet* March 2008;**73**(3):257–61.

105. Gibson JH, Williamson SL, Arbuckle S, Christodoulou J. X chromosome inactivation patterns in brain in Rett syndrome: implications for the disease phenotype. *Brain Dev* June 2005;**27**(4):266–70.

106. Klauck SM, Lindsay S, Beyer KS, Splitt M, Burn J, Poustka A. A mutation hot spot for nonspecific X-linked mental retardation in the MECP2 gene causes the PPM-X syndrome. *Am J Hum Genet* April 2002;**70**(4):1034–7.

107. Lindsay S, Splitt M, Edney S, Berney TP, Knight SJ, Davies KE, et al. PPM-X: a new X-linked mental retardation syndrome with psychosis, pyramidal signs, and macroorchidism maps to Xq28. *Am J Hum Genet* June 1996;**58**(6):1120–6.

108. Venkateswaran S, McMillan HJ, Doja A, Humphreys P. Adolescent onset cognitive regression and neuropsychiatric symptoms associated with the A140V MECP2 mutation. *Dev Med Child Neurol* January 2014;**56**(1):91–4.

109. Kankirawatana P, Leonard H, Ellaway C, Scurlock J, Mansour A, Makris CM, et al. Early progressive encephalopathy in boys and MECP2 mutations. *Neurology* July 11, 2006;**67**(1):164–6.

110. Topcu M, Akyerli C, Sayi A, Toruner GA, Kocoglu SR, Cimbis M, et al. Somatic mosaicism for a MECP2 mutation associated with classic Rett syndrome in a boy. *Eur J Hum Genet* January 2002;**10**(1):77–81.

111. Clayton-Smith J, Watson P, Ramsden S, Black GC. Somatic mutation in MECP2 as a non-fatal neurodevelopmental disorder in males. *Lancet* September 2, 2000;**356**(9232):830–2.

112. Schwartzman JS, Bernardino A, Nishimura A, Gomes RR, Zatz M. Rett syndrome in a boy with a 47,XXY karyotype confirmed by a rare mutation in the MECP2 gene. *Neuropediatrics* June 2001;**32**(3):162–4.

113. Amir RE, Sutton VR, Van den Veyver IB. Newborn screening and prenatal diagnosis for Rett syndrome: implications for therapy. *J Child Neurol* September 2005;**20**(9):779–83.

114. Jellinger K, Armstrong D, Zoghbi HY, Percy AK. Neuropathology of Rett syndrome. *Acta Neuropathol* 1988;**76**(2):142–58.

115. Armstrong D. Recent developments in neuropathology—electron microscopy—brain pathology. *Eur Child Adolesc Psychiatry* 1997;**6**(Suppl. 1):69—70.

116. Kaufmann WE, Johnston MV, Blue ME. MECP2 expression and function during brain development: implications for Rett syndrome's pathogenesis and clinical evolution. *Brain Dev* November 2005;**27**(Suppl. 1):S77—87.

117. Bauman ML, Kemper TL, Arin DM. Pervasive neuroanatomic abnormalities of the brain in three cases of Rett's syndrome. *Neurology* August 1995;**45**(8):1581—6.

118. Armstrong DD. Neuropathology of Rett syndrome. *Ment Retard Dev Disabil Res Rev* 2002;**8**(2):72—6.

119. Weng SM, McLeod F, Bailey ME, Cobb SR. Synaptic plasticity deficits in an experimental model of Rett syndrome: long-term potentiation saturation and its pharmacological reversal. *Neuroscience* April 28, 2011;**180**:314—21.

120. Chao HT, Zoghbi HY, Rosenmund C. MeCP2 controls excitatory synaptic strength by regulating glutamatergic synapse number. *Neuron* October 4, 2007;**56**(1):58—65.

121. Shahbazian M, Young J, Yuva-Paylor L, Spencer C, Antalffy B, Noebels J, et al. Mice with truncated MeCP2 recapitulate many Rett syndrome features and display hyperacetylation of histone H3. *Neuron* July 18, 2002;**35**(2):243—54.

122. Medrihan L, Tantalaki E, Aramuni G, Sargsyan V, Dudanova I, Missler M, et al. Early defects of GABAergic synapses in the brain stem of a MeCP2 mouse model of Rett syndrome. *J Neurophysiol* January 2008;**99**(1):112—21.

123. Kron M, Howell CJ, Adams IT, Ransbottom M, Christian D, Ogier M, et al. Brain activity mapping in Mecp2 mutant mice reveals functional deficits in forebrain circuits, including key nodes in the default mode network, that are reversed with ketamine treatment. *J Neurosci* October 3, 2012;**32**(40):13860—72.

124. Paterson DS, Thompson EG, Belliveau RA, Antalffy BA, Trachtenberg FL, Armstrong DD, et al. Serotonin transporter abnormality in the dorsal motor nucleus of the vagus in Rett syndrome: potential implications for clinical autonomic dysfunction. *J Neuropathol Exp Neurol* November 2005;**64**(11):1018—27.

125. Moretti P, Levenson JM, Battaglia F, Atkinson R, Teague R, Antalffy B, et al. Learning and memory and synaptic plasticity are impaired in a mouse model of Rett syndrome. *J Neurosci* January 4, 2006;**26**(1):319—27.

126. Kline DD, Ogier M, Kunze DL, Katz DM. Exogenous brain-derived neurotrophic factor rescues synaptic dysfunction in Mecp2-null mice. *J Neurosci* April 14, 2010;**30**(15):5303—10.

127. Kerr AM, Ravine D. Review article: breaking new ground with Rett syndrome. *J Intellect Disabil Res* November 2003;**47**(Pt 8):580—7.

128. Kudo S, Nomura Y, Segawa M, Fujita N, Nakao M, Dragich J, et al. Functional analyses of MeCP2 mutations associated with Rett syndrome using transient expression systems. *Brain Dev* December 2001;**23**(Suppl. 1):S165—73.

129. Ballestar E, Yusufzai TM, Wolffe AP. Effects of Rett syndrome mutations of the methyl-CpG binding domain of the transcriptional repressor MeCP2 on selectivity for association with methylated DNA. *Biochemistry* June 20, 2000;**39**(24):7100—6.

130. Larimore JL, Chapleau CA, Kudo S, Theibert A, Percy AK, Pozzo-Miller L. Bdnf overexpression in hippocampal neurons prevents dendritic atrophy caused by Rett-associated MECP2 mutations. *Neurobiol Dis* May 2009;**34**(2):199—211.

131. Wang H, Chan SA, Ogier M, Hellard D, Wang Q, Smith C, et al. Dysregulation of brain-derived neurotrophic factor expression and neurosecretory function in Mecp2 null mice. *J Neurosci* October 18, 2006;**26**(42):10911—5.

132. Sun YE, Wu H. The ups and downs of BDNF in Rett syndrome. *Neuron* February 2, 2006;**49**(3):321—3.

133. Chapleau CA, Calfa GD, Lane MC, Albertson AJ, Larimore JL, Kudo S, et al. Dendritic spine pathologies in hippocampal pyramidal neurons from Rett syndrome brain and after expression of Rett-associated MECP2 mutations. *Neurobiol Dis* August 2009;**35**(2):219—33.

134. Guy J, Gan J, Selfridge J, Cobb S, Bird A. Reversal of neurological defects in a mouse model of Rett syndrome. *Science* February 23, 2007;**315**(5815):1143—7.

135. Robinson L, Guy J, McKay L, Brockett E, Spike RC, Selfridge J, et al. Morphological and functional reversal of phenotypes in a mouse model of Rett syndrome. *Brain* September 2012;**135**(Pt 9):2699—710.

136. Calfa G, Percy AK, Pozzo-Miller L. Experimental models of Rett syndrome based on Mecp2 dysfunction. *Exp Biol Med (Maywood)* January 2011;**236**(1):3—19.

137. Gadalla KK, Bailey ME, Cobb SR. MeCP2 and Rett syndrome: reversibility and potential avenues for therapy. *Biochem J* October 1, 2011;**439**(1):1—14.

138. Samaco RC, Neul JL. Complexities of Rett syndrome and MeCP2. *J Neurosci* June 1, 2011;**31**(22):7951—9.

139. Rastegar M, Hotta A, Pasceri P, Makarem M, Cheung AY, Elliott S, et al. MECP2 isoform-specific vectors with regulated expression for Rett syndrome gene therapy. *PLoS One* 2009;**4**(8):e6810.

140. Casas-Delucchi CS, Becker A, Bolius JJ, Cardoso MC. Targeted manipulation of heterochromatin rescues MeCP2 Rett mutants and re-establishes higher order chromatin organization. *Nucleic Acids Res* December 2012;**40**(22):e176.

141. Hansen JC, Wexler BB, Rogers DJ, Hite KC, Panchenko T, Ajith S, et al. DNA binding restricts the intrinsic conformational flexibility of methyl CpG binding protein 2 (MeCP2). *J Biol Chem* May 27, 2011;**286**(21):18938—48.

142. Glaze DG, Percy AK, Motil KJ, Lane JB, Isaacs JS, Schultz RJ, et al. A study of the treatment of Rett syndrome with folate and betaine. *J Child Neurol* May 2009;**24**(5):551—6.

143. Sangkuhl K, Schulz A, Rompler H, Yun J, Wess J, Schoneberg T. Aminoglycoside-mediated rescue of a disease-causing nonsense mutation in the V2 vasopressin receptor gene in vitro and in vivo. *Hum Mol Genet* May 1, 2004;**13**(9):893—903.

144. Vecsler M, Ben Zeev B, Nudelman I, Anikster Y, Simon AJ, Amariglio N, et al. Ex vivo treatment with a novel synthetic aminoglycoside NB54 in primary fibroblasts from Rett syndrome patients suppresses MECP2 nonsense mutations. *PLoS One* 2011;**6**(6):e20733.

145. Samaco RC, Mandel-Brehm C, Chao HT, Ward CS, Fyffe-Maricich SL, Ren J, et al. Loss of MeCP2 in aminergic neurons causes cell-autonomous defects in neurotransmitter synthesis and specific behavioral abnormalities. *Proc Natl Acad Sci USA* December 22, 2009;**106**(51):21966—71.

146. Taneja P, Ogier M, Brooks-Harris G, Schmid DA, Katz DM, Nelson SB. Pathophysiology of locus ceruleus neurons in a mouse model of Rett syndrome. *J Neurosci* September 30, 2009;**29**(39):12187—95.

147. Zanella S, Doi A, Garcia 3rd AJ, Elsen F, Kirsch S, Wei AD, et al. When norepinephrine becomes a driver of breathing irregularities: how intermittent hypoxia fundamentally alters the modulatory response of the respiratory network. *J Neurosci* January 1, 2014;**34**(1):36—50.

148. Roux JC, Dura E, Moncla A, Mancini J, Villard L. Treatment with desipramine improves breathing and survival in a mouse model for Rett syndrome. *Eur J Neurosci* April 2007;**25**(7):1915—22.

149. Zanella S, Mebarek S, Lajard AM, Picard N, Dutschmann M, Hilaire G. Oral treatment with desipramine improves breathing and life span in Rett syndrome mouse model. *Respir Physiol Neurobiol* January 1, 2008;**160**(1):116—21.

150. Cassel S, Carouge D, Gensburger C, Anglard P, Burgun C, Dietrich JB, et al. Fluoxetine and cocaine induce the epigenetic factors MeCP2 and MBD1 in adult rat brain. *Mol Pharmacol* August 2006;**70**(2):487—92.

151. Wenk GL, Hauss-Wegrzyniak B. Altered cholinergic function in the basal forebrain of girls with Rett syndrome. *Neuropediatrics* June 1999;**30**(3):125–9.

152. Ricceri L, De Filippis B, Fuso A, Laviola G. Cholinergic hypofunction in MeCP2-308 mice: beneficial neurobehavioural effects of neonatal choline supplementation. *Behav Brain Res* August 10, 2011;**221**(2):623–9.

153. Blue ME, Kaufmann WE, Bressler J, Eyring C, O'Driscoll C, Naidu S, et al. Temporal and regional alterations in NMDA receptor expression in Mecp2-null mice. *Anat Rec (Hoboken)* October 2011;**294**(10):1624–34.

154. Young JI, Hong EP, Castle JC, Crespo-Barreto J, Bowman AB, Rose MF, et al. Regulation of RNA splicing by the methylation-dependent transcriptional repressor methyl-CpG binding protein 2. *Proc Natl Acad Sci USA* December 6, 2005;**102**(49):17551–8.

155. Durand S, Patrizi A, Quast KB, Hachigian L, Pavlyuk R, Saxena A, et al. NMDA receptor regulation prevents regression of visual cortical function in the absence of Mecp2. *Neuron* December 20, 2012;**76**(6):1078–90.

156. Voituron N, Hilaire G. The benzodiazepine Midazolam mitigates the breathing defects of Mecp2-deficient mice. *Respir Physiol Neurobiol* June 30, 2011;**177**(1):56–60.

157. Ogier M, Kron M, Katz DM. Neurotrophic factors in development and regulation of respiratory control. *Compr Physiol* July 2013;**3**(3):1125–34.

158. Zhou Z, Hong EJ, Cohen S, Zhao WN, Ho HY, Schmidt L, et al. Brain-specific phosphorylation of MeCP2 regulates activity-dependent Bdnf transcription, dendritic growth, and spine maturation. *Neuron* October 19, 2006;**52**(2):255–69.

159. Ben-Zeev B, Aharoni R, Nissenkorn A, Arnon R. Glatiramer acetate (GA, Copolymer-1) an hypothetical treatment option for Rett syndrome. *Med Hypotheses* February 2011;**76**(2):190–3.

160. Deogracias R, Yazdani M, Dekkers MP, Guy J, Ionescu MC, Vogt KE, et al. Fingolimod, a sphingosine-1 phosphate receptor modulator, increases BDNF levels and improves symptoms of a mouse model of Rett syndrome. *Proc Natl Acad Sci USA* August 28, 2012;**109**(35):14230–5.

161. Borrell-Pages M, Canals JM, Cordelieres FP, Parker JA, Pineda JR, Grange G, et al. Cystamine and cysteamine increase brain levels of BDNF in Huntington disease via HSJ1b and transglutaminase. *J Clin Invest* May 2006;**116**(5):1410–24.

162. Roux JC, Zala D, Panayotis N, Borges-Correia A, Saudou F, Villard L. Modification of Mecp2 dosage alters axonal transport through the Huntingtin/Hap1 pathway. *Neurobiol Dis* February 2012;**45**(2):786–95.

163. Amaral MD, Chapleau CA, Pozzo-Miller L. Transient receptor potential channels as novel effectors of brain-derived neurotrophic factor signaling: potential implications for Rett syndrome. *Pharmacol Ther* February 2007;**113**(2):394–409.

164. Schmid DA, Yang T, Ogier M, Adams I, Mirakhur Y, Wang Q, et al. A TrkB small molecule partial agonist rescues TrkB phosphorylation deficits and improves respiratory function in a mouse model of Rett syndrome. *J Neurosci* February 1, 2012;**32**(5):1803–10.

165. Itoh M, Ide S, Takashima S, Kudo S, Nomura Y, Segawa M, et al. Methyl CpG-binding protein 2 (a mutation of which causes Rett syndrome) directly regulates insulin-like growth factor binding protein 3 in mouse and human brains. *J Neuropathol Exp Neurol* February 2007;**66**(2):117–23.

166. Zala D, Colin E, Rangone H, Liot G, Humbert S, Saudou F. Phosphorylation of mutant huntingtin at S421 restores anterograde and retrograde transport in neurons. *Hum Mol Genet* December 15, 2008;**17**(24):3837–46.

167. Zhang Y, Mao RR, Chen ZF, Tian M, Tong DL, Gao ZR, et al. Deep-brain magnetic stimulation promotes adult hippocampal neurogenesis and alleviates stress-related behaviors in mouse models for neuropsychiatric disorders. *Mol Brain* 2014;**7**:11.

168. Tropea D, Giacometti E, Wilson NR, Beard C, McCurry C, Fu DD, et al. Partial reversal of Rett syndrome-like symptoms in MeCP2 mutant mice. *Proc Natl Acad Sci USA* February 10, 2009;**106**(6):2029–34.

169. Ballas N, Lioy DT, Grunseich C, Mandel G. Non-cell autonomous influence of MeCP2-deficient glia on neuronal dendritic morphology. *Nat Neurosci* March 2009;**12**(3):311–7.

170. Okabe Y, Takahashi T, Mitsumasu C, Kosai K, Tanaka E, Matsuishi T. Alterations of gene expression and glutamate clearance in astrocytes derived from an MeCP2-null mouse model of Rett syndrome. *PLoS One* 2012;**7**(4):e35354.

171. Lioy DT, Garg SK, Monaghan CE, Raber J, Foust KD, Kaspar BK, et al. A role for glia in the progression of Rett's syndrome. *Nature* July 28, 2011;**475**(7357):497–500.

172. De Filippis B, Fabbri A, Simone D, Canese R, Ricceri L, Malchiodi-Albedi F, et al. Modulation of RhoGTPases improves the behavioral phenotype and reverses astrocytic deficits in a mouse model of Rett syndrome. *Neuropsychopharmacology* April 2012;**37**(5):1152–63.

173. Derecki NC, Cronk JC, Lu Z, Xu E, Abbott SB, Guyenet PG, et al. Wild-type microglia arrest pathology in a mouse model of Rett syndrome. *Nature* April 5, 2012;**484**(7392):105–9.

174. Kriaucionis S, Paterson A, Curtis J, Guy J, Macleod N, Bird A. Gene expression analysis exposes mitochondrial abnormalities in a mouse model of Rett syndrome. *Mol Cell Biol* July 2006;**26**(13):5033–42.

175. Percy AK. Clinical trials and treatment prospects. *Ment Retard Dev Disabil Res Rev* 2002;**8**(2):106–11.

176. Haas RH, Rice MA, Trauner DA, Merritt TA, Opitz JM, Reynolds JF. Therapeutic effects of a ketogenic diet in rett syndrome. *Am J Med Genet* 1986;**25**(S1):225–46.

177. Nielsen JB, Lou HC, Andresen J. Biochemical and clinical effects of tyrosine and tryptophan in the Rett syndrome. *Brain Dev* 1990;**12**(1):143–7.

178. Zappella M. A double blind trial of bromocriptine in the Rett syndrome. *Brain Dev* 1990;**12**(1):148–50.

179. Percy AK, Glaze DG, Schultz RJ, Zoghbi HY, Williamson D, Frost Jr JD, et al. Rett syndrome: controlled study of an oral opiate antagonist, naltrexone. *Ann Neurol* April 1994;**35**(4):464–70.

180. Ellaway C, Williams K, Leonard H, Higgins G, Wilcken B, Christodoulou J. Rett syndrome: randomized controlled trial of L-carnitine. *J Child Neurol* March 1999;**14**(3):162–7.

181. Ellaway CJ, Peat J, Williams K, Leonard H, Christodoulou J. Medium-term open label trial of L-carnitine in Rett syndrome. *Brain Dev* December 2001;**23**(Suppl. 1):S85–9.

182. Goyal M, O'Riordan MA, Wiznitzer M. Effect of topiramate on seizures and respiratory dysrhythmia in Rett syndrome. *J Child Neurol* August 2004;**19**(8):588–91.

183. Freilinger M, Dunkler D, Lanator I, Item CB, Muhl A, Fowler B, et al. Effects of creatine supplementation in Rett syndrome: a randomized, placebo-controlled trial. *J Dev Behav Pediatr* July–August 2011;**32**(6):454–60.

184. Khwaja OS, Ho E, Barnes KV, O'Leary HM, Pereira LM, Finkelstein Y, et al. Safety, pharmacokinetics, and preliminary assessment of efficacy of mecasermin (recombinant human IGF-1) for the treatment of Rett syndrome. *Proc Natl Acad Sci USA* March 12, 2014;**111**(12):4596–601.

185. Pini G, Scusa MF, Congiu L, Benincasa A, Morescalchi P, Bottiglioni I, et al. IGF1 as a potential treatment for Rett syndrome: safety assessment in six Rett patients. *Autism Res Treat* 2012;**2012**:679801.

186. Pharmaceuticals N. *Neuren's NNZ-2566 successful in demonstrating clinical benefit in Rett syndrome phase 2 trial*. 2014. http://www.neurenpharma.com/IRM/Company/ShowPage.aspx/PDFs/1448-10000000/NeurensuccessfulinRettsyndromePhase2trial.

20

Fragile X Syndrome

Anne Hoffmann[1], Elizabeth Berry-Kravis[1,2]

[1]Department of Pediatrics, Rush University Medical Center, Chicago, IL, USA;
[2]Department of Neurological Sciences, and Biochemistry, Rush University Medical Center, Chicago, IL, USA

PREVALENCE AND GENETICS OF FRAGILE X SYNDROME AND FRAGILE X-ASSOCIATED DISORDERS

Fragile X syndrome (FXS) is the most common known single gene cause of intellectual disability (ID) and autism spectrum disorder (ASD), with an estimated frequency of about 1:4000–5000.[1] Prevalence varies somewhat between different populations, but the disorder affects all ethnic groups worldwide. Fragile X syndrome is one of a set of disorders, termed fragile X-associated disorders (FXDs), which arise from a trinucleotide repeat (CGG) expansion mutation in the promoter region of *fragile X mental retardation 1* gene (*FMR1*) as depicted in Figure 1. This CGG sequence is transcribed into the *FMR1* messenger ribonucleic acid (mRNA) but the sequence is located in the 5′-untranslated region of the mRNA, and thus the number of repeat units does not affect the sequence of the fragile X mental retardation protein (FMRP), the gene product of *FMR1*.[2]

Smaller expansions of the repeat sequence (55–200 CGG repeats) are termed a "premutation." Prevalence of the premutation has been shown to vary in different

Neuronal and Synaptic Dysfunction in Autism Spectrum Disorder and Intellectual Disability
http://dx.doi.org/10.1016/B978-0-12-800109-7.00020-0

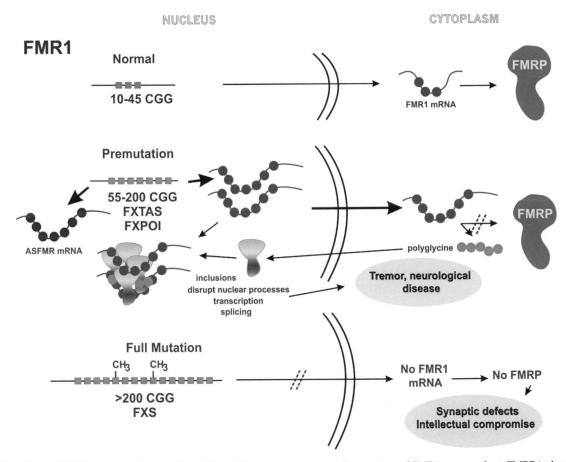

FIGURE 1	Normal *FMR1* gene function, location of the CGG repeat sequence, and expression of *FMR1* gene product, FMRP is depicted in the top panel. Effects of premutation-sized smaller CGG repeat expansion mutations, including increased production of CGG repeat-containing *FMR1* mRNA and *ASFMR* mRNA, and ribosomal stalling at the repeat sequence in the mRNA, leading to the polyglycine product of RAN as well as reduced production of FMRP are shown in the middle panel. Increases in CGG-containing mRNAs and polyglycine likely contribute to intranuclear inclusion formation and the neural toxicity that results in FXTAS. Effects of full mutation-sized larger expansions, which result in *FMR1* hypermethylation, gene silencing, and substantial reduction or absence of FMRP are shown in the lower panel. Lack of FMRP leads to synaptic plasticity deficits, ID, and FXS.

populations, but in the United States (US), two large studies estimated the frequency of the premutation to be about 1:151–1:209 in females and 1:430–1:468 in males.[3,4] The premutation is associated with risk for two well-defined adult-onset diseases: fragile X-associated tremor/ataxia syndrome (FXTAS) and fragile X-associated primary ovarian insufficiency (FXPOI). The mechanism for premutation-associated disease is thought to relate to a gain-of function RNA toxicity mechanism caused by elevated *FMR1* mRNA levels containing the expanded CGG sequence, although findings of elevated antisense *FMR1* transcripts (*ASFMR*) in premutation carriers[5] and polyglycine produced as a result of ribosomal stalling and repeat-mediated aberrant translation of the premutation at the ribosome[6] have suggested there may be multiple mechanisms of toxicity in *FMR1* premutation diseases (Figure 1). Indeed, individuals with a large premutation (>150 repeats) also have low FMRP levels

owing to repeat-mediated translational stalling and manifest symptoms milder than but overlapping with those observed in FXS.[2] Large full-mutation expansions in *FMR1* (>200 repeats) cause FXS, which results from the methylation and transcriptional silencing of the *FMR1* promoter with consequent loss or significant reduction of FMRP (Figure 1).[2] *FMR1* expansions tend to increase in size as they are passed from generation to generation, so FXDs affect families in multiple generations.

Adults with FXTAS present with tremor and/or ataxia, and may have executive dysfunction, neuropathy, parkinsonism, vestibular dysfunction, psychiatric symptoms such as anxiety, and in some cases autonomic dysfunction or dementia.[7] Clinically, patients often have multiple neurological symptoms and thus are difficult to categorize diagnostically. Fragile X-associated tremor/ataxia syndrome occurs in about 50% of male and 8–16% of female premutation carriers and the rate of progression varies, appears to be slower in females, and typically occurs over many years. Brain atrophy and increased signal in the deep white matter, splenium of the corpus callosum, and middle cerebellar peduncle (MCP sign) are seen on magnetic resonance imaging (MRI) scans, whereas the hallmark pathological finding is that of intranuclear inclusions in neurons throughout the brain and significant cerebellar Purkinje cell loss.[7] Diagnosis is accomplished through *FMR1* deoxyribonucleic acid (DNA) testing by polymerase chain reaction to identify the premutation expansion in a patient with suggestive symptoms and/or family history. Consistent with the RNA toxicity mechanism, the CGG repeat length in the premutation correlates with onset and severity of disease, MRI findings, and number of inclusions.[7] Treatment is supportive and symptom-based with beta blockers for tremor, L-DOPA for parkinsonism, antidepressants for anxiety, and donepezil or memantine for executive and cognitive problems showing some success in clinical cohort studies.[7]

Fragile X-associated primary ovarian insufficiency results in premature ovarian failure (POF) in up to 23% of women who are premutation carriers, and carriers experience menopause approximately 5 years earlier than noncarriers.[8] When women with POF are screened through reproductive endocrinology clinics, 11.5% with familial POF and 3.2% with sporadic POF are premutation carriers.[9–11] Even in carrier women who do not meet criteria for POF, reproductive aging milestones are also abnormal, with premutation carriers more likely to have short cycle lengths owing to a decrease in follicular phase length[12] elevated follicle-stimulating hormone (FSH) levels,[13] and lower anti-müllerian hormone levels.[14] Premutation carrier women have reduced fertility compared with noncarriers.[15] Increased rates of twinning occur in premutation women, which may result from elevations in FSH that occur as ovarian reserves decline.[16] This combined information led to the classification of the condition as a primary ovarian insufficiency (FXPOI). The onset and severity of FXPOI is nonlinearly associated with CGG repeat number, with the highest risk being present among PMC with midrange premutation repeats.[17] To date, the reason for this relationship and its implication with respect to the proposed RNA toxicity mechanism for ovarian disease is unclear.

Premutation carrier women may be at higher risk for atypical presentations of FXTAS and other medical problems not seen in male carriers, potentially owing to the presence of a second protective X chromosome.[18] Premutation women with ovarian insufficiency report higher rates of thyroid problems, depression, and anxiety.[19] Premutation women with definite or probable FXTAS have an increased prevalence of thyroid disease, hypertension, seizures, peripheral neuropathy, and fibromyalgia.[20] Premutation carrier women who do not

have FXTAS tend to have more symptoms of muscle pain and persistent paresthesias, and history of tremor. Premutation women who are daughters of men with FXTAS have a higher prevalence of neurological symptoms including tremor, balance issues, memory problems and dizziness, menopausal symptoms, sleep problems, and anxiety[21] compared with carrier women who did not have a father with FXTAS. In addition, one study has shown that 73% of women with FXTAS had at least one autoimmune disorder compared with 47% of premutation women without FXTAS and 32% of controls.[22] These disorders include autoimmune thyroid disease, fibromyalgia, irritable bowel syndrome, Raynaud phenomenon, rheumatoid arthritis, Sjögren syndrome, and systemic lupus erythematosus. There is some evidence that psychiatric disorders may also be prevalence among premutation carrier women. Data suggest that carrier women are frequently diagnosed or treated for depression, anxiety, or attention problems[18] and that the relationship of these problems to premutation carrier status appears to depend on the magnitude of life stress, which suggests a gene—environment effect. Accurate elucidation of risks associated with the premutation outside the well-defined syndromes of FXTAS and PXPOI await large population-based studies.

Alleles of 40—54 or 45—54 (depending on the study) CGG repeats are considered gray zone alleles. Some of these alleles are unstable and expand to premutation alleles in future generations. Presence and location of AGGs within the CGG repeat sequence define the instability and likelihood of expansion of these alleles.[23] The clinical significance of the gray zone expansion remains to be fully elucidated, although studies have shown a higher prevalence of gray zone carriers in both men[24] and women[25] with parkinsonism. The FXTAS phenotype has also been described in carriers of gray zone expansions.[26] The presence and magnitude of the risk for late-onset neurological disease in the gray zone population remain to be fully elucidated.

Individuals with FXS by definition have a full mutation, and intellectual and behavioral compromise result from the reduction or lack of FMRP in brain. Females with a full mutation are more variably and typically more mildly affected than males, owing to production of FMRP from the normal *FMR1* allele in cells expressing the nonmutated X chromosome. The severity of cognitive impairment in females with the full mutation is thought to be related to the activation ratio for the normal *FMR1* allele and the amount of expression of FMRP.[27] Males with mosaicism for a full and premutation or a partially unmethylated full mutation may also be mildly affected, with severity in this case also related to the amount of unmethylated DNA and FMRP levels.[27]

PHYSICAL AND MEDICAL FEATURES OF FXS

Physical Features

Physical features include macroorchidism in virtually all adult males with FXS. A characteristic pattern of facial features is seen in a percentage of individuals with FXS, including prominent ears, macrocephaly, long face, prominent jaw and forehead, midfacial hypoplasia, and high arched palate. Connective tissue laxity, leading to hyperextensible joints, flat feet, and soft skin is common in FXS but not present in all patients. Connective tissue laxity is thought to contribute to some of the medical issues seen in patients with FXS. Physical features are sufficiently variable that they cannot be used as indicators of which patients to screen for presence of FXS.

Medical Problems Associated with FXS

Recurrent Otitis Media

Recurrent otitis media (OM) is more common in FXS than in typically developing children, and 54.7% of males and 45.8% of females with FXS had recurrent OM, with 37.4% overall requiring pressure-equalizing (PE) tubes, in a study of medical problems in FXS based on data from 260 patients in the Fragile X Clinical and Research Consortium (FXCRC) database, a multicenter collaboration of FXS Clinics in the US (Table 1; Figure 2).[28] The FXCRC database frequency for recurrent OM was

similar to previous reports from smaller cohorts of children with FXS[29-31] and contrasts with a frequency of 15% in typically developing children and 38% in children with ID who do not have FXS.[29-31] In typically developing children, OM incidence is age-dependent, with frequencies of 21–64% in the first year of life and approximately 12.6% for 2- to 3-year-olds.[32] In FXS, the frequency of recurrent OM is also higher in early childhood, at 53.8% in children with FXS from age 0 to 3 years and 30% from age 4 to 5 years (Kidd et al.[28]).

It is speculated that children with FXS are susceptible to recurrent OM because they may have more collapsible Eustachian tubes, facial characteristics that affect the angle of the Eustachian tube, oromotor hypotonia, dyspraxia, and poor secretion control, all of which may lead to poor drainage of the middle ear, buildup of fluid, and increased likelihood of infection.[31] The long face and midfacial hypoplasia noted in individuals with FXS can also create structural impediments to drainage of the sinuses and increase the likelihood of recurrent sinusitis.

Strabismus and Visual Acuity

Children with FXS, have been reported to have a high prevalence of refractive errors ranging from 13% to 59%.[33-36] The variability is likely because of selection bias in populations studied and because children with FXS are difficult to evaluate for visual acuity owing to developmental delays, attention problems, anxiety, and sensory processing issues.[34] Prior studies reported a prevalence of strabismus in boys with FXS ranging from 4% to 57%. In the FXCRC Database cohort (Table 1; Figure 2),[28] the prevalence of strabismus in FXS was (16.4%), and particularly in boys (17.5%), it significantly increased from the population frequency in children of 2.6% to 4%.[31,35-39] Children with FXS appear to be at greater risk than the general population for eye disorders and warrant close and regular monitoring of ocular disorders, ocular motility, and visual acuity.

Seizures

Studies in the mouse model of FXS demonstrate immature dendritic connections and abnormal synaptic plasticity with excessive epileptiform bursts and proneness to audiogenic seizures in young animals.[40,41] Similar abnormal dendritic maturation is also observed in the brain from humans with FXS,[42] and likewise an increased frequency of seizures is found in individuals with FXS relative to the general population.[43]

Previous studies of FXS patient cohorts from epilepsy and neurology clinics reported prevalence rates for seizures of 14–44%,[44-52] whereas genetics clinics reported 9–27%.[53-56] Larger studies focused on individuals with FXS in the community or all patients at individual FXS clinics reported lower prevalence proportions overall,

TABLE 1   Frequency of Medical Problems in FXS

	FXS Males (FXCRC)	FXS Females (FXCRC)	FXS All (FXCRC)	FXS (Past Studies)	General Population
Seizures	12	3	10	15	1
Tics	5	7	6	15	4
Frequent ear infections	55	46	53	56	14
Strabismus/ lazy eye	18	13	16	30	3
Sleep problems	26	30	27	40	17
Sleep apnea	7	7	7	34	1
Loose stools	12	7	11		
GER	10	14	11	31	5
Mitral valve prolapse	1	2	1	55	1

All numbers are given as a percentage.
Data were adapted from Kidd et al.[28] Data from past studies in FXS are derived from the largest study published before the FXCRC Database study.

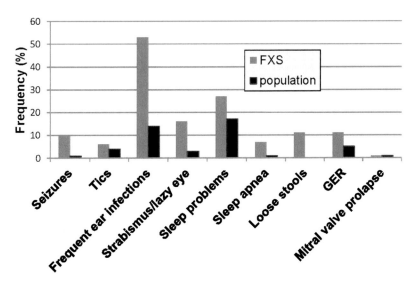

FIGURE 2 Frequency of medical problems in FXS (gray bars) relative to the general population of children (black bars). *Data derived from Ref. 28.*

ranging between 12% and 18%,[43,57−59] and with higher prevalence for males compared with females. In the FXCRC Database cohort (Table 1; Figure 2),[28] the prevalence of seizures was 10%, with a higher prevalence (12%) in males compared with females (3%). The available data suggest that the true population prevalence of seizure occurrence in individuals with FXS in minimally biased samples is likely between 10% and 15%.

Many children with FXS have abnormal EEGs without overt seizures.[43,45−48,50,59−61] Although some small studies have shown a predominance of generalized seizures,[44,50] larger studies have suggested that partial seizures are most common in FXS.[43,45−47,59,60] Likewise nearly half (45%) of patients with seizures in the FXCRC Database cohort had partial seizures. Both simple and complex partial seizures may occur,[59] and secondary generalization and status epilepticus can occur.[62,63] Seizures are easily controlled[43,48,49,51,56,59,60] and resolve during childhood in most individuals with FXS.

A study of a small cohort showed a trend toward an increased rate of seizures in individuals with FXS and autism (28%, compared with 12% with FXS alone).[64] A study of a large cohort from the National Fragile X Survey showed an increased frequency of autism in individuals with FXS and seizures, compared with an age- and gender-matched FXS group without seizures, which suggests a shared neurobiology resulting in seizure and autism propensity.[60] However, reading and thinking levels were not perceived as more impaired in the group with epilepsy than the matched group,[60] which suggests that the autism relationship may be specific and not result from generally lower cognition in those with seizures. The prevalence of seizures in individuals with autism and FXS was 16% in the FXCRC Database,[28] slightly higher than overall

seizure prevalence in FXS (10%) and consistent with prior literature suggesting an association. To date, secondary genetic risk factors for seizures or shared epilepsy/autism susceptibility in FXS are not known.

Stereotypies

Movement disorder is common in FXS, predominantly in the form of stereotypies such as hand flapping and hand movements, but also forehead rubbing, manipulating objects, and body movements.[65] Frequency of tics (6%) was not shown to be increased in FXS over the general population in the FXCRC database (Table 1; Figure 2).[66] Prior reports of higher rates of tics[67,68] likely reflect confusion between stereotypies and tics in parent reports, which can be challenging to distinguish without history and neurological exam data.

Sleep Problems

Sleep problems are observed in approximately 10−25% of typically developing children and adolescents,[69,70] but the prevalence is significantly higher in children with ID and autism, ranging from 36% to 73%.[71−75] An analysis of 90 children with FXS[76] found that nearly half of children with FXS had clinically significant sleep problems, regardless of whether they were receiving medication to improve sleep. A large-scale survey of 1295 children with FXS[77] showed a 32% rate of sleep difficulties, including difficulty falling asleep and frequent night awakenings. In the FXCRC Database, only 27% of parents of individuals with FXS reported sleep problems with little difference between males and females (Table 1; Figure 2).

Loud snoring and obstructive sleep apnea (OSA) have been reported in as high as 38% and 34%, respectively, of children with FXS. Results from the FXCRC database showed an overall lower prevalence of OSA of 7% of patients overall.[28] The reason for discrepancy in the prevalence between these studies is not known, but it appears that airway obstruction is more frequent in FXS than in the general population (Table 1; Figure 2).

Gastrointestinal Disorders

In the FXCRC Database, loose stools and gastroesophageal reflux GER were present in similar proportions (11%) of all individuals with FXS.[28] Comparison estimates from a similar-aged typically developing population[78] suggest that the prevalence of GER is increased in the FXS population (Table 1; Figure 2).

Mitral Valve Prolapse

Clinical findings of loose connective tissue in FXS have led to concerns that this may lead to mitral valve prolapse (MVP) and weakening of vessels in the form of aortic dilatation, as seen in Marfan and Ehlers–Danlos syndromes. In small case series, five of 23 adult patients had MVP on echocardiography[79]; one of 17 children had typical examination findings of MVP, but not on electrocardiography or echocardiography[80]; and three of 22 patients had abnormal echocardiographic evidence of MVP.[33] Loehr et al.[81] reported a high prevalence of MVP of 55% by echocardiography compared with the 0.8% prevalence observed based on clinician exam and history in the children and young adults in the FXCRC Database (Table 1; Figure 2).[28] Whether MVP increases as patients age into adulthood is unknown. Although MVP does not appear to be a frequent medical problem in children, a systematic study of MVP in a cohort of adults with FXS is needed.

Growth in FXS

In the FXCRC Database cohort, the overall birth weight was slightly higher than the general population[28]; however, the overall proportion of infants that were low birth weight was similar to that in the general population. The mean head circumference[82,83] and mean birth length[82–85] were not different from control populations. Mean gestational age was similar to the general population.

Two studies developed measurement curves for males with FXS that were compared to control anthropometric data[86] and unaffected relatives.[87] Height curves for FXS were higher at nearly every point in the prepubertal section of the curves, although height was lower in the postpubertal ages. In the FXCRC Database,[28] height for males was close to typically developing males until approximately postpuberty, when the height curve was decreased in comparison. Weight for males and females may be higher in FXS throughout childhood and adolescence and some children with FXS appear to have a genetic predisposition in the form of a Prader–Willi-like subphenotype.[88,89] Higher weights in cohorts of children and adolescents with FXS are likely also mediated by antipsychotic use for behavior.[90] Despite higher weights, cholesterol levels in individuals with FXS have been reported to be lower than population levels,[90] and there is a suggestion of other forms of metabolic dysregulation in the form of excessive insulin signaling and abnormal glucose homeostasis in FXS cellular models.[91] After birth, the head circumference tends to rise above the 50th percentile and continues to be larger than for males without FXS.[82,85,86,92–94]

DEVELOPMENTAL AND COGNITIVE CHARACTERISTICS OF FXS

Most males with fragile X syndrome (FXS) will meet criteria for mild to severe ID.[95] Average intelligence quotient (IQ) in adult males with FXS is 40–50, with a mental age of about of 5–6 years. Females with FXS are often less affected than males, with about 25% having cognitive impairment and others frequently being diagnosed with learning disabilities.[96] Average IQ in females is about 80, with a range from severe impairment to normal or even superior ability. There is a relatively consistent pattern of both intellectual weaknesses and strengths distinct to this disorder (Table 2). Females with FXS demonstrate many of the same deficits and skills as males, although the expression of these is often more subtle.[97] Most research indicates that this syndrome is associated with deficiencies in visuospatial skills, working memory, processing of sequential information, and attention.[97–100] However, along with these weaknesses, there are also relative strengths in simultaneous processing and long-term memory.

Visuospatial skills refer to the nonverbal ability to both understand and conceptualize visual information and spatial relationships while processing information. These are skills that would be used in tasks such as assembling puzzles, copying block designs, as well as

TABLE 2   Cognitive Strengths and Weaknesses in FXS

Domain	Strength	Weakness
Visuospatial skills		Visuo-construction
		Visuomotor (for males)
Attention		Shifting attention from previously correct response
Memory	Object memory	Working memory
	Visual memory	Sequencing
	Verbal memory	

Information taken from Cornish et al.[101,103] Munir et al.[104] Jakala et al.[110] Loesch et al.[111] Burack et al.[113] and Hodapp et al.[114]

drawing a specified image. Studies have found that males with FXS have specific deficits in visuo-construction and visuomotor skills, but not necessarily in visuospatial memory or visual perception.[101] This same visuo-construction deficit has also been found in females with FXS, although other visuospatial skills appear to be spared.[101]

At the cognitive level, attention is divided into multiple skills including sustained, selective, alternating, and divided. Deficits in attention are almost universal for individuals with fragile X and have been the subject of numerous studies. Even individuals with IQs that fall in the normal range typically exhibit impairments in this area.[102] Studies have found that deficits in attention are not global in nature, but rather depend on the task given. Tasks that require the individual to change attention from a previously correct pattern to a novel one are much more difficult.[103] This type of perseverative error has been found in toddlers through adults with FXS, which indicates that it is a pervasive issue in this disorder.[103–105] Compared with other developmental disabilities (e.g., Down syndrome, Williams syndrome), these studies demonstrate that individuals with FXS show a distinct pattern of attentional deficits, with significant weakness in areas requiring inhibitory control.

There is evidence that these attentional deficits may be attributable to a weakness in executive function.[103,104,106] Executive functions are high-order skills such as cognitive flexibility, planning, executing, and inhibition. There is growing evidence that this is a particular area of weakness for both males and females with FXS.[103,106–108]

Memory also has several subdomains, including working memory, short-term memory, long-term memory, and procedural memory. As in other cognitive processes, individuals with FXS demonstrate a pattern of strengths and weaknesses in areas of memory rather than an overall impairment. Working memory has received the most attention in research on FXS; it refers to information that is stored briefly so it can be manipulated in other processes (e.g., remembering the first sound in a novel word as it is decoded). Working memory is generally an area of weakness, and non-meaningful information is especially difficult for the individual to retain.[109] This tendency is also reflected in studies that found individuals with FXS struggled with retaining abstract information in short-term memory as well as sequencing of information.[110,111] In general, object memory and several types of visual memory are relatively strong for individuals with FXS.[110,111] Both males and females with FXS have a relative strength in visually presented meaningful stimuli.[110] In addition, verbal memory in general seems stronger than expected given the cognitive level of the individual. This pattern of strengths and weaknesses

within memory can be used to the advantage of individuals with FXS for academic and life-skills planning.

Sequencing is consistently problematic for individuals with FXS because it requires them to hold and manipulate information within their working memory, creating a significant cognitive load. Two studies found that males with FXS did significantly worse on the sequential subtests of the Kaufmann Assessment Battery for Children[112] compared with the simultaneous subtests.[113,114] This preference for gestalt processing is reflected in numerous clinical reports as well.[115,116]

COGNITIVE STRENGTHS AND WEAKNESSES IN FXS

Another aspect of cognition in FXS is the appearance of a cognitive decline after a certain age. Multiple early studies revealed that as individuals with FXS aged, their full-scale IQ scores would drop.[117–119] Standard scores on the Vineland Adaptive Behavior Scale for overall adaptive behavior as well as subdomains have also been shown to decline with age, in males more so than in females with FXS.[120] Decline in standard scores for intelligence and adaptive function is not the result of loss of skills or regression, but rather a failure to keep pace with the normal rate of intellectual development.

BEHAVIOR IN FXS

The behavioral phenotype in males with FXS covers a wide spectrum, although certain key behaviors are considered hallmarks of the disorder. These behaviors fall into the broad categories of attention, hyperarousal, anxiety, and aggression. As in other areas, females with FXS tend to follow the same general pattern of behavioral difficulties, but with milder symptomatology.

Attention disorders are often characterized by impulsivity as well as inattention. These behaviors are extremely common in FXS and result in a high rate of attention deficit hyperactivity disorder (ADHD) diagnoses. Some studies have found the incidence of ADHD in males with FXS to be as high as 73%.[30,121] For females, there is an increased risk of ADHD symptoms, although the rate of actual diagnosis of ADHD is lower, between about 30% and 63%.[97,108,122] For both genders, these rates are higher than what is found in populations with individuals with learning disabilities not related to FXS, and also does not seem to be attributable just to IQ or developmental level.[123,124] Impulsivity in boys with FXS does not seem to improve with age, which means that this behavior has the potential to present long-term challenges to the individual and their caregivers.[124]

Another key area of difficulty for individuals with FXS is anxiety. One study found that 86.2% of males with FXS and 76.9% of females with FXS met the criteria for an anxiety disorder.[125] Although individuals with FXS manifest high rates of generalized anxiety and of virtually all subtypes, the anxiety disorders most frequently found in the literature are specific phobias and social anxiety.[97,108,125] This social anxiety and consequent social avoidance appears to be present as early as preschool and continues through adulthood.[97,123,126] At its most severe, social avoidance can manifest itself as selective mutism, a condition in which an individual is unable to speak in certain environments. This condition was found in 28% of the individuals with FXS and is dramatically higher than the prevalence rate of less than 1% found in the general population.[125]

Arousal is the overall degree of alertness as well as the reaction to emotionally significant stimuli. It is regulated by the autonomic nervous system, which causes the heart rate to increase and avoidant behaviors to appear.[127] Thus hyperarousal occurs when an individual goes into a state of high arousal when presented with stimuli that would not provoke that reaction in other individual: for example, when presented with a disagreeable texture. This overreaction of the autonomic nervous system in individuals with FXS can be triggered by a wide range of situations, including noises, new environments, crowds, interpersonal distance, eye contact, and new people.[128] The effects of this hyperarousal are widespread: High levels of motor activity (e.g., running, jumping), stereotypic motor movements (e.g., hand flapping), gaze aversion, and perseverative behaviors are all frequently described as resulting from hyperarousal.[127–130] The perseverative behaviors can take many forms; perseverative speech is frequently noted in FXS and will be discussed in the language section. Perseverating on a certain movie, or part of a movie, as well as fixating on a particular theme (e.g., only being interested in movies that show one preferred character) is also common.[131] These extremely restricted interests are difficult to expand and cause difficulties in social interactions because the individual may be unwilling to deviate from preferred activities.

Aggression and self-injurious behavior (SIB) are often linked to hyperarousal as well. These problem behaviors are especially detrimental to family functioning because they can significantly impede an individual's ability to participate in daily activities. A large study used parental report to better define the rate of SIB found in the FXS population, with 41% of males and 17% of females described as having self-injured at some point in their lifetime.[132] Based on this examination, SIB typically appears fairly early in development, with the onset for most individuals (both male and female) occurring at age 1–3 years. There is a wide variety of types of SIBs,

including self-hitting, biting, pulling, picking, and scratching. Males with FXS who demonstrated SIBs were also more likely to have hyperactivity, attention problems, anxiety, autism, and sensory/sleep difficulties than a male with FXS and no SIBs.[132] Females with SIBs were also more likely to have autism, anxiety, and sensory difficulties.[132]

Aggression typically occurs later, mostly during the pubescent and postpubescent period. An FXS diagnosis carries with it an elevated risk of aggressive behaviors. One study found that approximately 25% of individuals with FXS were reported as having violent outbursts.[133] Another study found that 31% of caregivers of males with FXS and 17% of females reported being injured by individuals with FXS during the previous year. Of caregivers of males, there was a mean number of 16 injuries per year, with 2.7 being serious enough to require medical care.[134] Research indicates that a comorbid diagnosis of FXS and ASD is associated with a significantly higher rate of problem behaviors in adolescence and adulthood, including behaviors that are hurtful to others.[135] Interestingly, this study showed that both the group with FXS only and FXS and had better adaptive behaviors than the ASD-only group, which indicates that there may be a relationship between the FXS phenotype and the ability to compensate for individual weaknesses.

LANGUAGE IN FXS

Language development is globally delayed for most individuals with FXS. It is common for individuals with FXS to remain prelinguistic communicators, i.e., using gestures, vocalizations, and maybe a few single words, much later in life than is seen in typical development. Brady et al. used maternal reports to characterize the communication of 55 toddlers with FXS.[136] They found that of this group, 42 children were either nonverbal or minimally verbal at the time of the interview. Other studies found that a percentage of adolescents and adults with FXS may still be predominantly prelinguistic communicators.[137] However, most males and females with FXS will obtain spoken language at some point, and they will continue to gain language skills throughout the lifespan, albeit at a slower pace than typically developing individuals.[138,139]

In general, individuals with FXS have stronger receptive than expressive language skills. Although receptive language skills are usually below chronological age expectations, they are commensurate with nonverbal mental age.[140] This distinguishes FXS from other developmental disorders such as Down syndrome and autism. Both receptive vocabulary (understanding of words) and receptive syntax (comprehension of grammar and word combinations such as passive sentences) are relatively strong.[140] This contrasts to what is found in individuals with comorbid FXS and autism. Studies have found that individuals with FXS and ASD have receptive language skills below their nonverbal mental age, and that as ASD severity increases, so do the deficits in receptive vocabulary and grammar.[141,142]

Expressive language is delayed, with nonverbal mental age being a strong predictor of expressive vocabulary.[140] Expressive vocabulary is considered a relative strength for both male and female children with FXS. Some aspects of morphosyntax (i.e., combining words in the correct order and adding endings such as plurals and past tense) may also be a strength for individuals with FXS.[137] Studies looking at morphosyntax find that areas such as number agreement are stronger than expected, whereas areas such as the use of complex clauses are weaker. These strengths are particularly evident during narrative tasks as opposed to conversational tasks, most likely owing to the increased structure found in story-telling contexts.

Pragmatics is the most abstract form of language and one that is often the most problematic for individuals with developmental disabilities. Pragmatics refers to the way language functions in the real world, and what is required for people to interact successfully with others. Social interactions begin in the very early, prelinguistic period of development and rely on foundational skills, including engagement, reciprocity, and joint attention. As children age, the skills for communicative success evolve, and things such as topic maintenance, appropriate conversational turn-taking, following another person's conversational lead, and understanding of metaphorical and figurative language (e.g., nonliteral language such as "it's raining cats and dogs") become important.

Individuals with FXS show delays in pragmatic language early in development. Reciprocity refers to the back-and-forth sharing of facial expressions, vocalizations, and gestures between communication partners. This is an area of relative weakness in FXS, with evidence that young children with FXS have difficulty with reciprocating positive facial expressions.[138] Joint attention is the use of eye contact and gestures for purely social reasons, to share in an experience. This is a critical skill for overall language development and especially appropriate pragmatics. Joint attention in infants and toddlers with FXS is reduced, which may cause delays or abnormal development of behaviors such as pointing or following eye gaze, as well as decreased turn-taking.[143]

As children age, the development of theory of mind (the ability to understand how another person is feeling) takes place, which is a crucial step for acquiring more complicated pragmatic skills. A study looking at pragmatic language abilities in relation to theory of mind found that boys with FXS only performed similarly to a group of typically developing boys matched on nonverbal mental age.[144] In other words, the boys with FXS were following a delayed but not deviant path of pragmatic development. This contrasted with the group of boys who had a dual diagnosis of FXS and autism. That group displayed a deviant pattern more similar to boys with ASD only, with specific deficits in theory of mind.

Deficits in pragmatic skills continue to surface as individuals develop. Studies indicate that males with FXS demonstrate high rates of tangential (off-topic) language, overly literal interpretation of language, as well as decreased topic initiation and maintenance.[98,130] Repetitive language (also called perseverative) is a hallmark of FXS and one that causes significant social difficulty. This repetition can take several forms; it may be repeating a certain phrase over and over or it may be a refusal to allow conversation to move from a preferred topic. Conversational analysis of groups of men with FXS, autism, or intellectual deficits of unknown origin showed higher rates of repetitive speech at the sound, word, and phrase level for men with FXS than either of the other groups. Mazzocco et al. examined the conversational language of females with FXS and found several deficits in their ability to maintain a conversation during a short social interaction.[145] They had particular difficulty in extending a conversation using questions that logically followed the previous conversational turn, and also displayed fewer automatic comments such as introducing themselves at the beginning of a conversation.

It is clear that language development in FXS shows a global delay starting very early in life. This gap between individuals with FXS and their typically developing peers widens with time.[119] To maximize the potential of these individuals, it is crucial that they receive appropriate intervention as early as possible, including strong academic supports as they transition to the school system.

AUTISM IN FXS

Fragile X syndrome accounts for about 2–3% of all cases of ASD.[146,147] A variety of studies of FXS cohorts have suggested that about 18–67% of males and 20% of females with FXS meet criteria for ASD,[148,149] and it is generally thought that about half to two-thirds of males with FXS meet criteria for ASD based on *Diagnostic and Statistical Manual of Mental Disorders*, Fourth edition (DSM-IV) criteria.[150] *Diagnostic and Statistical Manual of Mental Disorders*, Fifth edition criteria have not been implemented for sufficient time to have estimates of the prevalence of ASD in FXS based on these criteria, although it is not thought that prevalence estimates will change much from past DSM IV–based data. Behavioral and neurological phenotypes common to FXS and ASD include social interactional and communication/language deficits, poor eye contact, repetitive motor movements such as stereotypies, unusual reactions to sensory input, including hypersensitivity (e.g., tactile defensiveness) and hyposensitivity (e.g., high tolerance for pain), cognitive strength in visual memory, increased prevalence of seizures relative to the general population (although peak incidence is in childhood in FXS and adolescence in ASD), macrocephaly, difficulties with regulation of attention, activity level, emotional behavior, and mood, often leading to additional diagnoses (e.g., ADHD, anxiety, mood disorder), other problematic behaviors (e.g., aggression, noncompliance, self-injury), and sleep problems. Some behavioral characteristics or symptoms are seen in both ASD and FXS, but for different underlying reasons. Individuals with FXS for example typically avoid eye contact directly,[151] looking away from people so as to help with coping with emotional discomfort that is driven by underlying social anxiety.[148,152] Thus, lack of social initiation and poor eye contact are thought to result mostly from anxiety[153] in FXS rather than a lack of social awareness or interest commonly seen in ASD, presumed at least in part to be a failure to recognize or process social cues such as eye gaze as a source of information or interaction.

Characteristics that tend to differ between the FXS and ASD phenotypes include a higher rate of ID in FXS than idiopathic ASD, significantly more severe motor coordination deficits in FXS than ASD, worse expressive than receptive language in FXS with the reverse pattern more likely in ASD, generally higher interest in socialization in FXS (although limited by anxiety), and better imitation skills in FXS than ASD. Individuals with FXS and ASD, relative to those with FXS alone, have less developed language skills, lower IQ and adaptive skills, more severe overall behavioral problems, and reduced social interaction.[150] Although individuals with FXS and ASD have a behavioral phenotype more similar to idiopathic ASD than those with FXS alone, these individuals have a characteristic pattern of ASD with higher levels of hyperarousal, social and generalized anxiety, and repetitive behaviors[151,153,154]

SUPPORTIVE TREATMENT OF FXS

Medical

The following conditions have been reported to be more common and clinically important in the FXS population: strabismus, recurrent OM, sleep, gastrointestinal problems, seizures, and weight gain.[28] Treatment of medical problems is important because these problems can affect development or behavior. The pediatrician should look for and ask about symptoms that might be related to these problems at routine yearly well-child visits, and should refer to specialists for further evaluation and management if needed. The type and timing of follow-up for these problems will depend on the severity and whether medication intervention is implemented.

Because children with FXS have expressive language delays, and recurrent OM may lead to conductive hearing loss and further language and articulation issues, it is important that all OM and/or any otologic issues be treated promptly and appropriately, with hearing monitoring and a relatively low threshold for early PE tube placement in children with FXS and recurrent OM.[155] It is important to recognize that children with FXS may not communicate pain well, and behavioral issues such as head banging may be a sign of pain from an acute OM. If chronically infected adenoids and tonsils become a problem, adenoidectomy and/or tonsillectomy may be performed at the same time the PE tubes are inserted.

It can be difficult to obtain good vision screening for children with FXS because of communication and behavioral issues. Children with FXS who cannot cooperate for standard vision screening should be referred to a professional who can obtain a good vision assessment yearly or every other year during childhood to ensure that any acuity issues are being addressed, so that these do not compound problems with reading and academics. When present, strabismus should be managed with eye patching, vision therapy, or surgery to avoid amblyopia and compounding of visual processing problems.

For concerns about episodes that might be seizures, an electroencephalogram (EEG) evaluation should be obtained along with neurology referral. Ambulatory EEG can be used to distinguish behavioral spells from seizures. Typically, patients would be treated after two documented seizures with anticonvulsants that are least likely to cause sedation or behavioral aggravation, with a plan to discontinue treatment after an individual with FXS is seizure-free for 2 years.

Children, especially those with ID, require adequate sleep for optimal development, learning, and functioning. Monitoring and managing OSA and other sleep problems is of particular importance in FXS, owing to their relationship to decrements in daytime performance and behavior.[156] The primary care physician should inquire about potential sleep problems in children with FXS at every well-child visit. Depending on the severity of the sleep problems, these may require behavioral or/and medical treatment or a referral to a sleep specialist. When symptoms of OSA are clearly present, management with tonsillectomy/adenoidectomy is indicated to prevent cognitive and behavioral aggravation. Sleep may also be affected by other environmental, health, and emotional factors, which should be addressed and treated accordingly.

Growth patterns identified in children with FXS suggest an increased risk for being overweight and for having somewhat diminished height in adulthood. It is important to encourage a healthy diet, food restriction when necessary, and exercise programs for 30–40 min four to five times a week to minimize problems associated with increased weight.

When GER is present, antacids should be used when needed to prevent pain, esophagitis, and resulting behavioral decompensation. Because individuals with FXS are not always able to describe heartburn, the only sign of GER may be behavioral outbursts occurring in patterns during the day in relation to meals, or sleep dysfunction with frequent night awakenings.

Some individuals with FXS benefit from orthotics or shoe inserts for foot pronation and flat feet to help with motor development when young, and to avoid leg pain and reduce gait problems when older.

Supportive Educational, Therapeutic, and Behavioral Management in FXS

There is a lack of peer-reviewed research on nonpharmacological interventions for individuals with FXS. Recommended practices are those that have been found successful by clinicians and teachers familiar with the population, and that play to the strengths of the phenotype. However, this is clearly an area that would benefit from additional research.

Therapeutic

Because of the global developmental delay most individuals with FXS display, it is likely that they will qualify for multiple services at a young age. Occupational therapy (OT), physical therapy (PT), and speech therapy should all be accessed at the maximum level allowed so as to maximize early growth. If verbal language is extremely delayed, families may find it beneficial to pursue another form of communication such as sign language or a picture exchange system to minimize frustration. Older individuals with FXS who are minimally verbal may find an electronic communication device or a communication program on an iPad helpful for communication.

Occupational therapy will often target both the fine-motor and sensory difficulties found in FXS. Fine-motor skills are often significantly delayed and OT may continue throughout the school years. If writing skills are delayed enough to inhibit performance at

school, it is recommended that individuals have access to a keyboard for typing or are allowed to dictate their responses.[157]

The hypotonia present in FXS will typically qualify an individual for PT, especially when younger. Physical therapy goals frequently focus on being able to navigate the home environment (for children aged less than 3 years) or school environment (for children aged over 3 years) safely. These could include things such as being able to climb the ladder to a slide on the playground or being able walk up the stairs to a classroom.

Therapy techniques that have been validated for autism are often helpful for FXS. However, it is important to modify them based on what is known about the FXS phenotype. For example, Applied Behavioral Analysis (ABA) approaches are systematic methods of behavioral modification that have been shown to be effective for individuals with autism.[158] This approach is often suggested as an intervention for individuals with FXS, but a common early goal in many ABA-based interventions is to increase eye contact. This is not appropriate for FXS because eye contact increases hyperarousal in FXS and decreases the ability to interact appropriately. Approaches used in autism also do not take advantage of the natural desire for social engagement found in FXS, a significant strength that should be used.

Educational

Inclusionary practices are recommended to the degree possible, which will provide better opportunities for the individual with FXS to benefit from peer modeling.[157,159] Because of the strength in imitation found in FXS, indirect teaching using peers can be an excellent tool for teaching. For inclusion to be successful, it is vital to provide the supports needed by the individual, a process that must be done systematically and consistently throughout the academic environment.

In general, individuals with FXS benefit from a structured approach in academics that relates to their areas of interest.[115,116,160] This could mean counting activities during which the individual counts a high-interest item, or targeting sight words from a preferred television program. Because individuals with FXS frequently display limited but intense interests, this is a simple way to increase engagement in an activity. Mathematics is often an academic weakness and visual and/or tactile strategies are useful for this area.

Visual memory strengths in FXS usually make reading approaches focused on sight words more successful.[160] The weaknesses in working memory and sequencing common to FXS make phonics-based approaches more frustrating and many individuals with FXS may struggle with them. Many individuals with

FXS are able to acquire some reading skills, and it is important for them to have consistent exposure to written content at the appropriate level to ensure that those skills are retained.

As individuals with FXS transition to higher levels of education, the gap between them and typical peers often widens. At the high school level, there is frequently a transition to vocational training as opposed to a strictly academic curriculum. The degree to which academics is continued depends on the needs of the individual; some may plan to attend a postgraduation academic program that would require additional academics.[157]

Throughout the school-age years, it is necessary to provide intentional and planned opportunities for socialization to ensure that interaction skills may continue to grow. Social goals should be included in the individualized education plan so that they can be targeted directly during the school day.

Behavioral

Although the behavioral phenotype of FXS is often challenging, some relatively simple strategies can be implemented to lessen their impact on daily functioning.

To manage anxiety, it is helpful to use visual schedules that provide a clear picture of when an activity will end and what will happen next.[116] Changes to routine and transitions are frequently problematic; extra support at these times can be extremely helpful. Social stories[161] are often useful for explaining changes, as well as what the appropriate behavior is in those situations.

Hyperarousal is an ongoing issue in FXS, and several strategies may be used to lessen its effect. Maintaining a calm environment will minimize the excessive stimuli that often result in hyperarousal.[162] This can involve minimizing extraneous noise from heating/cooling, dimming lights, and limiting excessive visual stimulation.

Sensory diets, which are a schedule of sensory breaks and activities designed to keep the individual regulated, can be developed with OT. Sensory diets are most effective when used to prevent hyperarousal from occurring, instead of being used reactively when the individual is already in a state of hyperarousal.[162]

Overall, it is important to bear in mind that there is a wide spectrum of abilities in FXS and that one approach will not be appropriate for every individual. These are general suggestions that may prove helpful in creating an initial therapy or academic plan, but will undoubtedly need to be altered to fit the strengths, weaknesses, and preferences of the individual. Individuals with FXS have been shown to display better behavioral and adaptive functioning when their environment and supportive programming is well matched to their needs,[163] and therefore a highly individualized behavioral, therapeutic, and educational intervention plan is needed both for home and school or work environments.

Psychopharmacology for Behavior

Because of the severity of behavior frequently seen in FXS and because behavior may prevent an individual with FXS from working or engaging in typical life activities and frequently causes a substantial burden for caregivers,[134,164] psychopharmacological treatment is often used to ameliorate behavioral symptoms in FXS. Medication for behavior may be employed because an individual with FXS is causing injury or property destruction and thus is a danger, because an individual is simply dysfunctional and cannot participate in normal life, or because it is perceived that an individual could perform better or be in more inclusive settings if behavior (e.g., attention) were better managed. Thus, although little to no formal clinical trial data regarding efficacy in FXS are available, psychopharmacologic treatment of ADHD symptoms, anxiety, hyperarousal, and irritable/aggressive behaviors with medications such as stimulants, selective serotonin reuptake inhibitors (SSRIs), alpha-agonists, and antipsychotics, respectively, is regularly employed for individuals with FXS in clinical settings (Table 3).[165–167] Indeed, in a reports from clinic data in the US, about 75% of males and 59% of females were treated at some time with medication for behavior.[167] The type of treatment needed varies with age because the behavioral phenotype tends to evolve with age, such that ADHD-like symptoms are more common in young children and anxiety and irritability/aggression increase during the adolescent years into young adulthood.[134] Thus, although there is overlap in behavioral symptoms and all classes of medication are used at all ages, males with FXS under age 18 years are most commonly treated with stimulants and/or alpha-agonists, and males over 18 years and females with FXS are most commonly treated with antidepressants.[165–168] Successful treatment of targeted behaviors in FXS in a clinic setting, as defined by stringent clinical criteria for behavioral improvement based on reports from two sources over 6 months' treatment duration, ranges from 53% to 62% for trials of different

TABLE 3　Percentage of Individuals with FXS Ever Treated with Medications in Different Psychopharmacological Classes at a Large Fragile X Clinic

Medication	Males	Females
Stimulant	57.6	35.2
SSRI	47.9	42
Antipsychotic	22.6	9.3
Alpha-Agonist	25.1	1.9

Data were derived from a retrospective chart review at the Rush University Medical Center Fragile-X Clinic (N = 257).[162]

classes of psychoactive medications (Figure 3).[134,166,167] In several studies, the rate of success improved with sequential trials of medications within a class to find the most effective and best tolerated medication, such that ultimately targeted behaviors were perceived as improved for about 73–77% of individuals with FXS receiving psychopharmacological treatment (Figure 3).[166,167] Because only data from clinic surveys are available, these response data are likely somewhat inflated owing to placebo responses.

However, available data suggest that psychopharmacology targeted toward ADHD-like anxiety and irritability symptoms in FXS can be helpful and appears to have

fairly high efficacy in a clinical setting, although several trials of medicines from a particular class may be needed to achieve successful treatment without problematic side effects. Most individual treatments that fail appear to do so because the medication is not helpful for the targeted symptom, although over a third of stimulant and antipsychotic trials fail because of side effects (Figure 3).[167] Side effects are a more frequent reason for medication discontinuance in children and adolescents with FXS than in adults, which is consistent with prior reports of similar effects.[58] Although behavior in FXS is often difficult to analyze and many patients have behaviors that fall into multiple categories and

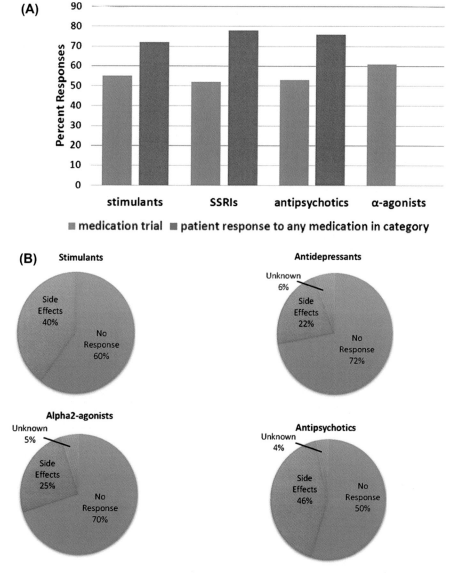

FIGURE 3   (A) Percentage of FXS patients in a clinical setting showing a clinical response to psychopharmacological intervention to a single medication trial or to any medication in a given category after potentially multiple trials of different medications in the category to optimize therapy. Stimulants were used for hyperactivity and attention problems, alpha-agonists for hyperactivity and hyperarousal, SSRIs for anxiety and mood symptoms, and antipsychotics for irritable and aggressive behaviors. (B) Frequency of reasons for failure of medications in different classes given as no response, side effects, or unknown. *Data for this figure were adapted from Berry-Kravis et al.[167]*

sometimes need treatment with a combination of medications to fully address their symptoms, the following subsections will address treatment based on common symptom complexes seen in FXS.

Attention, Hyperactivity, and Impulsivity

Stimulants are helpful in a clinical setting to target distractibility, hyperactivity, and impulsive behavior. A 67% response rate was seen with methylphenidate in 15 patients in the one placebo-controlled study evaluating stimulants in FXS.[169] This is consistent with the report that 73% of individuals with FXS responded without major side effects to some preparation of stimulant in a large FXS cohort in a clinical setting.[167] In another study, boys with FXS who received stimulants had better attention, lower motor activity levels, and higher academic test scores on medicated days versus unmedicated days, although levels of physiological arousal were unaffected by stimulant treatment.[170] Electrodermal studies measuring an enhanced sweat response to stimuli in children with FXS showed a decrease in response toward normal after stimulant treatment.[171]

Although adult males with FXS tend to be less overactive and more anxious, leading to a medication shift toward the use of antidepressants and antipsychotics, some individuals are still helped substantially by the use of stimulants, even into their thirties or forties. Taken together, currently available information suggests that stimulants are helpful in managing distractibility, hyperactivity, and impulsivity symptoms in a subgroup of boys and girls with FXS presenting with prominent difficulty in these behavioral domains.

In some individuals with FXS, stimulants exacerbate anxiety, irritability, or aggressive tendencies and must be abandoned. Indeed, 40% of stimulant trials in a clinical setting were reported to fail because of side effects, which mostly consisted of aggravation of anxiety/irritability/aggressiveness, but could occasionally include appetite suppression with occasional weight loss, stomach discomfort, lethargy, suppression of exuberance, and reduced speech output.[167] Stimulants now come in many different long-acting forms that may be useful in eliminating swings in mood and behavior during the day seen with multiple-dose regimens of fast-acting preparations. Stimulants may induce excessive side effects or may not be effective in children with FXS aged less than 5 or 6 years, although they may be effective if reintroduced at an older age. One study suggested that stimulant preparations in the two major classes, methylphenidate and amphetamine salts, have similar overall response rates and the same profile of reasons for failure.[167] Distinct groups of patients with FXS, however, may respond to or have side effects on only one class of stimulant, which suggests that both classes should

be tried before making a determination about stimulants are helpful for a given patient with FXS.

Alpha 2-agonists clonidine and guanfacine showed about 62% efficacy in a clinical setting in treating hyperactive, hyperaroused, hypersensitive, impulsive, and aggressive behaviors owing to overarousal in boys with FXS,[167] which is consistent with a survey study showing an 80% response rate for management of hyperarousal and hyperactivity.[172] Alpha 2-agonists may be particularly effective in young children who do not tolerate or respond to stimulants and can be helpful for sleep problems, although sedation can also be a problematic side effect. Sedation is often most prominent in the first few weeks after medication initiation and dose increases, and often abates after that. Extended-release preparations of both clonidine and guanfacine exist that can minimize sedation and eliminate the need for multiple daily doses of these agents.

Anxiety/Mood

Antidepressants are helpful in a clinical setting to target anxiety and mood symptoms, and to some extent perseverative behaviors. In a large clinic cohort study, 77% of individuals with FXS responded to at least one antidepressant without major side effects limiting treatment.[167] This is consistent with data from a self-report survey of effects of fluoxetine in adults with FXS, which revealed improvements in anxiety and mood in about 70% of treated individuals.[173] Selective serotonin reuptake inhibitors are the most commonly used form of treatment for females and adults with FXS[165–167] and appear to be particularly helpful for social anxiety and withdrawal in females with FXS. Fluoxetine has been previously reported to be successful for selective mutism in females with FXS and extreme shyness.[174] An unblinded prospective study of effects of sertraline in 12 children with FXS[175] showed improvement in emotional and behavioral parameters after starting sertraline, although some had to discontinue treatment because of disinhibition with increased impulsivity. Taken together, available studies suggest that SSRIs can be useful for management of anxiety and behavioral/emotional symptoms in individuals with FXS.

The predominant side effect of SSRIs in FXS is activation with an increase in hyperactivity and disinhibited behaviors, which may be more pronounced with fluoxetine, although nausea, diarrhea, and sedation are sometimes seen. Insomnia is uncommon as an SSRI side effect in FXS.[167] Less activating SSRIs, such as sertraline or escitalopram, may be better in individuals with FXS and higher levels of hyperactivity and impulsive behavior. For individuals who are too disinhibited with the use of SSRIs, other antidepressants such as venlafaxine may be successful and produce less disinhibition. Tricyclic antidepressants can also work well for bed wetting and sleep dysregulation,[176] although electrocardiograms must be monitored because sudden death, presumable resulting from to cardiac dysrhythmias, has been described in rare individuals with FXS. Bupropion, which increases dopamine levels more than other antidepressants, can help with both attention and mood/anxiety issues. Bupropion can precipitate seizures in at-risk individuals and therefore should not be used in individuals with FXS and active seizures. Trazodone can help with sleep dysregulation as well as anxiety.

Irritability/Aggression

Antipsychotics are generally reserved for individuals with FXS who exhibit more extreme behaviors, and use rates are thus lower than for stimulants and antidepressants. Antipsychotics were helpful in a clinical setting to target irritability and aggression in 76% of individuals with FXS who had treatment trials with one or multiple antipsychotics. The most problematic side effect of antipsychotics is weight gain, although nausea, vomiting, lethargy, and extrapyramidal symptoms can be seen infrequently, and although tardive dyskinesia was not seen in a large FXS clinic cohort treated with antipsychotics.[167] Risperidone was effective clinically in FXS with high response rates for aggressive behavior in older males with FXS, and other aberrant and undesired behaviors in young boys with FXS and autistic traits. This is consistent with the finding that risperidone is safe and effective for aggressive and aberrant behaviors in double-blind, placebo-controlled trials in individuals with autism.[177] Other atypical antipsychotics (quetiapine and ziprasidone) have less effect on weight and were helpful for aggressive behavior in some patients with excessive weight gain with risperidone or olanzapine. Aripiprazole also has less effect on weight and appears to have high response rates in individuals with FXS in clinic cohorts[166,167] and in an open-label trial,[178] for whom, because of its unique pharmacological profile, it may target multiple problematic areas including distractibility, aggressive and agitated behavior, and aberrant social behaviors. Some individuals with FXS, however, simply cannot tolerate aripiprazole because of side effects similar to those seen with stimulants, including aggravation of irritable and perseverative behaviors. This effect is not seen with other atypical antipsychotics, presumably because aripiprazole is the only atypical with partial dopamine agonist activity. Although the newer atypical antipsychotics are less sedating and have a more favorable motor side effect profile than older antipsychotics such as haloperidol and thioridazine, side effects, particularly weight gain in children more than adults,[179] are still more frequent for atypical antipsychotics than for other classes of medications (Figure 3).[167]

In summary, psychopharmacologic treatment of ADHD symptoms, anxiety, hyperarousal, and irritable/aggressive behaviors with medications such as stimulants, SSRIs, alpha-agonists, and antipsychotics, respectively, appears to be helpful in a clinical setting (Figure 3), but response is typically incomplete; and data from a National Survey on FXS showed that about 10–20% of respondents felt that medication was not helpful for the behavior problems treated in their child with FXS, whereas only about 40% felt the medication was helping a lot.[134] There is clearly an unmet need in FXS for better medications to treat behavior and for the development of treatments that target cognitive deficits. Thus, treatments that modify the underlying disorder would be a tremendously important advance.

EMERGING TARGETED TREATMENTS FOR FXS

Recent study of the neurobiology and synaptic mechanisms resulting from absence of FMRP in FXS has become an important window to future targeted treatments for FXS, ASD, and related neurodevelopmental disorders (NDDs).[58,150] The Fmr1 knockout mouse, which makes no functional FMRP, has been a critical resource to understand the role of FMRP in neurons, identify cellular targets for treatment, and explore effects of potential disease-modifying agents (see also Chapter 8). Fragile X mental retardation protein is an mRNA binding protein involved in the transport and translational regulation of a subset of dendritic mRNAs.[58] Fragile X mental retardation protein regulates (inhibits) dendritic protein translation in response to synaptic activation by group 1 metabotropic glutamate receptors (mGluR1 and mGluR5),[180] muscarinic (M1) acetylcholine receptors, and probably multiple Gq-linked receptors. Activation of these receptors results in signaling through ERK- and mTOR-dependent signaling pathways, ultimately resulting in loss of FMRP repressor function at the ribosome, and a pulse of new protein synthesis. Translation of multiple synaptic proteins is regulated by FMRP—for example, STEP and Arc—which are linked to AMPA receptor internalization.[181] Fragile X mental retardation protein also regulates activity of some pre- and postsynaptic ion channels such as BK and SLACK channels through direct protein–protein interactions.[90] These regulatory functions of FMRP appear to be critical for synaptic maturation and strength, because in the absence of FMRP (Figure 4), there is an elevation of levels of synaptic proteins usually controlled by FMRP, immature elongated dendritic spines,[182] abnormal spine density, abnormal synaptic plasticity including enhanced mGluR-activated hippocampal and cerebellar long-term depression, and

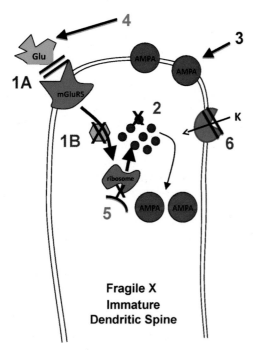

FIGURE 4 Diagram of mGluR (and other Gq-linked receptor)-activated signaling pathway for dendritic translation typically regulated by FMRP in an immature dendritic spine in FXS, showing excessive signaling through the translational activation pathway and enhanced dendritic translation in the absence of FMRP. Numbers in the diagram indicate potential categories of therapeutics that could target the pathway to reverse abnormal activity: (1) agents that reduce activity in signal transduction pathways leading from group 1 mGluR/other Gq-linked receptors to the FMRP regulated dendritic translational machinery (1A reagents acting outside the cell on receptors, 1B reagents acting inside the cell in the signaling pathway), (2) agents that reduce activity of individual proteins regulated by FMRP, (3) agents that increase expression and/or activity of surface AMPA receptors, (4) agents that modify activity of other receptors/proteins that interact with glutamate signaling, (5) agents that block or stall translation of mRNAs regulated by FMRP at the ribosome, and (6) agents that block channels that are overactive owing to a lack of direct protein interaction and modulation by FMRP. AMPA = α-amino-3-hydroxy-5-methyl-4-isoxazole propionic acid; mGluR = group 1 metabotropic glutamate receptors.

impaired LTP in hippocampus, cortex, and amygdala, and proneness to abnormal epileptiform discharges.[58,90] The morphological abnormalities and synaptic plasticity deficits found in the *fmr1* knockout mouse and the *Drosophila* model of FXS, in which there is loss of *dfmr1* (homolog of the *FMR1* gene in the *Drosophila* genome), are associated with numerous cognitive, behavioral, and electrophysiological phenotypes.[58,90]

The abnormalities observed in the absence of FMRP in the mouse model of FXS have led to the identification of treatment targets (Figure 4) directed at (1) reduction of excess activity in signal transduction pathways connecting group 1 mGluRs or other Gq-linked receptors to the dendritic translational machinery, (2) reduction of excessive activity of proteins normally regulated by FMRP, (3) increasing expression and activation of surface

AMPA receptors, (4) modification of activity of GABA and other receptors/proteins that regulate glutamate signaling or translational signaling pathways, and (5) using micro RNAs to block excessive translation of mRNAs normally regulated by FMRP.[58,90] Treatments aimed at all of these types of targets have shown success in reversing phenotypes in the *Fmr1* knockout mouse[183–185] and *dfxr* fly[186] models (Table 4) even in adulthood,[187] which suggests that there may not be an absolute developmental requirement for FMRP.

Successful preclinical testing in FXS models has led to early proof-of concept clinical trials and subsequent larger trials for some of the proposed targeted treatments (Table 4). Lithium, which is thought to reduce excess mGluR-dependent activation of translation by attenuating GSK3β activity and possibly phosphatidyl inositol turnover, resulted in significant improvement in behavioral scales, verbal memory, and abnormal ERK phosphorylation rates in lymphocytes in a 2-month pilot, open-label, proof-of-concept trial in children and young adults with FXS.[188] A pilot, placebo-controlled, crossover trial of minocycline, an antibiotic that inhibits overexpressed synaptic MMP9 in FXS models, conducted in children with FXS demonstrated mild global clinical improvement and reduction of blood MMP9 levels in responders.[189]

GABA-B agonist arbaclofen presumably lowers presynaptic glutamate release with resultant reduction of group 1 mGluR signaling. In a phase II double-blind, placebo-controlled, crossover trial,[190] arbaclofen showed improvement over placebo in the entire per protocol group for social withdrawal and parent nominated problem behaviors. However, a large phase III, placebo-controlled trial in adolescents and adults with FXS did not show benefits for arbaclofen over placebo in the primary outcome of social withdrawal. An additional phase III trial in children with FXS showed promise, but full analyses are pending. Acamprosate, currently approved by the Food and Drug Administration for alcohol withdrawal, with agonist properties at both GABA-A and GABA-B receptors, has shown promise for hyperactivity and social functioning in FXS in an open-label trial.[191] Acamprosate and GABA-A agonist ganaxolone are being tested in small placebo-controlled trials in FXS (clinicaltrials.gov).

Multiple negative modulators of the mGluR5 receptor (group 1 mGluR expressed throughout the brain) have been in trials in FXS. A single oral dose of fenobam[192] resulted in a significant improvement in abnormal prepulse inhibition compared with untreated control subjects with FXS. A phase II double-blind, placebo-controlled, crossover trial of AFQ056 in 30 adult males with FXS treated for 28 days, each with AFQ and placebo,[193] suggested improvement in maladaptive behavior in a post hoc analysis in the subgroup with

TABLE 4 Targeted Treatments in Development for FXS

Mechanism/Pathway Target (Number for Type of Mechanism in Figure 3)	Phase of Development			
	Preclinical	Phase I/Open Label	Phase II	Phase III
Block excess group 1 mGluR signaling directly by inhibiting mGluR5 receptor (1A)	MPEP	AFQ056	AFQ056	
	Fenobam	Fenobam	RO4917526	
	CTEP	STX107		
	AFQ056			
	STX107			
Block excess group 1 mGluR signaling by inhibiting pathway leading from receptor activation to protein translation (1B)	*Lithium*	*Lithium*	NNZ2566	
	PAK inhibitors	*Lovastatin*	Metadoxine	
	Lovastatin			
	GSK3B inhibitors			
	PIKE inhibitors			
	PI3K inhibitors			
	NNZ2566			
	Metadoxine			
	Bryostatin			
Block excess activity of protein produced to excess in absence of FMRP (2)	*Minocycline*	Rolipram	*Minocycline*	
	STEP inhibitors	*Minocycline*		
	Rolipram			
	PDE inhibitors			
Increase deficient AMPA receptor activity (3)	CX516		CX516	
Regulate signaling through nonglutamate receptors to reduce or balance group 1 mGluR or other abnormal receptor signaling resulting from absence of FMRP (4)	Baclofen	*Acamprosate*	Arbaclofen	Arbaclofen
	Arbaclofen	Ganaxolone	*Acamprosate*	
	Acamprosate	*Donepezil*	Ganaxolone	
	Ganaxolone		Metadoxine	
	Metadoxine		*Donepezil*	
Block excess synthesis of specific proteins with micro RNAs (5)	Mir-125a			
Regulate abnormal channel activity in absence of FMRP (6)	BK channel blockers	BK channel blockers		
	SLACK channel blockers			

Drug names in italics are those that are already approved by the Food and Drug Administration and on the market for an indication other than FXS. Mechanism of action of specific medications in the table: lithium decreases phosphatidylinositol turnover and GSK3B activity; lovastatin is an indirect ERK inhibitor; metodoxine reduces excess activation of ERK and AKT possibly through a GABA-mediated mechanism; NNZ-2256 reduces excess activation of ERK and AKT, Bryostatin is a protein kinase C epsilon inhibitor; minocycline reduces excess MMP9 activity; rolipram is a phosphodiesterase inhibitor, baclofen/arbaclofen are GABA-B agonists; acamprosate is a GABA-B and GABA-A agonist; ganaxolone is a GABA-A agonist; donepezil raises acetylcholine levels by inhibiting acetylcholinesterase; and mir-125a blocks PSD-95 translation at the ribosome.

full methylation of *FMR1*. Larger multinational trials of AFQ056 and RO4917523, another mGluR5-negative modulator from Roche, have not supported this behavioral outcome but have not addressed cognitive outcomes (clinicaltrials.gov).

Although many neuronal targets for treating the underlying disorder in FXS have been identified, and translational work has begun, there have been problems with demonstrating disease modification in early trials because there are still many uncertainties about how to demonstrate treatment effects optimally in a clinical trial setting.[90,194] Major trial design issues in FXS trials potentially include variable but narrow dosing windows, timing (age) and length of treatment necessary, the potential need for cognitive or behavioral interventions to see drug effects on synaptic plasticity in the form of learning, large placebo effects, and the lack of validated, sensitive biomarkers and functional outcome measures in FXS.[194] These trial design issues will need to be resolved to be able to demonstrate disease modification in FXS, but it is hoped that in the future treatment to reverse the underlying disorder will eventually replace or complement supportive treatment.

There is significant overlap in molecular and cellular pathways involving FMRP and those that include gene products associated with ASD.[27,58] This overlap falls into three broad categories: (1) defects in proteins in the signaling cascade for activation of FMRP-regulated translation such as SHANK, mTOR, PAK, and PTEN; (2) defects in proteins regulated directly by FMRP such as PSD95 and Arc; and (3) defects in proteins involved in the balance of activity in brain glutamate and GABA systems. Indeed, this pathway overlap has been supported by the findings that: (1) FMRP binds to one-third to one-half of all genes identified as associated with ASD in a meta-analysis of exome screening studies[195]; (2) FMRP target genes are more likely than other genes with similar expression patterns to contribute to ASD[196]; and (3) common variants in genes involved in postsynaptic regulation of FMRP (CAMK4, GRM1, and CYFIP1) are risk factors for ASD.[197] Treatments directed at mechanisms involving all of these overlap areas are being explored in FXS trials; if successful, progress in the development of targeted treatments for FXS may result in targeted treatments to reverse central nervous system defects and clinical manifestations of ASD, other NDDs, and ID.

References

1. Coffee B, Keith K, Albizua I, et al. Incidence of fragile X syndrome by newborn screening for methylated FMR1 DNA. *Am J Hum Genet* October 2009;**85**(4):503–14.
2. Willemsen R, Levenga J, Oostra BA. CGG repeat in the FMR1 gene: size matters. *Clin Genet* September 2011;**80**(3):214–25.
3. Seltzer MM, Baker MW, Hong J, Maenner M, Greenberg J, Mandel D. Prevalence of CGG expansions of the FMR1 gene in a US population-based sample. *Am J Med Genet* July 2012;**159B**(5):589–97.
4. Tassone F, Iong KP, Tong T-H, et al. FMR1 CGG allele size and prevalence ascertained through newborn screening in the United States. *Genome Med* December 21, 2012;**4**(12):100.
5. Ladd PD, Smith LE, Rabaia NA, et al. An antisense transcript spanning the CGG repeat region of FMR1 is upregulated in premutation carriers but silenced in full mutation individuals. *Hum Mol Genet* December 15, 2007;**16**(24):3174–87.
6. Iliff AJ, Renoux AJ, Krans A, Usdin K, Sutton MA, Todd PK. Impaired activity-dependent FMRP translation and enhanced mGluR-dependent LTD in Fragile X premutation mice. *Hum Mol Genet* April 15, 2013;**22**(6):1180–92.
7. Berry-Kravis E, Abrams L, Coffey SM, et al. Fragile X-associated tremor/ataxia syndrome: clinical features, genetics, and testing guidelines. *Mov Disord* October 31, 2007;**22**(14):2018–30. quiz 2140.
8. Allingham-Hawkins DJ, Babul-Hirji R, Chitayat D, et al. Fragile X premutation is a significant risk factor for premature ovarian failure: the International Collaborative POF in Fragile X study—preliminary data. *Am J Med Genet* April 2, 1999;**83**(4):322–5.
9. Bussani C, Papi L, Sestini R, et al. Premature ovarian failure and fragile X premutation: a study on 45 women. *Eur J Obstet Gynecol Reprod Biol* February 10, 2004;**112**(2):189–91.
10. Marozzi A, Vegetti W, Manfredini E, et al. Association between idiopathic premature ovarian failure and fragile X premutation. *Hum Reprod* January 2000;**15**(1):197–202.
11. Murray A, Webb J, Grimley S, Conway G, Jacobs P. Studies of FRAXA and FRAXE in women with premature ovarian failure. *J Med Genet* August 1998;**35**(8):637–40.
12. Welt CK, Smith PC, Taylor AE. Evidence of early ovarian aging in fragile X premutation carriers. *J Clin Endocrinol Metab* September 2004;**89**(9):4569–74.
13. Hundscheid RD, Braat DD, Kiemeney LA, Smits AP, Thomas CM. Increased serum FSH in female fragile X premutation carriers with either regular menstrual cycles or on oral contraceptives. *Hum Reprod* March 2001;**16**(3):457–62.
14. Rohr J, Allen EG, Charen K, et al. Anti-Mullerian hormone indicates early ovarian decline in fragile X mental retardation (FMR1) premutation carriers: a preliminary study. *Hum Reprod* May 2008;**23**(5):1220–5.
15. Allen EG, Sullivan AK, Marcus M, et al. Examination of reproductive aging milestones among women who carry the FMR1 premutation. *Hum Reprod* August 2007;**22**(8):2142–52.
16. Turner G, Robinson H, Wake S, Martin N. Dizygous twinning and premature menopause in fragile X syndrome. *Lancet* November 26, 1994;**344**(8935):1500.
17. Sullivan AK, Marcus M, Epstein MP, et al. Association of FMR1 repeat size with ovarian dysfunction. *Hum Reprod* February 2005;**20**(2):402–12.
18. Hagerman RJ, Berry-Kravis E, Kaufmann WE, et al. Advances in the treatment of fragile X syndrome. *Pediatrics* 2009;**123**(1):378–90.
19. Hunter JE, Rohr JK, Sherman SL. Co-occurring diagnoses among FMR1 premutation allele carriers. *Clin Genet* April 2010;**77**(4):374–81.
20. Coffey SM, Cook K, Tartaglia N, et al. Expanded clinical phenotype of women with the FMR1 premutation. *Am J Med Genet A* April 15, 2008;**146A**(8):1009–16.
21. Chonchaiya W, Nguyen DV, Au J, et al. Clinical involvement in daughters of men with fragile X-associated tremor ataxia syndrome. *Clin Genet* July 2010;**78**(1):38–46.
22. Winarni TI, Chonchaiya W, Sumekar TA, et al. Immune-mediated disorders among women carriers of fragile X premutation alleles. *Am J Med Genet A* October 2012;**158A**(10):2473–81.
23. Nolin SL, Sah S, Glicksman A, et al. Fragile X AGG analysis provides new risk predictions for 45–69 repeat alleles. *Am J Med Genet A* 2013;**161**(4):771–8.
24. Loesch DZ, Khaniani MS, Slater HR, et al. Small CGG repeat expansion alleles of FMR1 gene are associated with parkinsonism. *Clin Genet* 2009;**76**(5):471–6.
25. Hall DA, Berry-Kravis E, Zhang W, et al. FMR1 gray-zone alleles: association with Parkinson's disease in women? *Mov Disord* 2011;**26**(10):1900–6.
26. Hall D, Tassone F, Klepitskaya O, Leehey M. Fragile X—associated tremor ataxia syndrome in FMR1 gray zone allele carriers. *Mov Disord* 2012;**27**(2):297–301.
27. Loesch DZ, Huggins RM, Hagerman RJ. Phenotypic variation and FMRP levels in fragile X. *Ment Retard Dev Disabil Res Rev* 2004;**10**(1):31–41.
28. Kidd SALA, Barbouth D, et al. Fragile X syndrome: a review of associated medical problems. *Pediatrics* 2014;**134**(5):995–1005.

29. Hagerman RJ, Altshul-Stark D, McBogg P. Recurrent otitis media in the fragile X syndrome. *Am J Dis Child* 1987;**141**(2):184−7.

30. Hagerman RJ, Falkenstein AR. An association between recurrent otitis media in infancy and later hyperactivity. *Clin Pediatr (Phila)* 1987;**26**(5):253−7.

31. Hagerman RJ, Hagerman PJ. *Fragile X syndrome: diagnosis, treatment, and research.* JHU Press; 2002.

32. Hoffman HJ, Daly KA, Bainbridge KE, et al. Panel 1: epidemiology, natural history, and risk factors. *Otolaryngol Head Neck Surg* 2013;**148**(4 Suppl.):E1−25. http://dx.doi.org/10.1177/0194599812460984.

33. Alanay Y, Unal F, Turanli G, et al. A multidisciplinary approach to the management of individuals with fragile X syndrome. *J Intellect Disabil Res* 2007;**51**(Pt 2):151−61.

34. Hatton DD, Buckley E, Lachiewicz A, Roberts J. Ocular status of boys with fragile X syndrome: a prospective study. *J AAPOS* 1998;**2**(5):298−302.

35. Maino DM, Wesson M, Schlange D, Cibis G, Maino JH. Optometric findings in the fragile X syndrome. *Optom Vis Sci* 1991;**68**(8):634−40.

36. Van Splunder J, Stilma JS, Evenhuis HM. Visual performance in specific syndromes associated with intellectual disability. *Eur J Ophthalmol* 2003;**13**(6):566−74.

37. King RA, Hagerman RJ, Houghton M. Ocular findings in Fragile X syndrome. *Dev Brain Dysfunct* 1995;**8**(4−6):223−9.

38. Kleigman RN, Stanton B, Geme JS, Schor N, Behrman RE. *Nelson textbook of pediatrics.* 19th ed. Philadelphia: Elsevier Saunders; 2011.

39. Repka MX, Friedman DS, Katz J, Ibironke J, Giordano L, Tielsch JM. The prevalence of ocular structural disorders and nystagmus among preschool-aged children. *J AAPOS* April 2012;**16**(2):182−4.

40. Comery TA, Harris JB, Willems PJ, et al. Abnormal dendritic spines in fragile X knockout mice: maturation and pruning deficits. *Proc Natl Acad Sci USA* May 13, 1997;**94**(10):5401−4.

41. Musumeci SA, Bosco P, Calabrese G, et al. Audiogenic seizures susceptibility in transgenic mice with fragile X syndrome. *Epilepsia* January 2000;**41**(1):19−23.

42. Irwin SA, Patel B, Idupulapati M, et al. Abnormal dendritic spine characteristics in the temporal and visual cortices of patients with fragile-X syndrome: a quantitative examination. *Am J Med Genet* January 15, 2001;**98**(2):161−7.

43. Berry-Kravis E. Epilepsy in fragile X syndrome. *Dev Med Child Neurol* 2002;**44**(11):724−8.

44. Finelli PF, Pueschel SM, Padre-Mendoza T, O'Brien MM. Neurological findings in patients with the fragile-X syndrome. *J Neurol Neurosurg Psychiatry* 1985;**48**(2):150−3.

45. Incorpora G, Sorge G, Sorge A, Pavone L. Epilepsy in fragile X syndrome. *Brain Dev* 2002;**24**(8):766−9.

46. Kluger G, Bohm I, Laub MC, Waldenmaier C. Epilepsy and fragile X gene mutations. *Pediatr Neurol* 1996;**15**(4):358−60.

47. Musumeci SA, Ferri R, Colognola RM, Neri G, Sanfilippo S, Bergonzi P. Prevalence of a novel epileptogenic EEG pattern in the Martin-Bell syndrome. *Am J Med Genet* 1988;**30**(1−2):207−12.

48. Musumeci SA, Ferri R, Elia M, Colognola RM, Bergonzi P, Tassinari CA. Epilepsy and fragile X syndrome: a follow-up study. *Am J Med Genet* 1991;**38**(2−3):511−3.

49. Tondo M, Poo P, Naudo M, et al. Predisposition to epilepsy in fragile X syndrome: does the Val66Met polymorphism in the BDNF gene play a role? *Epilepsy Behav* 2011;**22**(3):581−3. http://dx.doi.org/10.1016/j.yebeh.2011.08.003. Epub 2011 Sep 3.

50. Vieregge P, Froster-Iskenius U. Clinico-neurological investigations in the fra(X) form of mental retardation. *J Neurol* 1989;**236**(2):85−92.

51. Wisniewski KE, French JH, Fernando S, et al. Fragile X syndrome: associated neurological abnormalities and developmental disabilities. *Ann Neurol* 1985;**18**(6):665−9.

52. Wisniewski KE, Segan SM, Miezejeski CM, Sersen EA, Rudelli RD. The Fra(X) syndrome: neurological, electrophysiological, and neuropathological abnormalities. *Am J Med Genet* 1991;**38**(2−3):476−80.

53. Bastaki LA, Hegazy F, Al-Heneidi MM, Turki N, Azab AS, Naguib KK. Fragile X syndrome: a clinico-genetic study of mentally retarded patients in Kuwait. *East Mediterr Health J* 2004;**10**(1−2):116−24.

54. Brodnum Nielsen K. Diagnosis of the fragile X syndrome (Martin-Bell syndrome). Clinical findings in 27 males with the fragile site at Xq28. *J Ment Defic Res* 1983;**27**(Pt 3):211−26.

55. Fryns JP. The fragile X syndrome. A study of 83 families. *Clin Genet* 1984;**26**(6):497−528.

56. Louhivuori V, Arvio M, Soronen P, Oksanen V, Paunio T, Castren ML. The Val66Met polymorphism in the BDNF gene is associated with epilepsy in fragile X syndrome. *Epilepsy Res* 2009;**85**(1):114−7. http://dx.doi.org/10.1016/j.eplepsyres.2009.01.005. Epub 2009 Apr 25.

57. Bailey DB, Raspa M, Olmsted M, Holiday DB. Co-occurring conditions associated with *FMR1* gene variations: Findings from a national parent survey. *Am J Med Genet* 2008;**146A**(16):2060.

58. Berry-Kravis E, Knox A, Hervey C. Targeted treatments for fragile X syndrome. *J Neurodev Disord* 2011;**3**(3):193−210. http://dx.doi.org/10.1007/978-3-642-21649-7_17. Epub 2011 Feb 19.

59. Musumeci SA, Hagerman RJ, Ferri R, et al. Epilepsy and EEG findings in males with fragile X syndrome. *Epilepsia* 1999;**40**(8):1092−9.

60. Berry-Kravis E, Raspa M, Loggin-Hester L, Bishop E, Holiday D, Bailey DB. Seizures in fragile X syndrome: characteristics and comorbid diagnoses. *Am J Intellect Dev Disabil* 2010;**115**(6):461−72. http://dx.doi.org/10.1352/1944-7558-115.6.461.

61. Sabaratnam M, Vroegop PG, Gangadharan SK. Epilepsy and EEG findings in 18 males with fragile X syndrome. *Seizure* 2001;**10**(1):60−3.

62. Di Bonaventura C, Mari F, Pierallini A, et al. Status epilepticus in a patient with fragile X syndrome: electro-clinical features and peri-ictal neuroimaging. *Epileptic Disord* 2006;**8**(3):195−9.

63. Gauthey M, Poloni CB, Ramelli GP, Roulet-Perez E, Korff CM. Status epilepticus in fragile X syndrome. *Epilepsia* 2010;**51**(12):2470−3. http://dx.doi.org/10.1111/j.1528-1167.2010.02761.x. Epub 2010 Nov 3.

64. Garcia-Nonell C, Ratera ER, Harris S, et al. Secondary medical diagnosis in fragile X syndrome with and without autism spectrum disorder. *Am J Med Genet A* 2008;**146A**(15):1911−6. http://dx.doi.org/10.1002/ajmg.a.32290.

65. Berry-Kravis E, Krause SE, Block SS, et al. Effect of CX516, an AMPA-modulating compound, on cognition and behavior in fragile X syndrome: a controlled trial. *J Child Adolesc Psychopharmacol* 2006;**16**(5):525−40.

66. Gadow KD, Nolan EE, Sprafkin J, Schwartz J. Tics and psychiatric comorbidity in children and adolescents. *Dev Med Child Neurol* May 2002;**44**(5):330−8.

67. Chonchaiya W, Tassone F, Ashwood P, et al. Autoimmune disease in mothers with the FMR1 premutation is associated with seizures in their children with fragile X syndrome. *Hum Genet* 2010;**128**(5):539−48. http://dx.doi.org/10.1007/s00439-010-0882-8. Epub 2010 Sep 1.

68. Gabis LV, Baruch YK, Jokel A, Raz R. Psychiatric and autistic comorbidity in fragile X syndrome across ages. *J Child Neurol* 2011;**26**(8):940−8. http://dx.doi.org/10.1177/0883073810395937. Epub 2011 Apr 27.

69. Mindell JA, Meltzer LJ, Carskadon MA, Chervin RD. Developmental aspects of sleep hygiene: findings from the 2004 National Sleep Foundation Sleep in America Poll. *Sleep Med* 2009;**10**(7):771−9. http://dx.doi.org/10.1016/j.sleep.2008.07.016. Epub 2009 Mar 12.

70. Owens JA, Witmans M. Sleep problems. *Curr Probl Pediatr Adolesc Health Care* 2004;**34**(4):154—79.

71. Goodlin-Jones BL, Tang K, Liu J, Anders TF. Sleep patterns in preschool-age children with autism, developmental delay, and typical development. *J Am Acad Child Adolesc Psychiatry* August 2008;**47**(8):930—8.

72. Krakowiak P, Goodlin-Jones B, Hertz-Picciotto I, Croen LA, Hansen RL. Sleep problems in children with autism spectrum disorders, developmental delays, and typical development: a population-based study. *J Sleep Res* June 2008;**17**(2):197—206.

73. Polimeni MA, Richdale AL, Francis AJ. A survey of sleep problems in autism, Asperger's disorder and typically developing children. *J Intellect Disabil Res* April 2005;**49**(Pt 4):260—8.

74. Richdale AL. Sleep problems in autism: prevalence, cause, and intervention. *Dev Med Child Neurol* 1999;**41**(1):60—6.

75. Robinson AM, Richdale AL. Sleep problems in children with an intellectual disability: parental perceptions of sleep problems, and views of treatment effectiveness. *Child Care Health Dev* March 2004;**30**(2):139—50.

76. Kronk R, Dahl R, Noll R. Caregiver reports of sleep problems on a convenience sample of children with fragile X syndrome. *Am J Intellect Dev Disabil* 2009;**114**(6):383—92. http://dx.doi.org/10.1352/1944-7588-114.6.383.

77. Kronk R, Bishop EE, Raspa M, Bickel JO, Mandel DA, Bailey Jr DB. Prevalence, nature, and correlates of sleep problems among children with fragile X syndrome based on a large scale parent survey. *Sleep* 2010;**33**(5):679—87.

78. Nelson SP, Chen EH, Syniar GM, Christoffel KK. Prevalence of symptoms of gastroesophageal reflux during childhood: a pediatric practice-based survey. Pediatric Practice Research Group. *Arch Pediatr Adolesc Med* February 2000;**154**(2):150—4.

79. Sreeram N, Wren C, Bhate M, Robertson P, Hunter S. Cardiac abnormalities in the fragile X syndrome. *Br Heart J* 1989;**61**(3):289—91.

80. Crabbe LS, Bensky AS, Hornstein L, Schwartz DC. Cardiovascular abnormalities in children with fragile X syndrome. *Pediatrics* 1993;**91**(4):714—5.

81. Loehr JP, Synhorst DP, Wolfe RR, Hagerman RJ. Aortic root dilatation and mitral valve prolapse in the fragile X syndrome. *Am J Med Genet* 1986;**23**(1—2):189—94.

82. Prouty LA, Rogers RC, Stevenson RE, et al. Fragile X syndrome: growth, development, and intellectual function. *Am J Med Genet* 1988;**30**(1—2):123—42.

83. Stevenson RE, Prouty LA, Dean JA. Fragile X syndrome I. Prenatal growth. *Proc Greenwood Genet Center* 1988;**7**:84—6.

84. Brondum Nielsen K. Growth pattern in boys with fragile X. *Am J Med Genet* 1988;**30**(1—2):143—7.

85. Lachiewicz AM, Dawson DV, Spiridigliozzi GA. Physical characteristics of young boys with fragile X syndrome: reasons for difficulties in making a diagnosis in young males. *Am J Med Genet* 2000;**92**(4):229—36.

86. Butler MG, Brunschwig A, Miller LK, Hagerman RJ. Standards for selected anthropometric measurements in males with the fragile X syndrome. *Pediatrics* 1992;**89**(6 Pt 1):1059—62.

87. Loesch DZ, Huggins RM, Hoang NH. Growth in stature in fragile X families: a mixed longitudinal study. *Am J Med Genet* 1995;**58**(3):249—56.

88. Beemer FA, Veenema H, de Pater JM. Cerebral gigantism (Sotos syndrome) in two patients with fra(X) chromosomes. *Am J Med Genet* 1986;**23**(1—2):221—6.

89. de Vries BB, Robinson H, Stolte-Dijkstra I, et al. General overgrowth in the fragile X syndrome: variability in the phenotypic expression of the *FMR1* gene mutation. *J Med Genet* 1995;**32**(10):764—9.

90. Berry-Kravis E. Mechanism-based treatments in neurodevelopmental disorders: fragile X syndrome. *Pediatr Neurol* May 2014;**50**(4):297—302.

91. Jacquemont S, Berry-Kravis E, Hagerman R, et al. The challenges of clinical trials in fragile X syndrome. *Psychopharmacology (Berl)* 2014;**231**(6):1237—50.

92. Meryash DL, Cronk CE, Sachs B, Gerald PS. An anthropometric study of males with the fragile-X syndrome. *Am J Med Genet* 1984;**17**(1):159—74.

93. Partington MW. The fragile X syndrome II: preliminary data on growth and development in males. *Am J Med Genet* 1984;**17**(1):175—94.

94. Thake A, Todd J, Bundey S, Webb T. Is it possible to make a clinical diagnosis of the fragile X syndrome in a boy? *Arch Dis Child* 1985;**60**(11):1001—7.

95. Kaufmann WE, Abrams MT, Chen W, Reiss AL. Genotype, molecular phenotype, and cognitive phenotype: correlations in fragile X syndrome. *Am J Med Genet* 1999;**83**(4):286.

96. de Vries BB, Wiegers AM, Smits AP, et al. Mental status of females with an FMR1 gene full mutation. *Am J Hum Genet* May 1996;**58**(5):1025.

97. Freund LS, Reiss AL, Abrams MT. Psychiatric disorders associated with fragile X in the young female. *Pediatrics* February 1993;**91**(2):321.

98. Sudhalter V, Cohen IL, Silverman W, Wolf-Schein EG. Conversational analyses of males with fragile X, down syndrome, and autism: comparison of the emergence of deviant language. *Am J Ment Retard* 1990;**94**.

99. Sudhalter V, Maranion M, Brooks P. Expressive semantic deficit in the productive language of males with fragile X syndrome. *Am J Med Genet* 1992;**43**(1—2):65—71.

100. Sudhalter V, Scarborough HS, Cohen IL. Syntactic delay and pragmatic deviance in the language of fragile X males. *Am J Med Genet* 1991;**38**(2—3):493.

101. Cornish KM, Munir F, Cross G. The nature of the spatial deficit in young females with Fragile-X syndrome: a neuropsychological and molecular perspective. *Neuropsychologia* November 1, 1998;**36**(11):1239.

102. Hagerman R, Kemper M, Hudson M. Learning disabilities and attentional problems in boys with the fragile X syndrome. *Am J Dis Child* 1985;**139**(7):674—8.

103. Cornish KM, Munir F, Cross G. Differential impact of the FMR-1 full mutation on memory and attention functioning: a neuropsychological perspective. *J Cogn Neurosci* 2001;**13**(1):144—50.

104. Munir F, Cornish KM, Wilding J. A neuropsychological profile of attention deficits in young males with fragile X syndrome. *Neuropsychologia* August 1, 2000;**38**(9):1261.

105. Scerif G, Cornish K, Wilding J, Driver J, Karmiloff-Smith A. Visual search in typically developing toddlers and toddlers with Fragile X or Williams syndrome. *Dev Sci* 2004;**7**(1):116.

106. Cornish K, Sudhalter V, Turk J. Attention and language in fragile X. *Ment Retard Dev Disabil Rev* 2004;**10**(1):11—6.

107. Bennetto L, Taylor AK, Pennington BF, Porter D, Hagerman RJ. Profile of cognitive functioning in women with the fragile X mutation. *Neuropsychology* 2001;**15**(2):290.

108. Mazzocco MM, Pennington BF, Hagerman RJ. The neurocognitive phenotype of female carriers of fragile X: additional evidence for specificity. *J Dev Behav Pediatr* 1993;**14**(5):328—35.

109. Munir F, Cornish KM, Wilding J. Nature of the working memory deficit in fragile-X syndrome. *Brain Cogn* December 2000;**44**(3):387.

110. Jakala P, Hanninen T, Ryynanen M, et al. Fragile-X: neuropsychological test performance, CGG triplet repeat lengths, and hippocampal volumes. *J Clin Invest* July 15, 1997;**100**(2):331.

111. Loesch DZ, Huggins RM, Bui QM, Epstein JL, Taylor AK, Hagerman RJ. Effect of the deficits of fragile X mental retardation protein on cognitive status of fragile X males and females assessed by robust pedigree analysis. *J Dev Behav Pediatr* 2002;**23**(6):416—23.

112. Kaufman AS. *K-ABC: Kaufman assessment battery for children: interpretive manual.* Circle Pines (MN): American Guidance Service; 1983.

113. Burack JA, Shulman C, Katzir E, Schaap T, Iarocci G, Amir PN. Cognitive and behavioural development of Israeli males with fragile X and down syndrome. *Int J Behav Dev* June 1999;**23**(2):519.

114. Hodapp RM, Leckman JF, Dykens EM, Sparrow SS, Zelinsky D, Ort S. K-ABC profiles in children with fragile X syndrome, down syndrome, and nonspecific mental retardation. *Am J Ment Retard* 1992;**97**.

115. Braden M. Behavior in the classroom. In: *Paper presented at: Greater Chicago Fragile X Fall Education Workshop*; 2014.

116. Stackhouse T, Scharfenaker S. A multidisciplinary approach to understanding hyperarousal in fragile X syndrome. In: *Paper presented at: International Fragile X Conference*; 2014.

117. Dykens EM, Hodapp RM, Leckman JF. Strengths and weaknesses in the intellectual functioning of males with fragile X syndrome. *Am J Ment Defic* 1987;**92**(2):234.

118. Fisch GS, Carpenter N, Holden JJA, et al. Longitudinal changes in cognitive and adaptive behavior in fragile X females: a prospective multicenter analysis. *Am J Med Genet* 1999;**83**(4):308.

119. Fisch GS, Simensen R, Tarleton J, et al. Longitudinal study of cognitive abilities and adaptive behavior levels in fragile X males: a prospective multicenter analysis. *Am J Med Genet* 1996;**64**(2):356.

120. Klaiman C, Quintin E-M, Jo B, et al. Longitudinal profiles of adaptive behavior in fragile X syndrome. *Pediatrics* 2014;**134**(2):315–24.

121. Baumgardner TL, Reiss AL, Freund LS, Abrams MT. Specification of the neurobehavioral phenotype in males with fragile X syndrome. *Pediatrics* May 1995;**95**(5):744.

122. Hagerman RJ, Jackson C, Amiri K, O'Connor R, Sobesky W, Silverman AC. Girls with fragile X syndrome: physical and neuro-cognitive status and outcome. *Pediatrics* 1992;**89**(3):395–400.

123. Borghgraef M, Fryns JP, Dlelkens A, Pyck K, Berghe H. Fragile (X) syndrome: a study of the psychological profile in 23 prepubertal patients. *Clin Genet* 1987;**32**(3):179.

124. Turk J. Fragile X syndrome and attentional deficits. *J Appl Res Intellect Disabil* 1998;**11**(3):175.

125. Cordeiro L, Ballinger E, Hagerman R, Hessl D. Clinical assessment of DSM-IV anxiety disorders in fragile X syndrome: prevalence and characterization. *J Neurodev Disord* 2011;**3**(1):57–67.

126. Reiss AL, Freund L, Abrams MT, Boehm C, Kazazian H. Neurobehavioral effects of the fragile X premutation in adult women: a controlled study. *Am J Hum Genet* 1993;**52**(5):884.

127. Boccia ML, Roberts JE. Behavior and autonomic nervous system function assessed via heart period measures: the case of hyperarousal in boys with fragile X syndrome. *Behav Res Methods Instrum Comput* 2000;**32**(1):5–10.

128. Cohen IL. A theoretical analysis of the role of hyperarousal in the learning and behavior of fragile X males. *Ment Retard Dev Disabil Rev* 1995;**1**(4):286–91.

129. Bailey DJ, Mesibov GB, Hatton DD, Clark RD, Roberts JE, Mayhew L. Autistic behavior in young boys with fragile x syndrome. *J Autism Dev Disord* December 1998;**28**(6):499.

130. Belser RC, Sudhalter V. Conversational characteristics of children with fragile X syndrome: repetitive speech. *J Info* 2001;**106**(1).

131. Hagerman RJ. *Fragile X syndrome. Management of genetic syndromes.* 2005.

132. Symons FJ, Byiers BJ, Raspa M, Bishop E, Bailey Jr DB. Self-injurious behavior and fragile X syndrome: findings from the national fragile X survey. *Am J Intellect Dev Disabil* 2010;**115**(6):473–81.

133. Merenstein SA, Sobesky WE, Taylor AK, Riddle JE, Tran HX, Hagerman RJ. Molecular-clinical correlations in males with an expanded FMR1 mutation. *Am J Med Genet* 1996;**64**(2):388–94.

134. Bailey DB, Raspa M, Bishop E, Olmsted M, Mallya UG, Berry-Kravis E. Medication utilization for targeted symptoms in children and adults with fragile X syndrome: US survey. *J Dev Behav Ped* February 2012;**33**(1):62–9.

135. Smith LE, Barker ET, Seltzer MM, Abbeduto L, Greenberg JS. Behavioral phenotype of fragile X syndrome in adolescence and adulthood. *Am J Intellect Dev Disabil* 2012;**117**(1):1.

136. Brady N, Skinner D, Roberts J, Hennon E. Communication in young children with fragile X syndrome: a qualitative study of mothers' perspectives. *Am J Speech Lang Pathol* 2006;**15**(4):353.

137. Levy Y, Gottesman R, Borochowitz Z, Frydman M, Sagi M. Language in boys with fragile X syndrome. *J Child Lang* 2006;**33**(1):125.

138. Roberts JE, Mirrett P, Anderson K, Burchinal M, Neebe E. Early communication, symbolic behavior, and social profiles of young males with fragile X syndrome. *Am J Speech Lang Pathol* 2002;**11**(3):295–304.

139. Roberts JE, Mirrett P, Burchinal M. Receptive and expressive communication development of young males with fragile X syndrome. *J Inf* 2001;**106**(3).

140. Abbeduto L, Hagerman RJ. Language and communication in fragile X syndrome. *Ment Ret Dev Dis Res Rev* November 1997;**3**(4):313.

141. Lewis P, Abbeduto L, Murphy M, et al. Cognitive, language and social-cognitive skills of individuals with fragile X syndrome with and without autism. *J Intellect Disabil Res* 2006;**50**(7):532–45.

142. McDuffie A, Kover S, Abbeduto L, Lewis P, Brown T. Profiles of receptive and expressive language abilities in boys with comorbid fragile X syndrome and autism. *Am J Intellect Dev Disabil* January 2012;**117**(1):18.

143. Murphy MM, Abbeduto L. Indirect genetic effects and the early language development of children with genetic mental retardation syndromes: the role of joint attention. *Infants Young Child* 2005;**18**(1):47–59.

144. Losh M, Martin GE, Klusek J, Hogan-Brown AL, Sideris J. Social communication and theory of mind in boys with autism and fragile X syndrome. *Front Psychol* 2012;**3**.

145. Mazzocco MM, Thompson L, Sudhalter V, Belser RC, Lesniak-Karpiak K, Ross JL. Language use in females with fragile X or turner syndrome during brief initial social interactions. *J Dev Behav Pediatr* 2006;**27**(4):319–28.

146. Ozonoff S, Heung K, Byrd R, Hansen R, Hertz-Picciotto I. The onset of autism: patterns of symptom emergence in the first years of life. *Autism Res* 2008;**1**(6):320–8.

147. *Double-blind, placebo-controlled proof of concept study in youth with fragile X syndrome.* 2015. clinicaltrials.gov [accessed 01.15].

148. Budimirovic DB, Bukelis I, Cox C, Gray RM, Tierney E, Kaufmann WE. Autism spectrum disorder in Fragile X syndrome: differential contribution of adaptive socialization and social withdrawal. *Am J Med Genet A* 2006;**140**(17):1814–26.

149. Kaufmann WE, Cortell R, Kau ASM, et al. Autism spectrum disorder in fragile X syndrome: communication, social interaction, and specific behaviors. *Am J Med Genet A* 2004;**129A**(3):225.

150. Wang LW, Berry-Kravis E, Hagerman RJ. Fragile X: leading the way for targeted treatments in autism. *Neurotherapeutics* July 2010;**7**(3):264–74.

151. De Sonia A, Visootsak J, Smith M, et al. *FXCRC analysis of arbaclofen responses in fragile X syndrome.* 2014. Orange County (CA).

152. www.clinicaltrials.gov; 2015 [accessed 21.01.15].

153. Talisa VB, Boyle L, Crafa D, Kaufmann WE. Autism and anxiety in males with fragile X syndrome: an exploratory analysis of neurobehavioral profiles from a parent survey. *Am J Med Genet* June 2014;**164A**(5):1198–203.

154. Abbeduto L, McDuffie A, Thurman AJ. The fragile X syndrome–autism comorbidity: what do we really know? *Front Genet* 2014;**5**.

155. Bennett KE, Haggard MP. Behaviour and cognitive outcomes from middle ear disease. *Arch Dis Child* 1999;**80**(1):28–35.

156. Goodlin-Jones B, Tang K, Liu J, Anders TF. Sleep problems, sleepiness and daytime behavior in preschool-age children. *J Child Psychol Psychiatry* December 2009;**50**(12):1532–40.

157. *Educational guidelines for fragile X syndrome: general. Consensus of the fragile X clinical & research consortium on clinical practices.* 2013.

158. Peters-Scheffer N, Didden R, Korzilius H, Sturmey P. A meta-analytic study on the effectiveness of comprehensive ABA-based early intervention programs for children with autism spectrum disorders. *Res Autism Spectrum Disord* 2011;**5**(1):60.

159. Braden M. Braden on behavior: navigating the road to inclusion. *Natl Fragile X Found Q* 2011;(41).

160. Riley K. Educational strategies in fragile X syndrome. In: *Greater Chicago Fragile X Fall Education Workshop*; 2013.

161. Gray CA, Garand JD. Social stories: improving responses of students with autism with accurate social information. *Focus Autistic Behav* 1993;**8**.

162. *Hyperarousal in fragile X syndrome. Consensus of the fragile X clinical & research consortium on clinical practices.* 2012.

163. Hessl D, Dyer-Friedman J, Glaser B, et al. The influence of environmental and genetic factors on behavior problems and autistic symptoms in boys and girls with fragile X syndrome. *Pediatrics* 2001;**108**(5):E88.

164. Bailey Jr DB, Raspa M, Bishop E, et al. Health and economic consequences of fragile X syndrome for caregivers. *J Dev Behav Pediatr* 2012;**33**(9):705–12.

165. Amaria R, Billeisen L, Hagerman R. Medication use in fragile X syndrome. *Ment Health Aspects Dev Disabil* 2001;**4**:143–7.

166. Berry-Kravis E, Potanos K. Psychopharmacology in fragile X syndrome—present and future. *Ment Retard Dev Disabil Rev* 2004;**10**(1):42–8.

167. Berry-Kravis E, Sumis A, Hervey C, Mathur S. Clinic-based retrospective analysis of psychopharmacology for behavior in fragile X syndrome. *Int J Pediatr* 2012;**2012**(5):11. Article ID 843016.

168. Berry-Kravis E, Grossman AW, Crnic LS, Greenough WT. Understanding fragile X syndrome. *Curr Paediatr* 2002;**12**(4):316–24.

169. Hagerman RJ, Murphy MA, Wittenberger MD. A controlled trial of stimulant medication in children with the fragile X syndrome. *Am J Med Genet* 1988;**30**(1–2):377–92.

170. Roberts JE, BDBBML. Psychophysiological measures of arousal: documentation of treatment effects and impact of disability. In: *8th International Fragile X Conference*; 2002. Chicago (IL).

171. Hagerman RJ, Miller LJ, McGrath-Clarke J, et al. Influence of stimulants on electrodermal studies in Fragile X syndrome. *Microsc Res Tech* 2002;**57**(3):168–73.

172. Hagerman R, Riddle J, Roberts L, Breese K, Fulton M. Survey of the efficacy of clonidine in fragile X syndrome. *Dev Brain Dysfunc* 1995;**8**(4–6):336–44.

173. Paribello C, Tao L, Folino A, et al. Open-label add-on treatment trial of minocycline in fragile X syndrome. *BMC Neurol* 2010;**10**(1):91.

174. Hagerman R, Hills J, Scharfenaker S, Lewis H. Fragile X syndrome and selective mutism. *Am J Med Genet* 1999;**83**(4):313–7.

175. Cohen JKK, Iacono T. Measuring emotion, behavior change and speech in individuals with fragile X syndrome whilst taking sertraline: a pilot of tools. In: *8th International Fragile X Conference*; 2002. Chicago (IL).

176. Hilton DK, Martin CA, Heffron WM, Hall BD, Johnson GL. Imipramine treatment of ADHD in a fragile X child. *J Am Acad Child Adolesc Psychiatry* 1991;**30**(5):831–4.

177. McCracken JT, McGough J, Shah B, et al. Risperidone in children with autism and serious behavioral problems. *N Engl J Med* 2002;**347**(5):314–21.

178. Erickson CA, Stigler KA, Wink LK, et al. A prospective open-label study of aripiprazole in fragile X syndrome. *Psychopharmacology (Berl)* 2011;**216**(1):85–90.

179. Berry-Kravis ENM, Levin R, Ooyang B. Effect of antipsychotic use on the prevalence of overweight/obesity in fragile X syndrome.

In: *Paper presented at: 14th International Fragile X Conference*; 2014. Orange County (CA).

180. Huber KM, Gallagher SM, Warren ST, Bear MF. Altered synaptic plasticity in a mouse model of fragile X mental retardation. *Proc Natl Acad Sci USA* June 28, 2002;**99**(11):7746–50.

181. Deng P-Y, Rotman Z, Blundon JA, et al. FMRP regulates neurotransmitter release and synaptic information transmission by modulating action potential duration via BK channels. *Neuron* March 20, 2013;**77**(4):696–711.

182. Grossman AW, Aldridge GM, Weiler IJ, Greenough WT. Local protein synthesis and spine morphogenesis: fragile X syndrome and beyond. *J Neurosci* July 05, 2006;**26**(27):7151–5.

183. Bilousova TV, Dansie L, Ngo M, et al. Minocycline promotes dendritic spine maturation and improves behavioural performance in the fragile X mouse model. *J Med Genet* March 2009;**46**(2):94–102.

184. Henderson C, Wijetunge L, Kinoshita MN, et al. Reversal of disease-related pathologies in the fragile X mouse model by selective activation of GABAB receptors with arbaclofen. *Sci Transl Med* September 19, 2012;**4**(152):152ra128.

185. Yuskaitis CJ, Mines MA, King MK, Sweatt JD, Miller CA, Jope RS. Lithium ameliorates altered glycogen synthase kinase-3 and behavior in a mouse model of fragile X syndrome. *Biochem Pharmacol* March 15, 2010;**79**(4):632–46.

186. McBride SMJ, Choi CH, Wang Y, et al. Pharmacological rescue of synaptic plasticity, courtship behavior, and mushroom body defects in a Drosophila model of fragile X syndrome. *Neuron* April 03, 2005;**45**(5):753–64.

187. Michalon A, Sidorov M, Ballard TM, et al. Chronic pharmacological mGlu5 inhibition corrects fragile X in adult mice. *Neuron* May 12, 2012;**74**(1):49–56.

188. Berry-Kravis E, Sumis A, Hervey C, et al. Open-label treatment trial of lithium to target the underlying defect in fragile X syndrome. *J Dev Behav Pediatr* August 2008;**29**(4):293–302.

189. Leigh MJS, Nguyen DV, Mu Y, et al. A randomized double-blind, placebo-controlled trial of minocycline in children and adolescents with fragile x syndrome. *J Dev Behav Pediatr* May 2013;**34**(3):147–55.

190. Berry-Kravis EM, Hessl D, Rathmell B, et al. Effects of STX209 (arbaclofen) on neurobehavioral function in children and adults with fragile X syndrome: a randomized, controlled, phase 2 trial. *Sci Transl Med* September 19, 2012;**4**(152):152ra127.

191. Erickson CA, Wink LK, Ray B, et al. Impact of acamprosate on behavior and brain-derived neurotrophic factor: an open-label study in youth with fragile X syndrome. *Psychopharmacology (Berl)* July 2013;**228**(1):75–84.

192. Berry-Kravis E, Hessl D, Coffey S, et al. A pilot open label, single dose trial of fenobam in adults with fragile X syndrome. *J Med Genet* May 2009;**46**(4):266–71.

193. Jacquemont S, Curie A, des Portes V, et al. Epigenetic modification of the *FMR1* gene in fragile X syndrome is associated with differential response to the mGluR5 antagonist AFQ056. *Sci Transl Med* February 05, 2011;**3**(64):64ra61.

194. Berry-Kravis E, Hessl D, Abbeduto L, et al. Outcome measures for clinical trials in fragile X syndrome. *J Dev Behav Pediatr* September 2013;**34**(7):508–22.

195. Iossifov I, Ronemus M, Levy D, et al. De novo gene disruptions in children on the autistic spectrum. *Neuron* May 26, 2012;**74**(2):285–99.

196. Steinberg J, Webber C. The roles of FMRP-regulated genes in autism spectrum disorder: single- and multiple-hit genetic etiologies. *Am J Hum Genet* July 11, 2013;**93**(5):825–39.

197. Waltes R, Duketis E, Knapp M, et al. Common variants in genes of the postsynaptic FMRP signalling pathway are risk factors for autism spectrum disorders. *Hum Genet* July 2014;**133**(6):781–92.

21

Phelan–McDermid Syndrome: Clinical Aspects

Katy Phelan[1], Luigi Boccuto[2], Sara Sarasua[2,3]

[1]Hayward Genetics Program and Department of Pediatrics, Tulane University School of Medicine, New Orleans, LA, USA; [2]Greenwood Genetic Center, Greenwood, SC, USA; [3]Clemson University, Clemson, SC, USA

INTRODUCTION

Phelan–McDermid syndrome (PMS) is a contiguous gene deletion syndrome resulting from haploinsufficiency of the distal long arm of chromosome 22. The commonly deleted region is identified as 22q13. The deletion size ranges from less than 100 kb to over 9 MB and the phenotype is variable. Key features of PMS include neonatal hypotonia, moderate to profound intellectual impairment, and absent or delayed speech.[1–3] Autism spectrum disorder (ASD) or autistic-like behavior is often present. The *SHANK3* gene has been identified as contributing to the neurological phenotype of PMS.[4,5] Minor dysmorphic features are common but the physical features are not clinically distinctive. The diagnosis of PMS must be confirmed by laboratory testing to demonstrate a chromosome deletion, gene disruption, or gene mutation.

INCIDENCE

According to the Phelan–McDermid syndrome Foundation, about 1200 cases have been diagnosed worldwide.[6] Nonetheless, the true incidence of this disorder remains unknown. The subtle clinical features cause PMS to be underdiagnosed or misdiagnosed. Individuals may be diagnosed with an ASD based on the neurobehavioral phenotype, or with cerebral palsy based on the lack of coordination.[1] Unless appropriate genetic testing is performed, the correct diagnosis will not be achieved.

DIAGNOSTIC TESTING

Cytogenetic analysis alone is insufficient to make the diagnosis of PMS owing to the large number of cases with deletion size below the detection threshold.

Although fluorescence *in situ* hybridization (FISH) studies can confirm the presence of a deletion of 22q13, a chromosomal microarray (CMA) is recommended to detect a deletion and rule out the possibility of an accompanying duplication which would suggest an unbalanced translocation or other structural chromosome abnormalities. Although it is more sensitive than high-resolution chromosome analysis in detecting microdeletions, CMA may fail to detect low-level mosaicism. The sensitivity depends on the type of microarray and the density of probes in the 22q13.3 region. Multiplex ligation-dependent probe amplification is a targeted method to identify cryptic deletions of 22q13.3 and confirm deletions identified by CMA. In an individual with features of PMS and a normal microarray, DNA sequencing may be necessary to detect a mutation of *SHANK3* or mutation of a different, as yet unidentified causative gene.

ETIOLOGY

The most common cause of PMS is loss of the distal segment of chromosome 22 which may result from a simple terminal deletion, an interstitial deletion, an unbalanced translocation, a ring chromosome, or other types of structural abnormalities. Loss-of-function mutations involving the *SHANK3* gene, which is localized to 22q13.3, may also lead to the phenotype of PMS.

Most individuals with PMS have terminal deletions in which there is one breakpoint in 22q13 and the segment distal to breakpoint is lost or deleted. Similar to other terminal deletion syndromes, the deletion of 22q13 in PMS is paternally derived in most cases. In studies of 56 and 33 individuals, Wilson et al.[5] and Luciani et al.[7] respectively, reported a preponderance of paternal deletions (69–74%) among informative cases. Bonaglia et al.[8] showed that 17 of 23 terminal deletions (74%) and two of two interstitial deletions (100%) were of paternal origin; a similar 73% of terminal deletions on paternal chromosome 22 were reported by Sarasua et al.[9] Interstitial deletions in which two breaks occur in the long arm of 22 with loss of the intervening segment are much less common than terminal deletions in PMS. The first interstitial deletion reported in PMS involved loss of 22q13.1q13.33 detected by chromosome analysis in an 18-year-old girl with developmental delay, hypotonia, and macrosomia.[10] A second child with a more proximal deletion of 22q13.1q13.2, detected cytogenetically and confirmed by FISH, was similarly affected with developmental delay, hypotonia, and accelerated growth.[11] Both children had speech delay, ptosis, epicanthal folds, long philtrum, and dysplastic ears.

Unbalanced translocations occur in about 20% of individuals with PMS. Parental FISH studies should be performed on metaphase chromosomes to identify familial rearrangements so that appropriate recurrence risk counseling can be provided. Multiplex families have been described with more than one child with PMS owing to malsegregation of a parental translocation.[8,12,13] Mother-to-son transmission of a direct insertion of band 7q21.2 into 22q13.3 with a submicroscopic deletion of 22q13 was reported by Slavotinek et al.[14] At age 26 years, the mother had limited intellectual ability, indistinct speech, and a large head. The son, who was also trisomic for 7q21.2, had neonatal hypotonia and global developmental delay. Other structural abnormalities, such as recombinant chromosome 22, have been described in patients with deletion of 22q13.[15,16] A recombinant chromosome 22 can result from meiotic crossing over within a parental inversion, resulting in deletion/duplication imbalance.

Since the first report of ring chromosome 22, or r(22), in 1968, over 100 cases have been described.[17] A ring chromosome typically forms when two breaks occur on chromosome 22, one on the distal long arm and one on the short arm or satellite region. The broken ends of the chromosome rejoin to form a circular structure, or ring, and the segments distal to the breaks are lost. The phenotype of ring 22 has been reviewed by several authors.[18–20] Key features are intellectual impairment, delayed motor development, hypotonia, lack of speech development, and minor dysmorphic features. Luciani et al.[7] found no gross phenotypic differences between simple deletions of 22q13 and ring 22 syndrome for similar-sized deletions, although individuals with simple deletions tended to be overgrown whereas those with r(22) often showed growth failure. Because rings are unstable during cell division, individuals are often mosaic with additional cell lines having lost, duplicated, or broken rings.

Mosaicism, in which an individual has two or more distinct populations of cells, is sometimes observed in individuals with PMS. Typically a mosaic individual will have a normal cell population and a second population with the deletion, although mosaicism with two abnormal cell lines has been described.[5,21] Mosaicism for a terminal deletion 22q13.2 was first detected in a 5-year-old girl who had abnormal skin pigmentation in addition to developmental delay, failure to thrive, dysmorphic features, and seizures.[22] Prenatal diagnosis of mosaic deletion of 22q13 was detected in a fetus with a cystic thymic tissue visualized by ultrasound[23] and in a pregnancy referred for increased risk of trisomy 21 by maternal serum screening.[21] In both cases mosaicism was confirmed by FISH after pregnancy termination. Parental mosaicism can lead to increased risk of producing offspring with PMS. A phenotypically normal mother with 6% mosaicism for deletion of 22q13 produced two offspring with PMS.[24] At least three cases of suspected gonadal mosaicism have been described, two of which inferred maternal mosaicism[25,26] and one which did not identify the parent of origin.[27]

Disruptions or mutations of the *SHANK3* gene can result in PMS. Disruption of *SHANK3* can occur when the breakpoint for a translocation, insertion, deletion, or other structural rearrangement occurs within the *SHANK3* gene, causing loss of gene function.[4,8,28] *De novo* nonsense mutations of *SHANK3* have also been reported in individuals with features of PMS.[29]

HISTORY

The first description of a pure deletion of 22q is credited to Watt et al.[15] who reported a 14-year-old boy with a recombinant chromosome 22 resulting from a maternal pericentric inversion. The recombinant chromosome was deleted for 22q12 and duplicated for p11-pter. The authors concluded that the duplication was not clinically significant. In 1988, several groups described individuals with simple terminal deletions of chromosome 22 detected by chromosome analysis. These included a 13-year-old boy with cognitive and motor delay, speech delay, bilateral epicanthal folds, and broad fingers and thumbs[30]; a 16-month-old boy with intellectual impairment, cortical blindness, and features of Goldenhar complex[31]; and a newborn male with neonatal hypotonia.[32] Mild dysmorphic features, severe speech delay, and hypotonia were reported in two children with terminal deletions of 22q[33] and in one child with an interstitial deletion.[10] Metabolic studies were used to show hemizygous deficiency of arylsulfatase A (*ARSA*) in a 7-month-old girl with hypotonia, full eyebrows, deep-set eyes, large ears, micrognathia, high arched palate, and subcutaneous syndactyly of toes 2 and 3, who had a deletion of 22q13.1.[34] Pseudodeficiency of *ARSA* was described in a patient (previously reported by Phelan et al.[32]) who inherited a pseudodeficiency allele from his mother and a *de novo* deletion of the paternal allele.[35]

Initial cases of 22q13 deletion were diagnosed on the basis of a cytogenetically visible loss of material from the distal portion of the long arm of chromosome 22. Deletions in these individuals were necessarily large, ie, greater than 3–4 MB, permitting detection at the microscope in prometaphase chromosome preparations. Later, fluorescence *in situ* hybridization, restriction fragment length polymorphism (RFLP) studies, and other molecular methods were used to confirm the results of chromosome analysis, detect cryptic changes involving chromosome 22, and map deletion size. Nesslinger et al.[36] summarized the features of seven

individuals with deletion of 22q13 and described a recognizable phenotype characterized by global developmental delay, severe delay in expressive speech, normal or accelerated growth, generalized hypotonia, and minor facial anomalies. RFLP analysis was used to map the size of the deletions and determine that the deletion in one patient was maternally inherited.

Several investigators used FISH to detect submicroscopic deletion and cryptic translocations involving chromosome 22.[37-41] Two children with hypotonia, developmental delay, and absent speech were serendipitously found to have cryptic deletions of 22q13 after one child was referred for FISH to rule out DiGeorge syndrome, and the other to rule out Angelman syndrome. Both deletions were paternally inherited.[42] A cryptic deletion of 22q13.3 was found in a boy initially thought to have FG syndrome based on congenital hypotonia, intellectual impairment, relative macrocephaly, and constipation.[43]

Disruption of the *SHANK3* gene by a *de novo* balanced translocation between 12q24.1 and 22q13 provided the first evidence that *SHANK3* has a role in the neurological phenotype of PMS.[4] The 4-year-old boy had hypotonia, mild intellectual impairment, severe speech delay, and mild dysmorphic facial features. The investigators determined that the breakpoint on chromosome 22 was within *SHANK3* exon 21, which suggested haploinsufficiency for *SHANK3* as a cause of some of the phenotypic features of 22q13.3 deletion syndrome. The following year, Anderlid et al.[44] reported the association between autism and loss of *SHANK3* in their description of a 100 kb deletion of 22q13 in a 33-year-old woman with mild intellectual impairment, speech delay, autistic features, mild facial dysmorphism, and deterioration in balance and daily living skills. The deletion resulted in disruption of the *PROSAP2* (*SHANK3*) gene and loss of *RABL2B* and *ACR*. A subsequent study of 56 patients with PMS showed that *SHANK3* was in the minimal deleted region in 45 informative individuals.[5] Similarly, an evaluation of 33 individuals with PMS, including 12 simple deletions, 17 rings, and four unbalanced translocations, reported that the minimal critical region included *SHANK3*, *ACR*, and *RABL2B*.[7] At least eight individuals with PMS resulting from cryptic interstitial deletions disrupting the *SHANK3* gene have been reported.[8,28,45,46] All of the individuals were reported to have developmental delay and impaired/absent speech, four had ASD, and six had normal to accelerated growth. In addition, several investigators described nonsyndromic autism with or without intellectual disability resulting from haploinsufficiency of *SHANK3* owing to deletion or mutation.[26,47,48]

Although it is agreed that *SHANK3* has a key role in the neurobehavioral phenotype of PMS, there have been reports of individuals with deletions that do not include *SHANK3* but share the phenotypic features. In 2008, Wilson et al.[49] described three individuals with interstitial deletions of 22q13 confirmed by microsatellite, FISH, and comparative genomic hybridization analysis to be proximal to *SHANK3*. Two unrelated children had intellectual impairment, severe speech delay, hypotonia, overgrowth with macrocephaly, and minor dysmorphic features. The deletion in the first child was about 3.58 MB, and in the second child, 4.15 MB. The second child inherited the deletion from his mother, who had mild speech delay, a long face, and macrocephaly. The investigators concluded that haploinsufficiency for genes other than *SHANK3* contribute to cognitive and language development and genes in the interstitial region may be more prone to nonpenetrance and variable expressivity than genes in the *SHANK3* region. A 0.72 MB interstitial deletion of 22q13.2 was observed in a 7.5-year-old boy described as having classic features of PMS plus an urticarial rash and elevated immunoglobulin E levels. Two genes within the deleted region (*NFAM1* and *TNFRSF13C*) are involved in immune function.[50] Disciglio et al.[51] described nine individuals with interstitial deletions of 22q13 ranging from 2.7 to 6.9 MB and overlapping the largest deletions in PMS. The investigators suggested that the interstitial deletion of 22q13 represents a new contiguous gene syndrome rather than the more parsimonious explanation that the interstitial deletion leads to a variable expression of PMS with other genes within the deleted region contributing to the phenotype.[52]

CLINICAL FEATURES

The classic features of PMS are neonatal hypotonia, developmental delay, speech impairment, and minor dysmorphic features.

Hypotonia: The first presenting symptom of PMS is neonatal hypotonia. Problems which may result from poor muscle tone include failure to thrive owing to poor feeding, reduced reflexes, difficulty speaking, and failure to achieve motor milestones. Failure to ask parents or caregivers about muscle tone in the newborn may cause neonatal hypotonia to be underreported in this syndrome. Infants evaluated for Prader–Willi syndrome and other disorders characterized by neonatal hypotonia should also be evaluated for PMS.[35]

Whereas some individuals with hypotonia in the newborn period develop normal tone or hypertonia in childhood or adolescence, other children may have an uncoordinated, ataxic gait which persists to adulthood. Neurological evaluation of 16 individuals from age 20 months to 45 years detected hypotonia of the limbs and trunk in all patients.[29] Hypotonia was scored as mild in seven individuals and moderate in nine.

Increased ankle tone, clonus, toe-walking, extensor signs, abnormal posturing of the upper extremities, and cortical thumbs were among the signs of upper motor neuron dysfunction observed in 9 of 16 individuals. Sarasua et al.[3] reported 82 of 110 cases (75%) with hypotonia with a different incidence in age groups. Interestingly, almost all patients aged under 5 years showed some signs of reduced muscular tone (41 of 45; 85%) whereas only 16 of 28 patients (57%) evaluated over age 10 years had hypotonia, which suggests a trend toward decreased incidence with older age (*p* value = 0.0428).

Hypotonia in PMS may affect the trunk, limbs, and/or face and is often accompanied by a series of correlated signs and symptoms such as ptosis, constipation, abnormal gait, and abnormal reflexes.[3,29] In many cases, neonatal hypotonia precedes by several years the onset of correlated symptoms, and the incidence of such neuromuscular symptoms may vary with age. Features decreasing in prevalence with increasing age include hypotonia, lax ligaments, hyperextensible joints, and hyporeflexia, whereas hyperreflexia increases in prevalence with age.[3]

Developmental Delay: The first individuals with PMS were diagnosed based on cytogenetically visible chromosome deletions and thus tended to represent the more severe end of the developmental spectrum. Initial reports described individuals as having "global developmental delay" and "moderate to profound mental retardation".[21,36] Later individuals with microdeletions detected by microarray techniques were described as having mild intellectual impairment. As mentioned previously, deletion size ranges from less than 100 kb to greater than 9 MB. Likewise, the developmental spectrum varies from mild delays to profound intellectual impairment with global developmental delay. The relationship between deletion size and development is complex because individuals with the same size deletion may be dramatically different in their levels of intellectual and motor development.[53] In general, major motor milestones will be delayed, with the child sitting up, rolling over, and walking later than unaffected peers. The gait is frequently ataxic and unsteady because of hypotonia, ligamentous laxity, and gross motor delay.[54] In a study of 201 individual with Phelan–McDermid syndrome, Sarasua et al.[3] found that the median age at walking was 22 months (range, 10–98 months). Toilet training was achieved by only 24% of individuals, with the age at attaining this skill ranging from 36 months to 20 years and a median age of 6.5 years.

Impaired Speech: Speech impairment ranges from the complete absence of speech to mild speech delay. Individuals may begin to make sounds at an appropriate age and then subsequently lose the ability to speak.[55] They may or may not regain the ability. Among individuals over age 3 years, Sarasua et al.[3] found that 50% of individuals had no speech. According to parent or caregiver reports, 27% had a vocabulary of 40 words or less, 10% had a vocabulary of 50 words or more or could use phrases, and 13% had a large vocabulary, used full sentences, or used speech as their primary form of communication. Speaking skills did not significantly improve with age and were inversely correlated with the level of developmental delay such that those with lower speech skills had a higher degree of developmental delay.[3] Webster et al.[56] summarized the communication profile in this syndrome as demonstrating severe to profound expressive language impairment, mild to moderate receptive language impairment, and mild to moderate problems with oral motor skills. Aggressive speech and communication therapies are recommended to aid individuals in reaching their potential for communication.[1]

Growth: Birth is typically at term; birth weight, length, and head circumference are appropriate for gestational age. Most individuals with PMS have normal growth parameters, with only 11% showing growth delay.[57] Although neonatal hypotonia is a frequent feature in PMS, it does not seem to frequently induce failure to thrive or major feeding issues affecting the growth curve.[1] Nesslinger et al.[36] observed that of their seven patients, all were of normal or accelerated growth, and noted that this was an unusual feature in a deletion syndrome because most deletions are associated with growth retardation. Three of their seven patients were macrocephalic, one was greater than the 95th percentile in height, and one had large hands and feet. Although most individuals are between the 5th and 95th percentile for stature, a tendency for decreasing height percentile with age has been reported.[3] Among those aged less than 5 years, 19% were greater than the 95th percentile for height and the mean height percentile was 68th. Mean height percentile decreased to 42nd for those between age 5 and 9 years and to the 35th percentile for those aged between 10 and 17 years. Macrocephaly has been reported to occur in 7—31% of individuals, and microcephaly in 6—13%.[3,20,29,57] Microcephaly was noted to be more common among those with short stature, and macrocephaly more common among those with tall stature.[3] The variability in head size does not reflect abnormalities in brain size or structure, although some minor malformations have been reported in certain brain areas in PMS (see neuroimaging findings).

Seizures: Early studies reported seizures to occur in about 25% of individuals with PMS and did not distinguish between febrile and nonfebrile seizures.[7,21,55] Soorya et al.[29] described seizure activity in 13 of 32 individuals (41%) by parent report. Of these, seven (22%) had febrile seizures only, four (13%) had nonfebrile seizures, and two (6%) had both febrile and nonfebrile seizures. In the seven individuals with febrile seizures only, four had normal EEG interpretations, two had not had an EEG study, and one was said to have an abnormal EEG but the interpretation was not available. In the six individuals with nonfebrile seizures (including four with nonfebrile only and two with both febrile and nonfebrile), five of six (83%) had generalized seizures and one had partial complex seizures. All of the individuals with nonfebrile seizures had abnormal EEG findings. Four of the 32 individuals had abnormal EEG findings without recognized seizures.[29] Although no characteristic EEG findings have been associated with PMS, a review of EEG recordings in six individuals ranging in age from 11 to 30 years found that all six patients demonstrated atypical results with multifocal paroxysmal abnormalities activated by sleep.[58]

In 2014, Sarasua et al. reported that the incidence of seizures in PMS increased with age. The overall incidence of seizures at any age was 27%, with an age-associated occurrence of 11% in those aged less than 5 years, 26% between age 5 and 9.9 years, 43% between age 10 and 17.9 years, and 60% between age 18 and 64 years. Seizures were also found to be three times more frequent among patients with a *de novo* deletion of the maternal 22 than the paternal 22; they are the only PMS feature to show a significant parent-of-origin effect.

In an investigation of copy number variants (CNVs) in 21 adults with Lennox—Gastaut (LG) syndrome or LG-like epilepsy, eight patients had one or more rare CNVs, including a 16-year-old boy with a *de novo* 800 kb deletion of 22q13.3.[59] The deleted region contained 37 genes, including *SHANK3*. Upon further examination, the patient had characteristic features of PMS: global developmental delay, severe speech delay, autistic behavior, increased tolerance to pain, hyperactivity, normal height, and long eyelashes. Although this is the first report in the literature of LG associated with PMS, the Phelan—McDermid Syndrome Foundation acknowledges that LG and LG-like epilepsy has been reported among their membership.

Craniofacial Features: Craniofacial findings are relatively subtle and there are no pathognomonic facial features for PMS (Figure 1). Data tabulated from nine surveys of individuals with PMS[3,7,20,29,36,53,55,60,61] are presented in Table 1. Long eyelashes, bulbous nose, epicanthal folds, flat midface, large and dysplastic ears, and periorbital fullness and high arched palate were described in over 50% of individuals. Wide nasal bridge, ptosis, dolichocephaly, full or puffy cheeks, and deep-set eyes were observed in 25—49% of patients. Macrocephaly, strabismus, long philtrum, and flat midface were observed in fewer than 25% of individuals. The subtle facial features of PMS make it difficult to arrive at a clinical diagnosis in the absence of a confirmatory laboratory test.

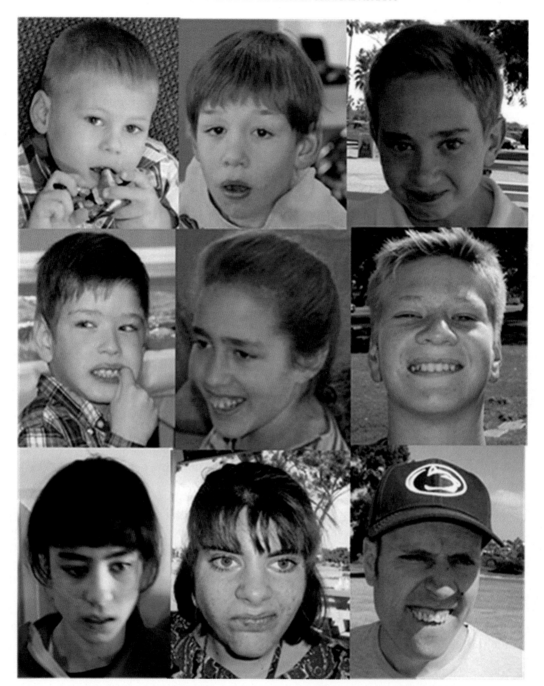

FIGURE 1   Facial features of individuals with Phelan–McDermid syndrome.

Neurobehavioral Features

Although the main neurological symptoms associated with PMS, hypotonia and seizures, have already been discussed, the clinical presentation of this condition may include a series of neurobehavioral issues that require a specific section of this chapter. Table 2 categorizes the main PMS neurobehavioral signs and symptoms according to the major system involved.

Autism: Prasad et al.[62] and Goizet et al.[63] associated autism with terminal deletion 22q13. In the first study three children displayed pervasive developmental behaviors within the autism spectrum whereas in the second study one child was diagnosed with autism and was noted to have a high threshold for pain. Autism and autistic-like behavior have repeatedly been observed in PMS, and estimates of the prevalence of ASD have been as high as 84%.[29] Sarasua et al.[3]

TABLE 1   Features Associated with Phelan—McDermid Syndrome[3,7,20,29,36,52,54,59,60]

≥75% Patients	≥50% Patients	≥25% Patients	<25% Patients
Global developmental delay	Decreased perspiration/ overheating	Wide nasal bridge	Lymphedema
Absent or severely delayed speech	Long eyelashes	Gastroesophageal reflux	Fifth finger clinodactyly
Hypotonia	Bulbous nose	2—3 syndactyly of toes	Lordosis/kyphosis
Mouthing or chewing nonfood items	Dysplastic toenails	Ptosis	Hearing loss
Decreased perception of pain	Hyperextensibility	Renal abnormalities	Macrocephaly
Normal or accelerated growth	Epicanthal folds	Dolichocephaly	Strabismus
	Large, fleshy hands	Seizures	Malocclusion/widely spaced teeth
	Autism/autistic-like behavior	Full, puffy cheeks	Long philtrum
	Flat midface	Deep-set eyes	Arachnoid cyst
	High arched palate		Precocious or delayed puberty
	Poorly formed/large ears		Cardiac defects
	Periorbital fullness		Hypothyroidism
			Flat midface

TABLE 2   Neurobehavioral Features in Phelan—McDermid Syndrome

Neuromotor System	Neurosensory System	Neurovegetative System	Behavior and Mood
Hypotonia	Decreased perception of pain	Decreased perspiration/ overheating	Autism spectrum disorder and autistic-like behavior
Seizures	Hypersensitivity to touch	Abnormal sleep patterns, sleep problems	Chewing nonfood items
Abnormal gait		Gastroesophageal reflux	Aggressive/impulsive behavior
Hypo- and/or hyperreflexia		Constipation	Biting, hair pulling, excessive crying and screaming
Cerebral palsy			Bipolar disorder

noticed that in older patients there is an increased incidence of both ASD and autism-like traits. In a preliminary attempt to characterize the autism features in the PMS, Oberman et al.[64] showed that patients had a complex behavioral phenotype, most notably characterized as mild to moderate generalized developmental delay/intellectual disability. As it relates to autism-specific symptoms, most of the individuals displayed persistent deficits in social communication, but only half met diagnostic criteria under the restricted, repetitive patterns of behavior, interests, or activities domain.

Other Behavioral and/or Mood Disorders: Parents of children with PMS report the occurrence of several behavioral issues (Table 2), usually starting during the second year of life. Other than the lack of verbal and nonverbal communication and social impairment, which are typical stigmata of ASD, patients often develop mouthing or chewing of nonfood items, aggressive behavior, impulsiveness, biting, hair pulling, and excessive screaming or crying. In older patients, more complex disorders may be present, such as anxiety, hyperactivity, bipolar disorder, and psychosis.[1–3,21,29,65–67] Nonfood chewing behavior has been reported in

44−85% of individuals and seems to become less frequent with age. It is probable that continuous chewing, along with other less frequent behavioral issues such as teeth grinding (24%) and tongue thrusting (15%), has an important role in some dental problems observed in PMS patients, such as malocclusion, teeth spacing, and crowding.[2,3] Other mood/behavioral problems show the same trend of becoming less common in older patients: biting themselves or others (reported in 46% of cases), hair pulling (41%), and excessive, prolonged crying (21%).[3]

Abnormal Reflexes: Sarasua et al.[3] showed a wide spectrum of reflex responses in individuals with PMS: Whereas roughly half of the cohort (52%) presented with normal reflexes, 31% of patients showed reduced reflex intensity or hyporeflexia, 15% had hyperreflexia, and in 2% both hyperreflexia and hyporeflexia at different locations in the same individual were reported.

Sensory Processing Abnormalities: Unusual responsiveness to environmental and sensory stimuli is a common feature of PMS: Lack of responsiveness to verbal or pain stimuli is accompanied by exaggerated reaction to tactile stimuli or overarousal to the environment.[66] Decreased perception of pain is arguably one of the most distinguishing neurologic traits in PMS, along with neonatal hypotonia; it has been reported in 77−92% of individuals and its incidence increases with age.[1,3,21,29] Hypersensitivity to touch is often considered to be part of the clinical presentation in patients with ASD and has been reported in 46% of PMS cases.[3]

Decreased Perspiration/Overheating: Many individuals with PMS have a tendency to become overheated or turn red easily (68%), accompanied by reduced perspiration (18−60%).[1,3,21,65] Pathogenic models have been proposed to explain these features, inferring a dysregulation at the hypothalamic level or, alternatively, an ectodermal dysplasia.

Sleep Problems: Sleep disturbances occur in 41−46% of individuals with PMS, affecting both children and adults.[3,29,66] Problems include difficulty getting to sleep at night and staying asleep; sleep apnea is uncommon. The average sleeping time may be limited to only 4 h per night, resulting in sleep deprivation and exacerbation of developmental disabilities and neurological symptoms.[1]

Neuroimaging Findings and Other Examinations: MRI scans have shown thin or morphologically atypical corpus callosum, delayed myelination, frontal lobe hypoplasia, cerebellar vermis hypoplasia, and mega cisterna magna with enlarged posterior fossa.[1,66,68] Malformations noted at the cerebellar level suggest candidate genes other than *SHANK3*, such as *MAPK8IP2/IB2* and *PLXNB2*. Both genes map in the terminal region of the 22q13 band, are highly expressed in cerebellar vermis, and have knockout mice models showing abnormalities in neuronal differentiation, dendritic arborization, and cerebellar fissure formation.[68−70]

Other neuroanatomical abnormalities reported in individuals with PMS are arachnoid cysts (about 15% of cases) and sacral dimple (13−50%). Arachnoid cysts may remain asymptomatic, especially if they are small in size, or they may be accompanied by a series of signs and symptoms of increased intracranial pressure, such as incessant crying bouts, irritability, severe headaches, cyclic vomiting, and seizures.[1,29]

Other Systems

Musculoskeletal: Over 50% of individuals had large fleshy hands with a puffy appearance of the hands possibly resulting, in some cases, from lymphedema which is seen in about 24% of individuals. Lymphedema more commonly affects the lower extremities than the upper extremities, and whereas it may be present in young children, it tends to worsen with age.[1] In one case, severe lymphedema led to ascites and pleural effusions, required repeated drainage and ultimately surgery in a 16-year-old girl with ring 22 and characteristic features of PMS.[71] Typical management strategies for lymphedema include massage and/or elevation of the affected limb, compressive stockings or bandages, and in more severe cases, the use of a compressive boot or sleeve which uses peristaltic motion to push excess fluid from the distal extremity toward the body.[1] Dysplastic toenails were reported in over 50% of individuals and suggest a possible ectodermal component to PMS. Over 25% had 2−3 syndactyly of the toes, and it has been found that about 20% of individuals with syndactyly of toes 2 and 3 have a parent who has the same feature.[1] Fewer than 25% were reported with fifth-finger clinodactyly and lordosis or kyphosis.

Genitourinary: Renal abnormalities are generally reported in about 25% of patients, although one study reported an incidence of 38%.[29] Abnormalities include renal agenesis, renal dysplasia, hydronephrosis, vesicoureteral reflux, horseshoe kidney, polycystic kidney, pyelectasis, duplicate kidney, and dilated renal pelvis.[3,29] Frequent urinary tract infections (UTIs) have also been reported in PMS[3] and specifically in ring 22.[20] Baseline renal and bladder ultrasound scans are recommended upon diagnosis of PMS to detect asymptomatic problems, and routine blood pressure measurements should be performed.[1,6] Kolevzon et al.[6] stressed that a prenatal sonogram is insufficient and should not be substituted for a postnatal ultrasound scan because renal development may not be complete at the time of fetal ultrasound imaging. The authors also recommend referral to a nephrologist or urologist for UTIs at a young age or recurrent UTIs. In addition, abnormal renal or bladder ultrasound imaging or high blood pressure should prompt urinalysis and blood tests to monitor kidney function.[6]

Cardiovascular: Cardiac abnormalities, including tricuspid valve regurgitation, atrial septal defect, patent ductus arteriosus, and total anomalous pulmonary return, occur in about 3–25% of individuals.[2,29,38,39,54] Some issues may be related to vascular/lymphatic dysfunction, such as lymphedema and large, fleshy hands, which have been reported in 22–24% and 53–63% of patients, respectively. Interestingly, the incidence of lymphedema appears to increase with age, whereas the incidence of large and fleshy hands decreases.[3,29] For both issues, however, an alternative pathogenic mechanism based on hypothyroidism has been proposed, although hypothyroidism has been reported in only about 6% of patients with PMS, and hyperthyroidism is present in some individuals.[3]

Gastrointestinal: Gastroesophageal reflux (GER) has been reported in about 33–44% of individuals with PMS.[1,3,29] The reflux may resolve by age 6–12 months and can be successfully managed with smaller meals, avoiding irritating food, elevating the head of the bed, sleeping on the left side, and avoiding meals within 2–3 h of bedtime.[1] Decreased sensitivity to pain may make the diagnosis of GER more complicated in adult patients with PMS.

Frequent constipation and/or diarrhea have been reported in 38–41% of individuals, sometimes with alternating episodes in the same patients.[29,52] In both cases increased fluid intake is recommended, either to replenish the hydro-saline lost caused by diarrhea or to help soften the stools in cases of recurrent constipation.[1] GER and constipation may share the same pathogenic mechanism with hypotonia and neurovegetative disorders (Table 2).

Cycling vomiting occurs in about 25% of PMS patients, with vomiting episodes every few months and often accompanied by headaches, lethargy, and/or dehydration. The co-occurrence of such signs suggests the possible implication of an arachnoid cyst.[1,2] Nutritional assessment may be appropriate for individuals with persistent GER and/or cyclic vomiting.

Ophthalmologic: Overall eye function appears to be usually intact in patients with PMS, although some rare cases of hyperopia, myopia, and cortical visual impairment have been reported.[1] The most recurrent ophthalmologic issues include ptosis, with an incidence ranging from 3% to 47%, and strabismus, reported in 23–35% of patients.[3,24,29,65] Both features might be related to hypotonia and therefore might have a neurologic, rather than ophthalmologic, etiology. Newborns with strabismus should undergo extensive eye examination and should be enrolled in routine yearly evaluations by age 3 years.[1] Treatment depends on the underlying cause and the severity of the strabismus. Glasses or eye drops are effective in some cases whereas patching the unaffected eye to strengthen the vision and the muscles in the misaligned eye is necessary in others.

Dental: The most frequently encountered dental problems in patients with PMS are malocclusion and crowding. Poor muscle tone, incessant chewing, bruxism, and tongue thrusting are contributing factors. Malocclusion is often accompanied by difficulty swallowing and drooling, which may contribute to difficulties in verbalization. GER and cyclic vomiting predispose the teeth to erosion.[2,24]

Dental treatment includes regular professional dental hygiene, routine brushing, and fluoride treatment. Routine dental examinations are important to monitor problems such as malocclusion, crowding, and accelerated tooth decay caused by poor enamel formation attributable to recurrent antibiotic therapy, acid reflux, and extended use of bottle feeding.[24] Oral-motor therapy is often necessary to alleviate chewing and swallowing problems along with orthodontic therapy to correct malocclusion. Because of the behavioral issues often associated with autistic traits, the dentist should consider prescribing a mouth guard for higher-functioning PMS children with severe bruxism or self-injurious behavior.

Dermatologic: Main dermatologic features in patients with PMS involve two ectodermal derivatives, the nails and the sweat glands, which suggests the possibility of an ectodermal dysplasia. Problems related to reduced sweating and perspiration have been discussed in the neurobehavioral section. Hypoplastic or dysplastic toenails are one of the most common physical traits in patients with PMS, with a prevalence ranging from 34% to 75%.[1–3,29,72] The toenails are thin and flaky, and tend to be ingrown.[1] The fingernails may also present with some degree of dysplasia, although their involvement is usually less common (23%, according to Sarasua et al.[3]).

Skin rashes (39%) and cellulitis (7%) are also relatively frequent dermatologic problems, and they tend to be more frequent in older patients.[3] A clinical report by Simenson et al.[50] described a patient with an interstitial 0.72 MB deletion in the chromosome 22q13.2 region, developmental delay, autistic behavior, seizures, mild dysmorphic features, urticarial rashes, and increased eosinophil count, and elevated levels of immunoglobulin E. The authors suggest that haploinsufficiency of the *NFAM1* and *TNFRSF13C* genes might be related to the high levels of circulating IgE and eventually to skin rashes.

Recurrent cellulitis has typically been reported in the legs, with the inflamed areas becoming hot, red, and tender. The inflammation appears to result from lymphedema, which shows the same trend of occurring more often in older patients with PMS. The large volume of fluid accumulated in lymphedematous limbs may make them more susceptible to infection. Accompanying symptoms are fever, chills or sweats, joint tenderness, and muscle aches.[1] Other less common skin problems have been reported in patients with PMS, including café-au-lait spots, hypopigmented areas, eczema, ringworm, hirsutism, and skin tags.[1]

Respiratory: Soorya et al.[29] reported 17 of 32 patients (53%) with a history of recurring infection of the upper respiratory tract, often associated with ear infections. In the literature, several types of respiratory infections have been diagnosed in patients with PMS, including pneumonia, respiratory syncytial virus, bronchitis, and bronchiolitis.[1] In young patients, respiratory problems may affect feeding and sleep, but they tend to subside as patients age. Treatment will be specific to the respiratory problem and may include a vaporizer, humidifier, inhaler, supplemental oxygen, ear tubes, and pharmacotherapy.[1]

Uncommon Medical Complications: There have been rare reports of medical complications associated with deletion 22q13 and it is not clear whether these are incidental or are caused by the deletion of chromosome 22. One case of diabetes insipidus was observed in a newborn girl with deletion of 22q13.31. Diabetes resolved at 27 months.[73] Atypical teratoid rhabdoid brain tumor (ATRT) has been described in four children: two with simple deletions and two with ring 22.[74–76] Molecular characterization of the tumor in one child with del(22) showed an acquired frameshift mutation of the *INI1* gene in addition to loss of the chromosome with the germline deletion of 22q13, resulting in homozygous inactivation of *INI1* and development of ATRT.[74] Immunohistochemical staining for expression of the INI1 protein in tumor cells from a child with r(22) showed loss of nuclear expression. The authors postulated that the ATRT may have resulted from loss of the ring 22 combined with a pathogenic mutation of *INI1* on the remaining chromosome 22.[75] The tumors were not characterized in the other two children.

Wilms tumor has been reported in a 22-month-old child with 22q13 deletion, who was known by prenatal ultrasound imaging to have a unilateral multicystic kidney.[77] The tumor affected the noncystic kidney. Two additional individuals with Wilms tumor and PMS are known to the Phelan–McDermid Syndrome Foundation.

There have been two cases of metachromatic leukodystrophy (MLD) in unrelated children who had deletions on one chromosome 22 and pathogenic mutation of *ARSA* on the nondeleted 22.[78,79] Coincidentally, one child had a *de novo* t(13;22) resulting in deletion of 22q13[78] and the other child had an unbalanced

translocation between 14q32.33 and 22q13.3.[79] Genetic evaluation of a third child, initially diagnosed with MLD based on low *ARSA* activity, revealed a *de novo* translocation between 16p11.2 and 22q13 with a 1.4 MB deletion of 22q including *ARSA* and *SHANK3*.[80] The child inherited an *ARSA* pseudodeficiency allele from a parent, both of whom were carriers of a pseudodeficiency allele. The authors stress the importance of a detailed genetic (cytogenetic/microarray) evaluation in patients with low *ARSA* activity and atypical or nonspecific clinical phenotypes.[80]

Fulminant autoimmune hepatitis requiring liver transplant was described in two unrelated females with deletions of 22q13.[81,82] Improved social interaction, sequential planning, and imitation was noted after liver transplant in the second child, which led to the suggestion that SHANK3 protein may have a role in immunological response. The *PIM3* protooncogene, which is about 775 kb proximal to *SHANK3*, was also within the deleted region, which led to the speculation that recovery from hepatic injury may be prolonged or prevented by haploinsufficiency of *PIM3*.[82]

INTELLECTUAL AND MOTOR REGRESSION

Loss of language skills with mental and physical deterioration is associated with ring chromosome 22,[19,83] although the incidence is not established. The first report of loss of speech in a simple deletion of 22q13 was in a 14-year-old girl with autism who acquired monosyllabic repetitions at age 7 months, then stopped talking at 8 months and did not verbalize again for 2 years.[63] Later, Manning et al.[55] reported developmental regression in 4 of 11 patients with PMS, two with loss of previously acquired motor skills and two with loss of language skills. Whereas loss of language skills early in childhood is well known to families affected by PMS,[1] the motor and mental deterioration described in adolescence and adulthood is not well understood and is of great concern.

Since 1995, 27 adults with PMS as a result of deletion of 22q13 have been described in detail in the literature. They range in age from age 17 to 70 years and include 10 males and 17 females. Table 3 summarizes the finding in 14 of 27 individuals who have experienced regression. Regression in a 33-year-old woman with a 100 kb deletion of 22q13 was first reported by Anderlid et al.[44] in 2002. At age 30 years, their patient had autistic features and a decline in speech. Her daily living functions were deteriorating as she had loss of balance, ataxic gait and became incontinent for urine. The authors questioned whether the decline in function was

TABLE 3 Regression in Adults with Phelan–McDermid Syndrome

Patient	Deletion	Features
33yo F[44]	100 kb	Age 30, decline in speech and decline in daily living skills; loss of balance, ataxic gait, incontinent for urine
46yo F[55]	22q13.3	Late-onset seizures, ataxia, decreased ambulation
43yo F[8]	8.1 MB	Age 39, frequent seizures; rapid motor and cognitive decline; unable to stand, walk, make eye contact; died from renal failure age 47
40yo F[8]	3.4 MB	Seizures, cortical tremors, speech decline at age 39
41yo M[8]	2 MB	Neurological deterioration; type 2 diabetes at age 34, 3 spontaneous pneumothorax episodes of left lung
48yo M[84]	1.8 MB	Age 45, general decline after pneumonia; no walking, feeding problems, seizures, low social interaction; died at age 48
17yo M[85] 24yo F[85] 43yo F[85] 46yo M[85] 51yo F[85]	76 kb 97 kb 1.7 MB 1.2 MB 3.4 MB	Regression and bipolar disorder in all; decline in expressive and receptive language; loss of balance and coordination; unable to use knife and fork
70yo F[27]	610 kb	Age 19, challenging, negativistic behavior; age 64, difficult behavior and sleep disturbance; abnormal posturing of hands, nonverbal, bipolar disorder
45yo M[29]	4.4 MB	Age 17, loss of language and toileting skills after move to residential program
38yo F[67]	22q13.3	Age 32, behavioral regression, decline in self-help skills; adult onset psychosis, major depressive disorder, catatonia

yo, years old; F, female; M, male.

a progressive process in the central nervous system or an early onset of dementia. Because this individual was the oldest reported case at the time, it was not known whether the regression was part of the 22q deletion phenotype.

Late-onset seizures, absent speech, ataxia, and decreased ambulation were reported in a 46-year-old woman.[55] The deletion was described cytogenetically with the breakpoint at 22q13.3, so it is presumed to be several megabases in size.

Three adults over age 40 years were reported by Bonaglia et al.[8] who concluded that all adults with PMS showed progressive clinical deterioration. Their first patient presented at age 43 years with a history of frequent epileptic seizures, even while taking medication. At age 39 years she experienced rapid motor and cognitive decline and was unable to stand, walk, or establish eye contact and she had markedly increased spastic tetraparesis. Right renal agenesis was diagnosed and she died of renal failure at age 47 years while in a vegetative state. Their second patient was diagnosed at

age 40 years but had a history of cortical tremors and speech decline beginning at age 39 years. The third patient, a 41-year-old man with neurological deterioration, developed type 2 diabetes at age 34 years and subsequently experienced three spontaneous pneumothorax episodes of the left lung.

Willemsen et al.[84] described a 48-year-old man who was diagnosed with hyperthyroidism at age 27 years. Since age 45 years he had general decline of function after hospitalization for pneumonia complicated by respiratory insufficiency. He could no longer walk and had feeding problems because of swallowing difficulties which required a feeding tube. Social interaction diminished and he developed seizures. He had a CT scan and an MRI scan which showed mild enlargement of cisterna magna and central atrophy. He died of pneumonia at age 49 years.

Denayer et al.[85] described seven individuals ranging in age from 5 to 51 years and found a high incidence of psychiatric disorders (particularly bipolar disorder) and attention-deficit disorder. The authors reported sudden decline after acute events, in addition to progressive loss of skills in all seven patients, even the 5-year-old. The patients experienced deterioration of language with age, particularly decline in receptive and expressive language or a regression in pronunciation; deterioration in balance and coordination; progressive rigidity of posture with shuffling gait; loss of the ability to do handwork and to eat with knife and fork; reduced eye contact; and diminished social interest. All of the adults were diagnosed with bipolar disorder.

The oldest individual with PMS described to date is a 70-year-old woman reported by Verhoeven et al.[86] She had been institutionalized at age 19 years, when she developed challenging, negativistic behaviors. She was reevaluated at age 64 years owing to difficult behavior and sleep disturbance. She had no speech, could not follow simple instructions, demonstrated abnormal posturing of the hands, and was diagnosed with bipolar disorder. The deletion size was 610 kb.

In 2013, Messias et al.[67] reported a 38-year-old woman with a history of hypotonia, seizures, developmental delay, and cerebral palsy. She had major depressive disorder with psychotic features and schizophrenia with catatonia. After her first psychiatric hospitalization at age 32 years, she began having behavioral regression with declining self-help skills, periods of confusion, detachment, incontinence, and loss of speech.

A clinical report from Hara et al.[87] describes a 25-year-old woman with significant neuromotor regression, seizures, and autistic behavior that led to the clinical suspicion of Rett syndrome. The genetic analyses, however, ruled out mutations in the major genes associated with this syndrome (*MECP2*, *CDKL5*, and *FOXG1*) and detected instead a *de novo* frameshift mutation in *SHANK3*. These findings highlight the effect of *SHANK3* mutations on neurodevelopmental regression and suggest PMS as a differential diagnosis in cases of suspected Rett syndrome.

Is regression a feature of PMS or did these particular patients have some underlying pathology that precipitated the regression? In some cases the regression occurred after some acute episode such as a prolonged epileptic state, pneumonia, septic shock, or an environmental change such as relocation to a group home.[29,84,85] As regression is observed in more individuals, it is apparent that there is not always a precipitating event. Even in children regression is noticeable but in a more subtle manner. Speech is delayed and children may acquire a few words and then lose those words, which suggests an onset of regression during childhood.[1] As more cases have been reported and more anecdotal date comes from the Phelan–McDermid Syndrome Foundation, where parents of adults described deterioration in speech, reduced physical activity, unexplained weight loss, increased muscle weakness, and onset of urinary incontinence, it seems apparent that regression is an inherent feature of this syndrome, although it does not affect all individuals.

GENOTYPE–PHENOTYPE CORRELATIONS

To understand the correlation between genes and phenotypes, a review of the 22q13 genomic region is useful. Figure 2 shows the distal 9 MB of chromosome 22 most commonly involved in PMS. This region encompasses the cytogenetic bands 22q13.2, 22q13.31, 22q13.32, and 22q13.33, as shown in the UCSC Genome Browser.[88] The 22q13.32 band is mostly gene poor whereas the other bands are gene rich. More than 200 genes, microRNAs, and regulatory elements are located in 22q13. Deletions of varying sizes will result in different complements of genes being deleted. Whereas many of the genes in this region are known, for many others the functions are still unknown. In addition to showing the locations of known genes, Figure 2 displays genes known to be associated with phenotypes (OMIM genes),[89] as well as region observed to be deleted or duplicated in typical humans (DGV),[90] and regions observed in patients with various phenotypes (Decipher).[91] There is almost a complete overlap in regions with observed deletions in typical populations as well as CNVs observed in individuals with significant phenotypes. Thus, it can be a challenge to determine whether an observed CNV in a patient is pathogenic or benign.

Challenges in Genotype Assessment: An ongoing challenge in medical genetics is the changing genomic technology and standards used to measure chromosomal imbalances.[3] The distal 100,000 base pairs consist of repetitive elements of the telomere and no known genes are listed in this region. The consensus chromosome build[88] hg19 released in 2009 describes chromosome 22 as having 51,304,566 base pairs, with the last approximate 100 kb containing no known genes. Build hg38, released in December 2013, lists chromosome 22 as having 50,818,468 base pairs, with the final approximate 100 kb having no known genes. When assessing reports in the literature, it is critical to note which reference build was used when comparing deletion sizes and locations across manuscripts. Furthermore, some genomic laboratories report coordinates for deletions using the first and last probe deleted whereas others will report the end of the chromosome for a terminal

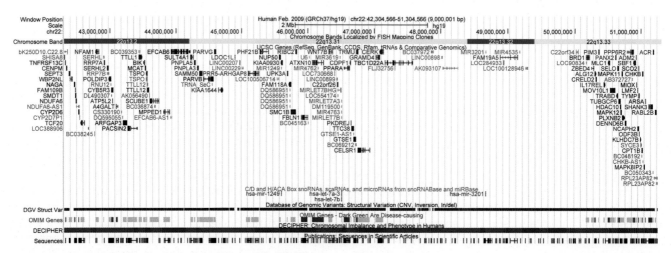

FIGURE 2   Distal region of 22q13 most commonly deleted in Phelan–McDermid syndrome. *The figure was produced using the UCSC Genome Browser[88] and the hg19 genome build.*

deletion. This can make the same sized deletion listed differ by 100 kb, yet convey the same level of accuracy. Note for instance, that for the coordinates of *SHANK3* in hg18 the RefSeq coordinates are Chr22:49,459,936-49,518,506. In hg19 the RefSeq coordinates are Chr22: 51,113,070-51,171,640. Finally, in hg38, the RefSeq coordinates are Chr22:50,674,642-50,733,212. In all cases the *SHANK3* gene is listed as being 58,570 base pairs in length, but its beginning and ending coordinates vary with the genome build.

To assess what is known about genotype–phenotype correlations in PMS, the literature was reviewed for studies that had deletion sizes spanning the full range typically observed in PMS and which addressed genotype–phenotype correlations statistically.[3,5,7,9,20,29,72] In addition, because of the rarity of interstitial deletions, two additional papers specifically addressing interstitial deletions were reviewed.[49,51] These studies are summarized in Table 4.

Across the studies examined, deletion sizes ranged from 67 kb to more than 10 MB. Whereas most were terminal deletions, some studies specifically addressed interstitial deletions.[3,49,51] In the case of terminal deletions, a finding of a correlation between larger deletion sizes and increased likelihood of disease or increased severity of disease would be supportive evidence of causal or contributory genes proximal to the terminus of the chromosome. Lack of an association between deletion size and a phenotype would be supportive evidence for the primary contributing genes to be located near the terminus. As in any study, larger sample sizes and large variability in deletion size improve the ability to distinguish associations between genomic regions and phenotypes. In the case of interstitial deletions, findings of phenotypes occurring in patients with interstitial, and not terminal, deletions contribute evidence for effects of genes located proximal to the terminus. In the case of PMS, much effort has been put into researching the effects of *SHANK3*, located near the terminus of 22q13.33. The reader is referred to chapter 10 of this volume (Verpelli and Schmeisser[92]) for an in-depth discussion of *SHANK3*. In the current review, the focus will be on evidence of loci proximal to *SHANK3* that may be associated with phenotypes of interest. The literature presents widely varying study designs and phenotypes examined. For the purpose of this review, eight features which were commonly assessed in the literature will be considered.

Developmental Delay: Developmental delay is present in nearly 100% of patients with PMS. Most investigators also observed an increase in severity of delay with increased deletion size.[3,5,7,9,20] Soorya et al.[29] found no correlation between deletion size and nonverbal intelligence quotient, but observed a correlation with gross motor skills. Patients with interstitial deletions reported by Wilson et al.[49] and Disciglio et al.[51] also had developmental delay. Wilson et al.[49] suggested future investigations of the 22q13.31 genes *CELSR*, *PLXNB2*, *SULT4A1*, *ATXN10*, and *PANX2* as potentially associated with developmental delay. Disciglio and coworkers[51] suggested the 22q13.31 genes *SULT4A1* and *PARVB* as potentially contributing to this phenotype. Sarasua et al.[72] suggested the genomic region of 22q13.31-q13.33 as being associated with late walking.

Speech and Language: Similarly, almost all patients were reported to have severely delayed or absent speech. Jeffries et al.[20] and Sarasua et al.[9] found significant correlation between increased deletion size and greater language impairment. Sarasua et al.[72] suggested a region near 22q13.2-q13.31 to be associated with speech. Jeffries et al.[20] suggested the 22q13.31 genes *CELSR1*, *PLXNB2*, *WNT7B*, *SULT4A1*, *ATXN10*, and *PANX2* to be potentially related to developmental delay and speech. Luciani et al.,[7] Wilson et al.,[5] and Soorya et al.[29] found no association between deletion size and speech/language delay. In particular, Soorya et al.[29] found no significant association with expressive or receptive language skills as measured on the Vineland Adaptive Behavior Scale (VABS). However, they found increased deletion size to be significantly associated with increased Autism Diagnostic Interview-Revised (ADI-R) qualitative abnormalities in communication score.

Autism: Two papers[20,29] found associations between increased deletion size and autism. Jeffries et al.[20] found increased deletion size to be correlated with increased autistic traits as measured with the Social Communication Questionnaire. Soorya et al.[29] found a significant association between increased deletion size and increased scores on ADI-R for reciprocal social interaction and abnormalities in communication. Deletion size was not significantly associated with restricted, repetitive, or stereotypical patterns or behavior. In addition, Soorya et al.[29] found that patients without autism had the smallest mean deletion sizes whereas those with autism had the largest mean deletion sizes. In contrast, Sarasua et al.[9,72] found that larger deletion sizes correlated with less likelihood of a parent report of an autism diagnosis. Among the interstitial deletion patients reported by Disciglio et al.[51] two of five patients were reported to have autism. Autism was not assessed in the study by Wilson et al.[49] of two interstitial patients. The varying sample sizes and diagnostic criteria make it difficult to understand the association between deletion size and autism. Taken together, the association of greater speech and language impairment with larger deletions and the finding of greater social and communication impairment with larger deletions, it may be that some domains of autism are more associated with proximal genomic regions than others (repetitive behaviors).

TABLE 4   Association between 22q13 Deletion Sizes and Selected Phenotypes as Reported in Literature[a]

Sample Size (Range of Deletion Sizes)	Global Developmental Delay	Autism	Speech/Language Delay	Growth	Hypotonia	Seizures
N = 33 (160 kb to 9 MB)[7]	Correlated with increased deletion size	Not examined	No correlation with deletion size	Not assessed statistically	Correlated; all patients with deletion >4 MB had hypotonia	No correlation with deletion size
N = 56 (130 kb to >9 MB)[5]	Correlated; authors suggest critical gene affecting neurological development in 130 kb region and more proximal	Not examined	Not correlated with deletion size	Increased head size correlated with deletion size	Correlated with deletion size	Not significantly correlated
N = 35 (67 kb to 10.2 MB)[20]	Correlated; authors suggest proximal genes contributory (CELSR, PLXNB2, SULT4A1, ATXN10, PANX2)	Significant correlation with increased autistic traits on Social Communication Questionnaire	Significant correlation with deletion size; authors suggest proximal genes contributory (CELSR, PLXNB2, SULT4A1, ATXN10, PANX2)	Not correlated with microcephaly or macrocephaly; stature not assessed	Not significantly correlated	Correlated
N = 2 (4.2–4.4 MB, interstitial)[49]	Present in both	Not examined	Both severely impaired	Tall stature and macrocephaly in both	Present in both	Seizures present in 1 patient with 22q13.2–q13.31 deletion
N = 71 (0.2–9 MB)[9]	Significantly correlated	Parent report of autism spectrum disorder associated with smaller deletions	Significant association between larger deletion size and fewer words	Deletion size associated with tall stature and large head circumference	Significant association with neonatal hypotonia	No association
N = 32 (SHANK3 point mutation –8.4 MB)[29]	No significant association with nonverbal intelligence quotient; significant association between decreased gross motor skills and increased deletion size	Significant association with scores on ADI-R. Larger mean deletion size for those with autism diagnosis than those without.	No association with language skills on the VABS; significant association with ADI-R qualitative abnormalities in communication score	Not addressed; macrocephaly more common in those with deletions > 5.3 MB; also present in 118-kb deletion and SHANK3 point mutation	No association	No association after correction for multiple testing, but significant at nominal P value
N = 9 (2.7–6.9 MB, all interstitial)[51]	Present in 9/9; authors suggest 22q13.31 region near SULT4A1 and PARVB (range of 44.15–45.19 hg19 region)	Present in 2/5	All had speech delay	4 of 8 had overgrowth; 5 of 9 had macrocephaly	7 of 9 have hypotonia	1 of 9 reports seizures
N = 70 (0.2–9.2)[72,b]	Not assessed	Interstitial region of lower risk	Region 22q13.2–13.31 associated with speech	Regions associated with macrocephaly, tall and short stature	22q13.31–q13.33 region associated with neonatal hypotonia	No association
N = 201 (0.2–9.2)[3,c]	Increased severity with increased deletion size					No association

[a]Published studies encompassing the full range (small–large) of deletion sizes and which conducted statistical examination of genotype–phenotype correlations are included in this review. In addition, two studies with interstitial deletions are included.[49,51]
[b]This study used the same sample as that published in Sarasua et al.[9] to identify specific genomic regions most associated with phenotypes.
[c]This study expands upon Sarasua et al.[72] to a total of 201 patients.

Growth: Growth was measured most commonly by stature or head circumference. Wilson et al.[5] found greater deletion sizes to be associated with macrocephaly, and Sarasua et al.[9,72] found an association with macrocephaly and stature. In particular, Sarasua et al.[72] found an association with specific 22q13.2 regions for short stature, 22q13.31-q13.32 regions for tall stature, and 22q13.31 regions for macrocephaly, and suggested *WNT7B* (mapping on 22q13.31) as a potential candidate gene for increased growth rate. Although Soorya et al.[29] did not specifically address macrocephaly, it appears to be more common in those with deletions greater than 5.3 MB, but was also present in a patient with a 118-kb deletion and a point mutation in *SHANK3*. Among those with interstitial deletions, both patients reported by Wilson et al.[49] had tall stature and macrocephaly whereas four of eight interstitial patients reported by Disciglio et al.[51] had overgrowth and five of nine had macrocephaly. These data point to a proximal genomic region, particularly around 22q13.31 associated with growth in these patients.

Dysmorphism: The general consensus of published reports is that patients with larger deletion sizes tend to have more dysmorphic features.[5,9,20,29] Commonly mentioned features include dysmorphic facial features such as a pointed chin, dolichocephaly, facial asymmetry, dental anomalies, and dysplastic toenails.

Hypotonia: Luciani et al.[7] and Wilson et al.[5] found a significant association between deletion size and hypotonia whereas Soorya et al.[29] and Jeffries et al.[20] found no association. Sarasua et al.[9] found a significant association with neonatal hypotonia (but not hypotonia later in life) and identified a genomic region of 22q13.31-q13.33 associated with neonatal hypotonia. In the interstitial cases, both interstitial patients reported by Wilson et al.[49] had hypotonia, and seven of nine interstitial patients reported by Disciglio et al.[51] had hypotonia. It is unclear whether hypotonia was obtained from physical examination, medical history, or neonatal records in the various studies; this uncertainly may cloud the association. Furthermore, muscle tone may change with age. Based on these studies, it appears that proximal genes in the 22q13.31-q13.33 region may contribute to muscle tone.

Seizures: Whereas Jeffries et al.[20] found a positive correlation between seizures and deletion size, no association was found by Luciani et al.,[7] Wilson et al.,[5] or Sarasua et al.[9,72] Soorya et al.[29] found a significant association between deletion size and seizures, but the association was no longer significant after correcting for multiple testing. One of two interstitial patients reported by Wilson et al.[49] and one of nine interstitial patients reported by Disciglio et al.[51] had seizures.

Summary of Genotype-Phenotype Correlations: Substantial evidence exists that genomic regions proximal to 22q13.33 may affect the PMS phenotype. The finding of a correlation with larger deletion sizes and more severe phenotypes, the presence of these phenotypes in individuals with interstitial deletions, the finding from segmental analysis which pinpointed regions of interest, and additional studies suggest that 22q13.31 in particular may contain genes that contribute to growth, dysmorphism, neurological features related to hypotonia, seizure, and developmental delay, speech and language, and autism.

DIFFERENTIAL DIAGNOSIS

PMS is characterized by vast phenotypical variability, and even the most recurrent features, such as global developmental delay, delayed or absent speech, and hypotonia, are relatively common in patients with neurodevelopmental disorders. The clinical heterogeneity reported in PMS presents physicians with a multitude of options for differential diagnosis. In some patients, dysmorphic traits might be minimal and overlooked, or even absent. In these patients, the behavioral problems may represent the sole clinical features and orient the diagnosis toward isolated, nonsyndromic autism.[1,2,47] Later in life, the onset of other neurobehavioral problems or minor dysmorphic features may lead the physician to reconsider the diagnosis.

Cerebral palsy shares several features with PMS: hypotonia, feeding difficulties, poor coordination, and subtle dysmorphic traits.[2,21,24] Individuals affected with Angelman syndrome or Rett syndrome present with global developmental delay, delayed or absent speech, regression, ataxic gait, seizures, and minor facial dysmorphism. In several cases for which the diagnosis of atypical Angelman syndrome has been proposed, a 22q13 deletion has been subsequently detected,[42] and a *de novo SHANK3* mutation has been identified in a female patient with Rett-like phenotype.[87] Other diagnoses carried by individuals subsequently shown to have PMS include velocardiofacial syndrome, Williams syndrome, Fragile X syndrome, FG syndrome, Smith—Magenis syndrome, and trichorhinophalangeal syndrome.[1,2,24]

The frequent use of chromosome microarray in the laboratory evaluation of individuals with developmental delay and the inclusion of *SHANK3* gene in the diagnostic panels of next-generation sequencing for intellectual disability and/or autism have increased the detection rate of PMS. However, the possibilities of small or balanced rearrangements affecting the 22q13 region, as well as the potential role of other genes than *SHANK3*, still make PMS a largely underdiagnosed condition.

References

1. Phelan MC, Stapleton GA, Rogers RC. 22q13 deletion syndrome: Phelan-McDermid syndrome. In: Cassidy SB, Allanson JE, editors. *The management of genetic syndromes*. Hoboken (NJ, USA): Wiley-Liss Inc.; 2010. p. 285−97.

2. Phelan K, McDermid HE. The 22q13.3 deletion syndrome (Phelan-McDermid syndrome). *Mol Syndromol* 2012;**2**(3−5):186−201.

3. Sarasua SM, Boccuto L, Sharp JL, Dwivedi A, Chen C-F, Rollins JD, et al. Clinical and genomic evaluation of 201 patients with Phelan-McDermid syndrome. *Hum Genet* 2014;**133**(7):847−59. http://dx.doi.org/10.1007/s00439-014-1423-7.

4. Bonaglia MC, Giorda R, Borgatti R, Felisari G, Gagliardi C, Selicorni A, et al. Disruption of the ProSAP2 gene in a t(12;22)(q24.1;q13.3) is associated with the 22q13.3 deletion syndrome. *Am J Hum Genet* 2001;**69**(2):261−8. http://dx.doi.org/10.1086/321293.

5. Wilson HL, Wong A, Shaw SR, Tse WY. Molecular characterisation of the 22q13 deletion syndrome supports the role of haploinsufficiency of SHANK3/PROSAP2 in the major neurological symptoms. *J Med Genet* 2003;**40**:575−84.

6. Kolevzon A, Angarita B, Bush L, Wang AT, Frank Y, Yang A, et al. Phelan-McDermid syndrome: a review of the literature and practice parameters for medical assessment and monitoring. *J Neurodev Disord* 2014;**6**(1):39. http://dx.doi.org/10.1186/1866-1955-6-39.

7. Luciani JJ, de Mas P, Depetris D, Mignon-Ravix C, Bottani A, Prieur M, et al. Telomeric 22q13 deletions resulting from rings, simple deletions, and translocations: cytogenetic, molecular, and clinical analyses of 32 new observations. *J Med Genet* 2003;**40**(9):690−6.

8. Bonaglia MC, Giorda R, Beri S, De Agostini C, Novara F, Fichera M, et al. Molecular mechanisms generating and stabilizing terminal 22q13 deletions in 44 subjects with Phelan/McDermid syndrome. *PLoS Genet* 2011;**7**(7):e1002173. http://dx.doi.org/10.1371/journal.pgen.1002173.

9. Sarasua SM, Dwivedi A, Boccuto L, Rollins JD, Chen C-F, Rogers RC, et al. Association between deletion size and important phenotypes expands the genomic region of interest in Phelan-McDermid syndrome (22q13 deletion syndrome). *J Med Genet* 2011;**48**(11):761−6. http://dx.doi.org/10.1136/jmedgenet-2011-100225.

10. Romain DR, Goldsmith J, Cairney H. Partial monosomy for chromosome 22 in a patient with del (22)(pter<-q13. 1::q13. 33->qter). *J Med Genet* 1990;**27**:588−9.

11. Fujita Y, Mochizuki D, Mori Y, Nakamoto N, Kobayashi M, Omi K, et al. Girl with accelerated growth, hearing loss, inner ear anomalies, delayed myelination of the brain, and del(22)(q13.1q13.2). *Am J Med Genet* 2000;**92**(3):195−9.

12. Rodríguez L, Martínez Guardia N, Herens C, Jamar M, Verloes A, López F, et al. Subtle trisomy 12q24.3 and subtle monosomy 22q13.3: three new cases and review. *Am J Med Genet A* 2003;**122A**(2):119−24. http://dx.doi.org/10.1002/ajmg.a.20243.

13. Su P-H, Chen J-Y, Chen S-J. Siblings with deletion 22q13.3 and trisomy 15q26 inherited from a maternally balanced translocation. *Pediatr Neonatol* 2011;**52**(5):287−9. http://dx.doi.org/10.1016/j.pedneo.2011.06.008.

14. Slavotinek A, Maher E, Gregory P, Rowlandson P, Huson SM. The phenotypic effects of chromosome rearrangement involving bands 7q21.3 and 22q13.3. *J Med Genet* 1997;**34**(10):857−61.

15. Watt JL, Olson IA, Johnston AW, Ross HS. A familial pericentric inversion of chromosome 22 with a recombinant subject illustrating a "pure" partial monosomy syndrome. *J Med Genet* 1985;**22**:283−7.

16. Tagaya M, Mizuno S, Hayakawa M, Yokotsuka T, Shimizu S, Fujimaki H. Recombination of a maternal pericentric inversion results in 22q13 deletion syndrome. *Clin Dysmorphol* 2008;**17**(1):19−21. http://dx.doi.org/10.1097/mcd.0b013e3281c1c81d.

17. Weleber RG, Hecht F. Ring-G chromosome, a new G-deletion syndrome? *Am J Dis Child* 1968;**115**:489−93.

18. Hunter AG, Ray M, Wang HS, Thompson DR. Phenotypic correlations in patients with ring chromosome 22. *Clin Genet* 1977;**12**(4):239−49.

19. Ishmael HA, Cataldi D, Begleiter ML, Pasztor LM, Dasouki MJ, Butler MG. Five new subjects with ring chromosome 22. *Clin Genet* 2003;**63**(5):410−4.

20. Jeffries AR, Curran S, Elmslie F, Sharma A, Wenger S, Hummel M, et al. Molecular and phenotypic characterization of ring chromosome 22. *Am J Med Genet A* 2005;**137**(2):139−47. http://dx.doi.org/10.1002/ajmg.a.30780.

21. Phelan MC, Rogers RC, Saul RA, Stapleton GA, Sweet K, McDermid H, et al. 22q13 deletion syndrome. *Am J Med Genet* 2001;**101**(2):91−9.

22. Yong YP, Knight LA, Yong MH, Lam S, Ho LY. Partial monosomy for chromosome 22 in a girl with mental retardation. *Singap Med J* 1997;**38**(2):85−6.

23. Riegel M, Baumer A, Wisser J, Acherman J, Schinzel A. Prenatal diagnosis of mosaicism for a del(22)(q13). *Prenat Diagn* 2000;**20**(1):76−9.

24. Phelan MC. Deletion 22q13.3 syndrome. *Orphanet J Rare Dis* 2008;**3**:14. http://dx.doi.org/10.1186/1750-1172-3-14.

25. Tabolacci E, Zollino M, Lecce R, Sangiorgi E, Gurrieri F, Leuzzi V, et al. Two brothers with 22q13 deletion syndrome and features suggestive of the Clark-Baraitser syndrome. *Clin Dysmorphol* 2005;**14**(3):127−32.

26. Moessner R, Marshall CR, Sutcliffe JS, Skaug J, Pinto D, Vincent J, et al. Contribution of SHANK3 mutations to autism spectrum disorder. *Am J Hum Genet* 2007;**81**(6):1289−97. http://dx.doi.org/10.1086/522590.

27. Verhoeven WM, Egger JI, Willemsen MH, de Leijer GJ, Kleefstra T. Phelan-McDermid syndrome in two adult brothers: atypical bipolar disorder as its psychopathological phenotype? *Neuropsychiatr Dis Treat* 2012;**8**:175−9. http://dx.doi.org/10.2147/ndt.S30506.

28. Macedoni-Lukšič M, Krgović D, Zagradišnik B, Kokalj-Vokač N. Deletion of the last exon of SHANK3 gene produces the full Phelan-McDermid phenotype: a case report. *Gene* 2013;**524**(2):386−9. http://dx.doi.org/10.1016/j.gene.2013.03.141.

29. Soorya L, Kolevzon A, Zweifach J, Lim T, Dobry Y, Schwartz L, et al. Prospective investigation of autism and genotype-phenotype correlations in 22q13 deletion syndrome and SHANK3 deficiency. *Mol Autism* 2013;**4**(1):18. http://dx.doi.org/10.1186/2040-2392-4-18.

30. Kirshenbaum G, Chmura M, Rhone DP. Long arm deletion of chromosome 22. *J Med Genet* 1988;**25**(11):780.

31. Herman GE, Greenberg F, Ledbetter DH. Multiple congenital anomaly/mental retardation (MCA/MR) syndrome with Goldenhar complex due to a terminal del(22q). *Am J Med Genet* 1988;**29**(4):909−15. http://dx.doi.org/10.1002/ajmg.1320290423.

32. Phelan MC, Rogers RC, Stevenson RE. A de novo terminal deletion of 22q. *Am J Hum Genet* 1988;**43**:A118.

33. Zwaigenbaum L, Siegel-Bartelt J, Teshima I, Ho C. Two patients with 22q13. 3 deletions have similar facies and developmental patterns. *Am J Hum Genet* 1990;**47**:A45.

34. Narahara K, Takahashi Y, Murakami M, Tsuji K, Yokoyama Y, Murakami R, et al. Terminal 22q deletion associated with a partial deficiency of arylsulphatase A. *J Med Genet* 1992;**29**(6):432−3.

35. Phelan MC, Thomas GR, Saul RA, Rogers RC, Taylor HA, Wenger DA, et al. Cytogenetic, biochemical, and molecular analyses of a 22q13 deletion. *Am J Med Genet* 1992;**43**(5):872−6. http://dx.doi.org/10.1002/ajmg.1320430524.

36. Nesslinger NJ, Gorski JL, Kurczynski TW, Shapira SK, Siegel-Bartelt J, Dumanski JP, et al. Clinical, cytogenetic, and molecular characterization of seven patients with deletions of chromosome 22q13.3. *Am J Hum Genet* 1994;**54**(3):464−72.

37. Flint J, Wilkie AO, Buckle VJ, Winter RM, Holland AJ, McDermid HE. The detection of subtelomeric chromosomal rearrangements in idiopathic mental retardation. *Nat Genet* 1995;**9**(2): 132–40. http://dx.doi.org/10.1038/ng0295-132.

38. Doheny KF, McDermid HE, Harum K, Thomas GH, Raymond GV. Cryptic terminal rearrangement of chromosome 22q13.32 detected by FISH in two unrelated patients. *J Med Genet* 1997;**34**(8):640–4.

39. Schröder K, Schuffenhauer S, Seidel H, Bartsch O, Blin N, Hinkel GK, et al. Deletion mapping by FISH with BACs in patients with partial monosomy 22q13. *Hum Genet* 1998;**102**(5):557–61.

40. Smith DP, Floyd M, Say B. Detection of a familial cryptic translocation by fluorescent in situ hybridisation. *J Med Genet* 1996;**33**(1):84.

41. Praphanphoj V, Goodman BK, Thomas GH, Raymond GV. Cryptic subtelomeric translocations in the 22q13 deletion syndrome. *J Med Genet* 2000;**37**(1):58–61.

42. Precht KS, Lese CM, Spiro RP, Huttenlocher PR, Johnston KM, Baker JC, et al. Two 22q telomere deletions serendipitously detected by FISH. *J Med Genet* 1998;**35**(11):939–42.

43. de Vries BB, Bitner-Glindzicz M, Knight SJ, Tyson J, MacDermont KD, Flint J, et al. A boy with a submicroscopic 22qter deletion, general overgrowth and features suggestive of FG syndrome. *Clin Genet* 2000;**58**(6):483–7.

44. Anderlid B-M, Schoumans J, Annerén G, Tapia-Paez I, Dumanski J, Blennow E, et al. FISH-mapping of a 100-kb terminal 22q13 deletion. *Hum Genet* 2002;**110**(5):439–43. http://dx.doi.org/10.1007/s00439-002-0713-7.

45. Delahaye A, Toutain A, Aboura A, Dupont C, Tabet AC, Benzacken B, et al. Chromosome 22q13.3 deletion syndrome with a de novo interstitial 22q13.3 cryptic deletion disrupting SHANK3. *Eur J Med Genet* 2009;**52**(5):328–32. http://dx.doi.org/10.1016/j.ejmg.2009.05.004.

46. Misceo D, Rødningen OK, Barøy T, Sorte H, Mellembakken JR, Strømme P, et al. A translocation between Xq21.33 and 22q13.33 causes an intragenic SHANK3 deletion in a woman with Phelan-McDermid syndrome and hypergonadotropic hypogonadism. *Am J Med Genet A* 2011;**155A**(2):403–8. http://dx.doi.org/10.1002/ajmg.a.33798.

47. Durand CM, Betancur C, Boeckers TM, Bockmann J, Chaste P, Fauchereau F, et al. Mutations in the gene encoding the synaptic scaffolding protein SHANK3 are associated with autism spectrum disorders. *Nat Genet* 2007;**39**(1):25–7. http://dx.doi.org/10.1038/ng1933.

48. Gauthier J, Spiegelman D, Piton A, Lafrenière RG, Laurent S, St-Onge J, et al. Novel de novo SHANK3 mutation in autistic patients. *Am J Med Genet B Neuropsychiatr Genet* 2009;**150B**(3): 421–4. http://dx.doi.org/10.1002/ajmg.b.30822.

49. Wilson HL, Crolla JA, Walker D, Artifoni L, Dallapiccola B, Takano T, et al. Interstitial 22q13 deletions: genes other than SHANK3 have major effects on cognitive and language development. *Eur J Hum Genet* 2008;**16**(11):1301–10. http://dx.doi.org/10.1038/ejhg.2008.107.

50. Simenson K, Õiglane-Shlik E, Teek R, Kuuse K, Õunap K. A patient with the classic features of Phelan-McDermid syndrome and a high immunoglobulin E level caused by a cryptic interstitial 0.72-MB deletion in the 22q13.2 region. *Am J Med Genet A* 2014; **164A**(3):806–9. http://dx.doi.org/10.1002/ajmg.a.36358.

51. Disciglio V, Rizzo Lo C, Mencarelli MA, Mucciolo M, Marozza A, Di Marco C, et al. Interstitial 22q13 deletions not involving SHANK3 gene: a new contiguous gene syndrome. *Am J Med Genet A* 2014;**164A**(7):1666–76. http://dx.doi.org/10.1002/ajmg.a.36513.

52. Phelan K, Boccuto L, Rogers RC, Sarasua SM, McDermid HE. Letter to the editor regarding Disciglio et al.: interstitial 22q13 deletions not involving SHANK3 gene: a new contiguous gene syndrome. *Am J Med Genet A* 2015;**167**(7):1679–80.

53. Dhar SU, del Gaudio D, German JR, Peters SU, Ou Z, Bader PI, et al. 22q13.3 deletion syndrome: clinical and molecular analysis using array CGH. *Am J Med Genet A* 2010;**152A**(3):573–81. http://dx.doi.org/10.1002/ajmg.a.33253.

54. Havens JM, Visootsak J, Phelan MC, Graham JM. 22q13 deletion syndrome: an update and review for the primary pediatrician. *Clin Pediatr (Phila)* 2004;**43**(1):43–53.

55. Manning MA, Cassidy SB, Clericuzio C, Cherry AM, Schwartz S, Hudgins L, et al. Terminal 22q deletion syndrome: a newly recognized cause of speech and language disability in the autism spectrum. *Pediatrics* 2004;**114**(2):451–7.

56. Webster KT, Raymond GV. 22q13 deletion syndrome: a report of the language function in two cases. *J Med Speech - Lang Pathol* 2004;**12**:42–6.

57. Rollins JD, Sarasua SM, Phelan K, DuPont BR, Rogers RC, Collins JS. Growth in Phelan-McDermid syndrome. *Am J Med Genet A* 2011;**155A**(9):2324–6. http://dx.doi.org/10.1002/ajmg.a.34158.

58. Figura MG, Coppola A, Bottitta M, Calabrese G, Grillo L, Luciano D, et al. Seizures and EEG pattern in the 22q13.3 deletion syndrome: clinical report of six Italian cases. *Seizure* 2014;**23**(9): 774–9. http://dx.doi.org/10.1016/j.seizure.2014.06.008.

59. Lund C, Brodtkorb E, Røsby O, Rødningen OK, Selmer KK. Copy number variants in adult patients with Lennox-Gastaut syndrome features. *Epilepsy Res* 2013;**105**(1–2):110–7. http://dx.doi.org/10.1016/j.eplepsyres.2013.01.009.

60. Koolen DA, Reardon W, Rosser EM, Lacombe D, Hurst JA, Law CJ, et al. Molecular characterisation of patients with subtelomeric 22q abnormalities using chromosome specific array-based comparative genomic hybridisation. *Eur J Hum Genet* 2005;**13**(9):1019–24. http://dx.doi.org/10.1038/sj.ejhg.5201456.

61. Lindquist SG, Kirchhoff M, Lundsteen C, Pedersen W, Erichsen G, Kristensen K, et al. Further delineation of the 22q13 deletion syndrome. *Clin Dysmorphol* 2005;**14**(2):55–60.

62. Prasad C, Prasad AN, Chodirker BN, Lee C, Dawson AK, Jocelyn LJ, et al. Genetic evaluation of pervasive developmental disorders: the terminal 22q13 deletion syndrome may represent a recognizable phenotype. *Clin Genet* 2000;**57**(2):103–9.

63. Goizet C, Excoffier E, Taine L, Taupiac E, Moneim El AA, Arveiler B, et al. Case with autistic syndrome and chromosome 22q13.3 deletion detected by FISH. *Am J Med Genet* 2000;**96**(6): 839–44.

64. Oberman LM, Boccuto L, Cascio L, Sarasua S, Kaufmann WE. Autism spectrum disorder in Phelan-McDermid syndrome: initial characterization and genotype-phenotype correlations. *Orphanet J Rare Dis* 2015;**10**(1):105. http://dx.doi.org/10.1186/s13023-015-0323-9.

65. Cusmano-Ozog K, Manning MA, Hoyme HE. 22q13.3 deletion syndrome: a recognizable malformation syndrome associated with marked speech and language delay. *Am J Med Genet C Semin Med Genet* 2007;**145C**(4):393–8. http://dx.doi.org/10.1002/ajmg.c.30155.

66. Philippe A, Boddaert N, Vaivre-Douret L, Robel L, Danon-Boileau L, Malan V, et al. Neurobehavioral profile and brain imaging study of the 22q13.3 deletion syndrome in childhood. *Pediatrics* 2008;**122**(2):e376–82. http://dx.doi.org/10.1542/peds.2007-2584.

67. Messias E, Kaley SN, McKelvey KD. Adult-onset psychosis and clinical genetics: a case of Phelan-McDermid syndrome. *J Neuropsychiatry Clin Neurosci* 2013;**25**(4):E27. http://dx.doi.org/10.1176/appi.neuropsych.12100241.

68. Aldinger KA, Kogan J, Kimonis V, Fernandez B, Horn D, Klopocki E, et al. Cerebellar and posterior fossa malformations in patients with autism-associated chromosome 22q13 terminal deletion. *Am J Med Genet A* 2013;**161A**(1):131–6. http://dx.doi.org/10.1002/ajmg.a.35700.

69. Friedel RH, Kerjan G, Rayburn H, Schüller U, Sotelo C, Tessier-Lavigne M, et al. Plexin-B2 controls the development of cerebellar granule cells. *J Neurosci* 2007;**27**(14):3921—32. http://dx.doi.org/10.1523/jneurosci.4710-06.2007.

70. Giza J, Urbanski MJ, Prestori F, Bandyopadhyay B, Yam A, Friedrich V, et al. Behavioral and cerebellar transmission deficits in mice lacking the autism-linked gene islet brain-2. *J Neurosci* 2010;**30**(44):14805—16. http://dx.doi.org/10.1523/jneurosci.1161-10.2010.

71. McGaughran J, Hadwen T, Clark R. Progressive edema leading to pleural effusions in a female with a ring chromosome 22 leading to a 22q13 deletion. *Clin Dysmorphol* 2010;**19**(1):28—9. http://dx.doi.org/10.1097/mcd.0b013e3283301f58.

72. Sarasua SM, Dwivedi A, Boccuto L, Chen C-F, Sharp JL, Rollins JD, et al. 22q13.2q13.32 genomic regions associated with severity of speech delay, developmental delay, and physical features in Phelan-McDermid syndrome. *Genet Med* 2014;**16**(4):318—28. http://dx.doi.org/10.1038/gim.2013.144.

73. Barakat AJ, Pearl PL, Acosta MT, Runkle BP. 22q13 deletion syndrome with central diabetes insipidus: a previously unreported association. *Clin Dysmorphol* 2004;**13**(3):191—4.

74. Sathyamoorthi S, Morales J, Bermudez J, McBride L, Luquette M, McGoey R, et al. Array analysis and molecular studies of INI1 in an infant with deletion 22q13 (Phelan-McDermid syndrome) and atypical teratoid/rhabdoid tumor. *Am J Med Genet A* 2009;**149A**(5):1067—9. http://dx.doi.org/10.1002/ajmg.a.32775.

75. Cho EH, Park JB, Kim JK. Atypical teratoid rhabdoid brain tumor in an infant with ring chromosome 22. *Korean J Pediatr* 2014;**57**(7):333—6. http://dx.doi.org/10.3345/kjp.2014.57.7.333.

76. Rubio A. March 1997 — 4 year old girl with ring chromosome 22 and brain tumor. *Brain Pathol* 1997;**7**(3):1027—8.

77. Kirkpatrick BE, El-Khechen D. A unique presentation of 22q13 deletion syndrome: multicystic kidney, orofacial clefting, and Wilms' tumor. *Clin Dysmorphol* 2011;**20**(1):53—4. http://dx.doi.org/10.1097/MCD.0b013e32833effb1.

78. Bisgaard A-M, Kirchhoff M, Nielsen JE, Kibaek M, Lund A, Schwartz M, et al. Chromosomal deletion unmasking a recessive disease: 22q13 deletion syndrome and metachromatic leukodystrophy. *Clin Genet* 2009;**75**(2):175—9. http://dx.doi.org/10.1111/j.1399-0004.2008.01113.x.

79. Zambrano RM. Unbalanced t(14;22) unmasks a recessive allele causing MLD in a child with Phelan-McDermid syndrome. In: *ACMG annual clinical genetics meeting. Nashville (TN)*; 2014. A231.

80. Artigalás O, Paskulin G, Riegel M, Burin M, Saraiva-Pereira ML, Maluf S, et al. A patient presenting a 22q13 deletion associated with an apparently balanced translocation t(16;22): an illustrative case in the investigation of patients with low ARSA activity. *Genet Mol Biol* 2012;**35**(2):424—7. http://dx.doi.org/10.1590/S1415-47572012000300007.

81. Tufano M, Corte Della C, Cirillo F, Spagnuolo MI, Candusso M, Melis D, et al. Fulminant autoimmune hepatitis in a girl with 22q13 deletion syndrome: a previously unreported association. *Eur J Pediatr* 2009;**168**(2):225—7. http://dx.doi.org/10.1007/s00431-008-0732-z.

82. Bartsch O, Schneider E, Damatova N, Weis R, Tufano M, Iorio R, et al. Fulminant hepatic failure requiring liver transplantation in 22q13.3 deletion syndrome. *Am J Med Genet A* 2010;**152A**(8):2099—102. http://dx.doi.org/10.1002/ajmg.a.33542.

83. Sovner R, Stone A, Fox C. Ring chromosome 22 and mood disorders. *J Intellect Disabil Res* 1996;**40**(Pt 1):82—6.

84. Willemsen MH, Rensen JHM, van Schronjenstein-Lantman de Valk HMJ, Hamel BCJ, Kleefstra T. Adult phenotypes in Angelman-and Rett-like syndromes. *Mol Syndromol* 2011;**2**:217—34. http://dx.doi.org/10.1159/000335661.

85. Denayer A, Van Esch H, de Ravel T, Frijns J-P, Van Buggenhout G, Vogels A, et al. Neuropsychopathology in 7 patients with the 22q13 deletion syndrome: presence of bipolar disorder and progressive loss of skills. *Mol Syndromol* 2012;**3**:14—20.

86. Verhoeven WMA, Egger JIM, Cohen-Snuijf R, Kant SG, de Leeuw N. Phelan-McDermid syndrome: clinical report of a 70-year-old woman. *Am J Med Genet A* 2013;**161A**(1):158—61. http://dx.doi.org/10.1002/ajmg.a.35597.

87. Hara M, Ohba C, Yamashita Y, Saitsu H, Matsumoto N, Matsuishi T. De novo SHANK3 mutation causes Rett syndrome-like phenotype in a female patient. *Am J Med Genet A* 2015;**167**(7):1593—6. http://dx.doi.org/10.1002/ajmg.a.36775.

88. Kent WJ, Sugnet CW, Furey TS, Roskin KM, Pringle TH, Zahler AM, et al. The human genome browser at UCSC. *Genome Res* 2002;**12**(6):996—1006. http://dx.doi.org/10.1101/gr.229102.

89. Amberger J, Bocchini CA, Scott AF, Hamosh A. McKusick's online mendelian inheritance in man (OMIM). *Nucleic Acids Res* 2009;**37**(Database issue):D793—6. http://dx.doi.org/10.1093/nar/gkn665.

90. MacDonald JR, Ziman R, Yuen RKC, Feuk L, Scherer SW. The database of genomic variants: a curated collection of structural variation in the human genome. *Nucleic Acids Res* 2014;**42**(Database issue):D986—92. http://dx.doi.org/10.1093/nar/gkt958.

91. Firth HV, Richards SM, Bevan AP, Clayton S, Corpas M, Rajan D, et al. DECIPHER: database of chromosomal imbalance and phenotype in humans using ensembl resources. *Am J Hum Genet* 2009;**84**(4):524—33. http://dx.doi.org/10.1016/j.ajhg.2009.03.010.

92. Verpelli C, Schmeisser MJ. SHANK3, SHANK2, and SHANK1 mutations in ID and ASD. In: Sala C, Verpelli C, editors. *Synaptic dysfunction in autism spectrum disorder and intellectual disability.* Elsevier; 2016.

22

Epilepsy Associated with ASD and Intellectual Disability

Carla Marini

Neurology Unit, Meyer Children's Hospital, Florence, Italy

INTRODUCTION

The relationship of autism to epilepsy has been an area of scientific interest for decades.

Initial studies of the relationship of autism to epilepsy and to electroencephalogram (EEG) abnormalities in the 1960s[1–3] were among the first to suggest that autism was a disorder of brain function.[4]

Autism spectrum disorder (ASD) is a biologically based neurodevelopmental disability characterized by a wide range of dysfunctions including communicative and social ability with repetitive, restricted, and stereotyped interests and behavior. Clinical presentation is heterogeneous with mild to severe impairment, perhaps reflecting multiple pathogenetic backgrounds. Ideally, the clinical diagnosis of autism should be reached by conducting an observation and patient examination and obtaining information from multiple sources such as parents and teachers. It requires the presence of full diagnostic criteria and differentiation from typical development, language delay, and other nonspectrum psychiatric disorders (*Diagnostic and Statistical Manual of Mental Disorders*, 5th edition).[5,6] To date, no diagnostic

biological markers or specific tests for ASD are available; thus, diagnosis depends on the individual clinician's interpretation of diagnostic criteria, which can be affected by multiple factors, most notably level of training and clinical expertise, and conceptualization of ASD. Generally, autism cannot be confidently diagnosed before age about 36 months, although early detection of at least some forms is possible. The term "ASD" is now commonly used to include children with autistic disorder and pervasive developmental disorders not otherwise specified, and those with Asperger syndrome.[4]

Epilepsy, which is characterized by the recurrence of seizures expression of neuronal hyperexcitability, is often associated with ASD.[7] The diagnostic category of epilepsy includes multiple seizure, epilepsy, and syndrome types.[8–10] Intellectual disability is also common in children with epilepsy. Population-based studies report that approximately a quarter of children with epilepsy also have some degree of intellectual disability.[11] The prevalence is highest in children with the youngest age at onset of epilepsy and in association with structural brain lesions. Intellectual disability is especially high in a group of epilepsy syndromes often referred to collectively as the epileptic encephalopathies (EE) because of their strong association with developmental and behavioral disabilities.[12,13] These syndromes include several disorders such as (but not limited to) West syndrome and Dravet, Ohtahara, and Lennox–Gastaut syndromes (see also Chapter 15).

Autism, ID, and epilepsy thus represent neurobiological disorders with clinical heterogeneity and with varying etiologies, pathophysiology, and outcome.

EPIDEMIOLOGY

Autism spectrum disorders are a heterogeneous group of disorders affecting approximately 1 in 1000 children.[14] The male:female ratio is estimated at 4:1, which may be partly explained by X-linked inheritance in some families.[15] Available data, arising from studies of large cohorts of patients with ASD, suggest that the co-occurrence of epilepsy and ASD is more than by chance.[16,17] A prospective study looking at the prevalence of epilepsy in 246 children with ASD revealed that 7.6% of children satisfying the criteria of infantile autism and 5% of those with an autistic condition had epilepsy.[16] Most had onset of seizures before age 1 year. There was no correlation between the age of onset of seizures, type of seizure, sex, mentality, and the outcome of epilepsy.[16] Instead, more recent studies show an increased risk of seizures in patients with a severe degree of ID, a family history with seizures, and tall stature.[17]

Nonetheless, percentages of the prevalence of epilepsy in ASD are variable, ranging from 5% to 46%.[18–23] Three main factors—age, cognitive level, and type of language disorder—account for such variability.[4] The prevalence of epilepsy is highest in studies that have included adolescents and young adults, individuals with moderate to severe mental retardation, those with motor deficits, and individuals with severe receptive language deficits. Percentages also vary depending on the inclusion of patients with only paroxysmal EEG abnormalities.[17,20] Autism spectrum disorder symptoms may occur in 15–35% of children with epilepsy.[24,25]

ETIOLOGY

The greater risk of recurrence of ASD and epilepsy in siblings than in the general population and the high concordance rate of monozygotic twins compared with dizygotic twins indicate that genetic factors have a major role in the pathogenesis of both disorders.[26–29] Furthermore, the association of autism with epilepsy or with EEG abnormalities suggests that these two disorders might share genetic factors in some cases or possibly pathophysiological mechanisms.[25,30] Over the past years, this comorbidity, termed autism–epilepsy phenotype (AEP), has been the object of clinical and genetic investigations.[18,25,31] Overall, genetic epidemiology studies suggest a polygenic inheritance, although the mechanism of inheritance and the AEP genes remain largely unknown.

A number of well-known genetic disorders share epilepsy, intellectual disability, and autism as prominent phenotypic features, including tuberous sclerosis, Rett syndrome (RTT), and fragile X (see also Chapters 7 and 8). In addition, mutations of several genes involved in neurodevelopment, including ARX, neuroligins, and neuropilin 2 have been identified in children with epilepsy, ID, ASD, or a combination of them. Mutations in both PRICKLE1 and SYN1 genes also predispose to epilepsy, autism, and abnormal behavior in both human and mice models (Table 1).[32,33] These two genes are implicated in synaptic function, which has led to the hypothesis that synaptic deregulation might be one of the shared pathophysiological mechanisms underlying both ASD and epilepsy.[32,33] The PTEN gene was identified, which encodes tumor suppressor dual-specificity phosphatase, might carry mutations in patients with ASD, seizures, and macrocephaly, which suggests its involvement in the pathogenesis of these disorders.[34,35]

Table 1 includes a list of the most relevant genes that when mutated can contribute to both disorders in some patients.

About 20% of patients with cognitive impairment, autistic clinical features, and epilepsy carry chromosomal abnormalities (Table 2).[36,37] The identification of chromosomal abnormalities is also important to identify new candidate genes for AEP. Indeed, the chromosomal deletion at 15q26.1 identified in a patient includes the alpha-2, 8-sialyltransferase 2 (ST8SIA2) gene, which is expressed in the developing brain and appears to have an important role in neuronal migration, axon guidance, and synaptic plasticity.[38,39] This case provides evidence that ST8SIA2 haploinsufficiency may have a role in neurobehavioral phenotypes.[38,39] Smaller and larger deletions of the 7q11.23, the Williams–Beuren syndrome region, implicate genes involved in mild facial phenotype, epilepsy, and autistic traits including HIP1 and YWHAG genes.[38,39]

Whole-exome sequencing (WES) and whole-genome sequencing (WGS) show promise as tools for identifying ASD and epilepsy risk genes as well as unreported mutations in known loci.[36,40] Recent WGS and WES studies of families with ASD detected genetic variants in unrecognized genes[41] and in genes previously associated with epilepsy including SCN2A and KCNQ2[42] (see also

TABLE 1   Known Genes Associated with ASD, ID, and Epilepsy

Gene	Locus	Gene Function	Phenotype	References
PCDH19	Xq22	Calcium-dependent cell–cell adhesion molecule	Only females, focal epilepsy, ID, ASD	[51,52]
CDKL5	Xq22.13	CDKL5; neural maturation and synaptogenesis interaction with MECP2	EOEE with IS, tonic, TC, focal and My seizures	[53–55]
MECP2	Xq28	Chromatin-associated protein; neural maturation and synaptogenesis	Rett syndrome	[57,58]
FOXG1	14q12	Developmental transcription factor with repressor activities	IS, EOEE, ASD, and Rett variant	[59]
PRICKLE1	12q12	Planar cell polarity signaling pathway; establishes cell polarity during embryonic development: destabilize synaptic homeostasis	ASD, ID, and epilepsy	[32]
SYN1	Xp11.23	Synapsin I, neuronal phosphoprotein associated with membranes of small synaptic vesicles; synaptic neurotransmission, neuronal development, synaptogenesis, maintenance of mature synapses, and plasticity	ASD, ID, and epilepsy	[33]
SYNGAP1	6p21.32	Brain-specific synaptic Ras GTP-ase activating protein AMPA receptor trafficking, excitatory synaptic transmission, and number of silent synapses	ASD, ID, and epilepsy	[69]
ARX	Xq21.3	Aristaless-related homeobox protein; GABAergic interneuron migration	IS, EOEE, and ASD	[70]
GABRG1	4p12	Member of GABA-A receptor gene family	ASD, ID, and epilepsy	[71]
NRXN1	2p16.3	Cell-surface receptor that binds neuroligins, forming Ca^{2+}-dependent trans-synaptic complex required for efficient neurotransmission and involved in formation of synaptic contacts	Severe early-onset epilepsy and autism	[72]
GRIN2A	16p13	Glutamate-activated ion channel permeable to Na^+, K^+, and Ca^{2+} and is found at excitatory synapses throughout brain.	EE (LKS and CSWSS) with global regression (>> language), autistic behaviors	[67,68]
SLC35A3	1p21.2	Nucleotide sugar transporter that transports UDP-N-acetylglucosamine (UDP-GlcNAc) from its site of synthesis in cytosol to its site of use in Golgi	ASD, ID, epilepsy, and arthrogryposis	[73]
TSC1	9q34;	Amartin; mTOR pathway	Tuberous sclerosis, epilepsy (>> IS), and autism	[74]
TSC2	16p.13	Tuberin; mTOR pathway	Tuberous sclerosis, epilepsy (>> IS), and autism	[75]
PTEN	10q23	Tumor suppressor dual-specificity phosphatase	ASD, seizures, macrocephaly autism	[34,35]

ASD, autism spectrum disorders; CSWSS, continuous slow waves of slow-sleep; EOEE, early-onset epileptic encephalopathy; EE, epileptic encephalopathy; ID, intellectual disability; IS, infantile spasms; LKS, Landau–Kleffner syndrome; My, myoclonic; TC, tonic–clonic seizures; >>, specially.

Chapter 15). Both genes encode for components of ion channels, which again highlights that the dysfunction of ion channels may underline several brain disorders from epilepsy to migraine and to autism. The extreme genetic heterogeneity and the uncertain mode of inheritance of both ASD and epilepsy have proven challenging for gene discovery, however.[43]

Table 2 reports recurrent chromosomal abnormalities.

EPILEPSIES AND SYNDROMES ASSOCIATED WITH ASD AND ID

The onset of seizures in ASD has a bimodal distribution, with one peak occurring before age 5 years and a later onset after age 10 years.[17,18,25,31]

There is no single unifying ASD-epilepsy phenotype, and seizures might be focal or generalized. One of the

TABLE 2   Frequent Chromosomal Abnormalities Associated with ASD, ID, and Epilepsy

Chromosomal segment	Clinical Features	Epilepsy
Del or dup 1q21.1	ASD, microcephaly	Generalized epilepsy
Del 2q23.1	ASD, macrocephaly, facial dysmorphic features	Generalized epilepsy
Del 7q11.23	Williams–Beuren syndrome	Both focal or generalized seizure
Del 15q13.3	ASD, ID	Generalized epilepsy with GTCS, absences, myoclonic; BRE
Del 15q26.1	ASD, ID	Both focal or generalized seizure
Del or dup 16p11.2	ASD, micro-macrocephaly, facial dysmorphic features	GTCS
Del or dup 16p13.11	ASD, micro-macrocephaly, congenital heart defects	Generalized epilepsy with GTCS, absences, myoclonic

ASD, autism spectrum disorder; BRE, benign Rolandic epilepsy; ID, intellectual disability; GTCS, tonic–clonic seizure.

earliest key observations was the relationship between infantile spasms, hypsarrhythmia, and ASD.[44] A Finnish study in 1981 found that 12.5% of 192 children with infantile spasms developed ASD.[45]

Fragile X syndrome (FXS) is the most frequent form of inherited intellectual disability and often presents with ASD and epilepsy. Fragile X results from an expanded triplet repeat in the FMR1 gene.[46] The *FMR1* gene codes for the fragile X mental retardation protein (FMRP), which is a messenger ribonucleic acid–binding protein abundant in the brain important for synaptic plasticity important for spine development and synaptic plasticity.[47] Fragile X mental retardation protein is also involved in axonal development, synapse formation, and the development and wiring of neuronal circuits[48] (see also Chapter 8). Evidence for a connection between the absence of Fmr1 and epileptogenesis was further supported by a study of neocortical circuits in FMRP knockout mice that found an increased intrinsic excitability in excitatory neurons from the knockout. In addition, dysregulation of glutamatergic neurons in fragile X syndrome can disrupt the normal actions of inhibitory GABAergic neurons and result in downregulation of GABA receptor subunits.[49,50]

There are also several rare neurodevelopmental disorders and EEs with mutations in known genes that in early childhood, during the course of the disease, might manifest autistic behaviors.[38,39]

- Mutations in *PCDH19* gene are clinically characterized by infantile onset of clusters of febrile focal seizures accompanied by later development of ID with various degrees of severity and ASD in about 50% of patients (Table 1).[51,52] It only affects females, whereas hemizygous males are unaffected carriers. The *PCDH19* gene is located on chromosome Xq21 and encodes for a calcium-dependent cell–cell adhesion molecule (see also Chapter 14).

- Mutations in the X-linked gene cyclin-dependent kinase-like 5 (*CDKL5*) cause a severe neurodevelopmental disorder with early-onset intractable seizures, severe developmental delay, autism, and often subsequent appearance of RTT-like features.[53,54] It affects girls more than boys. *CDKL5* is localized at excitatory synapses and contributes to correct dendritic spine structure and synapse activity[56] (Table 1).

- Rett syndrome is a postnatal progressive neurodevelopmental disorder that manifests in girls during early childhood. Symptoms appear over stages beginning at age 6–18 months and include loss of acquired speech, social skills, and purposeful use of the hands and motor skills. Patients typically develop profound cognitive impairment, and in addition to their characteristic clinical picture about 60% of females have epilepsy. Rett syndrome is caused by mutations in the gene encoding methyl-CpG binding protein 2 (MeCP2), a transcriptional regulator involved in chromatin remodeling and the modulation of ribonucleic acid splicing.[57] The precise mechanism by which loss of MeCP2 results in either epilepsy, ID, or ASD remains uncertain. Evidence suggests that alterations in cortical glutamatergic synaptic responses and excitatory connectivity resulting in a relative excess of inhibition compared with excitation may have an important role[58] (see also Chapter 7). Mutations of the *FOXG1* gene have also been associated with a form of congenital RETT syndrome with absent speech, stereotypies, and autism (Table 1).[57,59]

- Tuberous sclerosis complex (TSC) is a neurocutaneous syndrome characterized by benign tumors, early-onset epilepsy, intellectual disability, and autism. Some studies suggested that the combination of EEG discharges and tuber location is crucial to the development of ASD in children with tuberous sclerosis.[60] Tuberous sclerosis complex results from mutations of hamartin or tuberin (encoded by TSC1 and TSC2 genes). The exact mechanisms of epilepsy, ID, and ASD in TSC are still unknown, but alterations in trafficking of α-amino-3-hydroxy-5-methyl-4-isoxazolepropionic acid receptors and in expression of specific glutamate and GABA-A receptor subunits and decreases in the glutamate transporter GLT-1 all may contribute to imbalances in excitation and inhibition.[61,62]

- Mutations of the aristaless-related homeobox, X-linked (ARX) gene result in several clinical syndromes, all of which are associated with intellectual disability, ASD, and early-life seizures, most often infantile spasms. In animal models, ARX knockouts have reduced interneuron cell types and a variety of seizure types beginning in early life.[63]

In contrast to the increased risk for development of ASD in early-onset epilepsy, several studies reported the existence of a secondary peak of seizure onset in children with ASD during puberty. Deykin and MacMahon studied 183 children with ASD and found that the highest prevalence of seizures was in children between age 11 and 14 years.[64]

Conversely, whether subclinical epilepsy and epileptiform activity has adverse effects on cognition, language, and behavior is debated, as is the relation of autistic regression with an epileptiform EEG to Landau–Kleffner syndrome (LKS) and continuous spike waves in slow-sleep (CSWSS).[4] There is global regression in cognitive skills in CSWSS, whereas LKS is primarily characterized by early regression of language. Both CSWSS and LKS can share clinical manifestations that overlap with ASD.[4,65] Mutations in the GRIN2A gene have been associated with CSWSS and LKS (Table 1).[66,67]

MANAGEMENT AND TREATMENT OF SEIZURES AND AUTISTIC CLINICAL FEATURES

The best treatment to cure the core symptoms of ASD, including seizures, behavioral, and sleep disturbances, is, of course, based on the underlying etiology and pathophysiology, which are unfortunately unknown for most patients. Therefore, clinicians are left with the only possibility of improving arising symptoms including seizures, behavioral, and sleep problems.

Antiepileptic drugs (AEDs) are used to prevent seizure recurrence. There are no randomized control trials, cohort studies, or systematic reviews of case–control studies for any AEDs focusing on the control of seizure in the ASD population. A systematic review of efficacy of traditional and novel treatments for seizures has been published.[76] Table 3 summarizes the most

frequently used AEDs, dividing them into first- and second-line treatment. Effectiveness is reported evaluating clinical evidence of seizure control and improvement of behavioral and sleep disturbances. Valproic acid (VPA), carbamazepine, lamotrigine, and ethosuximide are reported to provide the best seizures control.[76–80] Other AEDs examined, including phenytoin, clonazepam, oxcarbazepine, topiramate, gabapentin, zonisamide, felbamate, and phenobarbital, were rated as significantly less beneficial for controlling seizures, with a less favorable effect on other clinical factors.[77–79]

One of the most salient questions is whether treatment with AEDs targeting the epileptiform activity can improve cognitive or behavioral functioning in children with autism. No large-scale controlled studies have been conducted to date to determine whether such interventions have a positive effect.

Antiepileptic drugs are also used to treat behavioral symptoms in autism, but with inconsistent results. An early open-label study of VPA[81] found improvement in aggression in children with autism, but a later placebo-controlled study showed no reduction in aggression using the same medication.[82] An open-label trial of levetiracetam showed significant improvement in emotional lability in children with autism compared with placebo.[83]

Traditional, non-AEDs treatments, including ketogenic diet, vagus nerve stimulator, and surgery, have proven effective in controlling seizures in a limited and highly selected number of patients.[84–86] Epilepsy surgery, for example, is straightforward for patients in whom epileptic foci are clearly visualized with magnetic resonance imaging, including tuberous sclerosis complex and tumors. Multiple subpial transections have been performed in some children with autistic clinical features related to seizures and paroxysmal activity on EEG recordings, but this type of surgery is uncommon and has unproven benefits.[76] Instead, immunomodulatory treatments, particularly steroids and intravenous immunoglobulin, seem to be more useful in patients with LKS and CSWSS.[87,88]

Individuals with seizures and ASD might have underlying metabolic conditions including disorders of energy, cholesterol, vitamin, gamma-aminobutyric acid, purine, pyrimidine, and amino acid metabolism and urea cycle disorders.[89] Identification and treatment of these disorders could improve the underlying metabolic derangements and potentially improve behavior and seizure frequency and/or severity in these individuals.[89]

Medications, especially atypical antipsychotic, may sometimes be necessary to ameliorate specific symptoms such as aggressive or self-injurious behavior. Conventional neuroleptic agents such as haloperidol and atypical antipsychotic ones including risperidone and aripiprazole have been used to treat the more aggressive and violent features of autistic patients.[90] Together with

TABLE 3   Most Common Therapies to Treat Seizures and Autistic Clinical Features

	Drugs/Treatment	Seizures and EEG	Behavioral Effect	Other Effects
AEDs first-line	Valproic acid	Broad-spectrum efficacy improves EEG	Mood stabilization	Improvement aggressive behaviors/irritability
	Ethosuximide	Efficacy > generalized seizure	Neutral	
	Carbamazepine	Efficacy > focal seizure	Mood stabilization	
	Lamotrigine	Broad-spectrum	Insufficient evidence	
	Levetiracetam	Broad-spectrum	Insufficient evidence	Improvement in emotional lability
AEDs second line	Phenytoin	Less beneficial		
	Clonazepam	Less beneficial		
	Oxcarbazepine	Less beneficial		
	Topiramate	Less beneficial	Insufficient evidence	
	Gabapentin	Less beneficial		
	Zonisamide	Less beneficial		
	Felbamate	Less beneficial		
	Phenobarbital	Less beneficial		
Neuroleptic	Haloperidol	Might decrease seizure threshold	Improvement aggressive behaviors/irritability	Sedation
	Olanzapine	Might decrease seizure threshold	Improvement aggressive behaviors/irritability	Sedation
	Quetiapine	Might decrease seizure threshold	Improvement aggressive behaviors/irritability	Sedation
	Risperidone	Might decrease seizure threshold	Improvement aggressive behaviors/irritability	Improvement obsessive compulsive disorders, repetitive behaviors, hyperactivity
	Aripiprazole	Might decrease seizure threshold	Improvement aggressive behaviors/irritability	Improvement of obsessive compulsive disorders, repetitive behaviors, hyperactivity
Other treatments	Melatonin ketogenic diet	Spectrum efficacy	Animal model modify complex social behaviors	Improvement sleep disturbance
	Vagus nerve stimulation	Broad spectrum efficacy	Insufficient evidence	
	Surgery	Efficacy > focal seizure	Insufficient evidence	
Etiology-based treatment	Metabolic disorders: multivitamins, biotin, Co-Q10, L-carnitine, folinic acid, N-acetylcysteine, pyridoxine, cobalamin	Broad spectrum efficacy	Behavioral improvement	
	Surgery	Efficacy > focal seizure	Insufficient evidence	

AEDs, antiepileptic drugs; >, greater.

pharmacological treatment, educational and behavioral therapies to promote conversational language and social interactions must be performed. The mainstay of therapy is early individualized intensive training either in the school or at home; visual supports are helpful in promoting language acquisition.

CONCLUSION

Autism spectrum disorder, ID, and epilepsy are closely related neurobiological disorders co-occurring in about a quarter of patients. Clinical, epidemiological, and genetic studies clearly demonstrate that they might share pathophysiological mechanisms.

A number of well-known genetic disorders share epilepsy, ID, and autism as prominent phenotypic features, including tuberous sclerosis, RTT, CDKL5 and PCDH19 gene-related EE, and fragile X. In addition, mutations of several genes involved in neurodevelopment, including ARX, neuroligins, and neuropilin 2, have been identified in children with epilepsy, ID, ASD, or a combination of them. It has been proposed that ID, ASD, and epilepsy can be understood as disorders of synaptic plasticity resulting in a developmental imbalance of excitation and inhibition. Indeed, many of these mutations cause abnormalities of synaptic plasticity that result in imbalances in excitation and inhibition in the developing brain. In addition to genetic abnormalities that disrupt synaptic plasticity, seizures and epileptogenesis in early life may affect synaptic plasticity and potentially contribute to ASD and ID. Early-life seizures may produce a variety of cellular and molecular changes in hippocampus that may contribute to the enhanced risk of ID and ASD in patients with early-life seizures and epilepsy. Abnormalities of synaptic plasticity resulting in imbalances of excitatory and inhibitory neurotransmission resulting either from genetic mutations or effects of early-life seizures may provide a common mechanism of epilepsy, ID, and ASD and provide a basis for understanding the frequent co-occurrence of these disorders. Although this concept of a shared pathophysiology can provide a broad framework with which to begin to understand the frequent association of epilepsy, ID, and autism, many questions remain unanswered. Continued research is essential to begin to address these and other gaps in our understanding of the neurobiological basis of the complex association between epilepsy and comorbid learning and behavior.

There are currently no guidelines for the treatment of seizures in individuals with ASD. Identifying and treating the underlying abnormalities could provide substantial benefit to the patients and improve seizures. For etiologies without specific treatments or when an etiological cause cannot be identified, there appear to be some AEDs that may be promising as first-line treatments, particularly lamotrigine, valproate, and levetiracetam.

References

1. Creak M, Pampiglione G. Clinical and EEG studies on a group of 35 psychotic children. *Dev Med Child Neurol* 1969;**11**(2):218–27.
2. Hutt SJ, Hutt C, Lee D, Ounsted C. A behavioural and electroencephalographic study of autistic children. *J Psychiatr Res* 1965;**3**(3):181–97.
3. Schain RJ, Yannet H. Infantile autism. An analysis of 50 cases and a consideration of certain relevant neurophysiologic concepts. *J Pediatr* 1960;**57**:560–7.
4. Tuchman R, Cuccaro M, Alessandri M. Autism and epilepsy: historical perspective. *Brain Dev* 2010;**32**(9):709–18.
5. American Psychiatric Association, editor. *Diagnostic and statistical manual of mental disorders (DSM-IV-TR)*. Washington (DC): American Psychiatric Association; 2000. p. 1–9.
6. World Health Organization, editor. *International classification of mental and behavioural disorders*. World Health Organization; 2007 [Chapter V].
7. Berg AT, Plioplys S, Tuchman R. Risk and correlates of autism spectrum disorder in children with epilepsy: a community-based study. *J Child Neurol* 2011;**26**(5):540–7.
8. Commission on Classification and Terminology of the International League Against Epilepsy. Proposal for revised classification of epilepsies and epileptic syndromes. *Epilepsia* 1989;**30**:389–99.
9. Commission on Classification and Terminology of the International League Against Epilepsy. Proposal for revised clinical and electroencephalographic classification of epileptic seizures. *Epilepsia* 1981;**22**:489–501.
10. Berg AT, Berkovic SF, Brodie MJ, Buchhalter J, Cross JH, van Emde Boas W, et al. Revised terminology and concepts for organization of seizures and epilepsies: report of the ILAE Commission on Classification and Terminology, 2005–2009. *Epilepsia* 2011;**51**(4):676–85.
11. Camfield C, Camfield P. Preventable and unpreventable causes of childhood-onset epilepsy plus mental retardation. *Pediatrics* 2007;**120**(1):e52–55.
12. Cross JH, Guerrini R. The epileptic encephalopathies. *Handb Clin Neurol* 2013;**111**:619–26.
13. Berg AT, Langfitt JT, Testa FM, Levy SR, DiMario F, Westerveld M, et al. Global cognitive function in children with epilepsy: a community-based study. *Epilepsia* 2008;**49**(4):608–14.
14. Rapin I. Autism. *N Engl J Med* 1997;**337**(2):97–104.
15. Jamain S, Quach H, Betancur C, Rastam M, Colineaux C, Gillberg IC, et al. Mutations of the X-linked genes encoding neuroligins NLGN3 and NLGN4 are associated with autism. *Nat Genet* 2003;**34**(1):27–9.
16. Wong V. Epilepsy in children with autistic spectrum disorder. *J Child Neurol* 1993;**8**(4):316–22.
17. Valvo G, Baldini S, Brachini F, Apicella F, Cosenza A, Ferrari AR, et al. Somatic overgrowth predisposes to seizures in autism spectrum disorders. *PLoS One* 2013;**8**(9):e75015.
18. Tuchman R, Rapin I. Epilepsy in autism. *Lancet Neurol* 2002;**1**(6):352–8.
19. Canitano R. Epilepsy in autism spectrum disorders. *Eur Child Adolesc Psychiatry* 2007;**16**(1):61–6.
20. Spence SJ, Schneider MT. The role of epilepsy and epileptiform EEGs in autism spectrum disorders. *Pediatr Res* 2009;**65**(6):599–606.
21. Hara H. Autism and epilepsy: a retrospective follow-up study. *Brain Dev* 2007;**29**(8):486–90.

22. Olsson I, Steffenburg S, Gillberg C. Epilepsy in autism and autistic-like conditions. A population-based study. *Arch Neurol* 1988;**45**(6): 666–8.

23. Mouridsen SE, Rich B, Isager T. Epilepsy in disintegrative psychosis and infantile autism: a long-term validation study. *Dev Med Child Neurol* 1999;**41**(2):110–4.

24. Saemundsen E, Ludvigsson P, Rafnsson V. Risk of autism spectrum disorders after infantile spasms: a population-based study nested in a cohort with seizures in the first year of life. *Epilepsia* 2008; **49**(11):1865–70.

25. Tuchman R, Moshe SL, Rapin I. Convulsing toward the pathophysiology of autism. *Brain Dev* 2009;**31**(2):95–103.

26. Steffenburg S, Gillberg C, Hellgren L, Andersson L, Gillberg IC, Jakobsson G, et al. A twin study of autism in Denmark, Finland, Iceland, Norway and Sweden. *J Child Psychol Psychiatry* 1989; **30**(3):405–16.

27. Bailey A, Le Couteur A, Gottesman I, Bolton P, Simonoff E, Yuzda E, et al. Autism as a strongly genetic disorder: evidence from a British twin study. *Psychol Med* 1995;**25**(1):63–77.

28. Abrahams BS, Geschwind DH. Advances in autism genetics: on the threshold of a new neurobiology. *Nat Rev Genet* 2008;**9**(5): 341–55.

29. Marini C, Scheffer IE, Crossland KM, Grinton BE, Phillips FL, McMahon JM, et al. Genetic architecture of idiopathic generalized epilepsy: clinical genetic analysis of 55 multiplex families. *Epilepsia* 2004;**45**(5):467–78.

30. Brooks-Kayal A. Epilepsy and autism spectrum disorders: are there common developmental mechanisms? *Brain Dev* 2010;**32**(9): 731–8.

31. Tuchman R, Cuccaro M. Epilepsy and autism: neurodevelopmental perspective. *Curr Neurol Neurosci Rep* 2011;**11**(4):428–34.

32. Paemka L, Mahajan VB, Skeie JM, Sowers LP, Ehaideb SN, Gonzalez-Alegre P, et al. PRICKLE1 interaction with SYNAPSIN I reveals a role in autism spectrum disorders. *PLoS One* 2013;**8**(12):e80737.

33. Fassio A, Patry L, Congia S, Onofri F, Piton A, Gauthier J, et al. SYN1 loss-of-function mutations in autism and partial epilepsy cause impaired synaptic function. *Hum Mol Genet* 2011;**20**(12): 2297–307.

34. Butler MG, Dasouki MJ, Zhou XP, Talebizadeh Z, Brown M, Takahashi TN, et al. Subset of individuals with autism spectrum disorders and extreme macrocephaly associated with germline PTEN tumour suppressor gene mutations. *J Med Genet* 2005; **42**(4):318–21.

35. Marchese M, Conti V, Valvo G, Moro F, Muratori F, Tancredi R, et al. Autism-epilepsy phenotype with macrocephaly suggests PTEN, but not GLIALCAM, genetic screening. *BMC Med Genet* 2014;**15**:26.

36. Poultney CS, Goldberg AP, Drapeau E, Kou Y, Harony-Nicolas H, Kajiwara Y, et al. Identification of small exonic CNV from whole-exome sequence data and application to autism spectrum disorder. *Am J Hum Genet* 2013;**93**(4):607–19.

37. Roberts JL, Hovanes K, Dasouki M, Manzardo AM, Butler MG. Chromosomal microarray analysis of consecutive individuals with autism spectrum disorders or learning disability presenting for genetic services. *Gene* 2014;**535**(1):70–8.

38. Kamien B, Harraway J, Lundie B, Smallhorne L, Gibbs V, Heath A, et al. Characterization of a 520 kb deletion on chromosome 15q26.1 including ST8SIA2 in a patient with behavioral disturbance, autism spectrum disorder, and epilepsy. *Am J Med Genet A* 2013; **4A**(3):782–8.

39. Fusco C, Micale L, Augello B, Teresa Pellico M, Menghini D, Alfieri P, et al. Smaller and larger deletions of the Williams Beuren syndrome region implicate genes involved in mild facial phenotype, epilepsy and autistic traits. *Eur J Hum Genet* 2013;**22**(1):64–70.

40. Rosti RO, Sadek AA, Vaux KK, Gleeson JG. The genetic landscape of autism spectrum disorders. *Dev Med Child Neurol* 2013;**56**(1): 12–8.

41. Yu TW, Chahrour MH, Coulter ME, Jiralerspong S, Okamura-Ikeda K, Ataman B, et al. Using whole-exome sequencing to identify inherited causes of autism. *Neuron* 2013;**77**(2):259–73.

42. Jiang YH, Yuen RK, Jin X, Wang M, Chen N, Wu X, et al. Detection of clinically relevant genetic variants in autism spectrum disorder by whole-genome sequencing. *Am J Hum Genet* 2013;**93**(2):249–63.

43. Liu L, Sabo A, Neale BM, Nagaswamy U, Stevens C, Lim E, et al. Analysis of rare, exonic variation amongst subjects with autism spectrum disorders and population controls. *PLoS Genet* 2013; **9**(4):e1003443.

44. Taft LT, Cohen HJ. Hypsarrhythmia and infantile autism: a clinical report. *J Autism Child Schizophr* 1971;**1**(3):327–36.

45. Riikonen R, Amnell G. Psychiatric disorders in children with earlier infantile spasms. *Dev Med Child Neurol* 1981;**23**(6):747–60.

46. Comery TA, Harris JB, Willems PJ, Oostra BA, Irwin SA, Weiler IJ, et al. Abnormal dendritic spines in fragile X knockout mice: maturation and pruning deficits. *Proc Natl Acad Sci USA* 1997;**94**(10): 5401–4.

47. Penagarikano O, Mulle JG, Warren ST. The pathophysiology of fragile x syndrome. *Annu Rev Genomics Hum Genet* 2007;**8**:109–29.

48. Brooks-Kayal A. Molecular mechanisms of cognitive and behavioral comorbidities of epilepsy in children. *Epilepsia* 2011;**52**(Suppl. 1): 13–20.

49. Gibson JR, Bartley AF, Hays SA, Huber KM. Imbalance of neocortical excitation and inhibition and altered UP states reflect network hyperexcitability in the mouse model of fragile X syndrome. *J Neurophysiol* 2008;**100**(5):2615–26.

50. D'Hulst C, De Geest N, Reeve SP, Van Dam D, De Deyn PP, Hassan BA, et al. Decreased expression of the GABAA receptor in fragile X syndrome. *Brain Res* 2006;**1121**(1):238–45.

51. Marini C, Darra F, Specchio N, Mei D, Terracciano A, Parmeggiani L, et al. Focal seizures with affective symptoms are a major feature of PCDH19 gene-related epilepsy. *Epilepsia* 2012; **53**(12):2111–9.

52. Dibbens LM, Tarpey PS, Hynes K, Bayly MA, Scheffer IE, Smith R, et al. X-linked protocadherin 19 mutations cause female-limited epilepsy and cognitive impairment. *Nat Genet* 2008;**40**(6):776–81.

53. Kalscheuer VM, Tao J, Donnelly A, Hollway G, Schwinger E, Kubart S, et al. Disruption of the serine/threonine kinase 9 gene causes severe X-linked infantile spasms and mental retardation. *Am J Hum Genet* 2003;**72**(6):1401–11.

54. Melani F, Mei D, Pisano T, Savasta S, Franzoni E, Ferrari AR, et al. CDKL5 gene-related epileptic encephalopathy: electroclinical findings in the first year of life. *Dev Med Child Neurol* 2011;**53**(4):354–60.

55. Weaving LS, Christodoulou J, Williamson SL, Friend KL, McKenzie OL, Archer H, et al. Mutations of CDKL5 cause a severe neurodevelopmental disorder with infantile spasms and mental retardation. *Am J Hum Genet* 2004;**75**(6):1079–93.

56. Ricciardi S, Ungaro F, Hambrock M, Rademacher N, Stefanelli G, Brambilla D, et al. CDKL5 ensures excitatory synapse stability by reinforcing NGL-1-PSD95 interaction in the postsynaptic compartment and is impaired in patient iPSC-derived neurons. *Nat Cell Biol* 2013;**14**(9):911–23.

57. Amir RE, Van den Veyver IB, Wan M, Tran CQ, Francke U, Zoghbi HY. Rett syndrome is caused by mutations in X-linked MECP2, encoding methyl-CpG-binding protein 2. *Nat Genet* 1999; **23**(2):185–8.

58. Dani VS, Chang Q, Maffei A, Turrigiano GG, Jaenisch R, Nelson SB. Reduced cortical activity due to a shift in the balance between excitation and inhibition in a mouse model of Rett syndrome. *Proc Natl Acad Sci USA* 2005;**102**(35):12560–5.

59. Ariani F, Hayek G, Rondinella D, Artuso R, Mencarelli MA, Spanhol-Rosseto A, et al. FOXG1 is responsible for the congenital variant of Rett syndrome. *Am J Hum Genet* 2008;**83**(1):89–93.

60. Curatolo P, Porfirio MC, Manzi B, Seri S. Autism in tuberous sclerosis. *Eur J Paediatr Neurol* 2004;**8**(6):327–32.

III. EXPERIMENTAL MODELS, CLINICAL AND PHARMACOLOGICAL ASPECTS OF MAJOR ASDS

61. White R, Hua Y, Scheithauer B, Lynch DR, Henske EP, Crino PB. Selective alterations in glutamate and GABA receptor subunit mRNA expression in dysplastic neurons and giant cells of cortical tubers. *Ann Neurol* 2001;**49**(1):67–78.

62. Wong M, Ess KC, Uhlmann EJ, Jansen LA, Li W, Crino PB, et al. Impaired glial glutamate transport in a mouse tuberous sclerosis epilepsy model. *Ann Neurol* 2003;**54**(2):251–6.

63. Marsh E, Fulp C, Gomez E, Nasrallah I, Minarcik J, Sudi J, et al. Targeted loss of Arx results in a developmental epilepsy mouse model and recapitulates the human phenotype in heterozygous females. *Brain* 2009;**132**(Pt 6):1563–76.

64. Uchino S, Waga C. SHANK3 as an autism spectrum disorder-associated gene. *Brain Dev* 2013;**35**(2):106–10.

65. Deykin EY, MacMahon B. The incidence of seizures among children with autistic symptoms. *Am J Psychiatry* 1979;**136**(10):1310–2.

66. Deonna T, Roulet E. Autistic spectrum disorder: evaluating a possible contributing or causal role of epilepsy. *Epilepsia* 2006;**47**(Suppl. 2):79–82.

67. Lemke JR, Lal D, Reinthaler EM, Steiner I, Nothnagel M, Alber M, et al. Mutations in GRIN2A cause idiopathic focal epilepsy with rolandic spikes. *Nat Genet* 2013;**45**(9):1067–72.

68. Lesca G, Rudolf G, Bruneau N, Lozovaya N, Labalme A, Boutry-Kryza N, et al. GRIN2A mutations in acquired epileptic aphasia and related childhood focal epilepsies and encephalopathies with speech and language dysfunction. *Nat Genet* 2013;**45**(9):1061–6.

69. Berryer MH, Hamdan FF, Klitten LL, Moller RS, Carmant L, Schwartzentruber J, et al. Mutations in SYNGAP1 cause intellectual disability, autism, and a specific form of epilepsy by inducing haploinsufficiency. *Hum Mutat* 2013;**34**(2):385–94.

70. Wallerstein R, Sugalski R, Cohn L, Jawetz R, Friez M. Expansion of the ARX spectrum. *Clin Neurol Neurosurg* 2008;**110**(6):631–4.

71. Kakinuma H, Ozaki M, Sato H, Takahashi H. Variation in GABA-A subunit gene copy number in an autistic patient with mosaic 4 p duplication (p12p16). *Am J Med Genet B Neuropsychiatr Genet* 2008;**147B**(6):973–5.

72. Harrison V, Connell L, Hayesmoore J, McParland J, Pike MG, Blair E. Compound heterozygous deletion of NRXN1 causing severe developmental delay with early onset epilepsy in two sisters. *Am J Med Genet A* 2011;**155A**(11):2826–31.

73. Edvardson S, Ashikov A, Jalas C, Sturiale L, Shaag A, Fedick A, et al. Mutations in SLC35A3 cause autism spectrum disorder, epilepsy and arthrogryposis. *J Med Genet* 2013;**50**(11):733–9.

74. van Slegtenhorst M, de Hoogt R, Hermans C, Nellist M, Janssen B, Verhoef S, et al. Identification of the tuberous sclerosis gene TSC1 on chromosome 9q34. *Science* 1997;**277**(5327):805–8.

75. Kandt RS, Haines JL, Smith M, Northrup H, Gardner RJ, Short MP, et al. Linkage of an important gene locus for tuberous sclerosis to a chromosome 16 marker for polycystic kidney disease. *Nat Genet* 1992;**2**(1):37–41.

76. Frye RE, Rossignol D, Casanova MF, Brown GL, Martin V, Edelson S, et al. A review of traditional and novel treatments for seizures in autism spectrum disorder: findings from a systematic review and expert panel. *Front Public Health* 2013;**13**:1–31.

77. Hirota T, Veenstra-Vanderweele J, Hollander E, Kishi T. Antiepileptic medications in autism spectrum disorder: a systematic review and meta-analysis. *J Autism Dev Disord* April 2014;**44**(4):948–57.

78. Frye RE, Sreenivasula S, Adams JB. Traditional and non-traditional treatments for autism spectrum disorder with seizures: an on-line survey. *BMC Pediatr* 2011;**18**:11–37.

79. Aman MG, Van Bourgondien ME, Wolford PL, Sarphare G. Psychotropic and anticonvulsant drugs in subjects with autism: prevalence and patterns of use. *J Am Acad Child Adolesc Psychiatry* 1995;**34**(12):1672–81.

80. Uvebrant P, Bauzienè R. Intractable epilepsy in children. The efficacy of lamotrigine treatment, including non-seizure-related benefits. *Neuropediatrics* 1994;**25**(6):284–9.

81. Hollander E, Dolgoff-Kaspar R, Cartwright C, Rawitt R, Novotny S. An open trial of divalproex sodium in autism spectrum disorders. *J Clin Psychiatry* 2001;**62**(7):530–4.

82. Hellings JA, Weckbaugh M, Nickel EJ, Cain SE, Zarcone JR, Reese RM, et al. A doubleblind, placebo-controlled study of valproate for aggression in youth with pervasive developmental disorders. *J Child Adolesc Psychopharmacol* 2005;**15**:682–92.

83. Rugino TA, Samsock TC. Levetiracetam in autistic children: an open-label study. *J Dev Behav Pediatr* 2002;**23**(4):225–30.

84. Ahn Y, Narous M, Tobias R, Rho JM, Mychasiuk R. The ketogenic diet modifies social and metabolic alterations identified in the prenatal valproic acid model of autism spectrum disorder. *Dev Neurosci* 2014;**36**(5):371–80.

85. Danielsson S, Rydenhag B, Uvebrant P, Nordborg C, Olsson I. Temporal Lobe Resections in Children with Epilepsy: Neuropsychiatric Status in Relation to Neuropathology and Seizure Outcome. *Epilepsy Behav* 2002;**3**(1):76–81.

86. Neville BG, Harkness WF, Cross JH, Cass HC, Burch VC, Lees JA, et al. Surgical treatment of severe autistic regression in childhood epilepsy. *Pediatr Neurol* 1997;**16**(2):137–40.

87. Stefanatos GA, Grover W, Geller E. Case study: corticosteroid treatment of language regression in pervasive developmental disorder. *J Am Acad Child Adolesc Psychiatry* 1995;**34**(8):1107–11.

88. Gupta SJ. Treatment of children with autism with intravenous immunoglobulin. *Child Neurol* March 1999;**14**(3):203–5.

89. Frye RE. Metabolic and mitochondrial disorders associated with epilepsy in children with autism spectrum disorder. *Epilepsy Behav* November 4, 2014;**47**:147–57 [Epub ahead of print].

90. Benvenuto A, Battan B, Porfirio MC, Curatolo P. Pharmacotherapy of autism spectrum disorders. *Brain Dev* February 2013;**35**(2):119–27.

Index

'*Note*: Page numbers followed by "f" indicate figures and "t" indicate tables.'